Handbook of Current **Diagnosis & Treatment**

A *Quick* Reference for the General Practitioner

Susan J. Friedman

Handbook of Current
Diagnosis & Treatment

A *Quick* Reference for the General Practitioner

Edited by
James O. Woolliscroft, MD
Professor of Internal Medicine
University of Michigan Medical School
Chief of Clinical Affairs
University of Michigan Hospitals
Ann Arbor, Michigan

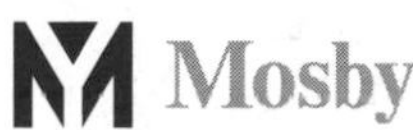

St. Louis Baltimore Boston Carlsbad Chicago Naples New York Philadelphia Portland
London Madrid Mexico City Singapore Sydney Tokyo Toronto Wiesbaden

Developed by Current Medicine, Inc., Philadelphia

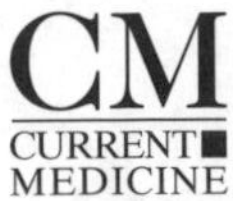

Current Medicine, Inc.
400 Market Street, Suite 700
Philadelphia, Pennsylvania 19106

Managing Editor: Lori J. Bainbridge
Developmental Editors: Barbara Cohen-Kligerman, Elise M. Paxson
Editorial Assistant: Scott Hurd
Art Director: Paul Fennessy
Designer: Mark Riches
Cover Design, Typesetting, and Layout: Patrick Ward
Illustration Director: Ann Saydlowski
Illustrators: Paul Bernson, Stuart Molloy, Yaron Tracz
Production: David Myers, Lori Holland
Indexer: Dorothy DiRienzi

Distribution rights for North America:
MOSBY-YEARBOOK, INC.
11830 Westline Industrial Drive
St. Louis, MO 63146

ISBN 1-57340-016-5
ISSN 1083-9658

Film supplied by Reed Technology and Information Services Inc.
Fort Washington, Pennsylvania, United States
Printed in Singapore by Imago Productions (FE) Ltd.
5 4 3 2 1

Section Editors

AIDS & Infectious diseases

Powel H. Kazanjian, MD
Assistant Professor
Department of Internal Medicine
University of Michigan Medical School
Ann Arbor, MI

Cardiology

Kim A. Eagle, MD
Associate Professor
Department of Internal Medicine
University of Michigan Medical School
Director, Clinical Cardiology
University of Michigan Medical Center
Ann Arbor, Michigan

Dermatology

Bruce R. Nelson, MD
Associate Professor
Department of Dermatology
University of Texas Medical School
Houston, Texas

Endocrinology & Metabolic disorders

Jamie Dananberg, MD
Assistant Professor
Department of Internal Medicine
University of Michigan Medical School
Ann Arbor, Michigan

Gastroenterology & Hepatology

Joseph C. Kolars, MD
Associate Professor
Associate Chair, Graduate Medical Education
Department of Internal Medicine
University of Michigan Medical School
Ann Arbor, Michigan

Hematology & Oncology

Paula L. Bockenstedt, MD
Assistant Professor
Department of Internal Medicine
Director, Adult Hemophilia and Coagulation Disorders Clinic
University of Michigan Medical School
Ann Arbor, Michigan

Nephrology

Richard D. Swartz, MD
Professor
Department of Internal Medicine
University of Michigan Medical School
Ann Arbor, Michigan

Neurology

Linda M. Selwa, MD
Clinical Assistant Professor
Department of Neurology
University of Michigan Medical School
Ann Arbor, Michigan

Psychiatry

Brent C. Williams, MD, MPH
Assistant Professor
Department of Internal Medicine
University of Michigan Medical School
Ann Arbor, Michigan

Contributors

James L. Abelson, MD, PhD
Assistant Professor
Department of Psychiatry
University of Michigan Medical School
Ann Arbor, Michigan

Mark A. Demitrack, MD
Assistant Professor
Department of Psychiatry
University of Michigan Medical School
Ann Arbor, Michigan

Joseph Himle, PhD
Lecturer
Department of Psychiatry
University of Michigan Medical School
Ann Arbor, Michigan

Michael D. Jibson, MD, PhD
Clinical Assistant Professor
Department of Psychiatry
University of Michigan Medical School
Ann Arbor, Michigan

Monica Starkman, MD, MS
Associate Professor
Department of Psychiatry
University of Michigan Medical School
Ann Arbor, Michigan

Elizabeth Young, MD
Associate Professor
Department of Psychiatry
University of Michigan Medical School
Ann Arbor, Michigan

Pulmonary disorders

Cyril M. Grum, MD
Associate Professor
Associate Chair, Undergraduate Education
Department of Internal Medicine
University of Michigan Medical School
Ann Arbor, Michigan

Rheumatology & Musculoskeletal disorders

Mark A. McQuillan, MD
Clinical Assistant Professor
Department of Internal Medicine
University of Michigan Medical School
Ann Arbor, Michigan

Preface

Information management is a challenge for modern physicians. Maintaining knowledge of current diagnostic and therapeutic developments, especially for clinical problems encountered less frequently, can be a formidable task. *Current Diagnosis and Treatment* is specifically structured to facilitate the busy clinician's access to current information on a wide variety of diseases. It is not designed to provide detailed explanations, but rather to remind the physician who needs to "brush up" on the diagnosis and management of a clinical entity.

The physical layout of each chapter is consistent throughout the book so that the clinician can rapidly access information on symptoms, signs, investigations, complications, differential diagnosis, etiology, and epidemiology on one page; and diet and lifestyle, pharmacologic and other treatments, management issues, prognosis, and recent references on the next page.

To maintain factual currency, regular revisions and updates of each topic are planned. As new topics germane to the North American practitioner are identified, spreads will be developed using the standard format. We welcome your suggestions for topics to include in future editions. The goal is to develop a "user friendly" clinically relevant reference for primary care physicians and other members of the healthcare team.

James O. Woolliscroft, MD
Ann Arbor, Michigan

Acknowledgments

The editor and contributors to this book are grateful to their colleagues in the United Kingdom who created the informational format on which this volume is based. We owe special thanks to Professor Roy Pounder and Dr. Mark Hamilton, editors, and their 13 section editors who supervised the extensive editing and peer-review process. We are also thankful to their 220 colleagues who acted as authors, editors, and academic referees and laid the foundation for this work.

Editors

Professor Roy Pounder
Professor of Medicine
Royal Free Hospital and Medical School
London, UK

Mark Hamilton, MD
Senior Registrar
University Department of Medicine
Royal Free Hospital
London, UK

Section editors

AIDS

Brian Gazzard, MD
Clinical Director, HIV/GUM Unit
Chelsea and Westminster Hospital
London, UK

Cardiology

Nigel Buller, MD
Consultant Cardiologist
Queen Elizabeth Hospital
Birmingham, UK

Dermatology

Malcolm Rustin, MD
Consultant Dermatologist
Royal Free Hospital
London, UK

Endocrinology

Professor John A.H. Wass
Director, Endocrine Unit
Radcliffe Infirmary and Nuffield Orthopaedic Centre
Oxford, UK
Linacre Fellow, Royal College of Physicians
London, UK

Gastroenterology

Professor Roy Pounder
Mark Hamilton, MD

Haematology

Professor H. Grant Prentice
Professor of Haematological Oncology
Royal Free Hospital and Medical School
London, UK

Hepatology

Andrew K. Burroughs, MD
Consultant Physician and Hepatologist
Royal Free Hospital
London, UK

Infectious diseases

Glyn R. Williams, MD
Consultant Physician in Infectious Diseases
Ayrshire Central Hospital
Irvine, UK

Nephrology

Paul Sweny, MD
NHS Consultant
Royal Free Hospital
London, UK

Neurology

Professor Anthony H.V. Schapira
Chairman and Professor of Neurology
Royal Free Hospital and Medical School
London, UK
Professor of Neurology
Institute of Neurology
London, UK

Psychiatry

Neil L. Holden, MD
Consultant Psychiatrist
Director of Postgraduate Education
Nottingham Healthcare NHS Trust
Nottingham, UK

Respiratory

Anthony J. Frew, MD
Senior Lecturer in Medicine
University of Southampton
Consultant Chest Physician
Southampton University Hospital
Southampton, UK

Rheumatology

Michael Doherty, MD
Reader and Consultant in Rheumatology
City Hospital
Nottingham, UK

Contents

xiii **Contents by specialty**
1 **How to use this book**

A

2 **Achalasia**
4 **Acne**
6 **Acromegaly**
8 **Acute crystal synovitis**
10 **Addison's disease**
12 **Adult respiratory distress syndrome**
14 **AIDS**
16 **AIDS-related lymphoma**
18 **Alcohol withdrawal syndrome**
delirium tremens
uncomplicated alcohol withdrawal
20 **Alopecia**
alopecia areata
chronic cutaneous lupus erythematosus
cicatricial alopecia
fungal infection
lichen planopilaris
noncicatricial alopecia
nonscarring
scarring
trichotillomania
22 **Anemia, aplastic**
24 **Anemia, megaloblastic**
26 **Anemia, pernicious**
28 **Angina pectoris, stable**
30 **Angina pectoris, unstable**
32 **Ankylosing spondylitis**
34 **Aortic dissection**
distal dissection
proximal dissection
36 **Aortic regurgitation**
38 **Aortic stenosis**
40 **Arthritis, psoriatic**
42 **Arthritis, rheumatoid**
44 **Arthritis, septic**
46 **Ascites**
spontaneous bacterial peritonitis
uncomplicated ascites
48 **Asthma**
50 **Asthma, occupational**
52 **Atrial septal defect**
ostium primum defect
ostium secundum defect
54 **Attempted suicide**
high risk of completed suicide
low risk of completed suicide

56 **Bacterial overgrowth of the small intestine**
58 **Bronchiectasis and cystic fibrosis**
60 **Bulimia nervosa**
62 **Bullous disorders**
bullous pemphigoid
dermatitis herpetiformis
pemphigus vulgaris

64 **Candidiasis, buccal and esophageal in AIDS**
66 **Cardiac failure and dilated cardiomyopathy**
68 **Cardiopulmonary resuscitation**
basic life support
advanced life support
70 **Celiac disease**
72 **Cerebral tumor**
74 **Cholangitis, primary sclerosing**
76 **Chronic fatigue syndrome**
78 **Chronic obstructive pulmonary disease**
80 **Cirrhosis, primary biliary**
82 **Colorectal cancer**
84 **Coma**
86 **Cranial arteritis**
88 **Crohn's disease**
90 **Cushing's syndrome**
92 **Cytomegalovirus infection in AIDS**

94 **Dementia**
96 **Depression and mania**
dysthymia
hypomania
major depression
mania
98 **Diabetes insipidus**
100 **Diabetes mellitus, insulin-dependent**
102 **Diabetes mellitus, non–insulin-dependent**
104 **Diabetic management in children**
106 **Diabetic management in pregnancy**
108 **Diabetic management in surgery**
110 **Dialysis**
continuous ambulatory peritoneal dialysis
hemodialysis
hemofiltration
home hemodialysis

Contents

112 **Diarrhea and HIV infection**
114 **Disseminated intravascular coagulation**
116 **Diverticular disease of the colon**
118 **Duodenal ulcer**
complicated ulcer
uncomplicated ulcer
120 **Dyslipoproteinemia**

122 **Eczema**
124 **Eisenmenger's complex**
126 **Encephalitis**
128 **Endocarditis**
acute endocarditis
culture-negative endocarditis
marasmic endocarditis
noninfective endocarditis
subacute endocarditis
130 **Epilepsy**
generalized epilepsy (absence, myoclonic, clonic, tonic, tonic-clonic, atonic)
partial epilepsy (simple, complex, secondary generalized)
132 **Erythema multiforme and Stevens–Johnson syndrome**
134 **Erythema nodosum**
136 **Esophageal carcinoma**
138 **Esophagitis**

140 **Female hypogonadotrophic hypogonadism**
142 **Fungal infections, invasive**
144 **Fungal nail infection**

146 **Gallstones, cholesterol**
complicated
uncomplicated
148 **Gastric cancer**
150 **Gastric ulceration**
152 **Gastrointestinal bleeding**
peptic ulcer
bleeding varices
154 **Glomerulonephritis**
non-proliferative glomerulonephritis
proliferative glomerulonephritis
endocapillary
extracapillary
156 **Gout**
158 **Gram-negative septicemia**
160 **Granulomatous lung disease**
bronchocentric granulomatosis
Churg–Strauss syndrome
lymphomatoid granulomatosis
Wegener's granulomatosis
162 **Growth abnormalities, short stature**
164 **Growth abnormalities, tall stature**
166 **Guillain–Barré syndrome**

H

168 **Heart block**
first-degree atrioventricular block
second-degree (Mobitz types I and II) atrioventricular block
third-degree (complete) atrioventricular block
170 **Hemolytic uremic syndrome**
hemolytic uremic syndrome
thrombotic thrombocytopenic purpura
172 **Hemophilia and von Willebrand's disease**
174 **Henoch–Schönlein purpura**
176 **Hepatic encephalopathy**
in chronic liver disease
in fulminant liver failure
178 **Hepatitis, acute viral**
180 **Hepatitis, chronic**
182 **Hepatocellular carcinoma**
184 **Herpes simplex infection**
cutaneous herpes
eczema herpeticum
genital herpes
herpes encephalitis
herpes meningitis
ocular herpes
orolabial herpes (cold sores)
primary gingivostomatitis
186 **Herpes zoster and varicella**
chickenpox
shingles
188 **Hodgkin's disease**
190 **Hypercalcemia**
192 **Hyperglycemic emergencies**
hyperglycemia
ketoacidosis
194 **Hyperkalemia and hypokalemia**
196 **Hypernatremia and hyponatremia**
198 **Hyperprolactinemia**
macroadenoma
200 **Hypertension**
202 **Hyperthyroidism**
204 **Hypertrophic cardiomyopathy**
206 **Hypocalcemia**

Contents

208 **Hypoglycemia**

210 **Hypopituitarism**
growth hormone deficiency
pituitary–adrenal axis deficiency
pituitary–gonadal axis deficiency
posterior pituitary deficiency
thyroid deficiency

212 **Hypothyroidism**
congenital hypothyroidism
iodine-deficient hypothyroidism

214 **Infections in hematological malignancy**

216 **Infectious diarrhea**

218 **Interstitial lung disease**

220 **Intracerebral hemorrhage**
cerebellar hemorrhage
subarachnoid hemorrhage

222 **Irritable bowel syndrome**

224 **Kaposi's sarcoma in AIDS**
gastrointestinal Kaposi's sarcoma
lymphatic Kaposi's sarcoma
mucocutaneous Kaposi's sarcoma
pulmonary Kaposi's sarcoma

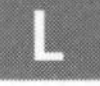

226 **Leptospirosis**
anicteric leptospirosis
icteric leptospirosis (Weil's syndrome)

228 **Leukemia, acute lymphoblastic in adults**

230 **Leukemia, acute lymphoblastic in children**

232 **Leukemia, acute myeloid**

234 **Leukemia, chronic lymphocytic**

236 **Leukemia, hairy cell**

238 **Liver failure, fulminant**

240 **Lung cancer**

242 **Lyme disease**

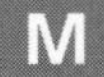

244 **Malaria**
complicated falciparum malaria
uncomplicated malaria

246 **Measles**

248 **Meningitis, bacterial**

250 **Meningitis, cryptococcal in AIDS**

252 **Migraine**
classic migraine (with aura)
cluster headache
common migraine (without aura)
hemiplegic migraine
ophthalmoplegic migraine
retinal migraine

254 **Mitral regurgitation**

256 **Mitral stenosis**

258 **Motor neuron disease**

260 **Multiple myeloma**

262 **Multiple sclerosis**
progressive multiple sclerosis
relapsing and remitting multiple sclerosis

264 **Myasthenia gravis**
early-onset myasthenia gravis
late-onset myasthenia gravis
seronegative myasthenia gravis
thymoma

266 ***Mycobacterium avium intracellulare* infection in AIDS**

268 **Myeloproliferative disorders**
chronic myeloid leukemia
essential thrombocythemia
polycythemia vera
primary myelofibrosis

270 **Myocardial infarction**

272 **Myositis, inflammatory**
dermatomyositis
polymyositis

N

274 **Nephropathies, tubulointerstitial**
acute interstitial nephritis
chronic interstitial nephritis

276 **Neuralgia, postherpetic**

278 **Neuralgia, trigeminal**

280 **Neuropathy, peripheral**
autonomic neuropathy
chronic inflammatory demyelinating polyradiculoneuropathy
focal/multifocal neuropathy
motor neuropathies
painful neuropathies
sensorimotor polyneuropathy
sensory polyneuropathy

282 **Non-Hodgkin's lymphoma**

284 **Obesity**

286 **Obsessive–compulsive disorder**

288 **Osteoarthritis**

290 **Ovarian failure**

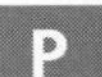

P

292 **Pancreatic cancer**

294 **Pancreatitis, acute**

296 **Pancreatitis, chronic**

298 **Panic and generalized anxiety disorder**

300 **Parkinson's disease**

302 **Parvovirus B19 infection**

304 **Pericarditis and tamponade**

306 **Personality disorders**
eccentric personality (paranoid/schizoid)
fearful personality (anancastic, anxious/avoidant, dependent)
flamboyant personality (dissocial, histrionic, impulsive/borderline)

308 **Pharyngitis**
coxsackie A virus
diphtheria
infectious mononucleosis
streptococcal infection (scarlet fever)

310 **Pheochromocytoma**

312 **Platelet disorders**
alloimmune thrombocytopenia (neonatal, posttransfusion)
bone marrow disorders
immune thrombocytopenia
platelet function defect
thrombotic thrombocytopenic purpura

314 **Pleural effusion**

316 ***Pneumocystis carinii* pneumonia in AIDS**

318 **Pneumonia**

320 **Polycystic kidney disease, autosomal-dominant**

322 **Polycystic ovarian disease**

324 **Polymyalgia rheumatica and giant-cell arteritis**

326 **Polymyositis**

328 **Postnatal mental illness**
mild depressive illness (neurotic or reactive)
puerperal psychosis (bipolar or manic-depressive)
severe depressive illness (unipolar)

330 **Prothrombotic states**

332 **Psoriasis**

334 **Pubertal abnormalities**
delayed puberty
precocious puberty
pseudoprecocious puberty

336 **Pulmonary complications of immunosuppression**

338 **Pulmonary embolism**

R

340 **Renal artery stenosis**
atherosclerotic disease
fibromuscular dysplasia

342 **Renal failure, acute**
postrenal acute renal failure
prerenal acute renal failure
renal acute renal failure

344 **Renal failure, chronic**

346 **Renal transplantation**

348 **Renal tubular acidosis**
distal renal tubular acidosis
hyporeninemic hypoaldosteronism
proximal renal tubular acidosis

350 **Restrictive cardiomyopathy and constrictive pericarditis**

352 **Rheumatic fever, acute**

354 **Rubella (German measles)**

S

356 **Sarcoidosis**

358 **Schizophrenia**

360 **Shock, acute hypotensive**

362 **Sickle cell disease**

364 **Skin infection**
abscesses
boils
carbuncles
cellulitis
erysipelas
impetigo
methicillin-resistant Staphylococcus aureus (MRSA)

366 **Sleep apnea, central hypoventilation, periodic breathing**
neuromuscular or chest-wall disease
periodic respiration

368 **Sleep apnea, obstructive**
central variant
laryngeal sleep apnea
obstructive sleep hypopnea
simple snoring
snoring with arousals from sleep

370 **Sleep disorders**
circadian sleep disorders
insomnia
narcoleptic syndrome
obstructive sleep apnea
parasomnias

Contents

372 **Spinal cord and cauda equina compression**

374 **Stroke**
cerebral infarction
primary intracerebral hemorrhage
subarachnoid hemorrhage

376 **Syndrome of inappropriate antidiuresis**

378 **Systemic lupus erythematosus**

380 **Systemic sclerosis**
diffuse cutaneous disease
limited cutaneous disease

T

382 **Tachycardia, supraventricular**
atrioventricular nodal re-entrant tachycardia
atrioventricular re-entrant tachycardia

384 **Tachycardia, ventricular**

386 **Testicular disorders**
adult male infertility
androgen deficiency
delayed puberty and hypogonadism
gynecomastia
male congenital adrenal hyperplasia
male pseudohermaphroditism
5α-reductase deficiency

388 **Thalassemia**

390 **Thyroid carcinoma**

392 **Toxic shock syndrome**
menstrual toxic shock syndrome
non-menstrual toxic shock syndrome

394 **Toxoplasmosis in AIDS**

396 **Transfusion medicine**
erythrocytes
fresh frozen plasma
platelets

398 **Transient ischemic attacks**

400 **Tremor**
cerebellar tremor
drug-induced tremor
drug-withdrawal tremor
dystonic tremor
essential tremor
exaggerated physiological tremor
focal tremor
hereditary tremor
idiopathic tremor
midbrain (rubral) tremor
neuropathic tremor
parkinsonian tremor

400 **Tremor *(continued)***
physiological tremor
primary orthostatic tremor
symptomatic tremor
task-specific action tremor
toxin-induced tremor

402 **Tuberculosis, extrapulmonary**

404 **Tuberculosis, pulmonary**

406 **Typhoid and paratyphoid fevers**

408 **Ulcerative colitis**

410 **Urinary tract infection**
lower urinary tract infection (cystitis, prostatitis)
upper urinary tract infection (pyelonephritis, renal abscess)

412 **Urticaria**
acute urticaria
chronic urticaria
urticarial vasculitis

414 **Variceal bleeding**

416 **Vasculitis, skin manifestations**

418 **Vasculitis, systemic**
large-artery vasculitis (giant-cell arteritis, Takayasu's arteritis)
medium-artery vasculitis (Kawasaki's disease, polyarteritis nodosa)
medium- or small-artery vasculitis (Churg–Strauss vasculitis, microscopic polyangiitis, Wegener's granulomatosis)
small-vessel vasculitis (essential mixed cryoglobulinemia, Henoch–Schönlein purpura, leukocytoclastic cutaneous vasculitis)

420 **Viral warts**
anogenital warts (condyloma acuminata, condyloma plana)
cutaneous warts ("butcher's," common, deep plantar, facial, mosaic, palmar/plantar, plane)

422 **Waldenström's macroglobulinemia**

424 **Wolff–Parkinson–White syndrome**

Z

426 **Zollinger–Ellison syndrome**

Index

429 **Index**

Contents by specialty

AIDS

14 AIDS
16 AIDS-related lymphoma
64 Candidiasis, buccal and esophageal in AIDS
92 Cytomegalovirus infection in AIDS
112 Diarrhea and HIV infection
224 Kaposi's sarcoma in AIDS
250 Meningitis, cryptococcal in AIDS
266 *Mycobacterium avium intracellulare* infection in AIDS
316 *Pneumocystis carinii* pneumonia in AIDS
336 Pulmonary complications of immunosuppression
394 Toxoplasmosis in AIDS

Cardiology

28 Angina pectoris, stable
30 Angina pectoris, unstable
34 Aortic dissection
36 Aortic regurgitation
38 Aortic stenosis
52 Atrial septal defect
66 Cardiac failure and dilated cardiomyopathy
68 Cardiopulmonary resuscitation
120 Dyslipoproteinemia
124 Eisenmenger's complex
128 Endocarditis
168 Heart block
200 Hypertension
204 Hypertrophic cardiomyopathy
254 Mitral regurgitation
256 Mitral stenosis
270 Myocardial infarction
304 Pericarditis and tamponade
338 Pulmonary embolism
350 Restrictive cardiomyopathy and constrictive pericarditis
360 Shock, acute hypotensive
382 Tachycardia, supraventricular
384 Tachycardia, ventricular
424 Wolff–Parkinson–White syndrome

Dermatology

4 Acne
20 Alopecia
40 Arthritis, psoriatic
62 Bullous disorders
122 Eczema
132 Erythema multiforme and Stevens–Johnson syndrome
134 Erythema nodosum
144 Fungal nail infection
224 Kaposi's sarcoma in AIDS
332 Psoriasis
364 Skin infection
412 Urticaria
416 Vasculitis, skin manifestations
420 Viral warts

Endocrinology & Metabolic disorders

6 Acromegaly
10 Addison's disease
90 Cushing's syndrome
98 Diabetes insipidus
100 Diabetes mellitus, insulin-dependent
102 Diabetes mellitus, non–insulin-dependent
104 Diabetic management in children
106 Diabetic management in pregnancy
108 Diabetic management in surgery
140 Female hypogonadotrophic hypogonadism
162 Growth abnormalities, short stature
164 Growth abnormalities, tall stature
190 Hypercalcemia
192 Hyperglycemic emergencies
194 Hyperkalemia and hypokalemia
196 Hypernatremia and hyponatremia
198 Hyperprolactinemia
202 Hyperthyroidism
206 Hypocalcemia
208 Hypoglycemia
210 Hypopituitarism
212 Hypothyroidism
284 Obesity
290 Ovarian failure
310 Pheochromocytoma
322 Polycystic ovarian disease
334 Pubertal abnormalities
348 Renal tubular acidosis
376 Syndrome of inappropriate diuresis
386 Testicular disorders
390 Thyroid carcinoma

Gastroenterology

2 Achalasia
26 Anemia, pernicious
56 Bacterial overgrowth of the small intestine
70 Celiac disease
82 Colorectal cancer
88 Crohn's disease
116 Diverticular disease of the colon
118 Duodenal ulcer

Contents by specialty

136 Esophageal carcinoma
138 Esophagitis
146 Gallstones, cholesterol
148 Gastric cancer
150 Gastric ulceration
152 Gastrointestinal bleeding
216 Infectious diarrhea
222 Irritable bowel syndrome
292 Pancreatic cancer
294 Pancreatitis, acute
296 Pancreatitis, chronic
408 Ulcerative colitis
426 Zollinger–Ellison syndrome

Hematology & Oncology

22 Anemia, aplastic
24 Anemia, megaloblastic
72 Cerebral tumor
82 Colorectal cancer
114 Disseminated intravascular coagulation
148 Gastric cancer
170 Hemolytic uremic syndrome
172 Hemophilia and von Willebrand's disease
182 Hepatocellular carcinoma
188 Hodgkin's disease
214 Infections in hematological malignancy
224 Kaposi's sarcoma in AIDS
228 Leukemia, acute lymphoblastic in adults
230 Leukemia, acute lymphoblastic in children
232 Leukemia, acute myeloid
234 Leukemia, chronic lymphocytic
236 Leukemia, hairy cell
240 Lung cancer
260 Multiple myeloma
268 Myeloproliferative disorders
282 Non-Hodgkin's lymphoma
292 Pancreatic cancer
312 Platelet disorders
330 Prothrombotic states
362 Sickle cell disease
388 Thalassemia
396 Transfusion medicine
422 Waldenström's macroglobulinemia

Hepatology

46 Ascites
74 Cholangitis, primary sclerosing
80 Cirrhosis, primary biliary
176 Hepatic encephalopathy
178 Hepatitis, acute viral
180 Hepatitis, chronic
182 Hepatocellular carcinoma
238 Liver failure, fulminant
414 Variceal bleeding

Infectious diseases

14 AIDS
44 Arthritis, septic
64 Candidiasis, buccal and esophageal in AIDS
76 Chronic fatigue syndrome
92 Cytomegalovirus infection in AIDS
126 Encephalitis
132 Erythema multiforme and Stevens–Johnson syndrome
134 Erythema nodosum
142 Fungal infections, invasive
158 Gram-negative septicemia
174 Henoch–Schönlein purpura
178 Hepatitis, acute viral
180 Hepatitis, chronic
184 Herpes simplex infection
186 Herpes zoster and varicella
216 Infectious diarrhea
226 Leptospirosis
242 Lyme disease
244 Malaria
246 Measles
248 Meningitis, bacterial
250 Meningitis, cryptococcal in AIDS
266 *Mycobacterium avium intracellulare* infection in AIDS
302 Parvovirus B19 infection
308 Pharyngitis
316 *Pneumocystis carinii* pneumonia in AIDS
352 Rheumatic fever, acute
354 Rubella (German measles)
364 Skin infection
392 Toxic shock syndrome
394 Toxoplasmosis in AIDS
402 Tuberculosis, extrapulmonary
404 Tuberculosis, pulmonary
406 Typhoid and paratyphoid fevers
410 Urinary tract infection

Nephrology

110 Dialysis
154 Glomerulonephritis
170 Hemolytic uremic syndrome

194 Hyperkalemia and hypokalemia
196 Hypernatremia and hyponatremia
274 Nephropathies, tubulointerstitial
320 Polycystic kidney disease, autosomal-dominant
340 Renal artery stenosis
342 Renal failure, acute
344 Renal failure, chronic
346 Renal transplantation
348 Renal tubular acidosis
410 Urinary tract infection

Neurology

72 Cerebral tumor
84 Coma
86 Cranial arteritis
94 Dementia
126 Encephalitis
130 Epilepsy
166 Guillain–Barré syndrome
220 Intracerebral hemorrhage
248 Meningitis, bacterial
252 Migraine
258 Motor neuron disease
262 Multiple sclerosis
264 Myasthenia gravis
276 Neuralgia, postherpetic
278 Neuralgia, trigeminal
280 Neuropathy, peripheral
300 Parkinson's disease
326 Polymyositis
370 Sleep disorders
372 Spinal cord and cauda equina compression
374 Stroke
388 Transient ischemic attacks
400 Tremor

Psychiatry

18 Alcohol withdrawal syndrome
54 Attempted suicide
60 Bulimia nervosa
96 Depression and mania
286 Obsessive–compulsive disorder
298 Panic and generalized anxiety disorder
306 Personality disorders
328 Postnatal mental illnes
358 Schizophrenia

Pulmonary disorders

12 Adult respiratory distress syndrome
48 Asthma
50 Asthma, occupational
58 Bronchiectasis and cystic fibrosis
78 Chronic obstructive pulmonary disease
160 Granulomatous lung disease
218 Interstitial lung disease
240 Lung canecr
314 Pleural effusion
318 Pneumonia
356 Sarcoidosis
366 Sleep apnea, central hypoventilation, periodic breathing
368 Sleep apnea, obstructive
404 Tuberculosis, pulmonary

Rheumatology & Muscular disorders

8 Acute crystal synovitis
32 Ankylosing spondylitis
40 Arthritis, psoriatic
42 Arthritis, rheumatoid
44 Arthritis, septic
86 Cranial arteritis
156 Gout
174 Henoch–Schönlein purpura
272 Myositis, inflammatory
288 Osteoarthritis
324 Polymyalgia rheumatica and giant-cell arteritis
352 Rheumatic fever, acute
378 Systemic lupus erythematosus
380 Systemic sclerosis
416 Vasculitis, skin manifestations
418 Vasculitis, systemic

Figure acknowledgments

We gratefully acknowledge the publishers and individuals who allowed us to use the following illustrations.

Page 64. Adapted with permission from Smith DE *et al.*: Itraconazole versus ketaconazole in the treatment of oral and oesophageal candidosis in patients infected with HIV. *AIDS* 1991, **5**:1367–1371.

Page 76. Adapted with permission from Ho-Yen DO: The epidemiology of post viral fatigue syndrome. *Scott Med J* 1988, **33**:368–369.

Page 84. Adapted with permission from Swash M, Oxberry J (eds): *Clinical Neurology*. Edinburgh: Churchill Livingstone; 1991:191.

Page 97. Adapted with permission from Kupfer DJ: Lessons to be learned from long-term treatment of affective disorder. *J Clin Psychiatry* 1991, **52 (suppl)**:12–16.

Page 106. Adapted with permission from Besser GM, Bodansky HJ, Cudworth AG: *Clinical Diabetes: An Illustrated Text*. London: Mosby–Wolfe, an imprint of Times Mirror International Publishers; 1995

Page 161. Adapted with permission from Hoffman GS *et al.*: Wegener granulomatosis: an analysis of 158 patients. *Ann Intern Med* 1992, **116**:488–498.

Page 198. Courtesy of Professor A Grossman, Department of Endocrinology, St Bartholomew's Hospital, London, UK.

Page 204. Reproduced with permission from Slade AKB, Saumarel RC, McKenna WJ: The arrythmogenic substrate – diagnostic and therapeutic implications: hypertrophic cardiomyopathy. *Eur Heart J* 1993, **14**:84–90.

Page 208. Adapted with permission from Frier BM, Fisher M (eds): *Hypoglycaemia and Diabetes*. London: Edward Arnold.

Page 236. Courtesy of Dr John Smith, Director, Wessex Regional Immunology Service Tenovus Laboratory, Southampton General Hospital.

Page 246. Adapted with permission from Ramsay M *et al.*: The epidemiology of measles in England and Wales. *Communicable Diseases Report* 1994, **4**:R141–R145.

Page 266. Reproduced with permission from Scolar A, French P, Miller R: *Mycobacterium avium intracellulare* infection in the acquired immunodeficiency syndrome. *Br J Hosp Med* 1991, **46**:295–300.

Page 274. Adapted with permission from Sweny P *et al.*: *The Kidney and its Disorders*. Oxford: Blackwell Scientific Publications; 1989.

Page 284. Adapted with permission from Garrow J: *Obesity and Related Diseases*. Edinburgh: Churchill Livingstone; 1988.

Page 293. Adapted with permission from Tsuchiya R: Resection of cancer of the pancreas – the Japanese experience. *Baillières Clin Gastroenterol* 1990, **4**:431–434.

Page 308. Adapted with permission from Gay NJ *et al.*: Age specific antibody prevalence to parvovirus B19: how many women are infected in pregnancy? *Communicable Diseases Report* 1994, **4**:R104–R107.

Page 340. Reproduced with permission from Stansby G *et al.*: Atherosclerotic renal artery stenosis. *Br J Hosp Med* 1993, **49**:388.

Page 364. Adapted with permission from Miller E *et al.*: Rubella surveillance to June 1994. *Communicable Diseases Report* 1994, **4**:R146–R152.

Page 390. Reproduced with permission from Franklyn JA, Sheppard MC: Thyroid nodules and thyroid cancer – diagnostic aspects. *Baillières Clin Endocrinol Metab* 1988, **2**:767.

Page 402. Adapted from *MMWR Morb Mortal Wkly Rep* 1992, **41**:58.

Page 402. Adapted from *MMWR Morb Mortal Wkly Rep* 1990, **39**:421–423.

Page 406. Reproduced with permission from Kennedy DH: Extrapulmonary tuberculosis. *Update* 1983, **27**:671–684.

How to use this book

This book provides current expert recommendations on the diagnosis and treatment of all major disorders throughout medicine in the form of tabular summaries. Essential guidelines on each of the topics have been condensed into two pages of vital information, summarizing the main procedures in diagnosis and management of each disorder to provide a quick and easy reference.

Each disorder is presented as a "spread" of two facing pages: the main procedures in diagnosis on the left and treatment options on the right.

Listed in the main column of the **Diagnosis** page are the common symptoms, signs, and complications of the disorder, with brief notes explaining their significance and probability of occurrence, together with details of investigations that can be used to aid diagnosis.

The pink side column contains information to help the reader evaluate the probability that an individual patient has the disorder. It may also include other information that could be useful in making a diagnosis (*e.g.*, classification or grading systems, comparison of different diagnostic methods).

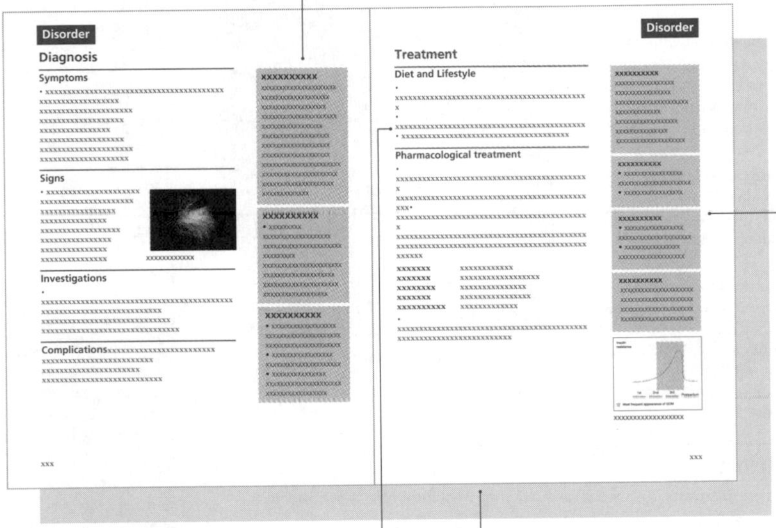

On the **Treatment** page, the main column contains information on lifestyle management and nonspecialist medical therapy of the disorder, with general information on specialist management when this is the main treatment.

Whenever possible under "Pharmacological treatment," guidelines are given on the standard dosage for commonly used drugs, with details of contraindications and precautions, main drug interactions, and main side effects. In each case, however, the manufacturer's drug data sheet should be consulted before any regimen is prescribed.

The main goals of treatment (*e.g.*, to cure, to palliate, to prevent), prognosis after treatment, precautions that the physician should take during and after treatment, and any other information that could help the clinician to make treatment decisions (*e.g.*, other nonpharmacological treatment options, special situations or groups of patients) are given in the blue side column. The key and general references at the end of this column provide the reader with further practical information.

Diagnosis

Symptoms

Dysphagia: usually perceived with both solid food and liquids [1].

Retrosternal chest pain: intermittent and variable duration, often related to eating.

Weight loss.

Regurgitation.

Nocturnal cough: related to regurgitation and aspiration.

Signs

• Usually no signs are manifest.

Evidence of weight loss.

Investigations

Radiography (plain film, erect): may show absence of air in gastric fundus or dilated esophagus with air-fluid level.

Radiography (barium swallow): shows delayed passage of contrast through cardia, absence of peristalsis (although "tertiary waves" may be prominent), or esophageal dilatation with "bird-beak" narrowing in the distal esophagus.

Upper gastrointestinal endoscopy: often normal; retained food or fluid may be encountered; increased resistance to passage of endoscope through cardia may be apparent.

Esophageal manometry: shows impaired relaxation of lower esophageal sphincter and absent peristalsis; may show prominent nonperistaltic (synchronous) contractions in esophageal body or elevated tonic pressure of lower esophageal sphincter [2].

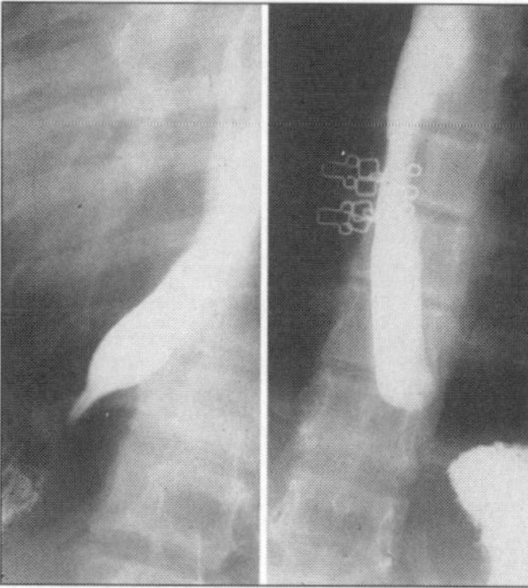

Delay of barium swallow due to spasm.

Complications

Respiratory complications: *e.g.*, cough, aspiration pneumonitis, in 10% of patients.

Esophageal carcinoma: possibly a late complication; very unusual.

Differential diagnosis

Benign or malignant esophageal stricture.

Gastric or other malignancy at cardia.

Aortic aneurysm compressing cardia.

Diffuse esophageal spasm.

Chagas' disease.

Hollow visceral neuropathy.

Etiology

• The underlying cause of the defect in the inhibitory innervation of the esophageal body and lower sphincter is unknown.

• Occasionally achalasia will occur as a paraneoplastic process; an occult malignancy should be considered promptly, particularly in older patients.

Epidemiology

• The annual incidence of achalasia is 1 in 100 000 adults.

• The male :female ratio is equal; achalasia may appear at any age in adult life.

• Although achalasia is more common in adults, the occurrence in children is well documented.

Diagnostic pitfalls

• The clinical features and radiography of "classic" achalasia are so characteristic that the existence of less typical presentations is not always appreciated; awareness of the following helps to minimize diagnostic errors:

• Early symptoms in some patients resemble those of gastroesophageal reflux.

• Abnormalities on barium swallow are sometimes subtle, so the diagnosis of achalasia is easily missed.

• Minor inflammation of the mucosa may be diagnosed as esophagitis at endoscopy when food retention in the esophagus is significant.

• In children especially, achalasia may be manifest with its respiratory complications.

• Despite clinical features and radiographs typical of achalasia, carcinoma or a peptic stricture should always be suspected when an endoscope cannot be passed through the cardia.

Treatment

Diet and lifestyle

• A soft diet with ingestion of meats and other solid food only if it has been ground into fine pieces.

Pharmacological treatment

• Nitrates and calcium antagonists (*e.g.*, nifedipine) reduce the lower esophageal sphincter pressure and may give short-term benefit before dilatation or surgery.

Nonpharmacological treatment

Dilatation of the cardia

• Endoscopic myotomy performed at the time of dilation using, for example, a Witzel balloon is the procedure of choice [3].

• Local injection therapy with botulinum toxin is also a consideration.

• Dysphagia is relieved in about two-thirds of patients after one attempt.

• A second attempt is usually worth while if the first attempt was unsuccessful.

• Complications include esophageal perforation in 2%–10% of patients; surgical repair is not always needed.

Surgery

• Cardiomyotomy through the thorax or abdomen or as a "minimal-access" procedure should be pursued if the endoscopic approach is unsuccessful.

Treatment aims

To restore acceptable swallowing.

Prognosis

• Relief of dysphagia and retrosternal pain can be achieved in >80% of patients.

Follow-up and management

• Symptomatic gastroesophageal reflux occurs in 5%–10% of patients after successful dilatation or cardiomyotomy; treatment with an H_2 receptor antagonist or proton pump inhibitor is usually successful.

Key references

1. Howard PJ *et al.*: Five year prospective study of the incidence, clinical features and diagnosis of achalasia in Edinburgh. *Gut* 1992, **33**:1011–1015.
2. Richter JE: Motility disorders of the esophagus. In *Textbook of Gastroenterology*. Edited by Yamada, T. Philadelphia: JB Lippincott; 1995:1182–1194.
3. Parkman HP *et al.*: Pneumatic dilatation or esophagomyotomy treatment for idiopathic achalasia: clinical outcomes and cost analysis. *Dig Dis Sci* 1993, **38**:75–85.

Diagnosis

Symptoms

Concern about appearance: even in cases that may be quite inconspicuous to the observer.

Social embarrassment.

Pain: from inflammatory papules, pustules, and cysts.

Signs

• Distribution is usually limited to the face, upper back, and chest, but acne can occur over the entire back and extend to the proximal arms in more severe cases.

• Lesions can be divided into inflammatory and noninflammatory.

Inflammatory

Papules.

Pustules.

Nodules and fluctuant cysts (nodulocystic acne).

Noninflammatory

Closed comedones (whiteheads).

Open comedones (blackheads).

Scars from resolved or treated areas of acne cysts.

Oily skin.

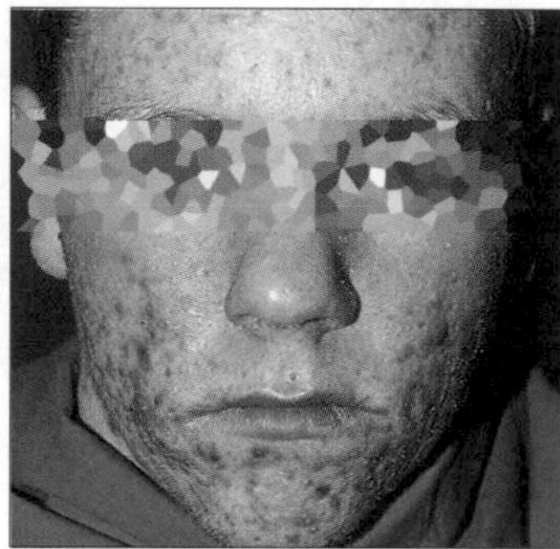

Moderate to severe facial acne.

Investigations

• Acne is a clinical diagnosis.

Culture: may be helpful to identify gram-negative folliculitis unresponsive to conventional acne treatment.

Biopsy: may be used to rule out other diseases in cases with an atypical presentation.

• Women with severe acne resistant to standard therapy or with hirsutism or menstrual irregularities may have underlying endocrine abnormalities; often the work-up is normal, but polycystic ovaries and ovarian or adrenal tumors may be present and need to be excluded as part of the work-up [1].

Complications

Scarring: from resolving lesions; "ice-pick" scarring or depressed atrophic plaques.

Hyperpigmented macules: from resolving comedones especially in patients with pigmented skin.

Keloids: especially on anterior chest and back.

Solid persistent inflammatory edema unresponsive to conventional treatment for acne: as a sequela [2].

Osteolytic bone lesions with musculoskeletal pain and septic fever: in cases of acne fulminans, a rare ulcerative form of acne [3,4].

Vaginal yeast infections: in patients treated with systemic antibiotics.

Aggressive cutaneous basal cell carcinomas/thyroid carcinomas: prone to develop in patients who have had superficial x-ray irradiation for treatment of acne in the past; such patients should be closely followed and educated.

Differential diagnosis

Rosacea
Facial flushing with periorbital pallor; can be purely telangiectatic, spares the face; granulomatous, papular, pustular or any combination.

Perioral dermatitis
Combination of eczematous patches and inflammatory papules around the mouth, most commonly in women.

Steroid acne
Multiple monomorphous inflammatory papules or pustules. Can occur from application of fluorinated topical steroids especially on face or in patients on systemic steroids (on chest, back, and shoulders).

Drugs
Can cause acneiform eruption, especially phenytoin and lithium.

Halogenoderma
From iodide, bromide, or chlorine.

Gram-negative folliculitis
Culture useful to differentiate from acne.

Excoriated acne
Can be incorrectly diagnosed as impetigo or factitial dermatitis.

Pyoderma faciale
Rapid development of indurated erythema and fluctuant abscesses on the face of young women.

Tumorous sclerosis
Angiofibromas often misdiagnosed as acne.

Acne fulminans
Severe sudden onset of painful inflammatory nodules mainly on the chest and back of adolescent boys common with associated leukocytosis, arthralgias, fever, and ulceration of the nodules.

Etiology

Defective keratinization that obstructs follicular outflow channels.

Increased sebum production (controlled by androgenic hormonal stimulation).

Inflammation: elevated population of *Propionibacterium acnes* within follicles behind obstructed follicular channels release lipases that act on triglycerides in sebum and release free fatty acids, which in turn causes inflammation; *P. acnes* also produces chemoattractants [5].

Epidemiology

Most common skin disease in the US.

85% of those between the ages of 12 and 25 are affected.

Peak incidence between ages 16 and 18.

Treatment

Diet and lifestyle

• Diet appears to have little effect on acne.

• Long-term exposure to chlorinated hydrocarbons, coal tar, machine oils, greases, lubricating oils, and dioxin can cause acneiform lesions [6].

• Pomade oils and comedogenic cosmetics should be avoided [7].

Pharmacological treatment

• Most treatments take 4 to 6 weeks of therapy before clinical improvement occurs [8].

For mild acne: topical treatment

Standard dosage Benzoyl peroxide, 2.5%–10%.
Tretinoin, 0.025%, 0.05%, 0.1% cream; 0.01%, 0.025%, 0.025% gel; 0.05% liquid. Apply as tolerated; increase to twice daily.

Contraindications None.

Special points *Retinoic acid:* needs to be increased as tolerated; many patients experience an initial flare-up of their acne.

Main drug interactions None.

Main side effects Drying, irritation and stinging, excessive skin peeling.

For mild acne: topical antibiotics

Standard dosage Clindamycin, 1% solution, gel, or lotion; erythromycin, 2% ointment, gel, or solution; meclocycline; tetracycline; benzamycin (3% erythromycin, 5% benzoyl peroxide); apply thin film to affected areas twice daily.

Contraindications None.

Main drug interactions None.

Main side effects Local irritation and mild scaliness; gels tend to be drying, ointments make skin feel "oily."

For moderate acne: oral antibiotics

Standard dosage Tetracycline, 1–2 g daily.
Erythromycin, 1 g daily.
Minocycline, 100–200 mg daily.
Trimethoprim-sulfamethoxazole, 1–2 tablets daily.

Contraindications *Tetracycline*: pregnancy and children under 12 years of age.
Erythromycin: patients taking terfenadine astemizole.

Special points *Tetracycline, minocyline*: may cause pseudotumor cerebri.
Minocycline: are acute hepatitis and liver failure, a Loffler-like syndrome, a lupus-like syndrome, and pustular folliculitis with eosinophilia (rare and often unrecognized side effects).

Main drug interactions *Erythromycin*: interacts with cytochrome P450; reported to decrease the effectiveness of oral contraceptives.

Main side effects *Tetracycline, minocycline*: nausea, vomiting, photosensitivity.
Erythromycin: severe gastric irritation.

For moderate or severe acne

Standard dosage Isotretinoin, 0.5–1 mg/kg daily in two doses with meals for 20 weeks.

Contraindications Pregnancy; caution in pre-existing renal or hepatic disease.

Special points Major fetal abnormalities have been reported; female patients in child-bearing years must use effective contraception during and at least 1 month after therapy.
Liver function tests and serum lipoprotein levels should be monitored monthly.

Main drug interactions Preparations containing high doses of vitamin A.

Main side effects Cheilitis of the lips; drying of nasal mucosa with mild epistaxis and conjunctivitis; fetal death and malformation; arthralgias; elevated liver enzymes and triglycerides.

Treatment aims

To reduce inflammatory lesions.
To prevent scarring and embarrassment.

Other treatments

Dermabrasion.
Chemical peels.
Triamcinolone injected into inflammatory papules.
Cryotherapy.
Punch grafting acne scars.
Comedo extraction.
Cyst incision and drainage.

Prognosis

Excellent with spontaneous remission after several years.

Excellent for nodulocystic acne treated with isotretinoin.

Acne sometimes persists into adulthood.

Follow-up and management

• Follow-up is crucial because rate of response to first-line agents is slow.

• Patient education is key to success.

• Isotretinoin should be considered early in severe cases unresponsive to first-line agents to prevent severe scarring.

Key references

1. Lucky AW: Hormonal correlates of acne and hirsutism. *Am J Med* 1995, **98**:89(S)–94(S).
2. Jungfer B, *et al.*: Solid persistent facial edema of acne: successful treatment with isotretinoin and ketotifen. *Dermatology* 1993, **187**:34–37.
3. Karvonen SL: Acne fulminans: report of clinical findings and treatment of twenty-four patients. *J Am Acad Dermatol* 1993, **28**:572–579.
4. Laasonen LS, *et al.*: Bone disease in adolescents with acne fulminans and severe cystic acne: radiologic and scintographic findings. *AJR Am J Roentgenol* 1994, **152**:1161–1165.
5. Pochi PE: The pathogenesis and treatment of acne. *Ann Rev Med* 1990, **41**:187–198.
6. Fischer AA: *Contact dermatitis*, edn 3. Philadelphia: Lea & Febiger; 1989:368–393; 486–514.
7. Plewig G, *et al.*: Pomade acne. *Arch Dermatol* 1970, **101**:580–584.
8. Drake LA, *et al.*: Guidelines of care for acne vulgaris. *J Am Acad Dermatol* 1990, **22**:676–680.

Diagnosis

Symptoms

General

Coarsening of facial features, enlargement of hands and feet.
Headache.
Sweating.
Musculoskeletal abnormalities: associated with joint degeneration.
Neuropathy: particularly carpal tunnel syndrome.
Sleep apnea: due to nasopharyngeal soft-tissue hypertrophy.

Local effects of pituitary tumor

Visual deterioration: due to chiasmal compression.
Hypopituitarism: hypothyroidism, gonadotropin deficiency, adrenal insufficiency.
Hyperprolactinemia: impaired libido, impotence, amenorrhea, galactorrhea.

Signs

General

Large hands and feet with soft tissue overgrowth.
Coarse features and frontal bossing.
Prognathism and dental separation.
Hypertension: in 30% of patients.
Carpal tunnel syndrome: in 40%.
Multinodular goiter: in 10%.
Gigantism and eunuchoid features: if disease was manifest during childhood.

Local effects of pituitary tumor

Decreased visual acuity.
Visual field defects.
Optic atrophy.
Hypopituitarism: loss of body hair, hypothyroidism.
Hyperprolactinemia: galactorrhea.

Investigations [1]

Tests of growth hormone secretion: diagnosis can be established by failure of growth hormone suppression to undetectable concentrations (<1 mU/L) during oral glucose tolerance test; may also show impaired glucose tolerance (in 40% of patients) or diabetes mellitus (in 20%); confirmed by raised level of insulin-like growth factor 1.
Pituitary function tests: thyroid function; pituitary–gonadal axis (luteinizing hormone, follicle-stimulating hormone, estradiol, testosterone); 09.00 h cortisol (dynamic testing with insulin tolerance test may be indicated); serum prolactin (raised in 30%).
Lateral skull radiography: shows thickened skull, enlarged frontal sinuses, abnormal pituitary fossa.
MRI or CT of pituitary fossa.
Visual field test: Goldmann perimetry.

Complications

Coronary artery disease and cardiac failure: high prevalence of hypertension and diabetes mellitus are significant risk factors.
Respiratory disease: small airway function abnormal; additional extrathoracic upper airway obstruction (macroglossia, goiter, nasopharyngeal soft-tissue hypertrophy); mortality significantly increased.
Arthropathies: frequent; contribute significantly to overall morbidity.
Hypercalciuria: in 50% of patients.
Hypercalcemia: in 5% of patients.
Renal stones: occasionally.
Colorectal polyps: increased incidence, although association between acromegaly and colonic malignancy inferred but so far unproven [2].

Differential diagnosis

- The facial appearance and enlargement of the hands and feet are characteristic for acromegaly.

Pseudoacromegaly (severe hypothyroidism).

Etiology

- Causes include the following:

Pituitary growth hormone producing-adenoma in 99% of patients.

Occasionally, excess secretion of growth hormone-releasing hormone from neuro-endocrine tumors (gut, pancreas, lung) or from hypothalamic ganglioneuromas.

- An association has been found with multiple endocrine neoplasia type 1 syndrome.

Epidemiology

- The annual incidence is 2.8–4.0 in one million.
- The prevalence is 40–60 in one million.
- Up to 600 new patients are afflicted with acromegaly annually in the US.

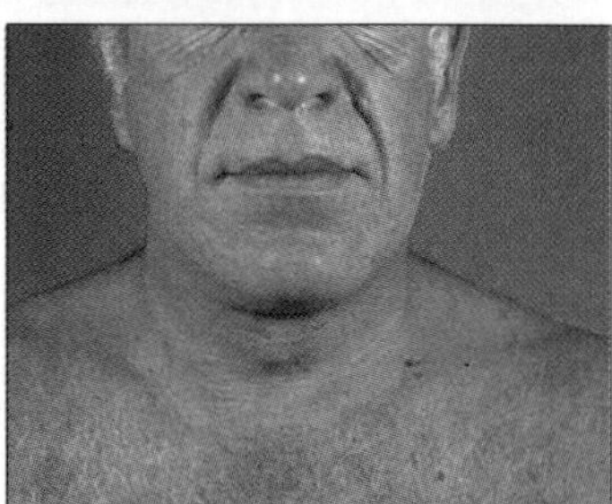

Typical coarse features of acromegaly.

Treatment

Diet and lifestyle

• Unless the patient suffers from diabetes mellitus or hyperlipidemia, no special dietary precautions are necessary.

• Measures to reduce known vascular risk factors (stopping smoking, controlling hypertension and diabetes, and normalizing lipids) are paramount from the outset.

Pharmacological treatment [1]

• Octreotide may be used when growth hormone concentrations remain >5 mU/L after surgery or in elderly patients as first-line treatment.

• Bromocriptine reduces growth hormone concentrations in some patients.

Standard dosage Octreotide, 100 µg s.c. 3 times daily.
Bromocriptine, 1.25 mg at night initially, increasing to 20–30 mg daily over a period of weeks as necessary.

Contraindications *Octreotide*: pregnancy and breast-feeding.
Bromocriptine: sensitivity to ergot alkaloids, porphyria.

Special points *Octreotide*: growth hormone may be further suppressed in some cases by a dose of 200 µg 3 times daily; little gain from further dose increases.
Bromocriptine: if effective, treatment costs much reduced.

Main drug interactions *Octreotide*: may alter insulin and hypoglycemic drug needs in patients with diabetes mellitus.
Bromocriptine: dopamine antagonists (*e.g.*, metoclopramide) interfere with action.

Main side effects *Octreotide*: local transient discomfort at injection site, which can be minimized by warming the solution before administration; colicky abdominal pain, diarrhea, nausea, bloating, flatulence, which usually resolve during first 2–3 weeks of treatment; gallstones, gastritis (long-term).
Bromocriptine: nausea, vomiting, headache, nasal congestion, postural hypotension, digital vasospasm, constipation.

Nonpharmacological treatment

Transsphenoidal surgery

• This is the treatment of choice.

• Cure rates of 40%–90% have been achieved, but variability of results may depend on parameters used to assess cure.

• The probability of success is influenced by preoperative growth hormone concentrations, tumor size and invasion.

Pituitary radiotherapy

• Radiotherapy is indicated for patients declining or unfit for surgery or for those not adequately treated by surgery.

• The greatest decrease in growth hormone concentration occurs during the first 2 years.

• Continued decrease in growth hormone concentration is seen for many years.

• Increasing development of hypopituitarism is seen.

Treatment aims

To relieve symptoms.

To reduce growth hormone concentrations to <5 mU/L.

To treat local effects of pituitary tumor.

To maintain normal pituitary function.

Prognosis [3]

• Patients with long-standing acromegaly have twice the mortality of the general population.

• Reduction of the serum growth hormone concentration to <5 mU/L is associated with mortality similar to that of the general population.

Follow-up and management

• Patients with acromegaly need lifelong follow-up to assess the response to treatment and to determine the function of the normal pituitary gland.

Key references

1. Acromegaly Therapy Consensus Development Panel: Benefits versus risks of medical treatment for acromegaly. *Am J Med* 1994, **97**:468-473.
2. Ezzat S, Melmed S: Are patients with acromegaly at increased risk for neoplasia? *J Clin Endocrinol Metab* 1991, **72**:245–249.
3. Bates AS, *et al.*: An audit of outcome of treatment in acromegaly. *Q J Med* 1993, **86**:293–299.

Diagnosis

Symptoms

• Symptoms develop rapidly, often becoming maximal within 4–12 h of onset.

• Usual sites are knee or wrist for pseudogout and first metatarsophalangeal joint, mid- or hindfoot, knee, or wrist for gout [1].

• Usually, only one or a few joints are involved; polyarticular attacks are rare.

Severe pain: "worst ever."

Stiffness, tenderness, swelling.

Fever and systemic upset: particularly with large- or multiple-joint involvement.

Signs

Overlying erythema: later desquamation.

Red hot joint: *i.e.*, periarticular and articular inflammation; always suggests crystals or sepsis.

Tense effusion, increased warmth, marked joint-line and periarticular tenderness, restricted movement with stress pain: *i.e.*, florid synovitis.

Pyrexia: possible confusion, especially in elderly patients.

Turbid or blood-stained aspirated fluid: high cell count, >95% polymorphs.

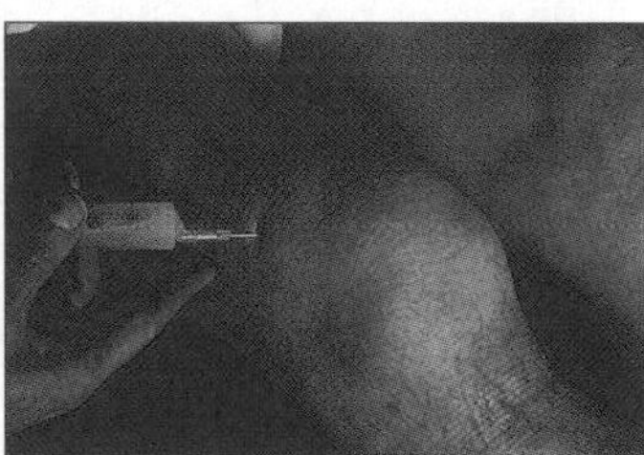

Turbid synovial fluid aspirated from acute knee

Investigations

Diagnostic: synovial fluid analysis

Compensated polarized light microscopy: usual method of crystal identification:
monosodium urate crystals: strong (negative) birefringence, needle-shaped, 2–25 µm long, easily identified;
calcium pyrophosphate dihydrate crystals: weak (positive) birefringence, rhomboid, 2–10 µm long, more difficult to identify;
other crystals (cholesterol, oxalate, injected steroid) rare.

Gram stain and culture: essential to exclude sepsis.

Supportive but nondiagnostic

Radiography: to detect chondrocalcinosis (pseudogout); osteophyte, sclerosis, cysts, joint-space narrowing (pseudogout, gout); para-articular erosion (gout); although characteristic, such changes are not always present.

ESR, CRP measurement: usually raised.

Serum uric acid measurement: often but not always raised in gout.

Disease associations

• These should be considered after diagnosis and acute management.

Metabolic screening: calcium, alkaline phosphatase, ferritin, magnesium; if patient is <55 years or has polyarticular chondrocalcinosis (pseudogout).

Urea (BUN), creatinine measurement: for renal impairment in primary or secondary gout.

Lipoprotein measurement, liver function tests: in primary and alcohol-associated gout.

Complications

Cluster attacks: one attack triggers attacks at other sites.

Joint rupture: with associated soft-tissue inflammation.

Nerve entrapment: due to acute soft-tissue swelling (most often median nerve).

Differential diagnosis

Septic arthritis: sepsis usually superimposes on abnormal, previously symptomatic joint.

Other crystal synovitis.

• Acute crystal synovitis and septic arthritis may coexist.

• More than one crystal type may be present ("mixed crystal deposition").

Etiology

Causes of primary gout

Inherited renal undersecretion of uric acid (in most patients).

Inherited overproduction of uric acid (rare).

Obesity, excess alcohol intake (mainly beer).

Inherited crystal nucleation or growth-promoting tissue factors.

Causes of secondary gout

Chronic diuretic treatment.

Chronic renal impairment.

Lead poisoning (in "moonshine" drinkers).

Causes of pseudogout

Sporadic isolated chondrocalcinosis, pyrophosphate arthropathy (osteoarthritis subset).

Familial predisposition (unusual).

Metabolic predisposition (rare): hemochromatosis, hypomagnesemia, hyperparathyroidism, hypophosphatasemia.

Triggering factors

Local trauma, intercurrent acute illness, surgery, initiation of drug treatment, *e.g.*, allopurinol (gout), thyroxine (pseudogout), parenteral fluids, joint lavage.

• "Shedding" of preformed (previously asymptomatic) crystals initiates acute attack.

Epidemiology

• Crystal synovitis is the most common cause of acute monoarthritis in middle-aged and elderly patients.

• Before the age of 65, more men than women present with gout (mainly primary).

• After the age of 65, as many men as women present with gout (mainly secondary).

• Patients with pseudogout are predominantly elderly, with as many men as women.

• Pseudogout is rare in patients <55 years (suggests familial or metabolic predisposition).

Treatment

Diet and lifestyle

• No special precautions are necessary.

Pharmacological treatment

Oral NSAIDs

• Simple analgesics may be effective with other treatments, but quick-acting NSAIDs are generally preferred (*see* Gout *for further details*) [1,2].

Colchicine

• Colchicine is effective in any crystal synovitis, but it should be used only for very resistant attacks because of toxicity [1].

Standard dosage	Colchicine, 1 mg, then 0.5 mg orally every 6 h until pain controlled or side effects develop (maximum, 6 mg) in first 24 h; then maximum dose of 0.6 mg 3 times daily.
Contraindications	Renal or hepatic impairment, dehydration.
Special points	Never given parenterally; not to be given again within 7 days.
Main drug interactions	None.
Main side effects	Severe nausea, vomiting, watery diarrhea.

Intra-articular steroids

• Steroids are indicated for problematic attacks (large joints, polyarticular involvement, elderly ill patient) or if oral agents are contraindicated.

• They usually reduce synovitis within 24–48 h.

• The dose should be varied according to joint size; doses listed here are for the knee [2].

Standard dosage	Methylprednisolone, 60 mg. Triamcinolone hexacetonide, 60 mg. Triamcinolone acetonide, 60 mg.
Contraindications	Coexistent sepsis.
Special points	Aseptic technique and single-dose vial should be used.
Main drug interactions	None.
Main side effects	Facial flushing, local skin or fat atrophy (mainly fluoridated steroids), exacerbation of pain (temporary), sepsis (rare).

Nonpharmacological treatment

Local physical measures

• The following are the first line of treatment and must be done early:

Aspiration: to reduce intracapsular hypertension (often temporary).

Local heat or cold: may ameliorate pain and swelling.

Resting support (possibly with splintage): to ease symptoms.

Elevation: to reduce edema.

Early rehabilitation (active movement, mobilization, graded exercise): to maintain muscle and range of movement.

• Prolonged immobilization should be avoided: regular passive movement should punctuate assisted rest.

Lavage

• Lavage is indicated for the following:

Florid, large joint synovitis unresponsive after 48 h to aspiration, steroid injection, and oral medications.

Large loculated effusion (inhibiting effective aspiration).

Coexistent sepsis.

Treatment aims

To relieve pain.

To reduce intra-articular hypertension.

To avoid muscle wasting or capsular restriction.

Prognosis

• Acute attacks resolve spontaneously, even without treatment, within 1–3 weeks.

• Although prolonged florid synovitis is potentially detrimental, most episodes settle with no apparent resulting damage.

• Incomplete recovery of muscle strength or bulk is the most common problem.

Follow-up and management

• Long-term interventions should be instituted only after an acute attack of gout has settled.

• Metabolic screening for pseudogout should be undertaken if appropriate.

• Patients with associated chronic pyrophosphate arthropathy should be advised about alteration of adverse mechanical factors, reduction in obesity, appropriate exercise, and use of symptomatic agents.

Key references

1. Star VL, Hockberg MC: Prevention and management of gout. *Drugs* 1993, **45**:212–222.
2. Tan N, Lertratanakul W, Barr WG: Acute gouty arthritis: modern approaches to an ancient disease. *Postgrad Med* 1993, **94**:73–75;78;83–84.

Diagnosis

Symptoms

• Onset is usually insidious.

Dizziness and syncope.

Weakness, fatigue, weight loss: common.

Gastrointestinal symptoms: in ~50% of patients.

Pigmentation, persistent tan after holiday, increase in normal skin pigmentation: common.

Mental changes.

Symmetrical musculoskeletal pain: in 10%.

Acute back pain: in anticoagulated patients; rare.

Signs

Postural hypotension.

Hypotension: usually systolic blood pressure <110 mm Hg.

Generalized pigmentation: common; extensor and exposed skin should be checked.

Buccal pigmentation: usually manifest with generalized pigmentation.

Scar pigmentation: only scars inflicted after onset of Addison's disease.

Signs of organ-specific autoimmune disease: *e.g.*, vitiligo, thyroid signs.

Hyponatremia: inability to excrete water due to raised antidiuretic hormone concentration and glucocorticoid effect on renal tubule (common).

Hyperkalemia: usually mild (normal in 40% of patients).

Hypercalcemia: in 10% of patients.

Hypoglycemia: sometimes seen in children or undernourished patients.

Investigations

Chest radiography: to check for tuberculosis.

Blood count and film: eosinophilia, macrocytosis with coexistent vitamin B_{12} deficiency, normocytic anemia after volume replacement.

Serum cortisol measurement: concentration usually <7 μg/dL; may be 7–18 μg/dL during stress; >18 μg/dL makes diagnosis improbable.

Plasma corticotropic hormone (ACTH) measurement: concentration usually >80 ng/L (sample must be collected, put on ice, centrifuged, and frozen immediately).

Plasma renin activity and aldosterone measurement: high renin, low aldosterone concentrations.

Cosyntropin stimulation test: cosyntropin, 250 μg i.v.; cortisol measured at 0, 30, and 60 min (normal rise >20 μg/dL); may not distinguish primary from secondary adrenal failure [1].

Insulin hypoglycemia test: under control conditions, 0.15 U/kg insulin is injected and serum glucose is monitored until <40 mg/dL. Samples for cortisol and ACTH measurement are drawn at baseline, during, and 30 and 60 min after hypoglycemia to differentiate primary from secondary adrenal failure.

Complications

Death: if diagnosis missed, if patient not given extra steroids in stress situations, or if replacement steroids not taken; hydrocortisone must be given before thyroxine when hypothyroidism and Addison's disease coexist (Schmidt's syndrome).

Associated autoimmune endocrine failure: vitamin B_{12} deficiency, hypothyroidism, hypoparathyroidism.

Differential diagnosis

Secondary adrenal insufficiency: low corticotropic hormone, cortisol response to insulin hypoglycemia.

Other causes of pigmentation: *e.g.*, hemochromatosis.

Etiology

• Causes include the following:

Autoimmune adrenalitis: cortex atrophy only, with antiadrenal antibodies (>80%) [2].

Tuberculosis: whole-gland involvement, calcification on radiography or CT (less common now).

• Rare causes include the following (80%–90% of both adrenals must be affected):

Adrenal hemorrhage: usually in anticoagulated or septicemic patients.

Adrenoleukodystrophy.

Amyloidosis.

Congenital adrenal hyperplasia.

Drugs: *e.g.*, ketoconazole.

Familial glucocorticoid deficiency: adrenocorticotropic hormone receptor mutation.

Glucocorticosteriod receptor defects.

Hemochromatosis.

HIV-related adrenalitis.

Metastases.

Sarcoidosis.

Epidemiology

• The incidence of Addison's disease is estimated to be 40–60 in one million.

• The female :male ratio is 2 :1.

Treatment

Diet and lifestyle

• Patients should always carry a steroid-warning card, Medicalert bracelet, and "emergency pack" (hydrocortisone, 100 mg ampule, with saline solution, green needle, and 2-mL syringe).

• Patients and partners should be taught how to give an i.m. injection in case of vomiting or coma.

• Patients should be educated about the need for extra hydrocortisone in case of illness or physical stress (surgery or fever).

• Patients should have 24-h direct access to a specialist endocrine center.

Pharmacological treatment

For acutely ill or hypotensive patients

• If the diagnosis is suspected, action must be taken immediately.

• In previously undiagnosed disease, blood should be drawn for cortisol and corticotropic hormone measurement.

Hydrocortisone, 100 mg i.v. bolus.

0.9% saline 1-L bolus initially in 1h followed by 0.9% saline infusion.

20% glucose i.v. bolus to correct hypoglycemia.

• Inotropic agents are usually not effective [3].

Continued treatment

Standard dosage	Hydrocortisone, 100 mg i.m. every 6 h until clinical improvement; patients in intensive care units or on anti-coagulants can be treated by 100 mg in 50 mL saline solution at 2 mg/h i.v. infusion.
Contraindications	None.
Special points	When conscious and taking fluids orally, most patients can be converted to oral hydrocortisone. Prednisolone and dexamethasone sometimes used instead. Patients receiving large doses of hydrocortisone do not usually require mineralocorticoid replacement. Patients on standard oral replacements with hydrocortisone may need fludrocortisone.
Main drug interactions	None.
Main side effects	Short-term treatment at these doses rarely has side effects, but diabetes mellitus and psychosis must be considered [4].

Treatment aims

To alleviate symptoms and restore circulating mineralosteroid and corticosteroids to physiological levels.

Prognosis

• Patients have a normal life expectancy if adequately treated.

• Adrenal function is rarely recovered.

Follow-up and management

• Electrolytes should be monitored periodically and with illness.

• Plasma renin activity may be monitored 2 h after fludrocortisone dose.

• Long-term management includes referral to a specialist endocrine unit; hydrocortisone, 15 mg orally on waking and 10 mg in the evening before 19.00 h (dose and frequency vary); and fludrocortisone, 0.1–0.2 mg daily.

Key references

1. Oelkers W, Diederich S, Bahr V: Diagnosis and therapy surveillance in Addison's disease: rapid adrenocorticotrophin (ACTH) test and measurement of plasma ACTH, renin activity, and aldosterone. *J Clin Endocrinol Metab* 1992, **75**:259–264.
2. De Bellis A, *et al.*: Remission of subclinical adrenocortical failure in subjects with adrenal autoantibodies. *J Clin Endocrinol Metab* 1993, **76**:1002–1007.
3. Werbel SS, Ober, KP: Acute adrenal insufficiency. *Endocrinol Metab Clin North Am* 1993, **22**:303–328.
4. Ur E, *et al.* Mania in association with hydrocortisone replacement for Addison's disease. *Postgrad Med J* 1992, **68**:41–43.

Adult respiratory distress syndrome

Diagnosis [1]

Symptoms

Dyspnea: variable severity, developing abruptly or gradual onset some days after initial insult.

Signs

Tachypnea: rapid and shallow.

Warmth and peripheral vasodilatation.

Signs of pulmonary edema: on auscultation.

Other signs of underlying disease.

• Cyanosis may or may not be apparent.

Investigations

Chest radiography: for bilateral pulmonary infiltrates; to confirm pulmonary edema in presence of predisposing condition.

Pulmonary artery catheterization: to measure pulmonary artery occlusion pressure (normally <15 mm Hg) to exclude cardiogenic edema.

Arterial blood gas analysis: refractory hypoxemia unresponsive to increased inspired oxygen concentration (partial arterial oxygen pressure <70 mm Hg breathing 40% oxygen, arterial–alveolar oxygen tension ratio <0.25); low total respiratory compliance (<30 ml/cm H_2O).

Fiberoptic bronchoscopy and lavage or biopsy, upper respiratory tract cultures, CT and nuclear imaging, specialized blood tests (*e.g.*, plasma amylase): to establish underlying condition.

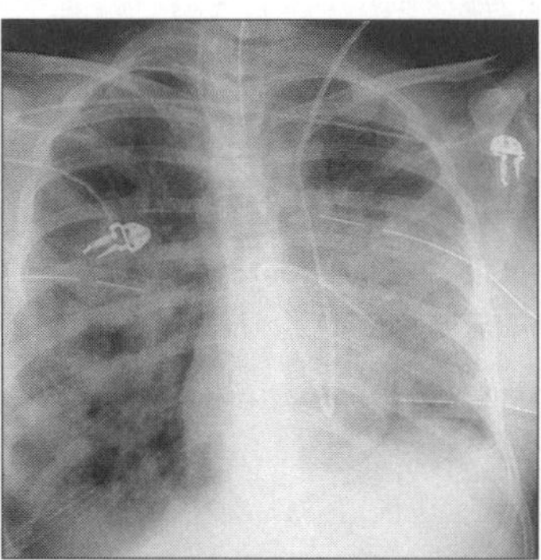

Typical chest radiograph appearance of established adult respiratory distress syndrome, showing pneumothoraces, position of endotracheal tube, intercostal chest drains, and pulmonary artery flotation catheter.

Complications [2]

Death.

Multisystem organ failure: especially renal failure.

Sepsis.

Shock.

Barotrauma: from mechanical ventilation (*e.g.*, pneumothorax).

Debilitation in period after intensive care: survivors usually recover fully within 12 months [3].

Differential diagnosis

• The diagnostic criteria exclude other diagnoses.

Etiology [4]

• Causes include the following:

Sepsis from any cause.

Bacterial, viral, or drug-induced pneumonia.

Massive burns or major trauma.

Aspiration of gastric contents.

Inhalation of toxic fumes.

Trauma resulting in direct pulmonary contusion.

Oxygen toxicity.

Disseminated intravascular coagulation.

Massive hemorrhage or multiple transfusion.

Pre-eclampsia.

Amniotic fluid embolism.

Acute pancreatitis.

Head injury or raised intracranial pressure.

Intravenous drug abuse.

Epidemiology

• Adult respiratory distress syndrome has an incidence of approximately 1.5 cases per 100 000 persons in the US, although cases of acute lung injury not meeting the diagnostic criteria occur much more often.

• The prevalence varies according to the predisposing illness (2%–25%).

Pathophysiology

• Adult respiratory distress syndrome may be the pulmonary manifestation of a pan-endothelial insult resulting from the activation of many humoral and cellular events.

• It is uniformly characterized by increased permeability of the alveolar–capillary membrane, leading to pulmonary edema.

• Deranged cellular use of oxygen occurs as part of the syndrome and may result in widespread multiorgan failure of variable severity.

Treatment

Diet and lifestyle

• Patients need nutritional support by parenteral or enteral route while on the ventilator.

Pharmacological treatment [5,6]

• Underlying conditions should be fully investigated and steps taken to correct any reversible disorders.

• Nosocomial infection and supra-added sepsis should be managed aggressively.

• Vasopressor, inotropic, and chronotropic agents should be used to support circulation and urine output.

• Enteral nutrition should be given when possible.

Nonpharmacological treatment [5,6]

• The involvement of multiple organ systems in the disease process means that supportive measures are not confined to the respiratory system.

• All patients with severe lung injury and established adult respiratory distress syndrome should be managed in the intensive care unit.

• Full respiratory and invasive hemodynamic monitoring and urinary catheterization are needed.

Respiratory support

• The aim is to maintain oxygen saturation at approximately 90% using continuous positive airways pressure applied via a face mask or mechanical ventilation.

• New techniques (*e.g.*, pressure-controlled, inverse-ratio ventilation) are aimed at recruiting collapsed alveoli while reducing peak airway pressures (and therefore the risk of barotrauma) and raising mean airway pressures (thereby improving oxygenation).

Cardiac and circulatory support

• The aim is to maximize oxygen delivery to tissues.

• Hemoglobin should be maintained at 10–12 g/dL, with a hematocrit of 30%–35%.

• Cardiac output and oxygen delivery should be measured and optimized by the judicious manipulation of filling pressures and the use of inotropic drugs.

Fluid balance

• The aim of manipulating fluid balance is to reduce circulating volume as much as possible in an effort to reduce further extravasation of edema into the alveoli.

• Pulmonary artery occlusion pressure should be maintained at 8–12 mm Hg.

• Diuretics may be needed to maintain urine output >0.5 mL/kg/h.

Treatment aims

To provide definitive treatment (if available) for the underlying condition.

To support affected systems, *e.g.*, respiratory and cardiovascular, until spontaneous resolution occurs, by optimizing oxygen delivery.

Prognosis

• Mortality depends on the underlying condition and is reported to be 40%–70%.

• 90% of survivors recover 90% of their premorbid lung function after 12 months and suffer little or no respiratory impairment.

• Supportive treatments carry appreciable morbidity (*e.g.*, pneumothorax, renal failure).

• Survivors are invariably debilitated after the prolonged stay in intensive care.

Follow-up and management

• The aim of follow-up is to maximize recovery from the effects of both the initial illness and the adult respiratory distress syndrome.

• Attention to physical rehabilitation, with nutritional advice, physical therapy, and controlled exercise when appropriate, is needed for patients.

Key references

1. Bernard GR, *et al.*: The American-European Consensus Conference on ARDS: definitions, mechanisms, relevant outcomes, and clinical trial coordination. *Am J Respir Crit Care Med* 1994, **149**:818–824.
2. Bone RC, *et al.*: Adult respiratory distress syndrome: sequence and importance of multiple organ failure. *Chest* 1992, **101**:320–326.
3. McHugh LG, *et al.*: Recovery of function in survivors of the acute respiratory distress syndrome. *Am J Respir Crit Care Med* 1994, **150**:90–94.
4. Hudson LD, *et al.*: Clinical risks for development of the acute respiratory distress syndrome. *Am J Respir Crit Care Med* 1995, **151**:293–301.
5. MacNaughton PD, Evans TW: Management of the adult respiratory distress syndrome. *Lancet* 1992, **339**:469–472.
6. Kollef MH, Schuster DP: The acute respiratory distress syndrome. *N Engl J Med* 1995, **332**:27–37.

Diagnosis

Definition

• AIDS is defined by progressive immunodeficiency without another cause, manifest by various conditions, including the following:

Opportunistic infections

Viral: cytomegalovirus.

Bacterial: *Mycobacterium avium intracellulare,* disseminated *M. tuberculosis,* recurrent *Salmonella* spp., pneumococcus.

Fungal: *Candida albicans, Cryptococcus neoformans, Histoplasma capsulatum, Aspergillus* spp.

Protozoan: *Pneumocystis carinii,* cryptosporidia, microsporidia, isospora (not diagnostic of AIDS).

Unusual tumors

Kaposi's sarcoma.

Non–T-cell lymphoma.

Invasive cervical carcinoma.

Neurological manifestations

AIDS dementia complex.

Vacuolar myelopathy.

Progressive multifocal leukoencephalopathy.

Symptoms

• Skin rashes (persistent and severe herpes simplex or zoster infection) occur during the asymptomatic period of 10 years or more after seroconversion.

Skin rash, temperature, lymphadenopathy (seroconversion illness): in 50% of patients.

Unexplained diarrhea, fever, marked asthenia, minor opportunistic infections: particularly oral candidiasis and oral hairy leukoplakia; in "pre-AIDS."

Signs

Skin rash.

Lymphadenopathy.

Oral candidiasis, oral hairy leukoplakia: in pre-AIDS.

Opportunistic infection: in AIDS.

Investigations

• In the asymptomatic phase, the diagnosis can be made only by HIV testing.

HIV test: antibodies to HIV (usually occurring within 3 months of exposure) measured by enzyme-linked immunosorbent assay, usually confirmed by second test or, less often, Western blot analysis to check pattern of antibody response.

CD4 lymphocyte count: used to assess immune function; normal value ~800×10^6/L; patients with <500×10^6/L will probably progress eventually; patients with <200×10^6/L at risk for developing various opportunistic infections.

Direct measurement of viral load using polymerase chain reaction or B DNA assay: useful for antiviral therapy.

Complications

Not applicable.

Differential diagnosis

Congenital immunodeficiency.

Iatrogenic immunodeficiency: *e.g.*, after bone-marrow transplantation.

HIV-antibody-negative CD4 lymphopenia: rare; different epidemiology from HIV infection.

Etiology

• AIDS is caused by infection by HIV.

• HIV leads to a progressive fall in T-helper (CD4) cells and a failure of T-cell proliferation after antigenic stimulation, even by T cells uninfected by HIV.

Epidemiology

• Geographically, three patterns of disease are seen:

North America and Western Europe

• Transmission is mainly among men having sex with men and among intravenous drug users, with only limited transmission vertically or among recipients of blood products (patients with hemophilia who received blood products between 1975 and 1984).

• In the UK, the peak transmission among men having sex with men was in the early 1980s. The number of heterosexual people and intravenous drug users in the US is increasing.

Sub-Saharan Africa

• The disease is predominantly a heterosexual epidemic, with major transmission vertically and through blood products.

Asia

• Transmission is sporadic, with introduction of the epidemic through blood products and visitors; although the disease is not widespread in these countries, an explosive increase in numbers is occurring, mainly by heterosexual transmission.

Treatment

Diet and lifestyle

Not applicable.

Pharmacological treatment

• Zidovudine (azidothymidine, AZT) prolongs life when given to patients with AIDS and prolongs disease-free survival in asymptomatic patients.

• The time at which treatment should be initiated and the use of combinations of the drugs remain controversial.

AZT

Standard dosage AZT, 200 mg 3 times daily.

Contraindications Bone-marrow suppression.

Special points None.

Main drug interactions Drugs with similar toxic profile.

Main side effects Bone-marrow suppression, headache, insomnia, occasionally myopathy.

Didanosine (ddI)

Standard dosage Didanosine, 200 mg twice daily.

Contraindications Previous pancreatitis.

Special points Indicated for patients intolerant of or unresponsive to AZT.

Main drug interactions Given in alkaline buffer, which may reduce absorption of compounds needing acidification in the stomach.

Main side effects Pancreatitis, peripheral neuropathy.

Dideoxycytosine (ddC)

Standard dosage Dideoxycytosine, 0.75 mg 3 times daily.

Contraindications Pre-existing peripheral neuropathy.

Special points Indicated for patients intolerant of or unresponsive to AZT.

Main drug interactions None known.

Main side effects Peripheral neuropathy, stomatitis.

Stavudine

Standard dosage Stavudine, 40 mg twice daily.

Contraindications Pre-existing peripheral neuropathy.

Special points Indicated for AZT, ddI or ddC intolerant patients or those who have not responded to these agents.

Main drug interactions None known.

Main side effects Peripheral neuropathy.

Treatment aims

To suppress viral replication.

To prevent immunologic decline.

To prolong life.

To prolong disease-free survival.

Prognosis

• 60% of patients progress to AIDS within 10 years of seroconversion.

• 5% remain well, with no evidence of immunological deterioration at this time.

• The median survival from AIDS diagnosis is 2 years.

Follow-up and management

• Asymptomatic patients with CD4 cell counts between 200 and 500 should have count measured 4 times a year to determine if antiviral therapy should be initiated.

• Patients with CD4 counts $<200 \times 10^6$/L should be reviewed every 3 months to determine changes in antiretroviral therapy and to review indications for prophylactic treatment against opportunistic infections.

General references

1. Alderson T: New directions for the anti-retroviral chemotherapy of AIDS – a basis for a pharmacological approach to treatment. *Biol Rev* 1993, **68**:265–289.
2. Hoth DF, *et al.*: HIV vaccine development: a progress report. *Ann Intern Med* 1994, **121**:603–611.
3. Pinching AJ: Immunological consequences of human immunodeficiency virus infection. *Review of Medical Microbiology* 1990, **1**:83–91.
4. Sheppard HW, Ascher MS: The natural history and pathogenesis of HIV infection. *Annu Rev Microbiol* 1992, **460**:533–564.
5. Weissman IL: AIDS: the whole body view. *Curr Biol* 1993, **30**:766–769.

Diagnosis

Symptoms

• Lymphoma B symptoms may be difficult to differentiate from other symptoms of HIV infection and AIDS.

Persistent, unilateral, and enlarging nodes: in 50% of patients.

Cough, shortness of breath.

Abdominal pain.

Headaches, focal neurological deficits.

Painful and ulcerated mucosal lesions.

Localized indurated skin nodule.

Weakness, weight loss, night sweats, fever.

Signs

Enlarged discrete rubbery nodes in **neck, axillae, or groins.**

Hepatosplenomegaly.

Enlarged retroperitoneal adenopathy.

Increased intracranial pressure, papilledema, focal neurological signs.

Mass involving unusual site: *e.g.*, pericardium.

Anemia, pyrexia, petechiae.

Investigations

Biopsy: to type lymphoma.

Complete blood count: baseline for treatment.

CT of chest, abdomen, and pelvis.

Lumbar puncture: high incidence of CSF involvement.

MRI, CT, CT-guided biopsy: of solitary brain lesion to detect cerebral lymphoma.

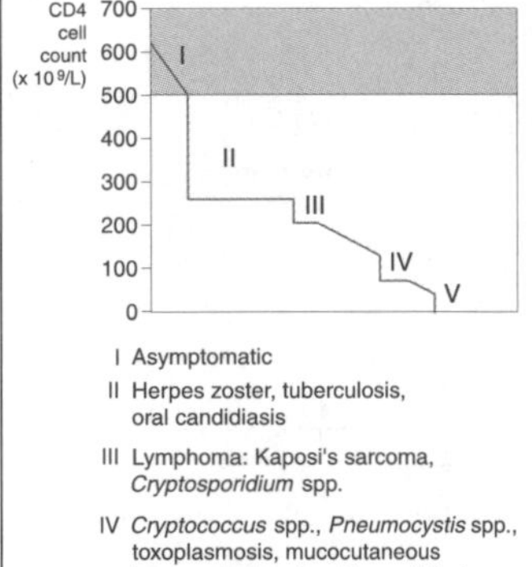

Relationship of CD4 cell count to clinical condition.

Complications

Poor bone-marrow reserve: because of infections or drugs.

Many opportunistic infections.

Differential diagnosis

Nodal

Persistent generalized lymphadenopathy.

Extranodal

Oral apthous ulcers, Kaposi's sarcoma.

Cerebral toxoplasmosis.

Systemic

Fever of unknown origin, *Mycobacterium avium intracellulare* or *M. tuberculosis* infection, HIV infection, drug reactions.

Etiology

Non-Hodgkin's lymphoma

• HIV-related immunosuppression may occur secondary to Epstein–Barr virus or other cytokines.

• Non-Hodgkin's lymphoma is seen in other immunosuppressed states: Wiskott–Aldrich syndrome (congenital), organ-transplant recipients.

Epidemiology

• Non-Hodgkin's lymphoma accounts for 3% of AIDS-defining diagnoses in HIV-positive patients; it is the AIDS-defining diagnosis in 60% of those in whom it occurs.

• It usually occurs with a low CD4 count (<200 × 10^6/L).

• It is seen equally in all risk groups.

• It is the most common AIDS-related malignancy in heterosexuals.

Pathology

B-cell non-Hodgkin's lymphoma

High grade: 90% small, noncleaved cells (65% immunoblastic, 25% Burkitt).

Low grade: occasionally, not related to AIDS.

Treatment

Diet and lifestyle

• No special precautions are necessary.

Pharmacological treatment

• Specialist supervision is needed.

• Discussion of treatment options with the patient is vital.

• Patients with good performance status and high CD4 counts are treated by conventional CHOP chemotherapy (cyclophosphamide, vincristine, adriamycin, prednisolone) or short-course high-dose multiple-agent regimens; traditional non-AIDS regimens may cause worsening of prognosis in poor-risk AIDS patients.

• Patients with poor performance status, low CD4 counts ($<100 \times 10^6$/L), and previous AIDS-defining diagnoses can receive low-dose CHOP or vincristine and bleomycin with steroids.

• CNS prophylaxis with intrathecal methotrexate is important because CNS involvement is frequent.

• All chemotherapy is immunosuppressive, depresses bone-marrow function, and may precipitate infection.

Treatment aims

To avoid overwhelming infection in good-risk patients receiving high-dose chemotherapy.

To maintain quality of life.

Other treatments

Radiotherapy

• This is useful in palliative treatment of nodal masses unresponsive to chemotherapy or when chemotherapy is not possible.

External beam radiotherapy for localized extranodal sites: *e.g.*, lymphoma of tonsil.

Whole-brain radiotherapy for cerebral lymphoma.

Bone-marrow support

With colony-stimulating factors.

Prognosis

• The median survival is <6 months (worse than for non–HIV-related non-Hodgkin's lymphoma, stage for stage).

• Factors associated with poor prognosis include having AIDS before diagnosis of lymphoma, poor performance status (<70% Karnofsky), having a CD4 count $<100 \times 10^6$/L.

• 50% of patients die of non-Hodgkin's lymphoma, 50% of AIDS-related problems.

• Burkitt's lymphoma responds better to chemotherapy than immunoblastic lymphoma does.

• The median survival for cerebral lymphoma is 4–8 weeks.

Follow-up and management

• Patients should be provided with psychological support and continuing care.

General references

1. Ioachim HL, *et al.*: Acquired immunodeficiency syndrome associated lymphomas. Clinical, pathologic, immunologic, and viral characteristics of 111 cases. *Hum Pathol* 1991, **22**:659–673.

2. Levine AM, *et al.*: Human immunodeficiency virus-related lymphoma. Prognostic factors predictive of survival. *Cancer* 1991, **68**:2466–2472.

3. Levine AM, *et al.*: Low dose chemotherapy with central nervous system prophylaxis and zidovudine maintenance in AIDS related lymphoma. A prospective multi-institutional trial. *JAMA* 1991, **266**:84–88.

Diagnosis

Symptoms and signs

Uncomplicated alcohol withdrawal

• Patients may continue to have physical signs and symptoms of long-term alcohol abuse (*e.g.*, peripheral neuropathy, calf tenderness, liver failure).

• Symptoms appear within several hours of reduction or cessation of alcohol intake and last 5–7 days.

Nausea or vomiting.

Anxiety, irritability, insomnia.

Illusions and poorly formed transient hallucinations.

Autonomic hyperactivity: *e.g.*, tachycardia, raised blood pressure.

Coarse tremor of hands, tongue, or eyelids.

Alcohol withdrawal delirium (delirium tremens)

• Symptoms develop 1–7 days after reduction or cessation of intake and last 2–3 days.

• The following features differentiate delirium tremens from uncomplicated alcohol withdrawal:

Disorientation and confusion.

Vivid hallucinations: visual, auditory, tactile.

Delusions.

Investigations

Routine

Full blood count: to identify anemia and macrocytosis.

Vitamin B_{12} and serum folate measurement: to detect deficiencies.

Electrolytes, glucose, blood urea nitrogen, creatinine, urinalysis: to assess level of hydration.

Serum magnesium and calcium: to detect deficiencies.

Liver function tests: to diagnose evidence of liver damage.

Chest radiography: to detect chest infections and cardiomyopathy.

Indicators of long-term excessive alcohol use

Alcohol history: most sensitive and important indicator; elicits amount and duration of intake and evidence of complications.

Mean cell volume measurement: raised volume 20% sensitive and nonspecific.

Gamma glutamyltransferase measurement: increased concentration 60% sensitive and nonspecific.

Complications

Tonic–clonic seizures.

Physical injury.

Wernicke's encephalopathy: acute onset, characterized by ataxia, ophthalmoplegia, and confusion; syndrome underdiagnosed but should be considered in all comatose patients.

Korsakoff's psychosis: irreversible brain damage; main defect is loss of recent memory, leading to confabulation.

Differential diagnosis

Withdrawal from sedatives (benzodiazepines, barbiturates).

Diabetic ketoacidosis.

Hypoglycemia.

Etiology

• Alcohol withdrawal syndrome is caused by stopping or reducing alcohol intake in patients dependent on alcohol.

Epidemiology

• Approximately 30 million Americans consume alcohol at dangerous levels.

• At least one in 10 ambulatory patients suffers from alcohol dependence.

• 25% of general hospital inpatients in the US are alcoholics.

Definitions

Safe level

• There is no single threshold between safe and hazardous drinking. The US Preventive Services Task Force and Surgeon General suggest ≤2 drinks/day as safe or moderate drinking [1].

Alcohol abuse

Regular daily intake of a large amount of alcohol.

Regular heavy drinking limited to weekends or in binges lasting weeks or months.

No evidence of withdrawal symptoms.

Alcohol dependence

Subjective awareness of a compulsion to drink.

Prominence of drink-seeking behavior.

Evidence of tolerance.

Presence of withdrawal symptoms after reduction or cessation of alcohol ingestion.

Use of alcohol to relieve or avoid development of withdrawal symptoms.

Social, psychological, and physical consequences of alcohol use.

Treatment

Diet and lifestyle

• No special precautions are necessary, beyond modifying alcoholic lifestyle.

Pharmacological treatment

• Pharmacological treatment is needed for patients showing evidence of alcohol withdrawal; treatment of alcohol abuse is not necessary.

Setting for treatment

• No evidence suggests that inpatient treatment is superior to outpatient treatment; inpatient treatment is, however, recommended for the following patients:

Those who may develop delirium tremens and severe withdrawal complications (fits, Wernicke's-Korsakoff's psychosis).

Those who are considered a high suicide risk.

Those who require respite from disorganized social settings.

Benzodiazepines

• These are the first-line treatment to relieve withdrawal symptoms and protect against complications [2,3].

Standard dosage	Chlordiazepoxide, 20–100 mg, or diazepam, 10–30 mg 4 times daily, gradually reduced over 7–10 days, then stopped.
Contraindications	Respiratory depression, acute pulmonary insufficiency.
Special points	Dose should be decreased if signs of oversedation or respiratory depression; long-term use to be avoided. Oxazepam (short-acting, no active metabolites) is agent of choice in liver failure. Patients in whom oral route is inadequate should be given slow i.v. diazepam emulsion according to manufacturer's current prescribing information.
Main drug interactions	Sedatives, cimetidine.
Main side effects	Drowsiness, ataxia, amnesia.

Thiamine

Standard dosage	*For uncomplicated alcohol withdrawal:* thiamine, 10–30 mg orally daily. *For imminent or diagnosed Wernicke's encephalopathy:* thiamine, 200–300 mg orally daily in divided doses or, if oral route inadequate, 200 mg i.m. or i.v. slowly (as two 100 mg/mL ampules); increased or repeated as necessary.
Contraindications	Known hypersensitivity to thiamine.
Main drug interactions	None.
Main side effects	Hypersensitivity reactions have been reported after repeated injections.

Adjunctive medications

Zinc vitamin: once or twice daily to facilitate alcohol metabolism.

Magnesium sulfate: if deficiency in patient with normal renal function; 50% magnesium sulfate, 2 mL i.m. every 6 h; may be given i.v.

Folic acid: 1 mg daily.

Treatment aims

To relieve withdrawal symptoms.

To prevent withdrawal complications.

To help patient to plan long-term goals.

Prognosis

• If the patient is adequately treated, in the absence of medical complications, the prognosis is good.

• 5%–20% of patients with delirium tremens die from complications, *e.g.*, infection, hypothermia, aspiration, and vascular collapse.

• Wernicke's encephalopathy, if untreated, can lead to irreversible brain damage.

Follow-up and management

• Individual patients' needs vary, and the regimen must be tailor-made.

• Anxiety and depressive illness must be excluded.

• Recently detoxified patients can be given long-term prophylactic treatment with thiamine, 10 mg daily.

• Disulfiram may be helpful in maintaining abstinence in some patients when combined with an organized outpatient treatment program.

Patient support

• Support should come from three sources: individual therapy (providing support, encouraging abstinence), group therapy (*e.g.*, Alcoholics Anonymous), and outpatient and day-hospital support.

Key references

1. Bradley KA, Donovan DM, Larson EB: How much is too much? Advising patients about safe levels of alcohol consumption. *Arch Intern Med* 1993, **153**:2734–2740.
2. Naik P, Lawton J: Pharmacological management of alcohol withdrawal: a review. *Br J Hosp Med* 1993, **50**:265–269.
3. Milhorn HT: Pharmacological management of acute abstinence syndromes. *Am Fam Phys* 1992, **45**:231–239.

Diagnosis

Symptoms and signs

• Alopecia is a clinical sign and needs to be classified as either scarring or nonscarring before an accurate diagnosis can be made.

Scarring (cicatricial alopecia)

Lichen planopilaris, kerion (fungal), dissecting cellulitis of the scalp, sarcoidosis, trauma (burns, chemical, direct trauma), localized secondary to fetal scalp monitor, aplasia cutis congenita.
Alopecia neoplastica: secondary to metastatic breast carcinoma.
Linear scleroderma, chronic cutaneous lupus (discoid lupus erythematosus).

Nonscarring (noncicatricial alopecia)

Alopecia areata, androgenetic alopecia, trichotillomania, telogen effluvium, anagen effluvium, tinea capitis ("ringworm").

Hair shaft disorders: monilethrix, trichorrhexis nodosa, trichorrhexis invaginata, pili torti, Menkes' kinky hair syndrome.

Alopecia areata [1]

Localized "ring shaped" area of diffuse or complete nonscarring alopecia: hallmarked by short, tapered "exclamation point" hairs.
Pitted or onychodystrophic nails: may be present.
Alopecia totalis (entire scalp) or alopecia universalis (entire body surface): may occur in rare instances.
Gray or depigmented hair: often regrows.

Alopecia areata, with deficient melanin in area of regrowth.

Spared pony tail growth in trichotillomania.

Trichotillomania (traumatic alopecia)

Incomplete nonscarring hair loss: hairs of unequal length in alopecic areas; most patients deny (or are unconscious of) pulling out hairs.

Lichen planopilaris

Lichen planus of the scalp: often no lichen planus elsewhere; cicatricial alopecia and follicular erythema within the alopecic areas.

Chronic cutaneous lupus erythematosus

Cicatricial alopecia with follicular prominence and plugging: frequent cutaneous involvement of the external pinnae (especially conchal bowl of the ears); may or may not be associated with systemic disease.

Fungal infection

Kerion.
Tinea capitis.

Investigations

Skin biopsy: diagnostic in cases of alopecia areata in which the clinical presentation is not classic.
Scalp biopsy: reveals follicular hemorrhage and empty follicles in trichotillomania.
Scalp biopsy: in lichen planopilaris; diagnostic in chronic cutaneous lupus erythematosus.
Fungal scrapings: often negative in kerion; can be helpful in tinea capitis along with culture.

Complications

Severe scarring: in kerions
Squamous cell carcinomas: in areas of cicatricial alopecia from lupus (rare).

Differential diagnosis

Alopecia areata
Androgenetic alopecia (diffuse in alopecia areata); trichotillomania; alopecia neoplastica.
Trichotillomania
Tinea capitis; alopecia areata; hair shaft disorders.
Lichen planopilaris
Pseudopelade; sarcoid; folliculitis decalvans.
Chronic cutaneous lupus
Necrobiosis lipoidica diabeticorum; sarcoid.
Kerion
Dissecting cellulitis of the scalp; folliculitis decalvans.
Tinea capitis
Alopecia areata; hair shaft disorders.

Etiology

Alopecia areata
Autoimmune [2,3]; rarely may be associated with thyroid disease, pernicious anemia, or vitiligo.
Trichotillomania
Psychological stresses.
Lichen planopilaris
Unknown.
Chronic cutaneous lupus
Autoimmune.

Epidemiology

75% of patients present before age 25.
Patients with Down syndrome, positive family history of alopecia areata, or atopy appear to be more prone; no consistent HLA genotypes have been identified.
Trichotillomania
Patients predominantly female.
Chronic cutaneous lupus
Appears to be more common in black women.
Fungal infections
Microsporum spp. infection is associated with animal contact and usually affects children.
Trichophyton tonsurans is the most common cause of tinea capitis in the US and usually occurs in school-age children.

Treatment

Diet and lifestyle

• Other than alteration of the underlying behavior of trichotillomania, there does not appear to be any role of diet and lifestyle.

Pharmacological treatment

Alopecia areata

• Alopecia areata usually resolves with no treatment but may be resistant to treatment.

• Potent topical steroids, intralesional steroids, topical irritants or allergens, and topical minoxidil have all been used successfully.

• Systemic steroids or cyclosporin have been effective but are often not used because of side effects.

Standard dosage Clobetasol propionate, 0.05% cream or ointment applied twice daily.
Triamcinolone acetonide, 10 mg/mL intralesionally every 2–4 weeks.

Contraindications Local infection, atrophy.

Special points Potent topical steroids: used over a large area can result in systemic absorption.

Main drug interaction None.

Main side effects Local steroid atrophy, steroid acne, systemic steroid absorption.

Trichotillomania

Psychiatric counseling.

Lichen planopilaris

Treatment is the same as for alopecia areata except irritants and allogens should be avoided.

Chronic cutaneous lupus

• After the condition is under control, alternative treatment should be substituted, *e.g.*, systemic antimalarial therapy, given by a specialist, and sunscreens and protective wear.

Standard dosage Intralesional triamcinolone, 10 mg/mL.

Contraindications None.

Special points Intralesional triamcinolone is only a local treatment; it does not affect systemic disease.

Main drug interaction None.

Main drug interaction Atrophy, hypopigmentation, systemic absorption.

Treatment aims

To arrest and reverse pathological hair loss.

Other treatments

Wigs to improve cosmesis.

Consider hair transplantation or hair-bearing flaps in cases of stable, limited cicatricial alopecia.

Prognosis

Alopecia areata

• In general, 50% of patients will have complete regrowth of localized areas in 1 year; approximately one third of patients never regrow hair.

• Scarring alopecia usually results even if treated.

Poor prognostic indicators as follows:

Early onset.

Severe initial involvement.

Total alopecia for more than 1 year.

Nail dystrophy.

Ophiasis pattern (alopecia around periphery of scalp).

Trichotillomania

Good with appropriate psychological counseling.

Lichen planopilaris

Poor even with treatment.

Chronic cutaneous lupus

Poor response in this chronic disease requiring long-term follow-up; antinuclear antibody (ANA)-negative patients can develop ANA-positive symptomatic systemic disease.

Follow-up and management

Every month at least in all diseases mentioned.

Key references

1. Nielson TA, Reichel M: Alopecia: diagnosis and management. *Am Fam Phys* 1995, **51**:1513–1522; 1527–1528.
2. Tobin DJ, Bystryn JC: Immunity to hair follicles in alopecia areata. *J Invest Dermatol* 1995, **104**(suppl 5):135–145.
3. McDonagh AJ, Messenger AG: The etiology and pathogenesis of alopecia areata. *J Dermatol Sci* 1994, **7**(suppl):S125–S135.

Anemia, aplastic

Diagnosis

Symptoms

• Symptoms and signs are due to and relate to the severity of the peripheral blood pancytopenia.

Fatigue, shortness of breath on exertion, headache, palpitation: symptoms of anemia.

Easy bruising and petechiae, gum bleeding, buccal hemorrhage, visual disturbance due to retinal hemorrhage: symptoms of thrombocytopenia.

Mouth and tongue ulcers: symptoms of infection due to leukopenia.

History of jaundice: may indicate posthepatitic aplasia or associated paroxysmal nocturnal hemoglobulinuria.

Signs

• Bleeding manifestations are usually more common than infection.

Pallor.

Ecchymoses, petechiae of skin and mouth, retinal hemorrhage.

Fever.

Mouth and tongue ulceration.

Pharyngitis, pneumonia.

Skin and perianal sepsis.

Skeletal, skin, and nail anomalies; short stature: may occur in congenital aplastic anemia.

• Spleen, liver, and lymph nodes are not enlarged.

Investigations

Full blood count and examination of blood film: show pancytopenia (isolated cytopenias may occur in early stages), macrocytosis, toxic granulation of neutrophils.

Reticulocyte count: shows absolute reticulocytopenia.

Bone-marrow aspiration and biopsy: shows hypocellular bone marrow, no abnormal infiltration, no increase in reticulin, colony-forming cells low or absent; cytogenetic studies to exclude preleukemia; in Fanconi's anemia, cultured peripheral blood lymphocytes show increased chromosomal breaks with DNA cross-linking agent (*e.g.*, diepoxybutane).

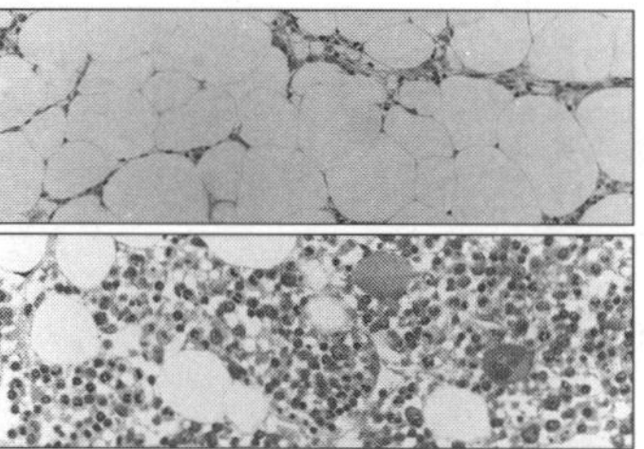

Aplastic anemia bone marrow (top), normal bone marrow (bottom).

Ham's test and urine hemosiderin analysis: classically negative in aplastic anemia and positive in paroxysmal nocturnal hemoglobulinuria (PNH), but a small proportion of PNH cells can be detected in up to 30% of patients with aplastic anemia.

Liver function tests and viral studies: to detect antecedent hepatitis; test for hepatitis A, B, and non-A, non-B (hepatitis C); Epstein–Barr virus; cytomegalovirus; and parvovirus B19 (parvovirus classically causes pure erythrocyte aplasia and can also cause pancytopenia associated with hemophagocytosis).

Chest and sinus radiography.

Hand and forearm radiography: may be abnormal in congenital aplastic anemia.

Abdominal ultrasonography: to exclude splenomegaly; anatomically displaced or abnormal kidneys in Fanconi's anemia.

Complications

Failure of random donor platelet transfusions to increase recipient's platelet count, increased bone-marrow graft rejection potential: due to sensitization to non-HLA antigens from multiple blood transfusions.

Late clonal evolution to myelodysplastic syndrome or acute myeloid leukemia in 10% of patients with aplastic anemia or paroxysmal nocturnal hemoglobulinuria in 10% of untransplanted patients.

Differential diagnosis

Hypoplastic myelodysplastic syndrome or hypoplastic acute myeloid leukemia in adults.

Hypoplastic acute lymphoblastic leukemia in children.

Hairy cell leukemia.

Other bone-marrow infiltration: *e.g.*, lymphoma, carcinoma, myelofibrosis.

Anorexia nervosa.

Severe infection: *e.g.*, tuberculosis, overwhelming gram-negative or gram-positive sepsis.

Etiology

Congenital causes

E.g., Fanconi anemia, dyskeratosis congenita.

Acquired causes

Idiopathic: in 75% of patients.

Drugs: *e.g.*, NSAIDs, gold, chloramphenicol, sulfonamides.

Chemicals: benzene, organic solvents, aniline dyes.

Viruses: hepatitis A, B, or non-A, non-B (hepatitis C) and other as yet unidentified viruses; Epstein–Barr virus.

Paroxysmal nocturnal hemoglobinuria: 25% of patients later develop aplastic anemia.

Rare causes

SLE, pregnancy.

Epidemiology

• The annual incidence in the United States is 2–8 per million.

• The male:female ratio is equal.

• Two peaks are seen in the age incidence for men: 15–25 years and >60 years; one peak for women: >60 years.

Treatment

Diet and lifestyle

• If neutrophils are <0.5 × 10^9/L, food should be well cooked and fresh fruit washed before consumption.

Pharmacological treatment

• Drugs are indicated for patients ineligible for bone-marrow transplantation.

• High-dose corticosteroids should be avoided because of toxicity (infection, hypertension, diabetes, avascular necrosis of bone) and lack of convincing benefit in aplastic anemia.

• Drugs that affect platelet function (aspirin, NSAIDs) or that may cause aplastic anemia must be avoided.

Antilymphocyte globulin (ALG) or antithymocyte globulin (ATG)

• Horse ATG should be used initially.

Standard dosage ATG, 10–20 mg/kg daily for 8–14 consecutive days followed by alternate day therapy for another 14 days.

Contraindications Hypersensitivity or severe systemic reaction to test dose, active infection, hemolytic paroxysmal nocturnal hemoglobinuria, SLE.

Special points Central line infusion to prevent thrombophlebitis; platelet transfusion before each dose; low-dose prednisone to prevent serum sickness.

Main drug interactions None.

Main side effects Anaphylaxis or allergic reactions (during infusion); serum sickness (7–14 days after starting treatment).

Cyclosporin

• Cyclosporin can be used after ALG or as a single agent.

Standard dosage Cyclosporin, 2.5 mg/kg orally twice daily for 3–6 months.

Contraindications Renal or liver impairment, breast feeding.

Special points Drug blood concentration, blood pressure, renal and liver function must be monitored regularly.

Main drug interactions Erythromycin, ketoconazole, aminoglycosides, vancomycin, amphotericin B, rifampin, phenytoin.

Main side effects Nephrotoxicity, nausea, tremor, hypertension, hypertrichosis, gum hypertrophy, hepatotoxicity.

Oxymetholone

• Oxymetholone is now used after ALG rather than as a single agent.

Standard dosage Oxymetholone, 2.5 mg/kg orally daily (0.5–1 mg/kg daily for Fanconi's anemia).

Contraindications Liver impairment, breast and prostate cancer, pregnancy; caution in children (behavioral problems) and elderly men (prostatic hypertrophy).

Special points Serum cholesterol concentration must be monitored.

Main drug interactions Other potentially hepatotoxic drugs, *e.g.*, erythromycin, rifampin, ketoconazole, cyclosporin.

Main side effects Reversible cholestatic jaundice, liver tumors, and peliosis hepatitis with long-term use, virilization in females, acne.

Treatment aims

To provide good supportive care (critical for survival of patient).

To treat fever promptly (broad-spectrum i.v. antibiotics), routine oral antifungal prophylaxis.

Other treatments

Allogeneic bone-marrow transplantation: treatment of choice for patients who have severe aplastic anemia, are <45 years, and have an HLA-identical sibling donor.

Bone-marrow transplantation from an HLA-matched volunteer donor: if patient has very severe aplastic anemia, is <30 years, and has no HLA-identical sibling [1,2].

• Hematopoietic growth factors such as granulocyte-colony stimulating factor (CSF), granulocyte macrophage-CSF, interleukin-3, and interleukin-6 have little effect in aplastic anemia, apart from a transient increase in neutrophil count in some patients. Serious toxicity may occur in aplastic anemia patients [3].

Prognosis

• After bone-marrow transplantation from an HLA-identical identical sibling, at least 70%–80% of patients are long-term survivors and can be considered cured of their disease.

• Response to antilymphocyte globulin or cyclosporin occurs in 50%–70% (rarely before 3–6 months), but relapse and later clonal disorders may occur.

Follow-up and management

• Long-term monitoring is needed for clonal disorders and relapse.

Key references

1. Soutar RL, King DJ: Bone marrow transplantation. *BMJ* 1995, **310**:31–36.
2. Storb R, Champlin RE: Bone marrow transplantation for severe aplastic anemia. *Bone Marrow Transplant* 1991, **8**:69–72.
3. Marsh JCW, *et al.*: Haemopoietic growth factors in aplastic anemia: a cautionary note. *Lancet* 1994, **344**:172–173.

Diagnosis

Symptoms

• Many patients have no symptoms; the disease is suspected on routine blood count.

Dyspnea on exertion, tiredness, headache.

Painful tongue.

Paraesthesias in feet, difficulty walking: vitamin B_{12} deficiency only.

Infertility.

Signs

Pallor of mucous membranes: if hemoglobin concentration <9 g/dL.

Mild jaundice.

"Beefy red" glossitis.

Signs of vitamin B_{12} neuropathy: if present.

Investigations [1,2]

General

Blood count: raised mean cell volume (>100 fL), reduced erythrocyte count, hemoglobin, and hematocrit, low reticulocyte count, reduced leukocyte and platelet counts (in severely anemic patients).

Blood film: shows oval macrocytes, hypersegmented neutrophils (>5 nuclear lobes).

Bone-marrow analysis: in severely anemic patients the bone marrow is hypercellular with increased proportion of early cells, many dying cells, megaloblastic erythroblasts, giant and abnormally shaped metamyelocytes, and hypersegmented megakaryocytes.

Bone marrow with megaloblastic anemia.

Serum indirect bilirubin and lactic dehydrogenase measurement: concentrations raised.

Direct Coombs test: complement only, positive in some patients.

Tests for disseminated intravascular coagulation or intravascular hemolysis: positive in some patients.

Tests for vitamin B_{12} (B_{12}) or folate deficiency: serum B_{12} low in B_{12} deficiency, normal or slightly low in folate deficiency; serum folate normal or raised in B_{12} deficiency, low in folate deficiency; erythrocyte folate normal or low in B_{12} deficiency, low in folate deficiency.

Deoxyuridine suppression, serum homocysteine and methylmalonic acid measurement: additional tests performed in some laboratories for B_{12} or folate deficiency [3].

Special

Diet history: to exclude veganism, low folate intake.

Schilling test: for B_{12} absorption.

Serum analysis: for intrinsic factor and parietal cell antibodies.

Fiberoptic endoscopy: for gastric biopsy, exclusion of gastric polyps, carcinoma in pernicious anemia.

Contrast radiography: to detect gastric atrophy, neoplasm (pernicious anemia), or small intestinal lesions.

Endoscopy and jejunal biopsy: if gluten-induced enteropathy is suspected in patients with folate deficiency.

Complications

Neuropathy: due to B_{12} deficiency.

Neural tube defects in fetus: risk reduced by folate treatment.

Carcinoma of stomach: in pernicious anemia.

Differential diagnosis

Other causes of macrocytosis [1,2]

Alcoholism, liver disease, hypothyroidism, aplastic anemia, myelodysplasia, acute myeloid leukemia, myeloma, reticulocytosis.

Other causes of megaloblastic anemia

Nitrous oxide anesthesia.

Transcobalamin II deficiency.

Antifolate drugs: methotrexate, pyrimethamine (reversed by folinic acid), co-trimoxazole.

Drugs inhibiting DNA synthesis: cytosine arabinoside, hydroxyurea, 6-mercaptopurine, azathioprine, 5-fluorouracil.

Congenital abnormalities of vitamin B_{12} or folate metabolism.

Congenital abnormalities of DNA synthesis: *e.g.*, orotic aciduria.

Etiology

Causes of vitamin B_{12} deficiency [1]

Diet deficiency: *e.g.*, in vegans.

Pernicious anemia.

Congenital intrinsic factor deficiency.

Total or subtotal gastrectomy.

Atrophic gastritis, gastric bypass.

Blind loop syndrome.

Ileal resection or abnormality: *e.g.*, Crohn's disease.

HIV infection.

Drugs: *e.g.*, metformin.

Specific malabsorption with proteinuria.

Fish tapeworm.

Causes of folate deficiency [1,2]

Dietary deficiency: poor-quality diet, goat's milk, specialized diets.

Malabsorption: gluten-induced enteropathy, tropical sprue, congenital.

Increased turnover: pregnancy, prematurity, hemolytic anemias, myelofibrosis, widespread inflammatory or malignant diseases.

Increased losses: congestive heart failure, hemodialysis or peritoneal dialysis.

Uncertain: anticonvulsant treatment.

Epidemiology

• The occurrence of megaloblastic anemia relates to diet (*e.g.*, Hindu communities, where veganism is common; poor people, in whom dietary folate intake is reduced).

• For pernicious anemia, the peak age of incidence is 60 years.

• The female:male ratio is 1.6:1.

Treatment

Diet and lifestyle

• The quality of the diet must be increased in patients with dietary folate deficiency.

Pharmacological treatment [1,2]

For vitamin B_{12} deficiency

Standard dosage Hydroxocobalamin, 1 mg i.m. 6 times in 2-3 weeks, then 1 mg every 3 months or 100-200 μg i.m. monthly.

Contraindications Rare hypersensitivity.

Special points No evidence suggests that more frequent doses are needed for B_{12} neuropathy.

Main drug interactions None.

Main side effects Gout and significant hypokalemia a few days after commencing treatment.

For folate deficiency

Standard dosage Folic acid, 5 mg orally daily for 4 months, then 5 mg daily or weekly as needed.

Contraindications B_{12} deficiency, malignancy (unless deficiency is clinically important).

Special points B_{12} deficiency must be excluded because B_{12} neuropathy could be precipitated or aggravated.

Main drug interactions None.

Main side effects None.

• Folic acid should be used as prophylaxis in pregnancy (300-400 μg daily; 5 mg daily if previous neural defect in fetus), and also in renal dialysis.

• In women of childbearing age, folate intake should be increased to at least 400 μg daily by diet or folate supplement.

• For premature babies (birth weight <1500 g), folic acid, 1 mg daily, is indicated.

Treatment aims

To correct anemia by replenishing body stores of vitamin.

To correct underlying disease.

To restore normal neurological status (vitamin B_{12} deficiency).

Other treatments

• Packed erythrocyte transfusion should be used only if essential: removal of equivalent volume of plasma in patients with congestive heart failure.

Prognosis

• Prognosis depends mainly on the underlying cause.

• Life expectancy is reduced slightly in patients with pernicious anemia because of the risk of carcinoma of the stomach.

Follow-up and management

• Patients with pernicious anemia should have annual clinical review and blood count.

• Routine endoscopy is not recommended.

• Patients having total gastrectomy or ileal resection need prophylactic hydroxocobalamin, 1 mg every 3 months, from the time of surgery for life.

Key references

1. Anthony AC: Megaloblastic anaemias. In *Hematology. Basic Principles and Practice*. Edited by Hoffman R, *et al*. New York: Churchill Livingstone; 1991:392–422.

2. Savage DG, Lindenbaum J: Folate–cobalamin interactions. In *Folate in Health & Disease*. Edited by Baily L. New York: Marcel Dekker; 1994:237–285.

3. Hoffbrand AV, Jackson BFA: The deoxyuridine suppression test and cobalamin–folate interrelations. *Br J Haematol* 1993, **85**:232–237.

Diagnosis

Symptoms

• Possibly no symptoms are apparent (vitamin B_{12} deficiency or atrophic gastritis may be an incidental finding).

• Symptoms are usually due to anemia or complications of vitamin B_{12} deficiency.

Shortness of breath, lethargy.

Sore tongue: glossitis in 50% of patients.

Parasthesias: due to peripheral neuropathy.

Gait disturbance: due to myelopathy (subacute combined degeneration of spinal cord).

Depression.

Impaired memory.

Signs

Mucosal pallor: reflecting anemia.

Glossitis.

Mild splenomegaly.

Signs of other organ-specific autoimmune disease: *e.g.*, hypothyroidism.

Peripheral sensory neuropathy with absent reflexes.

Pyramidal or long-tract signs.

Extensor plantars.

Loss of joint position sense.

Investigations

Hematology: for macrocytic anemia (mean corpuscular volume >100 fL), leukopenia or thrombocytopenia, hypersegmented neutrophils on blood film.

Bone-marrow analysis: megaloblastic changes with maturation arrest.

Liver function test: increased bilirubin due to ineffective erythropoiesis.

Serum vitamin B_{12} measurement: to detect low concentrations (normal, >160 ng/L).

Schilling test: abnormal part I test using ^{58}Co-labeled vitamin B_{12} (<10% urinary excretion); part II corrects to normal after administration of intrinsic factor.

Serum gastrin measurement: raised concentration in pernicious anemia (normal <100 pmol/L).

Pentagastrin or histamine-fast analysis: shows achlorhydria.

Endoscopy and biopsy: for atrophic gastritis on endoscopy and histological assessment of stage of gastritis.

Complications

Gastric carcinoid and enterochromaffin cell hyperplasia: associated with marked reflex rise in serum gastrin due to intragastric anacidity; 2%–9% prevalence of gastric carcinoid in patients with pernicious anemia [1].

Gastric carcinoma: 1%–7% increased risk in patients with pernicious anemia [2].

Peripheral sensory neuropathy, subacute combined degeneration of spinal cord: affects pyramidal tracts, causing spastic paraparesis and bladder involvement, and dorsal columns, causing sensory ataxia and impaired joint position sense.

High-output cardiac failure, myocardial ischemia: in severe anemia.

Differential diagnosis

Type B chronic gastritis related to *Helicobacter pylori* infection.

Other causes of vitamin B_{12} deficiency: *e.g.*, dietary deficiency in vegans, terminal ileitis (Crohn's disease), terminal ileal resection, blind loop syndromes, small bowel diverticula or bacterial overgrowth, postgastrectomy states, pelvic irradiation.

Etiology

• Pernicious anemia is an organ-specific autoimmune disease, with a strong association with other organ-specific autoimmune diseases, especially thyroid disease.

Epidemiology

• Pernicious anemia occurs more often in female patients than in male.

• Pernicious anemia is common in all races and countries.

Immunology

• Antigastric parietal-cell antibodies (probably involved in pathogenesis) occur in 70%–90% of patients, anti-intrinsic factor antibodies in 50%–70%.

• Antibodies have been shown to be directed against membrane-bound hydrogen/potassium ATPase pump, resulting in blockade of hydrochloric acid secretion and correlating with concentrations of gastric parietal-cell antibodies.

Treatment

Diet and lifestyle

• No special precautions are necessary for uncomplicated disease.

Pharmacological treatment

Standard dosage Hydroxocobalamin, 1 mg i.m. 6 times in 2–3 weeks, then 1 mg every 3 months.

Contraindications None.

Special points Can cause initial hypokalemia and folate deficiency in patients with marked vitamin B_{12} deficiency; chloride and folic acid supplements are advisable.

Main drug interactions None.

Main side effects None.

Treatment aims

To prevent neurological complications.

To correct anemia.

Prognosis

• Despite the small risk of gastric carcinoid or carcinoma, life expectancy is little altered in patients with uncomplicated disease [1,2].

• Gastric carcinoids have a good prognosis, with no reported cases of carcinoid syndrome in these patients and a low reported incidence of local or regional spread.

Follow-up and management

• The cost of endoscopic surveillance has been shown to outweigh the benefit of screening for the few patients who are found to have unsuspected malignancy; it should probably be reserved for patients who develop symptoms.

• Regular vitamin B_{12} supplementation in outpatients must be ensured.

Key references

1. Born K, *et al.*: Gastric endocrine cell hyperplasia and carcinoid tumors in pernicious anemia. *Gastroenterology* 1985, **88**:638–648.

2. Lechago J, Correa P: Prolonged achlorhydria and gastric neoplasia: is there a causal relationship? *Gastroenterology* 1993, **104**:1554–1557.

Angina pectoris, stable

Diagnosis

Symptoms

Chest discomfort: brought on by physical exertion or emotions, *e.g.*, anger, excitement; repeatable in onset, rapid resolution with rest, worse in cold weather and after meals; heavy, constricting, crushing, not sharp, often described as unpleasant rather than painful; may radiate down inner aspects of arms or into neck or jaw, rarely radiates into epigastrium or back. May cause effort dyspnea only, particularly in the elderly.

Signs

• Typically no signs are manifest, but patients should be examined for evidence of the following:

Hyperlipidemia.

Hypertension.

Left ventricular outflow obstruction: *i.e.*, aortic stenosis, hypertrophic cardiomyopathy.

Diabetes.

Previous myocardial damage.

Investigations

Full blood count: anemia aggravates angina.

Resting ECG: to detect left ventricular hypertrophy or past myocardial infarction.

Chest radiography: to check heart size and pulmonary vasculature.

Exercise stress test: to precipitate symptoms, to document workload at onset, and to record any associated ECG abnormality (planar ST segment depression or arrhythmia).

Thallium myocardial perfusion imaging: mainly used when conventional exercise stress test cannot be done or when ECG cannot be interpreted (*e.g.*, left bundle branch block); thallium administered during exercise or pharmacological stress test delineates an area of myocardial hypoperfusion; re-imaging after rest shows redistribution unless infarction has occurred. Alternative is exercise-stress or pharmacological-stress echocardiography. Ischemia manifest as wall motion abnormality such as hypokinesis, akinesis, or dyskinesis in region that is normal or mildly hypokinetic at rest.

Coronary angiography: gold standard; provides detailed anatomical information about site and severity of luminal narrowing but does not show atherosclerosis itself or functional importance of anatomical occlusive disease; prerequisite for consideration of angioplasty or surgery.

Complications

Unstable angina.

Acute myocardial infarction.

Arrhythmias.

Death.

Differential diagnosis

Cardiac

Pericarditis.

Myocardial infarction.

Aortic dissection.

Noncardiac

Esophageal spasm.

Reflux esophagitis.

Peptic ulceration.

Musculoskeletal pain.

Cervical spondylosis.

Da Costa's syndrome.

Etiology

Causes

Coronary atherosclerosis in 99% of patients.

Aortic stenosis.

Hypertrophic cardiomyopathy.

Arteritis.

Risk factors

Family history.

Smoking.

Diabetes.

Hypertension.

Hyperlipidemia.

Obesity.

Post menopause

Epidemiology

• Coronary atherosclerosis is endemic in industrialized countries, but the incidence is decreasing.

• In the US, more than 500 000 myocardial infarctions per year.

• No accurate figures are available for the prevalence of angina pectoris, but, in people aged >30 years, it is >2.6%.

Treatment

Diet and lifestyle

- Exercise should be encouraged, obesity corrected, and cigarette smoking stopped.
- Diet low in fat and cholesterol is critical.

Pharmacological treatment

- All patients should be screened for hyperlipidemia and treated as appropriate, including dietary and drug treatment as indicated [1].
- Hypertension and diabetes should be managed aggressively.
- An individual patient may, at different stages, need medical treatment, percutaneous transluminal coronary angioplasty, and coronary artery bypass grafting.

Nitrates

- For patients with mild symptoms, short-acting sublingual nitrates may be sufficient (including prophylactic use).
- With long-acting oral nitrates, tolerance is common, so a nitrate-free period should be provided.

Standard dosage Sublingual or oral nitrates or nitrate patches, dose depends on agent.

Contraindications Hypotension.

Special points Glyceryl trinitrate tablets have a limited shelf life.

Main drug interactions Reduced effect of sublingual preparations with drugs causing dry mouth (*e.g.*, disopyramide, tricyclic antidepressants, atropine); hypotension with other vasodilators; reduced heparin effect with glyceryl trinitrate.

Main side effects Headache, postural hypotension.

Beta blockers

- Beta blockers are the mainstay of regular antianginal treatment.

Standard dosage Depends on agent.

Contraindications Atrioventricular conduction defects, heart failure, asthma; caution in diabetes (masks symptoms of hypoglycemia), peripheral vascular disease.

Special points May be usefully combined with short- and long-acting nitrates and calcium antagonists.

Main drug interactions Increased risk of hypotension, bradycardia, and atrioventricular block with many agents.

Main side effects Lethargy, impotence, bronchospasm, cold extremities.

Calcium antagonists

- Calcium antagonists are useful in patients in whom beta blockers are contraindicated or who cannot tolerate beta blockers; in such cases, a calcium antagonist with negative chronotropic action should be prescribed (*e.g.*, diltiazem, verapamil).
- If used in the setting of an impaired ventricle, a calcium antagonist without negative inotropic activity should be prescribed (*e.g.*, amlodipine).

Standard dosage Depends on agent. Once-a-day preparations preferred.

Contraindications Depend on chronotropic and inotropic effect.

Main drug interactions Increased hypotensive effect with many agents; increased risk of atrioventricular block when negatively chronotropic agents combined with many agents (*e.g.*, beta blockers); increased effect of some antiepileptics (*e.g.*, phenytoin, carbamazepine).

Main side effects Headache, edema, flushing.

Antiplatelet agents

- Aspirin has a controversial role in primary prevention, but all patients with obstructive arterial disease benefit from long-term medium doses, so aspirin should be omitted only if strongly contraindicated [2].

Treatment aims

To control symptoms and restore normal exercise tolerance.

To prevent disease progression (myocardial infarction and death).

To improve prognosis.

Other treatments

Percutaneous transluminal coronary angioplasty

- This is complementary to drug treatment and surgery, but no improvement in survival has been shown.
- Best results are achieved in discrete single-vessel coronary artery disease.
- The restenosis rate is ~30% at 6 months.

Coronary artery bypass grafting

- This has prognostic value in patients with left main-stem coronary stenosis or three-vessel coronary artery disease and impaired left ventricular function.
- The risk of surgery is largely related to the degree of impairment of left ventricular function.

Prognosis

- 14% of patients with newly diagnosed angina pectoris progress to unstable angina, myocardial infarction, or death within 1 year.
- Mortality at coronary artery bypass grafting with normal ventricular function is 1%.

Follow-up and management

- Atherosclerosis is a progressive disease with no cure, so follow-up is important.
- Risk factor modification is an essential part of management.

Key references

1. Working Party of the Joint Audit Committee of the British Cardiac Society and the Royal College of Physicians of London: The investigation and management of stable angina. *J R Coll Physicians Lond* 1993, **27**:267–273.
2. Antiplatelet Trialists' Collaboration: Collaborative overview of randomised trials of antiplatelet therapy. I: Prevention of death, myocardial infarction, and stroke by prolonged antiplatelet therapy in various categories of patients. *BMJ* 1994, **308**:81–106.

Diagnosis

Symptoms

Angina occurring at rest or on trivial provocation.

Signs

• During pain, autonomic manifestations may occur, *e.g.*, the following:

Sweating.

Pallor.

Tachycardia.

Investigations

Full blood count: anemia aggravates angina; leukocytosis suggests infarction.

Cardiac enzyme measurement: to exclude infarction, creatine kinase MB preferable.

ECG: at rest and during pain to document phasic change, typically ST segment depression.

Chest radiography: to assess heart size and pulmonary vasculature.

Echocardiography: to assess ventricular function and to exclude differential diagnosis, *e.g.*, aortic stenosis, aortic regurgitation, hypertrophic cardiomyopathy with obstruction.

Coronary angiography: if pain does not settle with bed rest, to assess for further treatment (coronary artery bypass grafting or percutaneous transluminal coronary angiography); usually identifies "culprit" lesion [1].

Complications

Myocardial infarction.

Ventricular tachycardia, ventricular fibrillation.

Differential diagnosis

Cardiac

Myocardial infarction.

Aortic dissection.

Pericarditis.

Acute myocarditis.

Noncardiac

Pulmonary embolism.

Etiology

• Unstable angina is caused by rupture of a lipid-laden, macrophage-rich, atherosclerotic plaque; rupture occurs when circumferential tension exceeds the tensile strength of the fibrous cap [2].

• Exposure of blood to the ruptured plaque leads to activation of platelets and coagulation system, with consequent thrombosis and coronary artery spasm; in the setting of unstable angina, vessel occlusion is either transient or incomplete.

Epidemiology

• 14% of patients with newly diagnosed stable angina progress to unstable angina, myocardial infarction, or death within 1 year.

Treatment

Diet and lifestyle

• Patients should be hospitalized, with strict bed rest, possibly with sedation.

Pharmacological treatment

• Patients should be admitted to a high-dependency or coronary care unit and have continuous ECG monitoring.

Antiplatelet agents

Standard dosage	Aspirin, 300 mg initially, 75 mg daily maintenance.
Contraindications	Hypersensitivity.
Special points	Dipyridamole should be used if patient is allergic to aspirin.
Main drug interactions	Warfarin.
Main side effects	Gastric erosion.

Anticoagulants

Standard dosage	Heparin i.v. continuous infusion, dose adjusted according to activated partial thromboplastin time.
Contraindications	Gastrointestinal bleeding, recent major surgery, hemorrhagic stroke.
Main drug interactions	Reduced effect with glyceryl trinitrate.
Main side effects	Bleeding, rarely thrombocytopenia.

Nitrates

• Nitrates are used to reduce coronary artery spasm at the site of plaque rupture and enhance collateral blood flow.

Standard dosage	Nitroglycerine or isosorbide i.v. infusion, starting at 20–30 μg/min, adjusted according to symptoms.
Contraindications	Severe symptomatic hypotension.
Special points	Patients may develop drug tolerance.
Main drug interactions	Reduced heparin effect.
Main side effects	Hypotension, headache.

Beta blockers

Standard dosage	Depends on agent.
Contraindications	Atrioventricular conduction defects, heart failure, asthma; caution in diabetes (masks symptoms of hypoglycemia), peripheral vascular disease.
Special points	May be usefully combined with short- and long-acting nitrates.
Main drug interactions	Increased risk of hypotension, bradycardia, and atrioventricular block with many agents.
Main side effects	Lethargy, impotence, bronchospasm, cold extremities.

Calcium antagonists

• Calcium antagonists are useful in patients in whom beta blockers are contraindicated or who cannot tolerate beta blockers; in such cases, a calcium antagonist with negative chronotropic action should be prescribed (*e.g.*, diltiazem).

• If used in the setting of an impaired ventricle, a calcium antagonist without negative inotropic activity should be prescribed (*e.g.*, amlodipine).

Standard dosage	Depends on agent. Once-a-day agents preferred.
Contraindications	Depend on chronotropic and inotropic effect.
Main drug interactions	Increased hypotensive effect with many agents; increased risk of atrioventricular block when negatively chronotropic agents combined with many agents (*e.g.*, beta blockers); increased effect of some antiepileptics (*e.g.*, phenytoin, carbamazepine).
Main side effects	Headache, edema, flushing.

Treatment aims

To prevent complications, while allowing healing of the ruptured plaque.

Other treatments

Revascularization

• Unstable angina is a medical emergency: patients whose symptoms do not resolve rapidly on full medical treatment should be transferred to a cardiothoracic center for coronary angiography with a view to revascularization.

• The choice between percutaneous transluminal coronary angiography and coronary artery bypass surgery depends on the anatomical substrate of the unstable plaque and the presence or absence of additional disease. Both procedures carry an increased risk if performed in the setting of unstable symptoms.

Prognosis

• In hospital, the mortality is 1%; nonfatal myocardial infarction is 8%.

Follow-up and management

• After the ruptured plaque has healed, the patient's symptoms depend on the degree of fixed luminal obstruction; the patient should be investigated and managed as for angina pectoris [3].

Key references

1. McMurray J, Rankin A: Treatment of myocardial infarction, unstable angina and angina pectoris. *BMJ* 1994, **309**:1343–1350.
2. MacIsaac IA, Thomas JD, Topol EJ: Toward the quiescent coronary plaque. *J Am Coll Cardiol* 1993, **22**:1228–1241.
3. Braunwald E, *et al.*: Unstable angina: diagnosis and management. In *Clinical Practice Guideline*, Number 10. Rockville, MD: US Dept of Health and Human Services; 1994. [Agency for Health Care Policy and Research Publication 94–0602.]

Ankylosing spondylitis

Diagnosis

Symptoms

• Symptoms usually begin during the third decade, although some patients present in their teens and a few in their 30s [1].

• Onset is insidious, not associated with trauma.

Back pain and stiffness: worse in morning, improving with exercise, deteriorating with rest.

Peripheral joint symptoms: in 40%; affecting particularly shoulders, hips, knees.

Fatigue.

Uveitis and other stigmata of the spondylarthropathies: *e.g.*, related to psoriatic spondylitis, reactive arthropathy, enteropathic arthritis.

Signs

• Signs may be nonexistent or minimal.

Decreased mobility of lumbar spine, reduced chest expansion, poor mobility of cervical spine.

Decreased mobility of hips and shoulders, knee synovitis, Achilles tendinitis, dactylitis, psoriasis, psoriatic nail change.

Evidence of uveitis: during active attack.

Increasing stoop: with disease progression.

Anemia of chronic disease: particularly in patients with peripheral joint involvement.

Investigations

Radiography of pelvis: reveals sacroiliitis (sacroiliac change may be minimal, moderate, or severe), juxta-articular sclerosis and erosions, lumbar spine changes, calcification, cervical spine involvement.

ESR, plasma viscosity, CRP measurement: raised values in 50% of patients; laboratory changes may be absent even in severely ill patients.

Complications

Hip deterioration: ~20% of patients who develop the disease in their teens or early 20s need one or two new hips within 15 years of disease onset.

Knee involvement: occasionally results in need for total knee replacement.

Deteriorating vision: resulting from persistent uveitis.

Spinal fracture: can occur as a result of osteoporotic changes associated with spinal fusion; resulting spinal-cord injury can be catastrophic.

Cauda equina syndrome: rare.

Differential diagnosis

Reactive arthropathy (Reiter's syndrome) [2], psoriatic arthropathy, inflammatory bowel disease.

Nonspecific back pain (much more common): radiography differentiates the two.

Other causes of peripheral joint disease with coincidental back pain [3].

Etiology [1]

• Ankylosing spondylitis is the result of interplay between HLA B27 and other genes and environmental triggers.

• Environmental triggers probably include agents recognized in other forms of reactive arthropathy (*e.g.*, *Chlamydia* spp., ureaplasma, *Campylobacter*, *Shigella*, *Yersinia*, and *Salmonella* spp., and other gram-negative organisms) [2].

Epidemiology

• Ankylosing spondylitis occurs in 0.5% of the population in communities where HLA B27 is prevalent (northern Europe, United States, Asia, Central America).

• The male:female ratio is 2.5:1 overall, 3:1 in teenagers, and 1.5:1 with onset in the late 20s.

Treatment

Diet and lifestyle

• Exercise is of paramount importance [4].

• Attention to posture throughout the day and night is essential.

• Hydrotherapy and physical therapy are needed as an initial introduction to a lifelong exercise program.

• Patients and family members must understand the concept of treatment, and literature should be available describing the precise exercise program needed.

• Patients should avoid smoking.

Pharmacological treatment

• NSAIDs are needed by 80% of patients [4].

Standard dosage	Indomethacin, 75 mg slow release once or twice daily; dose and frequency titrated against patient's needs.
Contraindications	Active peptic ulcer disease, indomethacin intolerance (alternative NSAID should be tried); caution in elderly patients, those on anticoagulants, and those with past history of gastrointestinal bleed or perforation.
Main drug interactions	Warfarin and other anticoagulants.
Main side effects	CNS disturbance, gastrointestinal problems.

• Sulfasalazine may be useful in patients with peripheral joint involvement but may have little effect on spinal disease [4,5].

Treatment aims

To allow a good night's sleep.

To decrease morning stiffness (pharmacological treatment).

To enable patient to follow the important exercise program.

To maintain good function and posture.

Prognosis

• Outcome is determined by genetic and environmental factors.

• Although the disease does not burn out, most patients can follow a normal social, family, and professional life.

• Up to 10% of patients have relentless progression, with deteriorating posture and spinal fusion, needing spinal surgery.

• Patients with early age of onset and lower educational or social status may be at most risk of severe disease.

Follow-up and management

• After the patient has become stable, visits every 6–12 months to the rheumatologist suffice.

• For patients with severe disease, specialist inpatient management may be appropriate.

Patient support

Spondylitis Association of America
PO Box 5872
Sherman Oaks, CA 91413

Key references

1. Gran JT, Husby G: The epidemiology of ankylosing spondylitis. *Semin Arthritis Rheum* 1993, **22**:319–334.
2. Hughes RA, Keat AC: Reiter's syndrome and reactive arthritis: a current view. *Semin Arthritis Rheum* 1994, **24**:190–210.
3. Leirisalo-Repo M: Enteropathic arthritis, Whipple's disease juvenile spondyloarthropathy and uveitis. *Curr Opin Rheumatol* 1994, **6**:385–390.
4. Creemers MC, *et al.*: Treatment of seronegative spondyloarthropathies. *Semin Arthritis Rheum* 1994, **24**:71–81.
5. Dougados M, *et al.*: Sulfasalazine in the treatment of spondyloarthropathy. A randomized multi-center double-blind placebo controlled study. *Arthritis Rheum* 1995, **38**:618–627.

Aortic dissection

Diagnosis

Symptoms

Severe back or chest pain: tearing quality; sudden onset; back pain associated with dissection of descending thoracic aorta [1].

Neck or jaw pain: may indicate involvement of aortic arch.

Nausea, vomiting, sweating.

Syncope.

Dyspnea: resulting from pulmonary edema.

Paraplegia.

Abdominal pain.

Signs

General

Hypertension.
Mild pyrexia.

Proximal dissection

Loss of upper limb pulses or differential limb blood pressure.
Aortic regurgitation.
Cardiac tamponade.
Neurological deficit.

Hypotension: often associated with cardiac tamponade.

Distal dissection

Lower limb ischemia.
Hypertension.
Oliguria or anuria.

• The distinction between proximal and distal dissection should not be based solely on clinical criteria.

Investigations

ECG: to detect acute myocardial infarction and hypertensive changes.

Chest radiography: for widening of mediastinum, pleural effusion, pericardial effusion.

Echocardiography: to detect flap in ascending aorta, presence of aortic regurgitation, and pericardial effusion.

Transesophageal echocardiography: to detect true and false channel, presence and extent of intimal flap in thoracic aorta, relationship to coronary ostia, pericardial effusion, presence of aortic regurgitation.
Advantages: rapid diagnosis; can be performed in intensive care unit.
Disadvantages: needs sedation; may precipitate hypertensive reaction; proximal aortic arch not well visualized [2,3].

CT or MRI: to detect presence and extent of intimal flap, true and false channel, pericardial effusion, extension of dissection to abdominal aorta [2,3].
Advantages: visualization of entire aorta; identification of visceral jeopardy; noninvasive.
Disadvantages: time-consuming; unsuitable for unstable patients who must be moved from intensive care.

Contrast angiography: largely superseded by above investigations, although some centers still prefer coronary angiography before surgical intervention.

Complications

Death.
Aortic rupture.
Stroke.
Paraplegia.
Ischemic bowel.
Renal infarction.
Limb ischemia.
Acute myocardial infarction.

Differential diagnosis

Acute myocardial infarction.
Acute myocardial ischemia.
Acute aortic regurgitation.
Thoracic aortic aneurysm.
Musculoskeletal chest pain.
Pulmonary embolism.
Pericarditis.

Etiology

• The underlying disease process is cystic medial necrosis of the aorta.
• Related processes include the following:
Hypertension (in most patients).
Marfan syndrome.
Atheroma.
Pregnancy.

Epidemiology

• The annual incidence of acute aortic dissection is ~5–10 in one million population.
• 80%–90% of patients are >60 years old.

Classification

DeBakey classification

Type I: tear in ascending aorta, with dissection extending into arch and descending aorta.
Type II: tear and dissection localized to ascending aorta.
Type III: originates in descending aorta, usually propagating distally for a variable distance.

Stanford classification

Type A: includes all proximal dissections and distal dissections that extend proximally to involve the arch and ascending aorta.
Type B: all other distal dissections without proximal extension.

Acute versus chronic

Acute: symptom onset within 2 weeks.
Chronic: symptom onset longer than 2 weeks.

Treatment

Diet and lifestyle

• After surgical repair, patients are generally advised to avoid circumstances that cause an acute rise in blood pressure, *e.g.*, lifting or carrying heavy objects or weights.

Pharmacological treatment

• Treatment for patients with acute type A dissections is primarily surgical.

• Pharmacological treatment is usually reserved for patients with type B dissections.

• All patients require chronic medical therapy to control hypertension.

Emergency treatment

• In addition to bed rest and arterial blood pressure monitoring, patients should be treated by oral beta blockade to reduce the rate of blood pressure rise and sodium nitroprusside to maintain systolic blood pressure at 100–120 mm Hg.

Subsequent treatment

• Long-term management of hypertension is necessary, with medication (oral beta blockade, calcium antagonism, angiotensin-converting enzyme inhibition) to reduce blood pressure and the rate of rise of blood pressure; systolic blood pressure of 130–140 mm Hg or less is the aim. *See* Hypertension *for details.*

Non-pharmacological treatment

Indications for surgery

Type A dissection.

Type B dissection: limb ischemia, renal compromise, aortic rupture, extension of dissection to proximal aorta.

Types of surgery

Excision of intimal tear.

Obliteration of proximal false lumen.

Resuturing of aorta, possibly with interposition graft.

Resuspension of aortic valve in patients with aortic regurgitation secondary to proximal extent of dissection.

Aortic valve replacement.

Composite aortic graft (with attached mechanical aortic valve replacement) and reimplantation of coronary arteries; operation of choice in patients with Marfan syndrome.

Interposition aortic graft to descending aorta (vital organ perfusion may arise from false lumen, which may need to be left open at its proximal or distal end).

Complications of surgery

Death.

Bleeding.

Infection.

Renal failure.

Spinal-cord ischemia with paraplegia.

Progressive aortic regurgitation.

Aneurysm formation.

Redissection.

Acute myocardial infarction.

Treatment aims

To provide analgesia and sedation.

To stabilize dissection flap.

To treat underlying condition, usually systemic hypertension.

Prognosis

• Prognostic data from patients with untreated aortic dissection are sparse.

• In patients with type A dissection, mortality is ~60% after nonsurgical treatment (inpatient: 1 month) and 15%–30% after surgical treatment.

• In patients with type B dissection, 1-month mortality is <10% after nonsurgical treatment.

Follow-up and management

• Follow-up should be under the supervision of a cardiologist.

• Regular MRI or transesophageal echocardiography is advised to screen for aneurysm formation.

Key references

1. Guilmet D *et al.*: Aortic dissection: anatomic types and surgical approaches. *J Cardiovasc Surg Torino* 1993, **34**:23–32.
2. Nienaber CA *et al.*: The diagnosis of thoracic aortic dissection by noninvasive imaging procedures. *N Engl J Med* 1993, **328**:1–9.
3. Cigarroa JE, *et al.*: Diagnostic imaging in the evaluation of suspected aortic dissection. *N Engl J Med* 1993, **328**:35–43.

Diagnosis

Symptoms

• Many patients are asymptomatic.

Dyspnea and fatigue: due to left ventricular impairment and low cardiac output initially on exertion.

Symptoms of left ventricular failure: later.

Angina: less common than in aortic stenosis; usually indicates coronary artery disease.

Signs

Pulse

Large volume, rapid fall with low diastolic pressure: "collapsing."

Head nodding in time with pulse: Musset's sign.

Visible pulsation in neck: Corrigan's sign.

Capillary pulsation in fingernails: Quincke's sign.

A booming sound heard over femorals: "pistol-shot femorals."

Systolic and diastolic murmur: produced by compression of femorals by stethoscope; Duroziez's sign.

Heart

• Heart sounds are usually normal.

Forceful, displaced, "heaving" apex: may be seen and felt.

Ejection click: in early systole with bicuspid valve.

Third heart sound: in early diastole with left ventricular failure.

High-frequency early diastolic murmur: maximal at left sternal edge in expiration.

Ejection systolic murmur: resulting from increased flow across valve.

Low-frequency mid-diastolic murmur (Austin Flint): at apex, similar to murmur of mitral stenosis but without preceding opening snap.

Pulmonary hypertension, loud pulmonary component of second heart sound: in advanced cases.

Investigations

Chest radiography: usually normal in mild aortic regurgitation; possibly valvular calcification; cardiomegaly almost always in severe aortic regurgitation; possibly pulmonary venous congestion after left ventricular failure.

ECG: signs of left ventricular hypertrophy and strain (increased QRS amplitude and ST/T wave changes in precordial leads) and left atrial hypertrophy (wide P wave in lead II and biphasic P in lead V_1).

Echocardiography: for left ventricular size and function; valve may appear normal; fluttering on anterior leaflet of mitral valve and early closure of mitral valve in diastole indicate important aortic regurgitation; may also give useful information on state of aortic root.

Doppler ultrasonography: best method of detecting aortic regurgitation.

Cardiac catheterization: essential when coronary artery disease suspected (*e.g.*, in patients >40 years) and when severity of aortic regurgitation doubted; injection of contrast into aortic root gives information on degree of regurgitation and state of aortic root (presence of dilatation, dissection, root abscesses).

MRI: for assessment of aortic root.

Complications

Cardiac failure: most important cause of disability and death.

Infective endocarditis: should be considered in patients with unexplained illness; may lead to sudden and catastrophic aortic regurgitation.

Arrhythmias: ventricular tachycardia, usually indicating left ventricular failure.

Differential diagnosis

Pulmonary regurgitation: usually accompanying signs of pulmonary hypertension; echo-Doppler examination should resolve the issue.

Patent ductus arteriosus: continuous murmur heard well to the left of sternum; again, echo-Doppler is definitive investigation.

Etiology

• Causes include the following:

Rheumatic disorder in 30% of patients: *e.g.*, coexistent mitral valve disease.

Aortic root dilatation in 20%: *e.g.*, aortic dissection (frequently leads to aortic regurgitation, an indication for urgent surgery) or degeneration of aortic media (frequently idiopathic but may underlie more generalized conditions, *e.g.*, Marfan syndrome, Ehler–Danlos syndrome, osteogenesis imperfecta).

Inflammations in 10%: *e.g.*, rheumatoid arthritis, syphilis, ankylosing spondylitis, Reiter's syndrome.

Bicuspid valve in 15%: usually causes stenosis, can become regurgitant (bicuspid valves present in 1% of population).

Infective endocarditis in 20%: may occur on a bicuspid valve, leading to rupture of a valve cusp.

Epidemiology

• Aortic regurgitation is one of the most common valve lesions.

Treatment

Diet and lifestyle

• Competitive sport should be discouraged.

Pharmacological treatment

Antibiotic prophylaxis

• Prophylaxis is needed against infective endocarditis in asymptomatic patients with known aortic regurgitation; it is particularly important before dental procedures. *See* Endocarditis *for specific details.*

Vasodilatation [1,2]

• Surgery is the main treatment, but angiotensin-converting enzyme (ACE) inhibitors have a role in reducing systemic vascular resistance and decreasing aortic regurgitation. For patients unable to take ACE inhibitors nifedipine, a calcium channel blocker, is a reasonable alternative [1].

Standard dosage	Captopril, 6.25 mg test dose, then 25 mg twice daily.
Contraindications	Hypotension, severe left ventricular impairment, renal failure; extreme caution with coexistent aortic stenosis.
Main drug interactions	Increased hypotensive effect with beta blockers, diuretics, calcium antagonists.
Main side effects	Hypotension, renal failure.

Nonpharmacological treatment

• Surgery is the main form of treatment for aortic regurgitation [3].

• Aortic valve with or without root replacement is indicated for onset of symptoms, increased heart size, and change in ECG, all of which indicate onset of left ventricular dysfunction. By echocardiography, end-systolic left ventricular diameter greater than 55 mm may be used to determine operative timing in patients with no or minimal symptoms.

Treatment aims

To prevent or delay deterioration of left ventricular function and relieve symptoms of dyspnea and fatigue.

Prognosis

• Prognosis depends mainly on the underlying condition and left ventricular function.

• Rheumatic aortic regurgitation, if detected early, has an excellent prognosis.

• Acute aortic regurgitation due to a dissection or endocarditis is fatal unless treated promptly.

• Patients with an underlying collagen disorder, *e.g.*, Marfan syndrome, have a poor prognosis.

Follow-up and management

• Patients with aortic regurgitation should be seen at regular intervals in a cardiology clinic; signs of deteriorating left ventricular function should be vigorously sought by follow-up echocardiography.

• Patients who have had valve replacement should also be seen regularly and monitored for signs of failure of the aortic valve prosthesis (particularly in patients with biological valves) and endocarditis.

Key references

1. Scognamiglio R, *et al.*: Long-term nifedipine unloading therapy in asymtpomatic patients with chronic severe aortic regurgitation. *J Am Coll Cardiol* 1990, **16**:424–429.
2. Greenberg B, *et al.*: Long-term vasodilator therapy of chronic aortic insufficiency. A randomized double-blinded, placebo-controlled clinical trial. *Circulation* 1988, **78**:92–103.
3. Bonow RO, *et al.*: Survival and functional results after valve replacement for aortic regurgitation 1976 to 1983; impact of preoperative left ventricular function. *Circulation* 1985, **72**:1244–1256.

Diagnosis

Symptoms [1,2]

• Many patients are asymptomatic.

Angina: in ~70% of adult patients.

Syncope: in ~25% of patients, during or immediately after exercise.

Dyspnea: common presenting symptom; severe dyspnea, paroxysmal nocturnal dyspnea, and orthopnea late manifestations indicating left ventricular dysfunction.

Signs [1,2]

Pulse

• The pulse is normal in mild aortic stenosis (gradient <50 mm Hg).

Slow rise with diminished "volume," sometimes with "notch" on upstroke ("anacrotic"): indicating severe aortic stenosis; with associated aortic regurgitation, double pulse may be felt ("bisferious").

Heart

Undisplaced, "thrusting" apex beat: thrill may be palpable at base of heart.

Delayed or absent aortic component in second heart sound: in severe aortic stenosis and calcified valves, respectively.

Added sounds: ejection click may be heard at apex in bicuspid aortic valve; fourth heart sound may be heard in severe aortic stenosis; third sound implies impaired left ventricular function.

Murmurs: midsystolic, rough; best heard at base of heart in second right interspace but often heard anywhere over precordium, almost always radiating to neck in severe aortic stenosis, increased in expiration; may be very soft with poor left ventricular function and low cardiac output.

Investigations

ECG: usually shows left ventricular hypertrophy, possibly left axis deviation, later left atrial hypertrophy (negative P wave in V_1), conduction abnormalities due to calcification of conducting tissues (first-degree heart block, left bundle branch block).

Chest radiography: may show cardiac enlargement, poststenotic dilatation of aorta, calcification of aortic valve (particularly in older patients).

Echocardiography: normal valve appearance excludes significant aortic stenosis in adults; also helps to define level of obstruction (*i.e.*, valvar, supravalvar, subvalvar); left ventricular function can also be assessed; Doppler examination permits determination of peak gradient across the valve.

Cardiac catheterization: necessary if coronary artery disease suspected or diagnosis doubted; aortography useful in presence of concomitant aortic regurgitation; retrograde crossing of valve indicated only if echocardiography inadequate; gradient obtained using this method is peak-to-peak, 10–15 mm Hg less than peak instantaneous gradient measured by Doppler examination.

Complications

Sudden death: in 10%–20% of adults and 1% of children.

Cardiac failure: indicates poor prognosis unless valve replaced.

Arrhythmias and conduction abnormalities: ventricular arrhythmias more common than supraventricular arrhythmias; heart block may occur because of calcification of conducting tissues.

Systemic embolization: caused by deposits breaking off valve apparatus or by concomitant aortic atheroma.

Infective endocarditis: should be considered in patients with aortic stenosis who present with unexplained illness.

Differential diagnosis

Aortic sclerosis: old age, normal pulse character, echocardiogram with mild thickening of leaflets without restricted motion or gradient.

Flow murmur (pregnancy, anemia, thyrotoxicosis): large-volume pulse, normal echocardiogram, no gradient.

Mitral regurgitation: pansystolic murmur, no radiation to neck, mitral valve abnormality on echo-Doppler examination.

Hypertrophic cardiomyopathy: late systolic murmur, jerky pulse, echocardiogram showing left ventricular hypertrophy, asymmetric septal hypertrophy, systolic anterior motion of mitral valve.

Ventricular septal defect: pansystolic murmur at left sternal edge with thrill, jet detected on Doppler examination.

Etiology

Congenital: bicuspid or unicuspid valve

• The disease is usually manifest in early childhood or adolescence.

• It may be associated with other congenital abnormalities (coarctation of aorta and patent ductus arteriosus).

• Subvalvar stenosis is more common in boys and accounts for 10% of congenital cases.

• Supravalvar aortic stenosis is rare, usually a component of Williams syndrome.

Acquired

• The disease can be calcific (calcified bicuspid or tricuspid aortic valves manifest in adults) or rheumatic (rarely isolated; usually accompanies rheumatic mitral valve disease).

Epidemiology

• Valvar aortic stenosis is the most common valve lesion in adults in industrialized countries.

• 70% of patients suffer from calcific stenosis (60% bicuspid, 10% tricuspid), 15% rheumatic, and 15% other forms.

Treatment

Diet and lifestyle

• Patients must avoid strenuous exercise and competitive sports.

Pharmacological treatment

• Drug treatment has no place in the treatment of aortic stenosis, but patients should be given antibiotic prophylaxis against infective endocarditis (*see* Endocarditis *for details*).

Nonpharmacological treatment

Surgery

• Surgery is mandatory for symptomatic patients.

• It should be considered in asymptomatic patients objectively with severe aortic stenosis (peak-to-peak gradient >50 mm Hg) [3]. Efforts to objectively exclude symptoms in sedentary patients who report no symptoms may be useful, *e.g.*, gentle treadmill test.

• Age alone is not a contraindication.

• Patients with severe aortic stenosis should have valve replacement early to avoid deterioration in left ventricular function.

Balloon valvuloplasty

• This is useful in infants (in whom the results of surgery are poor) and in children and young adults (in whom the valve apparatus is not calcified).

• It should only be considered in adults when surgery is contraindicated [4].

Treatment aims

To replace valve before left ventricular dysfunction occurs.

Prognosis

• Up to 20% of patients with severe congestive aortic stenosis die during childhood, mainly because of progressive heart failure.

• In adults, the 5-year survival rate is 40%.

• The prognosis after surgery depends on age and left ventricular function.

Follow-up and management

• Patients with mild to moderate aortic stenosis should be monitored for increasing severity.

• Patients who have had valve replacement should be monitored for failure of the valve prosthesis (particularly biological valves) and endocarditis.

Key references

1. Braunwald E: Valvular Heart Disease. In *Heart Disease* edn 4. Edited by Braunwald E. Philadelphia: WB Saunders; 1992:1007–1077.
2. Selzer A: Changing aspects of the natural history of valvular aortic stenosis. *N Engl J Med* 1987, **317**:91–98.
3. Kennedy KD, *et al.*: Natural history of moderate aortic stenosis. *J Am Coll Cardiol* 1991, **17**:13–19.
4. Bernard Y, *et al.*: Long-term results of percutaneous aortic valvuloplasty compared with aortic valve replacement in patients more than 75 years old. *J Am Coll Cardiol* 1992, **20**:796–801.

Diagnosis

Symptoms and signs

Any form of psoriasis or a history compatible with psoriasis.

Skin lesions: possibly years after arthritis (family history of psoriasis may be suggestive).

Peripheral polyarthritis: frequently symmetrical; may be indistinguishable from rheumatoid arthritis, involving small joints of hands and feet, wrists, ankles, knees, and elbows.

Inflammatory oligoarthritis: mainly lower limbs, asymmetrical.

Inflammatory involvement of distal interphalangeal joints: nearly always with psoriatic nail changes.

Asymmetrical spondylitis and sacroiliitis, insertion enthesopathy, *e.g.*, of Achilles tendon, plantar fascia, musculotendinous insertions around pelvis.

Mutilating arthritis: with telescoping of fingers and toes (rare).

Dactylitis: "sausage" digits.

- Rheumatoid nodules and other extra-articular features are absent.

Investigations

Blood tests: rheumatoid factor absent; biochemical response to active disease similar to rheumatoid arthritis; ESR or plasma viscosity best guide to activity.

Radiography: shows asymmetrical small joint changes, tendency to ankylosis, osteolysis with pencil-in-cup deformity, whittling terminal phalanges (especially hallux); enthesitis; asymmetrical sacroiliitis and syndesmophytes.

Complications

Amyloidosis, exfoliation of skin: rare.

Differential diagnosis

Rheumatoid arthritis.

Reactive (Reiter's syndrome).

Etiology

- Psoriatic arthritis has a genetic component: HLA B27 positive in 71% of patients with psoriatic spondylitis, 32% in distal joint group.
- It may be triggered by trauma.

Epidemiology

- 5%–8% of patients with psoriasis have psoriatic arthritis.
- The male:female ratio is equal, but more men have the distal-joint and spondylitic forms.
- Juvenile psoriatic arthritis is rare; it is found in groups similar to those of adult disease.

Classification

Classic psoriatic arthritis: involving predominantly distal interphalangeal joints of hands and feet, in 5% of patients.

Arthritis mutilans: with sacroiliitis, in 5%.

Symmetrical polyarthritis: resembling rheumatoid arthritis but with negative serum rheumatoid factor, in 15%.

Asymmetrical, pauci-articular, small joint involvement: with "sausage" digits, in 70%.

Ankylosing spondylitis: with or without peripheral arthritis, in 5%.

Associated features

Palmar-plantar pustulosis: sternoclavicular hyperostosis, chronic sterile multifocal osteomyelitis, hyperostosis of spine and peripheral arthritis.

Eye lesions: conjunctivitis in 20% of patients; iritis in 7%.

Edema: unilateral.

HIV infection: exacerbates psoriatic but not rheumatoid arthritis.

Keratoderma blenorrhagica of Reiter's syndrome: may develop into psoriasis vulgaris.

Treatment

Diet and lifestyle

- Activity should be encouraged.
- No special diet is necessary.

Pharmacological treatment

Principles

For psoriasis (simple cases): topical steroids, coal tar (*see* Psoriasis *for further details*).

For arthritis (simple cases): NSAIDs, analgesics [1].

For severe cases: second-line treatment according to severity of each system.

Second line for arthritis alone

Standard dosage — Sulfasalazine, 1 g twice daily.
Sodium aurothiomalate, 10 mg i.m. test dose, then 50 mg increase weekly to 1 g, then spaced out to monthly maintenance.

Contraindications — *Sulfasalazine:* hypersensitivity to sulfonamides or salicylates.
Sodium aurothiomalate: pregnancy, lactation, renal or hepatic disease, history of blood dyscrasias, exfoliative dermatitis, or SLE; caution in elderly patients, urticaria, eczema, colitis.

Special points — *Sulfasalazine:* full blood count initially and monthly for first 3 months, liver function tests also monthly for first 3 months.
Sodium aurothiomalate: urine test for protein before injection, skin inspection for rash; full blood count and urine checks monthly.
Antimalarials, *e.g.*, chloroquine, hydroxychloroquine, can also be used.

Main drug interactions — *Sodium aurothiomalate:* aspirin.

Main side effects — *Sulfasalazine:* nausea (dose must be reduced), reversible azoospermia, bone-marrow suppression.
Sodium aurothiomalate: proteinuria, bone-marrow suppression, dermatitis.

Second line for arthritis and skin involvement

- Treatment should be given under specialist supervision [1].

Standard dosage — Methotrexate, azathioprine, possibly etretinate, or possibly cyclosporin A.

Contraindications — *Methotrexate:* liver damage, excess alcohol intake, pregnancy.
Azathioprine: pregnancy.
Etretinate: hepatic and renal impairment, pregnancy.
Cyclosporin: renal impairment.

Special points — *Methotrexate:* regular blood tests (full blood count, liver function).

Main drug interactions — *Methotrexate:* NSAIDs, co-trimoxazole, phenytoin, retinoids, diuretics.
Azathioprine: allopurinol, rifampin.
Etretinate: anticoagulants, methotrexate.
Cyclosporin: angiotensin-converting enzyme inhibitors, NSAIDs.

Main side effects — *Methotrexate:* bone-marrow suppression, liver damage, nausea and vomiting, stomatitis.
Azathioprine: bone-marrow suppression.
Etretinate: fetal malformation, cheilosis, hypercholesterolemia.
Cyclosporin: impaired renal function, nausea.

Treatment aims

To relieve pain and stiffness.

To achieve full functional capacity.

To prevent progression of arthritis.

To minimize skin lesions.

Prognosis

- Prognosis is usually good.
- A few patients are disabled.

Follow-up and management

- A few patients need regular review.
- Second-line drugs need blood monitoring.

Orthopedic guidelines

- Psoriatic arthritis has the same indications as other arthropathies.
- It has no more infective complications than other diseases.
- Physicians should consult with medical, physical therapy, and occupational therapy staff.
- Early postoperative mobilization is advised.

Key reference

1. Pioro MH, Cash JM: Treatment of refractory psoriatic arthritis. *Rheum Dis Clin North Am* 1995, **21**:129–149.

Diagnosis

Symptoms

Painful, swollen, warm joints, with morning stiffness and impaired function: onset usually insidious, sometimes rapid; characteristically in hands or feet, occasionally monoarticular (most often in a knee); often accompanied by tiredness.

Signs

Articular

Warm, tender, swollen joints: decreased range of movement; peripheral joints most often affected; characteristic symmetry of involvement; proximal interphalangeal, metacarpophalangeal, wrist, and metatarsophalangeal joints usually affected.

Extra-articular

Bursitis: *e.g.*, olecranon.

Tenosynovitis.

Nodules: extensor surfaces.

Serositis: *e.g.*, pleurisy.

Keratoconjunctivitis sicca: secondary Sjögren's syndrome.

Vasculitis, scleritis.

Fibrosing alveolitis.

Investigations

• No single diagnostic test is available; the diagnosis relies on some or all of the following:

ESR, CRP, plasma viscosity measurement: for evidence of inflammation.

Immunology: rheumatoid factor positivity (not essential for diagnosis).

Radiography: initially shows periarticular osteoporosis, followed by erosions around affected joint.

Blood count: for anemia of chronic disease, thrombocytosis.

Serum immunoglobulin measurement: for polyclonal gammopathy.

• In addition, the duration of morning stiffness, level of functional impairment, and number of inflamed joints must be monitored in established disease.

Complications

• The following occur in patients with established disease and global decline in function or severe systemic malaise.

Widespread active synovitis.

Septic arthritis.

Systemic rheumatoid disease.

Iatrogenic problems: *e.g.*, NSAIDs and anemia, gold and renal impairment.

Atlantoaxial subluxation.

Non-Hodgkin's lymphoma: possible.

Amyloidosis.

Differential diagnosis

Seronegative spondylarthritis.

Reactive arthritis: gastrointestinal or sexually acquired.

Viral arthritis: *e.g.*, rubella, hepatitis B virus infection.

Septic polyarthritis: *e.g.*, staphylococcal or gonococcal infections.

Crystal polyarthritis: *e.g.*, gout.

Generalized nodal osteoarthritis: may have inflammatory component.

SLE.

Etiology

• The cause of rheumatoid arthritis is unknown, but the following have a role:

Genetic factors: subtypes of HLA DR4 and DR1.

Hormonal factors: remission during pregnancy; contraceptive pill protects from disease.

Epidemiology

• Rheumatoid arthritis is a significant disease that affects 1%–2% of the population.

• It is a chronic disease, with high prevalence and low incidence.

• It is a modern disease, with little evidence to indicate its presence >400 years ago.

• The female : male ratio is 3 : 1.

Treatment

Diet and lifestyle

• Activity should be encouraged, but heavy work intensifies joint inflammation.

• Physical therapy, taught exercise, and "joint protection" are helpful to maintain strength and function.

• Omega-3 fatty acids may reduce inflammation [1].

Pharmacological treatment

NSAIDs

• The response is variable and idiosyncratic; if one drug fails, another from a different group may be worth trying.

• The most commonly used drugs are diclofenac, ibuprofen, indomethacin, naproxen, and salicylate.

Standard dosage	Depends on drug used.
Contraindications	Caution in peptic ulceration, asthma, renal impairment, pregnancy, and elderly patients.
Special points	No influence on disease progression.
Main drug interactions	Diuretics, warfarin.
Main side effects	Dyspepsia, altered bowel habit, renal impairment, fluid retention.

Second-line agents

• These are increasingly started early in the disease process, particularly in patients who do not respond to NSAIDs or who respond partially but have evidence of active disease [2–4].

Standard dosage	Sulfasalazine, 2–3 g daily, with gradual build-up over 4 weeks. Methotrexate, 2.5–15 mg orally once weekly (not daily) [4,5].
Contraindications	*Sulfasalazine:* sulfonamide and salicylate hypersensitivity. *Methotrexate:* pregnancy, liver disease.
Special points	*Sulfasalazine:* full blood count every 4 weeks for 2 months, monthly for 2–3 months, then 3-monthly; liver function test at onset, monthly for 3 months, then 3-monthly. *Methotrexate:* full blood count monthly, liver function test 3-monthly; close monitoring in renal impairment; alcohol use should be avoided; NSAIDs must be used cautiously if at all.
Main drug interactions	*Sulfasalazine:* warfarin, co-trimoxazole. *Methotrexate:* co-trimoxazole, trimethoprim, phenytoin.
Main side effects	*Sulfasalazine:* nausea, vomiting, rashes, reversible azoospermia. *Methotrexate:* nausea, diarrhea, rash, pulmonary hypersensitivity, blood dyscrasias.

Other options [2,4,6]

Gold (oral or i.m.) [4].

Hydroxychloroquine.

Penicillamine.

Local steroids.

Systemic steroids: either induction before or adjunctive to second-line agents in poorly controlled disease [3].

Immunosuppressants: for severe articular or extra-articular disease.

Minocycline [6].

Nonpharmacological treatment

Physical therapy: during active disease.

Occupational therapy.

Surgery: synovectomies, arthroplasty, arthrodesis, tendon repair; for painful joints (particularly at night), functionally restricted joints, and joints that do not respond to other treatments.

Treatment aims

To decrease pain and symptoms and signs of inflammation.

To prevent progression of irreversible joint damage.

To monitor for and treat extra-articular manifestations.

To restrict disability and handicap.

Prognosis

• The prognosis is very variable.

• Poor prognostic markers include female sex, insidious onset, high-titer rheumatoid factor, low educational achievement, persistently raised ESR or CRP, and extra-articular manifestations [7].

Follow-up and management

• Second-line treatment must be monitored regularly.

• Stable disease needs occasional assessment for progressive functional decline.

• Active disease needs regular follow-up so that modifying the various treatment options can be considered.

• Care should be shared between primary care and hospital services.

Key references

1. Geusens P, *et al.*: Long term effect of omega 3 fatty acid supplementation in active rheumatoid arthritis; a 12 month double blind controlled study. *Arthritis Rheum* 1994, **37**:824–829.
2. Anonymous: Slow-acting antirheumatic drugs. *Drug Ther Bull* 1993, **31**:17–20.
3. Harris ED: Rheumatoid arthritis. Pathophysiology and implications for treatment. *N Engl J Med* 1990, **332**:1277–1289.
4. Wilke WS, *et al.*: Early aggressive therapy for rheumatoid arthritis concerns, descriptions and estimates of outcome. *Semin Arthritis Rheum* 1993, **23**:26–41.
5. Weinblatt ME, *et al.*: Methotrexate in rheumatoid arthritis. A five year prospective multi-center study. *Arthritis Rheum* 1994, **37**:1492–1498.
6. Kloppenburg M, *et al.*: Minocycline in active rheumatoid arthritis: a double blind placebo controlled trial. *Arthritis Rheum* 1994, **37**:629–636.
7. Tugwell P, *et al.*: End points in rheumatoid arthritis. *J Rheumatol* (suppl) 1994, **42**:2–8; 20–24.

Diagnosis

Symptoms

• Symptoms and signs are more difficult to interpret in the presence of pre-existing joint disease and may be muted in immunosuppressed or elderly patients [1].

• Polyarticular infection occurs in 10%–15% of patients [1–3].

Pain: most consistent feature; typically progressive; may be worse at night; with pre-existing joint disease, change or exacerbation of pain is an important warning sign [3].

Loss of function, limp: possibly presenting feature in children [2].

Fever: possibly only manifestation, particularly in elderly patients [3].

Signs

Swelling and local tenderness, pain and restriction of movement: most marked in previously fit younger patients [2].

Local erythema: possibly but often less marked than in crystal synovitis.

Fever: although temperature normal in up to one-third of patients.

Confusion: possibly prominent feature in elderly patients [3].

Investigations

• Most investigations are nonspecific, and results may be normal; a high index of suspicion is necessary to make the diagnosis [4].

• Adequate specimens must be obtained for microbiological examination before antimicrobial treatment is started.

Synovial fluid analysis: Gram stain positive in 50% of patients; culture positive in 75%; presence of leukocytes not diagnostic; crystals may coexist with sepsis.

Blood cultures: positive in 50% (may be presenting feature of subacute bacterial endocarditis).

Urogenital swabs: should be obtained if gonococcal infection suspected.

Plain radiography: usually unhelpful in early stages of infection [4].

Complications

Death: in up to 15%, especially elderly, immunosuppressed, and rheumatoid arthritis patients.

Loss of function of joint.

Loss of prosthesis.

Osteomyelitis: from direct spread.

Bacterial endocarditis, disseminated intravascular coagulation.

Differential diagnosis

Acute flare of inflammatory joint disease.

Crystal synovitis.

Hemarthrosis.

Etiology

• Pathogens depend on age and predisposing factors; most infections are due to *Staphylococcus aureus* and streptococci; in children <5 years, *Haemophilus influenzae* type b has been an important pathogen; gonococcal infection appears to be in decline but should be considered in sexually active patients.

• Spread is usually hematogenous; joint disease or blunt trauma may act to localize blood-borne pathogens.

• Direct inoculation during surgery, injection, or trauma occurs but is unusual.

• Risk factors include extremes of age, previous joint disease, diabetes mellitus, immunosuppression, prosthetic joint material, and corticosteroids.

Epidemiology

• The incidence of septic arthritis is unknown but is estimated to be 3–10 in 100 000 population.

Treatment

Diet and lifestyle

• No special precautions are necessary.

Pharmacological treatment

General principles

• A possible septic arthritis is a medical emergency and should be urgently referred to a specialist rheumatologist or an orthopedic surgeon.

• High-dose antibiotics are given i.v. for at least 2 weeks, then orally for at least a further 2–4 weeks, depending on the clinical response and presence of prosthesis.

• Antibiotics should be started only after appropriate specimens for culture have been obtained.

• Initially, a "best guess" choice of antibiotics is used, based on the most probable pathogen, patient's age, and sensitivities of pathogen; treatment is later tailored by the results of the Gram stain and culture.

Possible "best-guess" regimen

Child <5 years: cefotaxime and nafcillin [2].

Child >5 years, adult: nafcillin (with penicillin G if gonococcal infection likely) [1–3,5].

Immunosuppressed, prosthetic-joint patient: cefotaxime and floxacillin. Vancomycin i.v. for methicillin-resistant *Staphylococcus aureus*.

Specific drugs

Standard dosage	Nafcillin, 2 g i.v. every 4 h. Penicillin G, 4.8–9.6 g i.v. daily. Cefotaxime 3–6 g i.v. daily. Vancomycin, 1 g i.v. every 12 h.
Contraindications	Hypersensitivity.
Special points	Full blood count needed twice weekly. Aminopenicillin can be used instead of penicillin V for oral treatment.
Main drug interactions	None.
Main side effects	Rash, hypersensitivity reaction (rare), neutropenia (after prolonged treatment), diarrhea.

Treatment aims

To prevent septicemia or osteomyelitis.
To preserve joint function.
To resolve infection.

Other treatments

• Repeated medical aspiration with adequate drainage may be associated with better outcome than surgical drainage [6].

• Surgery is indicated for the following [7]:
Inability to drain medically.
Failure to improve on antibiotic or medical management.
Osteomyelitis.
Prosthetic joints (surgical drainage, debridement, or removal).

Prognosis

• The overall mortality is 15%.

• The prognosis is worse if treatment is delayed, in elderly patients with gram-positive infection, and in patients with predisposing joint or systemic disease.

• Infection of prosthetic material carries a particularly poor prognosis; revision or removal of the prosthesis is a common outcome.

Follow-up and management

• Patients with infected prostheses may need long-term suppressive antibiotic treatment, although, in most, revision surgery is delayed rather than prevented.

Key references

1. Goldenberg DL: Bacterial arthritis. *Curr Opin Rheumatol* 1994, **6**:394–400.
2. Shaw BA, Kasser JL: Acute septic arthritis in infancy and childhood. *Clin Orthop* 1990, **257**:212–225.
3. Esterhai JL Jr, Gelb I: Adult septic arthritis. *Orthop Clin North Am* 1991, **3**:503–514.
4. Hendrix RW, Fisher MR: Imaging of septic arthritis. *Clin Rheum Dis* 1986, **12**:459–487.
5. Norden C, *et al.*: Evaluation of new anti-infective drugs for the treatment of infectious arthritis in adults. *Clin Infect Dis* 1992, **15**(suppl):S167–S171.
6. Broy SB, Schmid FR: A comparison of medical drainage (needle aspiration) and surgical drainage (arthrotomy or arthroscopy) in the initial treatment of infected joints. *Clin Rheum Dis* 1986, **12**:501–522.
7. Parisien JS, Shaffer R: Arthroscopic management of pyarthrosis. *Clin Orthop* 1992, **275**:243–247.

Diagnosis

Symptoms

Uncomplicated ascites

Abdominal distension and discomfort.

Dyspnea: due to splinting of diaphragm.

Fatigue, encephalopathy, and other symptoms of chronic liver disease: may be present.

Spontaneous bacterial peritonitis

Pain, fever: in <50% of patients.

Deterioration in liver function, renal impairment, gastrointestinal hemorrhage, encephalopathy: may be present.

Signs

Uncomplicated ascites

Distension.

Shifting dullness on percussion of flanks, fluid wave.

Ballotable liver.

Spontaneous bacterial peritonitis

- Often no new clinical signs are manifest.

Fever, encephalopathy: more common than tenderness, rebound, rigidity.

Investigations

In all cases

Measurement of serum and ascitic albumin: to allow calculation of concentration gradient.
Cell count using ascites: >250 polymorphonuclear neutrophils/mL suggests peritonitis; lymphocyte predominance suggests tuberculosis or malignancy.
Cytologic study: of fluid to evaluate for malignancy.

Gram stain and culture of ascites: blood culture bottle inoculation; polymicrobial infections suggest perforation of the gastrointestinal tract.

Urine electrolytes analysis.

Serum electrolytes, blood urea nitrogen, creatinine.

Specific tests for selected presentations

Amylase measurement: concentration raised in pancreatic ascites.

Cholesterol or triglyceride measurement: concentration raised in chylous ascites.

Total protein: high in malignancy, tuberculosis, cardiac ascites.

Laparoscopy and biopsy: for tuberculosis.

Abdominal ultrasonography or CT: for malignant ascites.

Complications

Spontaneous bacterial peritonitis: most common in patients with high serum-ascites albumin gradients.

Pleural effusion.

Inguinal, femoral, or umbilical hernias.

Mesenteric venous thrombosis.

Renal failure.

Differential diagnosis

High serum-ascites albumin gradient (*i.e.*, ≥1.1 g/dL)
Portal hypertension.
Cirrhosis.
Cardiac ascites.
Fulminant hepatitis.
Budd-Chiari/veno-occlusive disease.
Myxedema.

Low serum-ascites albumin gradient (*i.e.*, <1.1 g/dL)
Peritoneal carcinomatosis.
Tuberculosis.
Pancreatic ascites.
Biliary ascites.
Nephrotic syndrome.

Chylous
Trauma and surgery, abdominal tuberculosis, lymphoma or other malignancy, filariasis.

Etiology

- Common causes include the following:

High serum-ascites albumin gradient
Overflow hypothesis: primary increase in renal sensitivity to aldosterone, causing sodium retention or volume expansion, ascites forming in abdomen because of portal hypertension and hypoalbuminemia.
Underfill hypothesis: fluid sequestration in abdomen, causing renal hypoperfusion and secondary hyperaldosteronism, renal retention of sodium to maintain circulating volume.
Vasodilatation hypothesis: overflow factors initiating and underfill factors perpetuating ascites.

Low serum-ascites albumin gradient
Increased capillary permeability.

Chylous
Lymphatic leakage.

Epidemiology

- 80% of patients with chronic liver disease develop ascites during their course (spontaneous bacterial peritonitis in 10%).

Treatment

Diet and lifestyle

• Patients should have a low-salt diet (<2 g daily) and maintain an adequate intake of calories.

• Bed rest during mobilization of ascites may lower renin–angiotensin concentrations.

Pharmacological treatment

For uncomplicated ascites

• Initially, treatment should involve spironolactone, with high-volume paracentesis reserved for patients with respiratory compromise or those with disease that is refractory to diuretic management.

• Furosemide can be added if no response is seen after 3 days and is more effective in patients with peripheral edema.

Standard dosage	Spironolactone, 100 mg daily, or furosemide, 40 mg daily, aiming for 1.0 kg of weight loss per day if pedal edema present and 0.5 kg per day if there is no pedal edema; dosage is increased slowly depending on diuresis to maximum spironolactone, 400 mg, or furosemide, 160 mg.
Contraindications	Renal failure.
Special points	Renal function should be watched carefully and diuretics decreased or witheld for any increase in creatinine of 0.5 mg/dL over baseline. Hyponatremia <122 mEq/L should be treated with fluid restriction. Hyperkalemia should be managed by a decrease in spironolactone or an increase in furosemide.
Main drug interactions	Diuretics and aminoglycosides may have increased nephrotoxicity in this context.
Main side effects	Hyponatremia, impaired renal function with raised creatinine, hyperkalemia [1]. For patients with gynecomastia from spironolactone, amiloride is an alternative (5–10 mg daily).

• High-volume paracentesis (removal of >6 L of ascites) should be done in cases refractory to diuretic management. Caution should be exercised in patients with renal dysfunction (creatinine >2.0 mg/dL). Intravenous albumin (10 g/L of ascites removed) administered to patients with elevated creatinine or those without pedal edema may protect against progressive renal dysfunction.

For functional renal failure

• Renal failure is often precipitated by infection, hemorrhage, hypotension, or overaggressive diuretic treatment; it may reverse after orthotopic liver transplantation.

• Treatment involves central venous monitoring, volume expansion, and treatment of precipitating factors; renal vasodilators are of no proven benefit.

For spontaneous bacterial peritonitis [2]

• 80% of organisms are aerobic gram-negative bacilli; 20% are nonenteric organisms.

• Cefotaxime or ceftizoxime is effective in up to 85%; ciprofloxacin and amoxicillin may be as effective, but gentamicin is potentially more toxic.

• Treatment should last 5–7 days.

• Antibiotic treatment is influenced by hospital sensitivities.

• Clearance of ascitic leukocytes should be checked after 3 days, and renal function should be monitored daily.

• Long-term antibiotic prophylaxis with antibiotics (*e.g.*, norfloxacin) may prevent recurrence.

Treatment aims

To reduce ascitic volume.

Other treatments

For diuretic-resistant ascites: orthotopic liver transplantation or, if contraindicated for surgical or medical reasons, jugulo-peritoneal shunt, regular abdominal paracentesis with albumin infusion, or transhepatic intravascular portal systemic stent shunt.

Prognosis

• 1-year and 5-year survival rates after development of ascites without renal impairment are 50% and 20%, respectively.

• 80% of patients respond to medical treatment.

• 30% develop functional renal failure within 24 months.

• When urine sodium is <5 mmol/L or diuretic-resistant ascites has developed, 1-year survival is <50%.

• Spontaneous bacterial peritonitis has a hospital mortality of up to 50%.

• >50% of survivors have a recurrence in the following year.

Follow-up and management

• Patients with uncomplicated ascites must be monitored using weight and fluid input and output charts daily.

• If no response is seen at maximum tolerated dose of diuretic, the development of hepatoma, portal-vein thrombosis, or spontaneous bacterial peritonitis must be excluded.

Key references

1. Arroyo V, *et al.*: Ascites, renal failure and electrolyte disorders in cirrhosis. Pathogenesis, diagnosis and treatment. In *Oxford Textbook of Clinical Hepatology.* Edited by McIntyre N, *et al.* Oxford: Oxford Medical Publications, 1991:429–470.
2. Bhuva M, Ganger D, Jensen D: Spontaneous bacterial peritonitis: an update on evaluation, management, and prevention. *Am J Med* 1994, **97**:169–175.

Diagnosis

Symptoms

Wheeze.

Breathlessness.

Chest tightness: not pain.

Cough: with or without sputum; may be the only symptom, especially in children.

• Symptom severity shows considerable temporal variation; they are often worse at night or in early morning.

Signs

Diffuse wheeze.

Use of accessory muscles of respiration: due to high negative intrapleural pressure or rapid respiratory rate.

Tachycardia: in severe attack.

Pulsus paradoxus: in severe attack.

Cyanosis or confusion: signs of impending respiratory arrest; wheeze may be absent.

Investigations

On presentation

Spirometry: forced expiratory volume in 1 s (FEV_1) and forced vital capacity; response to beta-2 agonist (>15% improvement in FEV_1 confirms reversible airflow obstruction; failure to improve does not exclude asthma).

Serial peak flow monitoring: early peak flow often low in asthma; >15% diurnal variation strongly suggests asthma, peak flow reduced after work or exposure to sensitizing agent.

Skin tests: to assess role of atopy (~50% of patients have positive immediate skin tests).

Steroid response test: >15% increase in FEV_1 after 2-week course of oral prednisone, 30 mg daily.

Airways hyperresponsiveness test: increased sensitivity to methacholine, shown by 20% fall in FEV_1 to abnormally small doses of nebulized methacholine.

For acute episodes

Spirometry or peak flow rate measurement: to assess severity.

Arterial blood gas analysis: partial oxygen pressure reduced; partial carbon dioxide pressure usually low in acute episode; rising or raised partial carbon dioxide pressure suggests exhaustion and impending respiratory arrest; different patterns in acute exacerbations of chronic obstructive pulmonary disease (*see* Chronic obstructive airway disease *for details*).

Chest radiography: to check for pneumothorax or pneumonia and to exclude heart failure.

ECG: if cause of breathlessness unclear.

Sputum culture: good samples often difficult to obtain; most exacerbations due to viral not bacterial infection.

Complications [1]

Respiratory arrest and death.

Pneumothorax.

Recurrent bronchial infection.

Irreversible airflow limitation.

Differential diagnosis

• The diagnosis is usually obvious and easily confirmed.

Acute or chronic bronchitis.

Irreversible airway obstruction (chronic obstructive pulmonary disease).

Rhinitis with postnasal drip.

Left ventricular failure.

Pulmonary embolism.

Etiology [2,3]

• Asthma has an important genetic component, which is inherited separately from the genetic tendency to atopy.

• ~50% of patients have associated atopic allergy, especially children.

• All grades of asthma show airway inflammation, with eosinophils, mononuclear cells, and epithelial desquamation.

• Viral infections are clearly linked to exacerbations of asthma and may be responsible for initiating asthma in patients with adult-onset disease.

• Exposure to environmental chemicals and pollution is blamed for the current increase in prevalence: clear evidence of a causal relationship is awaited.

Epidemiology

• The prevalence of asthma appears to be increasing in the US; an estimated 5%–10% of the population is asthmatic.

• Asthma is more common in children, and may remit as they grow.

Treatment

Diet and lifestyle

• Special diets are not usually needed; patients with salicylate or sulfite sensitivity should avoid foods containing salicylates or sulfites.

• Exercise is encouraged; swimming is often better tolerated than outdoor sports (exercise-induced asthma is triggered by cold dry air).

Pharmacological treatment [4]

Corticosteroids [5,6]

Standard dosage *Inhaled corticosteroids:* starting dose varies according to severity and corticosteroid formulation (*e.g.*, beclomethasone, 200–400 μg twice daily).
Oral corticosteroids: prednisone, 30 mg daily for 5 days; longer courses may be needed if improvement is slow; dose need not be tapered if course lasts <14 days.

Contraindications None.

Special points Rinsing mouth after inhaling steroids reduces risk of oropharyngeal side effects.
Spacer device should be used.

Main drug interactions None.

Main side effects *Inhaled steroids:* hoarse voice, oropharyngeal candidiasis.
Oral steroids: cushingoid features, especially osteoporosis, bruising, weight gain.

Xanthines

Standard dosage Theophylline, dose adjusted to give blood concentrations of 10–15 mg/L.

Contraindications Liver disease, heart disease, epilepsy, porphyria.

Special points Narrow therapeutic margin, so dose should be low initially and adjusted with aid of plasma drug concentrations.

Main drug interactions Plasma concentration increased with many other drugs, *e.g.*, antibiotics (ciprofloxacin, erythromycin), cimetidine, antidepressants, diltiazem, verapamil, fluconazole.

Main side effects Nausea, reflux esophagitis, tremor.

Short-acting beta-2 agonists

Standard dosage Depends on agent and device, *e.g.*, albuterol, terbutaline, 1–2 puffs as needed.

Contraindications None.

Special points Frequent use of short-acting beta-2 agonists suggests suboptimal control.

Main drug interactions Beta blockers must be avoided.

Main side effects Tremor.

For severe attacks [1]

Hospital admission.

Severity assessment (especially spirometry and blood gases).

Oxygen administration.

Bronchodilatation (nebulizer).

Oral prednisone administration.

Intravenous hydrocortisone administration.

Intravenous aminophylline administration.

Ventilation if patient is tired or weakening or if blood gases show rising arterial blood pressure.

Treatment aims

To find minimum level of treatment to suppress symptoms.
To enable patients to take responsibility for day-to-day management of the condition.
To enable patients to avoid days off work or school.
To reduce the frequency of exacerbations and to avoid hospital admissions.

Prognosis

• Many children with asthma experience spontaneous remission in their second decade of life.
• Adult-onset asthma rarely remits.
• Most asthmatic patients cope well with their disease and have a normal life expectancy.
• A few severely ill or unstable asthmatic patients are at risk of respiratory arrest; often, these patients need large doses of oral corticosteroids to control the disease.

Follow-up and management

• Exacerbations should be treated by the following:
Increased dose of inhaled corticosteroid.
Oral prednisone, 30 mg daily for 5–7 days.
Antibiotics if patient is febrile or sputum discoloured.
Increased dose of bronchodilators.

Key references

1. Corbridge TC, Hall JB: The assessment and management of adults with status asthmaticus. *Am J Respir Crit Care Med* 1995, **151**:1292–1316.
2. Djukanovic R, *et al.*: Mucosal inflammation in asthma. State of the art. *Am Rev Respir Dis* 1990, **142**:434–457.
3. Goldstein RA, *et al.*: NIH conference: asthma. *Ann Intern Med* 1994, **121**:698–708.
4. National Asthma Education Program—Expert Panel Report: *Guidelines for the Diagnosis and Management of Asthma.* Washington, D.C.: U.S. Department of Health and Human Services, Public Health Service, National Institutes of Health; 1991.
5. Chapman K, *et al.*: Effect of a short course of prednisone in the prevention of early relapse after the emergency room treatment of acute asthma. *N Engl J Med* 1991, **324**:788–794.
6. McFadden E, Jr: Dosages of corticosteroids in asthma. *Am Rev Respir Dis* 1993, **147**:1306–1310.

Diagnosis

Symptoms

Breathlessness at rest or on exertion, wheeze, worsening after work, improvement at weekends or during holidays.

Signs

Diffuse wheeze.

Use of accessory muscles of respiration: due to high negative intrapleural pressure or rapid respiratory rate.

Tachycardia: in severe attack.

Pulsus paradoxus: in severe attack.

Rhinitis.

Investigations [1]

Baseline spirometry: response to beta-2 agonist.

Bronchial hyper-responsiveness test: using methacholine PC_{20}.

Detailed peak flow monitoring: at work and on days off or vacations.

Detailed list of materials encountered in the workplace.

Serial measure of airway responsiveness.

Specific challenge tests: to confirm role of new agent in causing asthma or to determine responsible agent when several agents are present in the workplace.

Challenge test: >20% fall in forced expiratory volume in 1 s, with no such change on control day.

Bronchial response test: twofold increase, with no such change on control day.

Complications

Interstitial fibrosis.

Respiratory failure.

Chronic breathlessness.

Differential diagnosis

Asthma due to nonoccupational causes.

Other causes of breathlessness.

Irritant effect of chemical at work.

Etiology [2,3]

- Causes include the following:

Animal hair.
Laboratory animals.
Chemicals.
Food processing.
Enzymes (detergents).
Hairdressing.

Epidemiology

- The incidence of occupational asthma is increasing and now accounts for >50% of industrial lung disease.

Treatment

Diet and lifestyle

• Exposure should be reduced (to zero if possible) by moving to low-exposure zone, provision of personal respirator, or leaving employment.

Pharmacological treatment

• Treatment is the same as for other forms of asthma (*see* Asthma *for details*).

• All cases of occupational lung disease need specialist assessment to ensure that the correct diagnosis is reached and appropriate treatment instituted.

• Most patients need inhaled corticosteroids and bronchodilators.

Standard dosage	Beclomethasone, 400–800 µg daily.
Contraindications	None.
Special points	Rinsing of mouth after inhaling steroids reduces risk of oropharyngeal side effects. Spacer device should be used.
Main drug interactions	None.
Main side effects	Hoarse voice, oropharyngeal candidiasis.

Treatment aims

To control symptoms of asthma and restore normal levels of activity.

To reduce risk of developing chronic asthma.

Prognosis

• Most patients improve when withdrawn from exposure.

• >40% should have no residual signs or symptoms of asthma, but up to 30% have chronic persistent symptoms, despite full withdrawal from exposure.

• Persistent asthma is especially frequent with low molecular weight sensitizers but can also occur with high molecular weight (protein) antigens.

Follow-up and management

• Patients should be followed carefully to check whether asthma resolves with time.

• Regular radiographic monitoring is necessary for patients with interstitial fibrosis.

Key references

1. Chan-Yeung M, Malo JL: Occupational asthma. *N Engl J Med* 1995, **333**:107–112.
2. Bernstein IL, *et al.*, eds: *Asthma in the Workplace*. New York: Marcel Dekker; 1993.
3. Salvaggio JE: The impact of allergy and immunology on our expanding industrial environment. *J Allergy Clin Immunol* 1990, **85**:689–699.

Diagnosis

Symptoms

Ostium secundum defect [1–3]

- Patients are often asymptomatic in early life.
- Children may have increased incidence of chest infections.
- Symptoms increase with age: >70% of adults are symptomatic by 40 years.

Palpitation: indicating atrial arrythmias.
Dyspnea.
Productive cough: indicating recurrent chest infections.
Fatigue, ankle swelling: indicating right-sided congestive heart failure.
Symptoms of paradoxical emboli.

Ostium primum defect

- Patients will more probably develop symptoms and heart failure in childhood.

Failure to thrive.
Chest infections.
Poor development.

- In adults, in addition to the same symptoms as for secundum defect, the following occur:

Syncope: indicating heart block.
Symptoms of infective endocarditis.

Signs [1–3]

Ostium primum and secundum defects

- The following signs of pulmonary hypertension may be manifest:

Right ventricular hypertrophy, palpable pulmonary closure, pulmonary ejection click, early diastolic murmur of pulmonary regurgitation.

Normal or small-volume pulse.
Normal or raised venous pressure: raised pressure with pulmonary hypertension and right ventricular enlargement.
Prominent right ventricular impulse.
Widely split second sound in inspiration and expiration (fixed).
Ejection systolic flow murmur in pulmonary area and mid-diastolic tricuspid flow murmur: increased right-sided flows, louder on inspiration.

Ostium primum defect only

Pansystolic murmur at apex: indicating mitral regurgitation (mitral valve abnormal).

Investigations

ECG: for ostium secundum defect, shows right axis deviation, right bundle branch block; for ostium primum defect, shows left axis deviation, right bundle branch block, prolonged PR interval.
Chest radiography: for secundum and primum defects, shows moderate cardiac enlargement, small aortic knuckle, large pulmonary artery, pulmonary plethora.
Two-dimensional echocardiography: identifies precise anatomy in most patients; contrast studies may reveal site of shunting.
Cardiac catheterization: often unnecessary in diagnosis but may be used to assess shunt with saturation samples taken from right and left heart, right heart pressures, and pulmonary vascular resistance.

Complications

Atrial arrhythmias: atrial fibrillation most common.
Pulmonary hypertension and development of right ventricular disease.
Eisenmenger's syndrome with reversal of shunt.
Paradoxical embolus.
Infective endocarditis: in patients with ostium primum defect only.

Differential diagnosis

Uncomplicated ostium secundum defect
Mild pulmonary stenosis.

Atrial septal defect with pulmonary hypertension
Rheumatic mitral and tricuspid valve disease.
Mitral valve prolapse.
Primary pulmonary hypertension.
Cor pulmonale.

Etiology

- The cause is unknown.

Epidemiology

- Atrial septal defect constitutes 7% of all congenital heart disease and 30% of congenital heart disease in adults.
- The female : male ratio is 2 : 1.

Types

Ostium secundum
Defect of fossa ovalis (most common; 70% of all defects).

Ostium primum
Defect in septum inferior to fossa ovalis; may occur in isolation or as atrial component of atrioventricular septal defect.

Sinus venosus
Defect at base of superior vena cava/upper part of interatrial septum; often associated with anomalous pulmonary venous drainage.

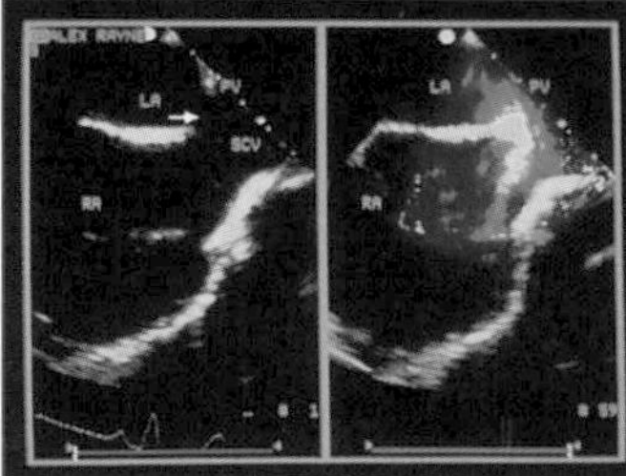

Sinus venosus atrial septal defect (*arrow*).

Treatment

Diet and lifestyle

• No special precautions are necessary.

Pharmacological treatment

• Drug treatment has a role only in the management of complications of the defect such as atrial fibrillation (antiarrhythmic agents), right ventricular failure (diuretics), and infective endocarditis of a primum defect (antibiotics).

Nonpharmacological treatment

• Treatment of the defect itself involves surgical closure or transcatheter delivery of an umbrella or clamshell device across the defect [4].

Ostium secundum defect

• Asymptomatic infants and children are usually followed, with closure advocated before the age of 10 years, if the pulmonary : systemic flow ratio is >1.5 : 1; the feasibility of device closure is determined on transthoracic and transesophageal echocardiography.

• If the child is unsuitable for transcatheter closure, surgical placement of pericardial or Dacron patch should be used.

• For adults, the debate continues on whether closure is worthwhile, but, if symptomatic with shunt >2 : 1, most experts advocate closure; transcatheter device closure may be feasible [5].

• Contraindications to closure are pulmonary vascular resistance >6 Woods units, and age >65 years with small shunt [5].

Ostium primum defect

• All patients with significant shunt, unless complicated by severe pulmonary vascular disease, should have surgical closure, with repair of associated mitral valve abnormalities.

Treatment aims

To prevent late-onset pulmonary hypertension.

To avoid right ventricular failure.

To reduce or delay incidence of atrial arrhythmias.

Prognosis

• In patients with ostium secundum defect, mortality of repair in an uncomplicated case is <1%; in older patients with rise in pulmonary vascular resistance, mortality is higher.

• Most patients with unoperated ostium primum defect die by the age of 30 years; operative mortality varies with the complexity of the defect but is usually 5%–10%.

Follow-up and management

• Patients must be observed for symptoms of atrial arrhythmias, developing pulmonary hypertension, and right ventricular failure.

• After repair of an ostium primum defect, heart block is possible.

Key references

1. Dexter L: Atrial septal defect. *Br Heart J* 1956, **18**:209–225.
2. Perloff JK: Atrial Septal Defect. In *The Clinical Recognition of Congenital Heart Disease*, edn 3. Edited by Perloff JK. Philadelphia: WB Saunders, 1987:272–349.
3. Liberthson RR: Atrial Septal Defect. In *Congenital Heart Disease: Diagnosis and Management in Children and Adults.* Boston: Little Brown; 1989:45–60.
4. Murphy JG: Long-term outcome after surgical repair of isolated atrial septal defect. *N Engl J Med* 1990, **323**:1645–1650.
5. Sutton MGS, Tajik AJ, McGoon DC: Atrial septal defect in patients aged 60 years or older: operative results and long-term postoperative follow-up. *Circulation* 1981, **64**:402–409.

Diagnosis

Symptoms and signs [1]

History: high risk of completed suicide

Presence or previous history of major mental illness: especially endogenous depression, mania, and schizophrenia.

Evidence of planning: time spent in preparation of the means of death, *e.g.*, buying and hoarding tablets, precautions taken against discovery or intervention by others, acts in anticipation of death, *e.g.*, making or updating will, writing suicide note.

Continuing wish to die: no help sought after attempt, continued wish to die after resuscitation, hopelessness.

Violent method chosen: *e.g.*, hanging, jumping from height.

History: low risk of completed suicide

No history or presence of major mental illnesses.

Little or no preparation or precautions: decision to attempt suicide taken within 1 h of the act or after ingestion of alcohol, act performed in front of another.

No continuing wish to die: help sought after act, no wish to die after resuscitation, optimism about future.

Nonviolent means: method perceived by patient as having a low risk of real harm; patients may not understand the toxic effects of drugs taken and may mistakenly consider acetaminophen and aspirin harmless because they are available over the counter and benzodiazepines dangerous because they are prescription-only drugs.

Mental state

• Orientation and memory must be checked first because the toxic effects of drugs or alcohol must be allowed to wear off before further assessment is attempted.

• An acute organic brain syndrome, including visual hallucinations can be caused by overdose of tricyclic antidepressants.

Features of major mental illness, especially endogenous depression or psychosis: patient should be asked about persistent low mood, worse in mornings, sleep disturbance with early morning wakening, appetite and weight loss, lack of energy, pessimism, low self-esteem, guilt, excessive worrying, delusions, and hallucinations.

Investigations

• Available databases should be checked for evidence of previous or present psychiatric care.

• Further history should be obtained from available informants.

• Physical investigations appropriate for the type of self-harm should be made.

Complications

• No overall physical complications are seen; complications depend on the nature of the self-harm.

Differential diagnosis

Self-cutting or self-damage to relieve tension: often multiple superficial cuts on forearms.

Self-mutilation in context of psychotic illness: especially schizophrenia.

Accidental ingestion of toxic substances: *e.g.*, tablets that look like sweets to children, weedkiller stored in a lemonade bottle.

Etiology

• Causes include the following:

High risk of completed suicide

Major depression, schizophrenia, mania.

Alcoholism and drug abuse.

Chronic physical ill health.

Recent bereavement.

Low risk of completed suicide

Poorly developed coping skills.

Relationship problems.

Social stressors.

Epidemiology [1]

• The low rate of suicide (11 per 100 000) makes prediction of an individual suicide very difficult.

• The rate of adolescent suicide is increasing in the US.

• Trends vary widely over time and across different cultures.

• Risk factors for completed suicide are older age, male sex, poor physical health, unemployment or retirement, being separated, widowed, or divorced, living alone.

• Patients at low risk of completed suicide are usually female, <45 years, from a low socioeconomic class, and living in urban areas with social deprivation and crowding.

Treatment

Diet and lifestyle

• High alcohol intake, social isolation, and lack of employment are all high risk factors for repetition of suicide attempts, so efforts should be made to change the lifestyle of the patients through therapeutic intervention.

Pharmacological treatment

• The physical consequences of self-harm must be treated first.

• Except in emergencies, psychotropic drugs should be given only for treatment of specific mental illness under close psychiatric supervision, usually as an inpatient.

• Tranquillizing drugs must be avoided unless absolutely necessary for the safety of patients or others.

• For the emergency management of violently mentally disturbed patients, a short-acting antipsychotic, *e.g.*, droperidol or haloperidol in 5 mg increments i.m. every 15 min, should be used until symptoms are controlled, unless seizures are a risk. An antiparkinsonian drug, *e.g.*, procyclidine, 5–10 mg i.m., can be added to avoid dystonic reactions. Drugs should not be given i.v. when the cause of the mental disturbance is not known.

• When seizures are a risk, a benzodiazepine, *e.g.*, diazepam in 5 mg increments i.v. or lorazepam, 2–5 mg i.m., can be used. Benzodiazepines must be avoided in patients with severe respiratory impairment. Antipsychotic agents and benzodiazepines combined have an additive tranquillizing effect.

Nonpharmacological treatment [1]

Counseling

• Most patients are cooperative, and many are not suffering from mental illness. Low-risk patients should be offered brief problem-orientated counseling, where available.

• Patients with alcohol or substance abuse problems should be referred to the relevant specialist services.

• Relationship therapy should be offered to patients with relationship problems if both partners are agreeable.

• Open access or a telephone help-line may be offered, if available.

Psychiatric referral [2]

• High-risk patients need psychiatric referral.

• Patients with major mental illness need urgent psychiatric treatment, usually on an inpatient basis.

Detention and emergency treatment [3]

• Patients threatening discharge who have not been assessed or who have been assessed and are considered to be at immediate risk may have to be detained for further assessment or treatment.

• If a patient refuses to talk, information to make an assessment must be obtained from other informants before the patient can be discharged.

• Compulsory detention in hospital must be considered in cases of psychiatric illness or serious suicide risk.

• Emergency action in the patient's best interest is legally sanctioned in virtually every state; failure to act may be construed as negligence.

Treatment aims

To treat any underlying mental disorder.

To help patient to solve problems and to provide support through current crisis.

To strengthen patient's future coping skills.

Prognosis

• Repetition occurs most often within the first 3 months of an episode.

• Repetition with increased suicidal intent may herald completed suicide.

• Long-term risk of completed suicide overall is ~1% at 1 year and ~2.8% at 8 years.

• ~7% of patients make 2 or more attempts, 2.5% 3 or more, and 1% 5 or more.

Follow-up and management

• Low-risk patients do not need special care.

• High-risk patients and those with mental illness need close monitoring.

Factors associated with repetition

• Factors that indicate a greater risk of repetition include previous psychiatric treatment, alcohol problems, previous deliberate self-harm, sociopathic traits, living alone, and unchanged problems and circumstances.

• Chronic repeaters invariably have severe personality difficulties, chaotic lifestyles, deprived backgrounds, and great difficulty in engaging in any form of therapy.

Dealing with violent mentally disturbed patients

• Aggressive patients are often frightened.

• Keep calm and gentle in voice and actions.

• Do not corner, crowd, or threaten the patient.

• Give clear explanations of what is happening.

• Do not see or leave the patient alone.

• Call for adequate extra staff, porters, security staff, or police as necessary backup.

Key references

1. Blumenthal SJ: A guide to risk factors, assessment, and treatment of suicidal patients. *Med Clin North Am* 1988, **72**:937–969.
2. Hoffman DP, Dubovsky SL: Depression and suicide assessment. *Emerg Med Clin North Am* 1991, **9**:107–121.
3. Anonymous: Management of behavioural emergencies. *Drug Ther Bull* 1991, **29**:62–64.

Bacterial overgrowth of the small intestine

Diagnosis

Definition

• This disorder is also known as *bacterial contamination of the small intestine*.

• Normally, the microflora of the small intestine consists of a small number of aerobic, Gram-positive organisms derived from the upper gastrointestinal tract. In bacterial overgrowth, these are replaced by anaerobic, facultative Gram-negative organisms, especially *Escherichia coli* and *Bacteroides* and *Clostridium* spp. at $>10^5$ colony-forming units/mL on culture [1].

• *Blind loop syndrome* refers to bacterial overgrowth of a portion of the intestinal tract excluded surgically (*e.g.*, by a Billroth II procedure) or due to fistualizations (*e.g.*, Crohn's disease).

Symptoms

Diarrhea, abdominal pain, weight loss, nausea, and vomiting.

• Many patients are asymptomatic and suffer no adverse effects.

• Bacterial overgrowth of the proximal small intestine tends to produce more marked symptoms than overgrowth of the distal small bowel.

Signs

Steatorrhea: bulky, oily stools.

Anemia: megaloblastic, secondary to vitamin B_{12} deficiency.

Ataxia, neuropathy: due to vitamin B_{12} deficiency.

Pouchitis: in ileal reservoirs and ileo-anal anastomoses, with occult or obvious blood loss.

Investigations

Full blood count: macrocytic anemia present in those with long-standing cases.

Vitamin B_{12} measurement: concentration low or normal.

Serum or erythrocyte folate measurement: concentration high or normal; "inverted" profile (*i.e.*, elevated folate with low B_{12}), suggestive but nonspecific marker.

Schilling test with intrinsic factor: absorption not corrected; also found in terminal ileal disease.

Spot test with Sudan red: marker for neutral stool fat.

3-day fecal fat collection: useful but unpopular test to quantify steatorrhea.

Barium follow-through: for jejunal diverticulosis, strictures, and fistulas; delayed transit of barium through small intestine indirect evidence of impaired motility.

Duodenal aspiration: for culture and strain identification; gold standard; presence of detectable concentrations of unconjugated bile acids and short chain fatty acids can provide useful adjunct, although these tests are not widely available; false-negative results do not exclude bacterial overgrowth distal to ligament of Treitz.

Duodenal biopsy: to assess villous architecture and exclude parasitic infestation (*i.e.*, giardiasis, Whipple's disease, celiac sprue).

Breath tests: simple, noninvasive, and increasingly available; early rise of breath hydrogen after lactulose or glucose, ^{14}C D-xylose or ^{14}C glycocholic acid.

Complications

• In patients with long-standing symptoms, complications result in chronic malnutrition and debility.

Secondary weight loss: if food exacerbates abdominal pain.

Subacute combined degeneration of spinal cord: after profound vitamin B_{12} deficiency (rare).

Dehydration.

Differential diagnosis

Celiac disease.

Chronic pancreatitis.

Crohn's disease

Infections: *Yersinia* or *Campylobacter* spp. (bacterial); *Giardia lamblia* (protozoan); *Ascaris* or *Strongyloides* spp. (helminthic); AIDS enteropathy (viral).

Etiology

• Causes are often multifactorial and poorly understood; they include the following:

Structural abnormalities

Jejunal diverticulosis.

Blind loop.

Adhesions.

Motility disorders

Autonomic neuropathy, as in insulin-dependent diabetes mellitus.

Progressive systemic sclerosis.

Postoperative ileus.

Excessive bacterial load

Diminished gastric acid production.

Incompetent ileocecal valve.

Incompetent pyloric valve.

Ileocolic fistula (Crohn's).

Impaired immunity

Raised intraluminal pH [2].

Gastric surgery or vagotomy.

Drugs: proton pump inhibitors [3,4].

Hypochlorhydria and associated states: *e.g.*, autoimmune gastritis, pernicious anemia, primary immunodeficiencies (especially IgA), protein or energy deficiency.

Acquired: *e.g.*, intensive chemo- or radiation therapy, malignancy, HIV infection.

• Malnutrition can cause bacterial overgrowth by impairing mucosal immunity, diminishing gastric acid production, altering goblet cell mucus production, and reducing the bacteriostatic properties of pancreatic exocrine secretions.

Epidemiology

• Prevalence studies are difficult because of the lack of a suitable screening test.

• Children and elderly people are particularly susceptible.

Treatment

Diet and lifestyle

• A high-protein, high-energy, high-fat diet is recommended.

• Vitamin supplementation, especially injections of vitamin B_{12} and fat-soluble vitamins (A, E, D, K), or oral iron may be beneficial.

• Total parenteral nutrition is rarely necessary.

Pharmacological treatment

• Treatment is often empirical, the diagnosis being made by observing improvement in symptoms and biochemical abnormalities after treatment.

Antibiotics

Standard dosage
Trimethoprim, 160 mg/sulfamethoxazole, 800 mg twice daily.
Metronidazole, 500 mg 3 times daily.
Tetracycline, 250 mg 4 times daily.
Ciprofloxacin, 500 mg twice daily (1-week course usually adequate).
2-week course may be adequate, but maintenance with alternating courses of two agents may be needed.

Contraindications
Trimethoprim/sulfamethoxazole: sensitivity to sulfa.
Metronidazole: pregnancy, lactation.
Tetracycline: renal insufficiency, children <12 years, lactation.
Ciprofloxacin: children or adolescents, glucose 6-phosphate dehydrogenase deficiency, epilepsy, lactation.

Special points
Metronidazole: Antabuse (disulfiram-like) effect with alcohol.
Tetracycline: permanent tooth discoloration if used during dental development.
Ciprofloxacin: causes arthropathy in immature animals.

Main drug interactions
Trimethoprim/sulfamethoxazole: potentiates anticoagulant effect of warfarin, prolongs half-life of phenytoin and sulfonylureas.
Metronidazole: potentiates warfarin.
Tetracyclines: calcium, magnesium, iron, and aluminum salts (*e.g.*, milk, antacids) impair absorption.
Ciprofloxacin: magnesium, aluminium salts inhibit absorption; theophylline levels raised; anticoagulants potentiated.

Main side effects
Metronidazole: metallic taste (meteorism), furred tongue, peripheral neuropathy with prolonged use.
Tetracyclines: gastrointestinal disturbances, photosensitive rash, hypersensitivity (rare).
Ciprofloxacin: gastrointestinal symptoms, rashes, restlessness, dizziness, pruritis, tremor, convulsions.

Treatment aims

To clear and prevent recurrence of bacterial overgrowth.

To reduce diarrhea.

To correct hematological abnormalities and secondary nutritional deficiencies.

Other treatments

Surgery to correct underlying anatomical abnormality; may cause prolonged post-operative ileus.

Prognosis

• The prognosis depends on the underlying disease: motility disorders have the worst prognosis.

Follow-up and management

• Regular infrequent outpatient follow-up may be needed to monitor for symptoms and to detect relapses early.

• Long term maintenance antibiotic treatment is only rarely needed, and surgical treatment may be definitive.

Key references

1. Kirsch M: Bacterial overgrowth. *Am J Gastroenterol* 1990, **85**:231–237.
2. Cook GC: Hypochlorhydria and vulnerability to intestinal infection. *Eur J Gastroenterol Hepatol* 1994, **6**:693–695.
3. Fried M, *et al.*: Duodenal bacterial overgrowth during treatment in outpatients with omeprazole. *Gut* 1994, **35**:23–26.
4. Larner AJ, Hamilton MIR: Infective complications of therapeutic gastric inhibition. *Aliment Pharmacol Ther* 1994, **8**:579–584.

Diagnosis

Symptoms

Bronchiectasis and cystic fibrosis

Cough, purulent, large-volume sputum, episodic fever or malaise, night sweats, nasal discharge, possibly with purulent sinusitis, dyspnea, recurrent hemoptysis, pleuritic chest pain.

Cystic fibrosis: additional symptoms

Diarrhea or steatorrhea, abdominal pain, constipation: in adults.

Meconium ileus: 10% of childhood presentations.

Failure to thrive: in children.

Prolonged neonatal jaundice, rectal prolapse.

Signs

Bronchiectasis and cystic fibrosis

Clubbing, rhonchi, coarse crackles, tachypnea, hyperinflation, signs of weight loss.

Cystic fibrosis: additional signs

Greasy smelly feces, steatorrhea, abdominal distension, poor growth.

Investigations

Sputum culture: for *Staphylococcus aureus*, *Haemophilus influenzae*, and *Pseudomonas* spp. (especially *P. aeruginosa* and *P. cepacia*) and to exclude active tuberculosis.

Sputum cytology: to exclude malignancy.

Serum immunoglobulin measurement.

Chest radiography: shows hyperinflation, crowded lung markings, and ring shadows.

High-resolution CT: shows ring and cystic lesions and bronchial wall thickening.

Sinus radiography: shows mucosal thickening and fluid levels.

Respiratory function tests: for obstructive or mixed ventilatory defect.

Aspergillus skin and precipitin tests.

Sweat test: to diagnose cystic fibrosis; sweat chloride >60 mmol/L in 98% of patients.

Gene analysis.

Complications

Bronchiectasis and cystic fibrosis

Infective exacerbations: viral or bacterial.

Pneumothorax.

Respiratory failure.

Cor pulmonale.

Empyema.

Chest pain: usually pleuritic, associated with an area of bronchiectasis.

Hemoptysis.

Metastatic spread of infection: now rare; brain abscess was classic complication.

Arthropathy: rheumatoid arthritis and nonspecific seronegative arthritis related to activity of disease.

Cystic fibrosis: additional complications [1]

Diabetes mellitus, biliary cirrhosis, heat exhaustion, intussusception in children, cholelithiasis, azoospermia, volvulus in children, esophageal reflux, distal intestinal obstruction syndrome.

Differential diagnosis

Bronchiectasis

Asthma.
Interstitial fibrosis.
Chronic bronchitis.
Lung carcinoma.
Sinusitis with chronic cough.

Cystic fibrosis

Celiac disease.

Etiology

- Bronchiectasis results from failure of the airway protective mechanisms, including mucociliary clearance mechanisms, and the inflammatory response [2].
- Further damage may be due to the host response and the infecting microbes.
- Causes include the following:

Bronchiectasis [3]

Impaired clearance: defective mucociliary clearance, congenital, bronchial obstruction, immunodeficiency.

Inflammation: inflammatory pneumonitis, fibrotic or granulomatous lung disease, previous severe infection, allergic aspergillosis.

Cystic fibrosis [4]

Gene (chromosome 7) mutations that produce abnormal cystic fibrosis transmembrane conductance regulator, causing viscid secretions.

Epidemiology [5]

- The estimated prevalence of bronchiectasis is declining with the advent of modern antibiotics.
- Cystic fibrosis is the most common serious inherited disease.
- In the US cystic fibrosis occurs in 1 of 2500 births.
- 1 in 25 people carries the abnormal gene.

Associated diseases

Rheumatoid arthritis.
Purulent sinusitis.
Allergic bronchopulmonary aspergillosis.
Malignancy.
Connective tissue disorders.
Vasculitis.
Infertility.
Primary ciliary dyskinesia.
Immune deficiency syndromes.

Treatment

Diet and lifestyle

• Adequate nutrition is important.

• Patients with cystic fibrosis need pancreatic supplements with snacks and meals, high energy intake to maintain weight, overnight nasogastric feeding or feeding gastrostomy, and fat-soluble vitamin supplements.

Pharmacological treatment [3]

General guidelines

• Treatment specific to the underlying cause includes the following:

Removal of foreign body or inspissated mucus.

Replacement of immunoglobulins: for panhypogammaglobulinemia, selective IgM and IgG, and possibly IgG_2 deficiency, but not for selective IgA deficiency (risk of anaphylaxis).

Treatment of associated conditions, *e.g.*, rheumatoid arthritis.

For bronchiectasis

Antibiotics: drug choice based on sputum culture; given either for exacerbations or at regular intervals; courses should last 2-3 weeks, and antimicrobial agents should be given in high doses; for patients colonized with *Pseudomonas* spp., specific antipseudomonal antibiotics should be given, including nebulized antibiotics, *e.g.*, gentamycin, for maintenance treatment between courses.

Bronchodilators: for patients with demonstrable airflow obstruction.

Steroids: improved morbidity in short term, but effects on prognosis not known; inhaled steroids recommended for patients with prominent or reversible airflow obstruction.

For cystic fibrosis [6–9]

Mucolytics: nebulized DNAase is effective in many patients with viscid sputum.

Lactulose, oral acetylcysteine, and oral meglumine diatrizoate: for distal intestinal obstruction syndrome.

Nasogastric aspiration and intravenous fluids.

Nonpharmacological treatment

Physical therapy

• Physical therapy is the main form of nonpharmacological treatment.

• Methods include postural drainage, deep cough, and forced expiratory maneuvers twice daily.

Other options

For hemoptysis: bed rest and antibiotics, selective embolization, intubation and balloon tamponade, or local resection.

For pneumothorax: aspiration, intercostal drainage, pleurodesis or partial pleurectomy (if recurrent or unresponsive).

For respiratory failure: supplemental oxygen therapy, nasal ventilation.

For nasal polyps: polypectomy.

For severe localized disease: surgery.

Lung or heart-lung transplantation, especially in cystic fibrosis.

Treatment aims

To minimize lung damage by limiting pulmonary infection and increasing clearance of pulmonary secretion.

Prognosis

• The prognosis of bronchiectasis depends on the severity of the disease.

• The median survival with cystic fibrosis is approximately 27 years in the US.

Follow-up and management

• All patients with moderate to severe bronchiectasis need regular care from a respiratory physician.

• All patients with cystic fibrosis should attend a recognized cystic fibrosis center.

Patient support

Counselling regarding lung transplantation, fears of dying, reproduction, etc.

Key references

1. diSant'Agnese P, Davis P: Cystic fibrosis in adults: 75 cases and a review of 232 cases in the literature. *Am J Med* 1979, **66**:121–322.
2. Barker AF, Bardana EJ: Bronchiectasis: update of an orphan disease. *Am Rev Respir Dis* 1988, **137**:969–978.
3. Weg J: Bronchiectasis. *Semin Respir Med* 1992, **13**:177–189.
4. Koch C, Hoiby N: Pathogenesis of cystic fibrosis. *Lancet* 1993, **341**:1065–1069.
5. Orenstein DM: Cystic fibrosis. *Curr Probl Pediatr* 1993, **23**:4–15.
6. Davis PB: Evolution of therapy for cystic fibrosis. *N Engl J Med* 1994, **331**:672–673.
7. Fiel SB: Clinical management of pulmonary disease in cystic fibrosis. *Lancet* 1993, **341**:1070–1074.
8. Hodson ME: Aerosolized dornase alfa (rhDNase) for therapy of cystic fibrosis. *Am J Respir Crit Care Med* 1995, **151**:S70–S74.
9. Fiel SB: Clinical management of pulmonary disease in cystic fibrosis. *Lancet* 1993, **341**:1070–1074.

Diagnosis

Symptoms

Behavior disguised because of shame and guilt.

Preoccupation with diets: in a woman of normal weight.

Vomiting: with atypical symptoms.

Edema: in young women.

Fullness and bloating after meals.

Preoccupation with constipation.

Amenorrhea or irregular menstruation.

Low mood, anxiety, drug or alcohol abuse.

Sports injury.

Signs

Tooth enamel loss, caries, prostheses.

Enlarged salivary glands.

Mouth abrasions.

Callus on dorsum of hand: Russell's sign, due to gag reflex causing a bite.

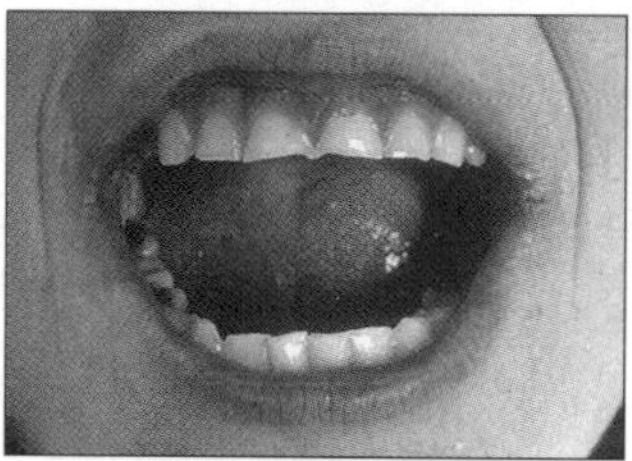

Loss of tooth substance in an 18-year-old girl who had vomited since the age of 15 years.

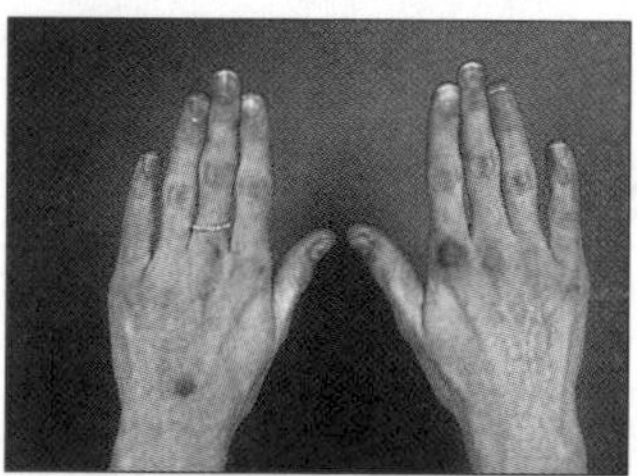

Callus on the back of the hand (Russell's sign).

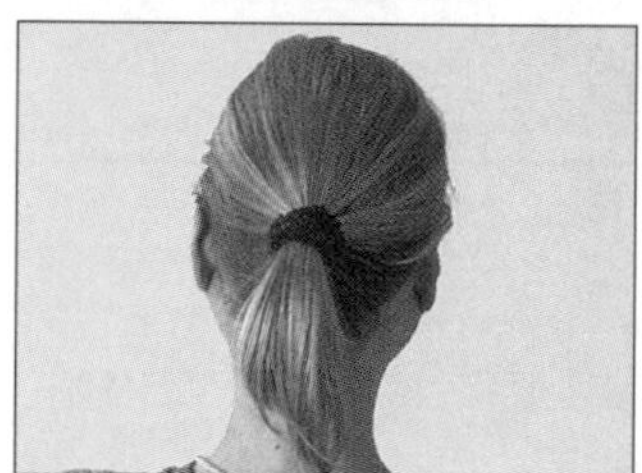

Salivary gland enlargement in a young woman vomiting twice each day.

Investigations

History: for psychological, nutritional, and weight-control measures.

Electrolytes: vomiting causes low potassium and high bicarbonate; laxatives cause low sodium, low potassium, and low bicarbonate; blood urea nitrogen increased with dehydration.

Complications

• Complications occur in <1% of sufferers.

Gastrointestinal bleeding.

Cardiac dysrhythmia.

Renal failure.

Differential diagnosis

• After the history has been obtained, it is characteristic.

Anorexia nervosa.

Depression.

Etiology [1]

• Causes include the following:

Dieting: risk increased 8-fold.

Psychosocial: poor parenting experiences, life events.

Genetic: family history of depression, obesity, and alcoholism.

Epidemiology [2]

• 3% of women between the ages of 15 and 25 years suffer from bulimia nervosa.

• The prevalence is increasing in generations born after 1950.

• The ratio of men to women is 1:10.

• Upper socioeconomic classes are disproportionately represented.

Treatment

Diet and lifestyle [3]

• Patients must be helped to eat a regular, well balanced diet; this is achieved by pharmacological and nonpharmacological treatment.

Pharmacological treatment [3–5]

• Drugs are less effective than psychological therapy but can produce a window of remission during which psychological therapy can begin.

Standard dosage	Fluoxetine, 60 mg.
Contraindications	Hypersensitivity, renal failure, lactation, unstable epilepsy; caution in liver failure, renal impairment, cardiac disease, diabetes, pregnancy.
Special points	Produces 20% abstinence rates.
Main drug interactions	Monoamine oxidase inhibitors, tryptophan, tricyclic antidepressants, lithium, flecainide, encainide, vinblastine, carbamazepine.
Main side effects	Asthenia, fever, neurological effects (including headache), pharyngitis, dyspnea, rash, nausea (paradoxically).

Nonpharmacological treatment [3,5]

• Psychological approaches are the treatment of choice because they are more effective in the short term, probably also in the long term, but 9–19 hourly sessions of specialist therapy may be needed. Self-treatment manuals are available.

• The effective components include the following:

Educational: nutritional, weight control.

Behavioral: food and purging diary, prescription of regular meals, stimulus control to limit meal size, distraction or relaxation to interrupt symptomatic behaviour.

Cognitive: modification of distorted beliefs about shape and weight, strengthening of coping resources, stress management, problem solving, communication and assertiveness skills.

• Abstinence rates of 50%–60% are achieved.

Treatment aims

To restore normal eating patterns.

To provide psychological support and treatment.

Prognosis

• 50%–60% of patients are asymptomatic after treatment.

• Relapse is common in the first year after treatment.

• 70% are asymptomatic after 2 years.

• Self-harm is common in the 30% of patients with borderline personality disorders (i.e. ~30% of these or ~10%–20% of all patients).

Follow-up and management

• 6-monthly follow-up is needed.

Key references

1. Johnson C, Connors ME, eds: *The Etiology and Treatment of Bulimia Nervosa: A Biopsychosocial Perspective*. New York: Basic Books; 1987.
2. Halmi K, ed: *Psychobiology and Treatment of Anorexia Nervosa and Bulimia Nervosa*. Washington DC: American Psychiatric Association Press; 1992.
3. American Psychiatric Association: Practice guidelines for eating disorders. *Am J Psychiatry* 1993, **150**:212–228.
4. Hoffman L, Halmi K: Psychopharmacology in the treatment of anorexia nervosa and bulimia nervosa. *Psychiatr Clin North Am* 1993, **16**:767–778.
5. Mitchell JE, Raymond N, Specker S: A review of the controlled trials of pharmacotherapy and psychotherapy in the treatment of bulimia nervosa. *Int J Eat Disord* 1993, **14**:229–247.

Diagnosis

Symptoms

Pemphigus vulgaris
Painful oral ulcers.
Erosions of mucous membranes.
Weeping, uncomfortable skin erosions.

Bullous pemphigoid
Large, tense blisters on the skin: gradually expanding and uncomfortable.
Oral symptoms: occur rarely.

Dermatitis herpetiformis
Intense, severe, pruritis: seemingly out of proportion to the sparse clinical signs.

Signs [1,2]

Pemphigus vulgaris
Oral ulcerations and gingivitis: often sole manifestation of disease and precede skin involvement.
Flaccid blisters: rupture easily.

Bullous pemphigoid
Large, tense blisters: often on urticarial or erythematous bases in elderly patients.
Oral involvement: only in one third of patients.

Dermatitis herpetiformis
Groups of papules and vesicles: on an erythematous base; often excoriated with a predilection for the extensor surfaces of the extremities and buttocks.

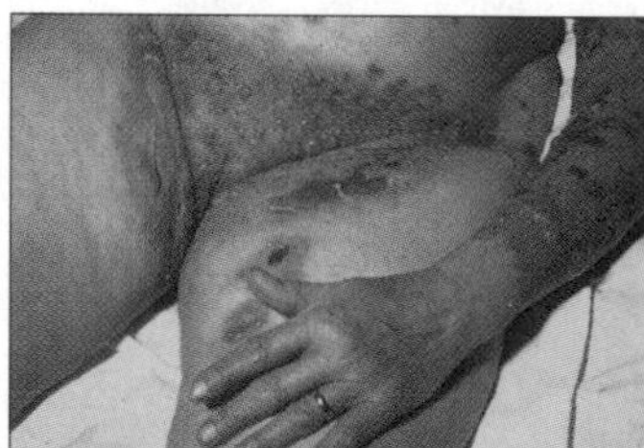

Bullous pemphigoid.

Investigations

Pemphigus vulgaris
Biopsy: of perilesional skin to detect directed acantholysis (intraepidermal blister).
Direct immunofluorescence: to detect IgG and C3 directed at keratinocyte cell membranes (intraepidermal band).

Bullous pemphigoid
Biopsy: of perilesional skin to detect subepidermal split; many eosinophils.
Direct immunofluorescence: IgG and C3 directed at the dermoepidermal junction (linear band at base of epidermis).

Dermatitis herpetiformis
Biopsy: of perilesional skin to detect papillary dermal neutrophilic abscesses (subepidermal).
Direct immunofluorescence: to detect granular deposits of IgA and C3 in the dermal papillary tips.

Complications

Pemphigus vulgaris
Secondary bacterial infection: in denuded areas.
Fluid and electrolyte imbalance: in severe cases.
Sepsis: in severe cases (especially immunosuppressed patients).

Bullous pemphigoid
Underlying occult malignancy: controversial association.

Dermatitis herpetiformis
Gluten sensitive enteropathy: in approximately 90% of cases.
Lymphoma: possible increased incidence, especially in jejunum.

Differential diagnosis
Infections: *e.g.*, varicella zoster, herpes simplex, zosteriform herpes simplex, bullous impetigo.
Bullous bite reaction (insect bites).
Drug-induced pemphigus: *e.g.*, d-penicillamine.
Epidermolysis bullosa.
Porphyria cutanea tarda.
Pseudo–porphyria cutanea tarda.
Sweat gland necrosis.
Diabetic bullosis.
Bullous cellulitis.
Pompholyx.
Cicatricial pemphigoid.
Urticaria pigmentosa.
Bullous fixed drug reaction.

Etiology [3–5]

Pemphigus vulgaris
Molecular immunopathogenesis: autoantibody against transmembrane cadherin family of intercellular adhesion molecules (desmoglein desmosomal component).

Bullous pemphigoid
Molecular immunopathogenesis: autoantibody against proteins on the basilar keratinocyte that anchor keratin intermediate filaments to the basement membrane by a hemidesmosone (bullous pemphigoid antigen 1, a 230-kD intracellular protein, and bullous pemphigoid antigen 2, a 180-kD transmembrane protein).

Dermatitis herpetiformis
Molecular immunopathogenesis plus HLA-B8 and DW3-associated autoimmune disorder; also associated with gluten-sensitive enteropathy.

Epidemiology

Pemphigus vulgaris
More common in patients with Jewish or Mediterranean heritage; much rarer than bullous pemphigoid.

Bullous pemphigoid
Most common in patients 60–70 years of age (less common variant can occur in children).
- 75% of treated patients have remission after approximately 5 years.

Dermatitis herpetiformis
Onset between 2–4 decades of life.
Annual incidence of 1:100,000 in Scandinavian patients.
Usually chronic when untreated.

Treatment

Diet and lifestyle

• Dietary measures applicable only in dermatitis herpetiformis, in which a gluten-free diet may be curative.

• Wound care of open erosions is essential to prevent secondary infection in all bullous diseases.

Pharmacological treatment

• Treatment should be administered by a specialist with experience in treating bullous disorders.

• Topical steroids are the mainstay of therapy for pemphigus vulgaris.

Systemic steroids (the dosage may vary depending on severity of disease, clinical response, and concomitant use of other agents).

Standard dosage
Prednisone, 80–160 mg orally, daily initially to control; then 40–60 mg daily; then, taper as tolerated to a maintenance dose of 5–10 mg daily.
Cyclophosphamide, 100–200 mg orally daily.
Azathioprine, 100–200 mg orally daily.
Gold sodium thiomalate, 10 mg i.m. initial test dose; followed by 25 mg at weeks 2 and 3; then 25–50 mg i.m. every week.
Dapsone, 100 mg orally, daily; may have to increase dose up to 400 mg daily; can often lower the dose in patients on gluten-free diet [6,7].

Contraindications
Prednisone: gastric ulcers, underlying infections, hypertension, diabetes, history of tuberculosis.
Cyclophosphamide, azathioprine: pregnancy.
Gold: pregnancy.
Dapsone: pregnancy.

Special points
Only those physicians with experience and training to monitor these diseases and the drugs used to treat them should follow-up these patients.

Main drug interactions
Azathioprine: allopurinol enhances effect and increases toxicity.

Main side effects
Prednisone: weight gain, hypertension, diabetes, fragile skin, decreased wound healing, adrenal suppression.
Cyclophosphamide, azathioprine: bone marrow suppression, hemorrhagic cystitis, potential for malignancy.
Dapsone: gastrointestinal upset (common), hemolytic anemia in patients with glucose-6-phosphate dehydrogenase deficiency, agranulocytosis, methemoglobinemia; peripheral neuropathy.

Other treatments

Plasmapheresis.

Extracorporeal immunoabsorption of autoantibodies.

Treatment aims

To relieve pain and heal wounds.
To prevent secondary infection.
To suppress disease activity with lowest possible dose of drug.

Prognosis

Pemphigus vulgaris
Mortality rate less than 10% today.
•Patients do very well with close control and monitoring of this chronic disease.

Bullous pemphigoid
Usually self-limited, with remission in 75% of patients in 3–6 years.
Mortality rate of 10%–20% related to systemic steroid treatment.

Dermatitis herpetiformis
Chronic course when untreated, with temporary remission.
Appears to be a risk of bowel lymphoma.
•Response to dapsone is dramatic; pruritis and skin lesions resolve within the first week of therapy.

Follow-up and management

Long-term follow-up by a specialist is advised.

Key references

1. Crosby DL, Diaz LA: Introduction. *Dermatol Clin* 1993, **2**:373–378.
2. Guidice GJ, Diaz LA: New laboratory methods in the investigation of bullous diseases. *Dermatol Clin* 1993,**2**:419–427.
3. Giudice GJ, *et al.*: Development of an ELISA to detect anti-BP180 autoantibodies in bullous pemphigoid and herpes gestationis. *J Invest Dermatol* 1994, **102**:878–881.
4. Klatte DH, Jones JC: Purification of the 230kD bullous pemphigoid antigen (BP230) from bovine tongue mucosa: structural analyses and assessment of BP230 tissue distribution using a monoclonal antibody. *J Invest Dermatol* 1994, **102**:39–44.
5. Beutner EH, Jordon RE: Demonstration of skin antibodies in sera of pemphigus vulgaris patients by indirect immunofluorescent staining. *Proc Soc Exp Biol Med* 1964, **117**:505–510.
6. Zuidema J, *et al.*: Clinical pharmacokinetics of dapsone. *Clin Pharmacokinet* 1986, **11**:299–315.
7. Stern RS: Systemic dapsone. *Arch Dermatol* 1993, **129**:301–303.

Diagnosis

Symptoms

• 30% of patients are asymptomatic.

Altered taste sensation.

Oral discomfort or pain.

Coated mouth or tongue.

Dysphagia.

Odynophagia.

Loss of appetite.

Signs

Angular cheilitis.

Intraoral removable white plaques, with erythematous underlying mucosa.

Intraoral mucosal ulceration or erythema.

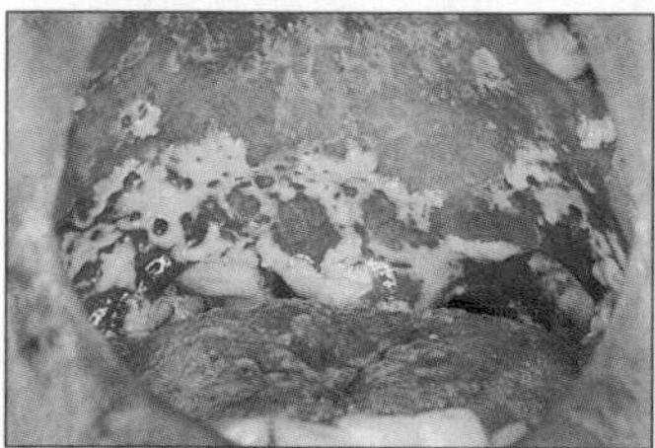

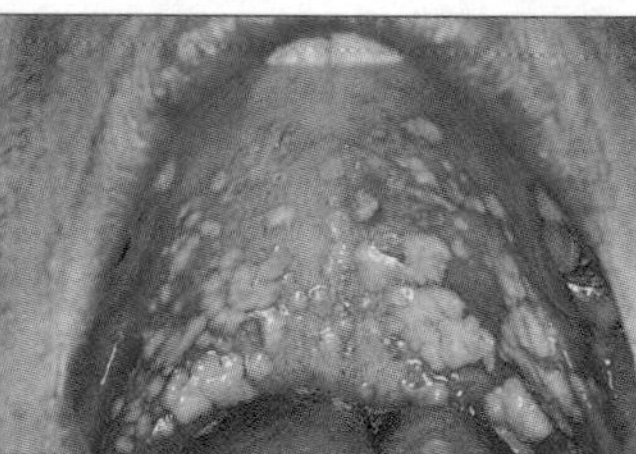

Curdish white plaques of pseudomembranous candidiasis.

Investigations

Buccal candidiasis

• The diagnosis is usually obvious without further investigation.

Direct microscopy: direct staining of mouth scraping with hydrogen peroxide or Gram stain rapidly confirms presence of fungal hyphae.

Mouth swab or washings: to determine sensitivity of *Candida* spp.

Esophageal candidiasis

Fiberoptic endoscopy: allows direct visualization of esophageal involvement, with biopsy confirming diagnosis; should be considered gold standard.

Barium-swallow radiography: can highlight linear filling defects.

Complications

Oral ulceration.

Weight loss: secondary to depressed appetite.

Esophageal obstruction: rarely, secondary to overgrowth of *Candida* spp. (systemic dissemination unusual).

Differential diagnosis

Oral hairy leukoplakia.

HIV-related gingivitis, peridontitis, herpes simplex, or giant aphthous ulcers.

Cytomegalovirus ulceration, Kaposi's sarcoma, or lymphoma.

Etiology

• Candidiasis is the overgrowth and invasion of mucosal surfaces by *Candida albicans* or occasionally other *Candida* spp. The emergence of clinical disease is related to the loss of cell-mediated immunity and not to the presence of more virulent *Candida* strains.

• In HIV infection, buccal candidiasis is often seen when the number of circulating CD4 lymphocytes is $<350 \times 10^6$/L, and esophageal candidiasis is seen when CD4 cells are $<250 \times 10^6$/L.

Epidemiology

• *Candida albicans* is a normal commensal of the mouth and can be cultured from 30% of the population.

• Although both buccal and esophageal candidiasis have been described during acute primary infection with HIV, they are generally associated with moderate to severe immunodeficiency 4–10 years after initial infection.

• 90% of HIV-infected patients develop candidiasis at some stage of their illness.

• Esophageal, bronchopulmonary, or invasive candidiasis is classified as an AIDS-defining opportunistic infection.

Treatment

Diet and lifestyle

No special precautions are necessary.

Pharmacological treatment

Topical antifungals

• Nystatin and clotrimazole are of benefit in cases of buccal candidiasis; however, they do not treat any esophageal involvement.

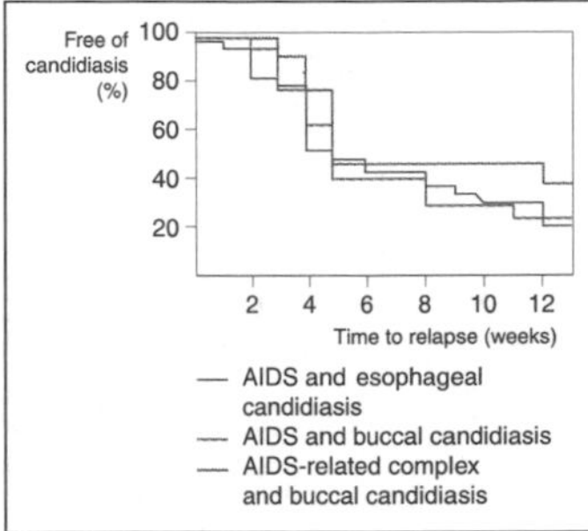

Patients free of relapse after clinical and mycological clearance.

Fluconazole

• Fluconazole is effective for oral and esophageal candidiasis. Improvement results in 3–5 days. It is predominantly renally excreted so the patient does not suffer from hepatic metabolism problems.

Standard dosage Fluconazole, 100–400 mg daily for 1–3 weeks.

Contraindications Azole hypersensitivity.

Special points Reduced dose in patients with renal impairment.

Main drug interactions Pentamidine, amphotericin-induced nephrotoxicity may impair renal excretion.

Main side effects Abnormalities in liver function (higher doses), rashes.

Itraconazole

• Itraconazole is used in patients who cannot tolerate fluconazole (70% response rates at 1 week and 90% at 1 month) but less hepatotoxic than ketoconazole.

Standard dosage Itraconazole, 200 mg daily for 1–4 weeks.

Contraindications Azole hypersensitivity.

Special points An oral suspension is available in some countries on a compassionate basis, with better absorption features.

Main drug interactions Decreased absorption with antacids, cimetidine, or omeprazole; increased metabolism with rifampicin, rifabutin, or phenytoin.

Main side effects Rash, nausea.

Treatment aims

To suppress *Candida albicans* overgrowth.

Prognosis

• 59% of patients with pseudomembranous candidiasis develop an AIDS diagnosis within 3 months.

• ~80% of patients with acute *Pneumocystis carinii* pneumonia also have oral candidiasis.

• 80% of patients with a successfully treated episode of oral or esophageal candidiasis relapse within 3 months.

Follow-up and management

• Patients often relapse after treatment, so detecting relapses early is important; they are often mild and easily treated over time.

• As immunodeficiency worsens, episodes become more frequent and less responsive to treatment; occasionally, continuous suppressive doses of an azole or courses of intravenous amphotericin are needed.

Causes of treatment failure

Poor drug absorption.

Increased metabolism or excretion from other drugs.

Candida albicans developing drug resistance.

Nonalbicans species or dual infection.

Immunodeficiency too severe for drug treatment alone to work.

General references

1. Klein RS, *et al.*: Oral candidiasis in high risk patients as the initial manifestation of the acquired immunodeficiency syndrome. *N Engl J Med* 1984, **311**:354-358.
2. Laine L, *et al.*: Fluconazole compared with ketoconazole for the treatment of *Candida* esophagitis in AIDS. A randomized trial. *Ann Intern Med* 1992, **117**:655–660.
3. Miyasaki SH, *et al.*: The identification and tracking of *Candida albicans* isolates from oral lesions in HIV-seropositive individuals. *J Acquir Immun Defic Syndr* 1992, **5**:1039–1046.
4. Smith DE, *et al.*: Itraconazole versus ketoconazole in the treatment of oral and oesophageal candidosis in patients infected with HIV. *AIDS* 1991, **5**:1367–1371.

Diagnosis

Symptoms

• Dilated cardiomyopathy starts as asymptomatic left ventricular dysfunction.

• Cardiac failure is defined as symptomatic left ventricular dysfunction.

Exertional fatigue, dyspnea, ankle edema: major symptoms.

Nocturia, urinary frequency, chest discomfort: less common symptoms.

Signs

Cardiac failure

• Cardiac failure can be free of objective signs.

Edema, raised jugular venous pressure, lung crepitations: signs of fluid retention.

Cold clammy skin, low blood pressure: signs of impaired perfusion.

Displaced left ventricular apex, right ventricular heave, third or fourth heart sound, functional mitral or tricuspid regurgitation, tachycardia: signs of ventricular dysfunction.

Underlying disorder

Valvular disease.

Atherosclerotic vascular disease.

Severe hypertension.

Severe anemia or volume overload: *e.g.*, arteriovenous shunt.

Pathological arrhythmia.

Evidence of generalized myopathy or poisoning.

Investigations

Chest radiography, echocardiography, cardiopulmonary exercise testing: to confirm diagnosis.

ECG: to look for underlying cause, *e.g.*, ischemia or infarction, left ventricular hypertrophy, arrhythmia, other causes of pathological Q-waves.

Echocardiography: to look for valvular disease; differentiates globally impaired left ventricle (*e.g.*, dilated cardiomyopathy) from segmental dysfunction (*e.g.*, ischemic heart disease).

Blood tests: for rare causes, *e.g.*, hypocalcemic cardiomyopathy, thyroid heart disease, iron-storage diseases, anemia, heavy metal poisons, amyloid (serum electrophoresis, rectal biopsy), sarcoid (serum angiotensin-converting enzyme, Kveim test).

Coronary angiography: occasionally, to identify ischemic heart failure.

Ventricular biopsy: rarely, for specific myocarditis, especially viral.

Radionuclide ventriculography or echocardiography: for ejection fraction, to quantitate severity of systolic dysfunction.

24-h Holter ECG monitoring: for ventricular arrhythmias.

Blood tests: for associated disease; renal, liver, and electrolyte disturbances common.

Complications

Atrial and ventricular brady- and tachyarrhythmias: especially atrial fibrillation and ventricular tachycardia.

Peripheral emboli, postural hypotension.

Renal failure.

Hepatic congestion and dysfunction.

Poor gastrointestinal absorption.

Muscle wasting, tissue abnormalities, oxidative enzyme depletion, early fatigue.

Pulmonary congestion, nonasthmatic bronchial constriction, respiratory muscle weakness.

Pulmonary hypertension and right ventricular failure: rare.

Differential diagnosis

Chronic lung disease.

Psychogenic dyspnea.

Etiology

• Causes include the following:

Ischemic heart disease: in 40–70% of patients.

Hypertension: in 10–30%.

Idiopathic, alcoholic, puerperal, or familial dilated cardiomyopathy: in 10–20%.

Valvular heart disease: in 5–10%.

Post-viral myocarditis: possibly in 1–10% (but presumed cause for many idiopathic).

HIV-related.

Epidemiology

• 1% of the general adult population suffers from cardiac failure or dilated cardiomyopathy.

• The incidence increases with age (>10% in people aged 80 years or more).

Treatment

Diet and lifestyle

• Patients should be encouraged to restrict sodium and alcohol intake and to maintain ideal weight. Advanced disease may require fluid restriction.

• Patients with stable moderate cardiac failure should undertake exercise training; patients with unstable cardiac failure or intercurrent illness should rest.

Pharmacological treatment

Diuretics

• Patients with fluid retention should be given thiazides for mild disease, loop diuretics for moderate disease, or combinations of loop, thiazide, and potassium-sparing agents for severe cardiac failure; metolazone is particularly effective with loop diuretics.

Standard dosage Depends on degree of fluid retention.

Contraindications Renal failure, hypokalemia (both relative).

Main drug interactions Low potassium with digoxin.

Main side effects Hypokalemia, renal impairment.

Angiotensin-converting enzyme inhibitors

• These are used for symptomatic heart failure without contraindications and asymptomatic left ventricular dysfunction in some patients (*e.g.*, after myocardial infarction).

Standard dosage Higher doses, *e.g.*, captopril 25 to 50 mg 3 times daily, or enalapril, 10 mg twice daily.

Contraindications Worsening renal function, allergy, severe cough.

Main drug interactions Hyperkalemia with potassium-sparing agents.

Main side effects Cough, renal failure.

Digoxin

• Digoxin is used to control ventricular response rate in atrial fibrillation; its role in sinus rhythm is controversial.

Standard dosage Digoxin, 0.0625–0.25 mg daily.

Contraindications Renal failure.

Special points Serum concentrations must be monitored.

Main drug interactions Diuretic-induced low potassium.

Main side effects Arrhythmias, nausea, visual disturbances.

Beta blockers and partial beta agonists

• These are indicated only for selected patients in specialist units.

Standard dosage Slow-dose increments.

Contraindications Worsening cardiac failure, heart block, asthma.

Main drug interactions Other bradycardic agents (digoxin, some calcium antagonists).

Main side effects Worsening cardiac failure, heart block.

Sympathomimetics and phosphodiesterase inhibitors

• Such agents are indicated only for acute short-term support, not for chronic oral administration.

• No beneficial effect has been found in ambulatory patients.

• They interact with monoamine oxidase inhibitors.

• They can cause ventricular arrhythmias.

Antiarrhythmics

• With the exception of digoxin, antiarrythmics are advisable only in symptomatic life-threatening arrhythmias. Amiodarone is probably the best choice (implantable defibrillators are an expensive alternative).

Standard dosage Amiodarone, 100–200 mg daily.

Contraindications Severe heart failure, heart block.

Main drug interactions Digoxin, warfarin doses must be reduced.

Main side effects Proarrhythmic effects, worsening heart failure, liver and lung toxicity, thyroid dysfunction.

Treatment aims

To alleviate symptoms.

To delay disease progression.

To reduce mortality.

Other treatments

Coronary bypass grafting: in selected patients with severe coronary disease.

Heart transplantation: for younger patients with severe left ventricular disease; organ supply remains inadequate for demand.

Myoplasty.

Prognosis

• Adverse prognostic features include the following:

Old age.
Low ejection fraction.
Poor exercise tolerance.
Ischemic origin.
Ventricular arrhythmias.
Reduced heart rate variability.
High plasma noradrenaline concentration.
Low serum sodium concentration.

• The annual mortality is 50% in patients with severe heart failure and 10%–20% in patients with mild to moderate heart failure.

Follow-up and management

• Life-long regular review is needed.

Key references

1. Cohn JN *et al.*: A comparison of enalapril with hydralazine-isosorbide dinitrate in the treatment of chronic congestive heart failure. *N Engl J Med* 1991, **325**:303–310.
2. CONSENSUS Trial Study Group: Effects of enalapril on mortality in severe congestive heart failure: results of the Co-operative North Scandinavian Enalapril Survival Study. *N Engl J Med* 1987, **316**:1429–1435.
3. Pfeffer MA *et al.*: Effect of captopril on mortality and morbidity in patients with left ventricular dysfunction after myocardial infarction. Results of the Survival and Ventricular Enlargement trial. *N Engl J Med* 1992, **327**:669–677.
4. SOLVD Investigators: Effect of enalapril on survival in patients with reduced left ventricular ejection fractions and congestive heart failure. *N Engl J Med* 1991, **325**:293–302.
5. Kasper EK, *et al.*: The causes of dilated cardiomyopathy: a clinicopathologic review of 673 cases. *J Am Coll Cardiol* 1994, **23**:568–590.

Basic life support

Definition

• The term "basic life support" refers to maintaining an airway and supporting breathing and the circulation without equipment [1].

• This is a practical skill, and training must be sought.

• Health-care professionals should also have more complex skills, including the use of airway adjuncts, *e.g.*, Guedel airway plus face-mask (with or without a non-return valve) or bag-mask ventilation and two-rescuer resuscitation.

Safety for the rescuer

• No evidence is available for the transmission of HIV or hepatitis B virus during mouth-to-mouth ventilation.

• Up to 70% of cardiac arrests occur in the home and involve people who are known to the rescuer.

• In the hospital, if patients are suspected or known to have an infection, mouth-to-mouth ventilation should not be attempted; airway adjuncts should be available for use.

Assessment [1]

Approach

• Safety for the rescuer and the patient must be assessed.

Responsiveness

• The rescuer should gently shake the patient's shoulders and ask loudly "Are you all right?"

• If the patient is unresponsive, the rescuer should call for help.

• The airway is opened by the combined maneuver of head tilt and chin lift; in most cases, this alone lifts the tongue from the back of the throat.

• If neck injury is likely, a chin lift or jaw thrust must be performed without moving the head or neck to open the airway.

• Any obvious obstruction should be removed from the mouth.

• Well fitting dentures should be left in place because these help to maintain a mouth seal during ventilation.

Breathing

• After opening the airway, the rescuer should look for chest movements, listen for breath sounds at the mouth, and feel for exhaled air with the cheek.

• These must be done for 5s before deciding that breathing is absent.

Pulse

• The best pulse to feel in any emergency is the carotid.

• This should be palpated for 5s to ensure that circulation is absent.

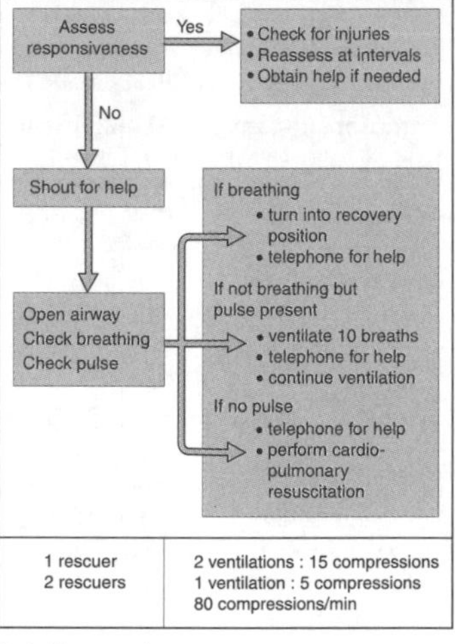

Basic life support.

Action

For respiratory arrest

• If the patient is not breathing but a pulse is present, 10 breaths/min expired-air ventilation must be given.

• The pulse must be checked again after every 10 breaths, and full cardiopulmonary resuscitation instituted if the pulse disappears.

For cardiorespiratory arrest

• If the patient is unconscious, not breathing, and the pulse is absent, ventilation and initiation of chest compression are needed at a rate of 2 breaths: 15 compressions, with 80 compressions/min (single rescuer).

• Chances are remote that effective spontaneous cardiac action will be restored without other techniques of advanced life support (including defibrillation), so time should not be wasted by further checks for the presence of a pulse [2].

• If, however, the patient makes a movement or takes a spontaneous breath, the carotid pulse should be checked to establish whether the heart is beating, taking no more than 5s, and breathing should be checked.

• Otherwise, resuscitation must not be interrupted [3].

Advanced life support

Defibrillation

• Electrical defibrillation is the only effective method of terminating ventricular fibrillation, a lethal rhythm disturbance, and of restoring a perfusing cardiac rhythm.

• The success of electrical defibrillation depends on time and the metabolic state of the myocardium.

• The delay in the administration of defibrillating shocks should be minimal.

• If the first three shocks, at 200J, 200J, and 360J, can be delivered quickly (within 30–45s), the sequence should not be interrupted by basic life support.

• If the time to charge a manual defibrillator or to confirm that the rhythm is still ventricular fibrillation is likely to be unduly prolonged, one or two sequences of basic life support should be administered between shocks.

• The prospects of success decrease relatively rapidly over a few minutes after cardiac arrest.

• Basic life support is unlikely to improve the odds of successful defibrillation; its value is in maintaining some cerebral perfusion and in slowing myocardial deterioration.

• After repeating the loops 3 times, different paddle position, a different defibrillator, and other antiarrythmic drugs (*e.g.*, amiodarone, lidocaine, bretylium tosylate) are still worth considering for refractory ventricular fibrillation.

• The position of the defibrillation paddles influences current flow through the myocardium; one electrode should be placed below the second intercostal space midclavicular line on the right and the other just outside the usual position of the cardiac apex (V_4-V_5).

Precordial thump

• The precordial thump is recommended for patients in ventricular fibrillation, pulseless ventricular tachycardia, or asystole.

• The application of a precordial thump takes only 2–3s and should not cause a significant delay in the application of electric defibrillation; it should be used only when advanced life support is available.

Pharmacological treatment

Indications

For ventricular fibrillation and pulseless ventricular tachycardia: epinephrine.

For asystole: adrenaline, atropine.

For electromechanical dissociation: treatment of cause (*e.g.*, hypovolemia, tension pneumothorax, cardiac tamponade, pulmonary embolism, drug overdose or intoxication, hypothermia, electrolyte imbalance); consideration of routine pressor agents, calcium chloride, alkalizing agents, or high-dose adrenaline (one or more of these may be of value in some circumstances).

For prolonged resuscitation or according to blood gas analysis: sodium bicarbonate.

Specific drugs

Adrenaline, 1 mg i.v. (10 ml 1 : 10 000 solution); should be followed by 10 sequences of 5 compressions : 1 ventilation; high-dose epinephrine (5 mg) should be considered in asystole and electromechanical dissociation, although value unproven if no response after 3 cycles.

Atropine, 3mg.

Sodium bicarbonate, 50mmol (50ml 8.4% solution).

Calcium chloride, 1g (10ml 10% solution).

• A large peripheral or central vein should be the standard route, with rapid infusion.

• The endotracheal route should be used only if an i.v. line cannot be established, in which case, double or triple doses of adrenaline or atropine should be given through an endotracheal tube.

Treatment aims

To resuscitate the patient.

To enhance basic life support (adrenaline).

Prognosis

• Survival from cardiac arrest is greatest when the event is witnessed, when a bystander starts resuscitation, when the heart arrests in ventricular fibrillation, or when defibrillation is carried out at an early stage [4].

Follow-up and management

• After resuscitation, patients should be observed, monitored, and treated in an intensive care unit.

• Patients must be checked by assessment of responsiveness, airway, breathing, circulation, and blood pressure; arterial blood gas and electrolyte measurements should be taken; chest radiography is advised.

Training

• Doctors need regular formal practical training in resuscitation.

• Advanced life support courses are available through local American Heart Association affiliates and most large emergency departments.

Key references

1. Emergency Cardiac Care Committee and Subcommittees, American Heart Association: Guidelines for cardiopulmonary resuscitation and emergency cardiac care. *JAMA* 1992, **268**:2172–2298.
2. O'Nunain S, Ruskin J: Cardiac arrest. *Lancet* 1993, **341**:1631–1647.
3. Cohen TJ: A comparison of active compression-decompression CPR with standard CPR for cardiac arrests in the hospital. *N Engl J Med* 1993, **329**:1918–1921.
4. Lombardi G: Outcome of out of hospital cardiac arrest in New York City. *JAMA* 1994, **271**:678–683.

Diagnosis

Symptoms

• Only 50% of patients present with the classic symptoms of diarrhea associated with malabsorption. Many are detected because of anemia (especially iron or folate deficiency) [1].

Symptoms of steatorrhea: foul-smelling stools, difficult to flush away.

Weight loss: common.

Failure to thrive, vomiting, or diarrhea: in infants.

Short stature, lassitude, irritability: in children.

Diarrhea, malabsorption, lassitude, infertility, constipation: in adults.

Signs

Short stature, fine skin, clubbing, evidence of weight loss [2].

Pallor: anemia due to iron or folic acid deficiency.

Calcium deficiency: with possible tetany.

Investigations

Initial

Full blood count, serum iron, ferritin, or folate, and erythrocyte folate measurement: to identify microcytic (iron deficiency) or macrocytic (folic acid deficiency) anemia or a dimorphic pattern of anemia due to both.

Vitamin B_{12} measurement: concentration frequently low but rarely abnormal.

Serum calcium and magnesium measurement: concentration possibly depressed.

Specific

Circulating antibody (antigliadin, antiendomysial) measurement: concentrations always raised; may be used as a screening test, particularly in children.

Fecal fat estimation: 3-day fecal fat excretion >7 g/day in patients ingesting at least 100 g fat daily (infrequently used).

Upper gastrointestinal endoscopy with biopsy of duodenum or proximal jejunum: reveals short (or absent) villi, intraepithelial lymphocytes, and crypt hyperplasia; for unequivocal diagnosis, at least six biopsy specimens should be obtained; celiac disease confirmed when biopsies return to normal on a gluten-free diet.

Contrast radiography: small bowel follow-through to assess small intestine; poor sensitivity, luminal dilation, and altered mucosal folds often observed.

Complications

Anemia: due to iron or folic acid deficiency.

Osteomalacia, osteoporosis: due to hypocalcemia (tetany and seizures due to exacerbation by magnesium deficiency).

Ulcerative jejunitis: rare, possibly early manifestation of malignancy.

Small-intestinal lymphoma: T-cell lymphoma complicating 5%–10% of cases; may be manifest as unexplained small intestinal perforation.

Wernicke's encephalopathy or Korsakoff's psychosis: due to acute or prolonged vitamin B_1 (thiamine) deficiency.

Differential diagnosis

Diarrhea

Irritable bowel syndrome.

Giardiasis.

Inflammatory bowel disease.

Laxative abuse.

Chronic pancreatitis.

Tropical sprue.

Zollinger–Ellison syndrome.

Failure to thrive

Cow's milk allergy.

Cystic fibrosis.

Postinfective mucosal damage.

Shwachman syndrome (inherited pancreatic insufficiency).

Nutritional deficiencies

Inadequate dietary intake.

Small-bowel bacterial overgrowth syndrome.

Etiology

• In northern Europeans, 98% of cases of celiac disease are associated with the extended haplotype HLA B8, DR3, DQ2, although, in southern Europeans, HLA DR5/7, DQ2 accounts for one-third of cases.

• 10%–20% of first-degree relatives of probands are similarly affected.

• Family history often reveals a Celtic ancestry [3].

Epidemiology

• Accurate data relating to the incidence and prevalence of celiac sprue in the US are lacking.

• The prevalence of celiac disease in the UK is particularly high (1 in 1200 people, rising to 1 in 300 around Galway Bay in Ireland).

• Slightly more women than men suffer from celiac disease; an association with anemia due to menstruation and pregnancy is possible.

• The incidence of presentation has three peaks:

infancy (9–36 months), on introduction of foods containing gluten;

third decade, frequently manifest as severe anemia of pregnancy;

fifth decade, normally manifest with a specific nutritional deficiency *e.g.*, iron, folic acid, or calcium.

Treatment

Diet and lifestyle

• A gluten-free diet is the mainstay of treatment and involves avoiding products containing wheat, rye, barley, or oats. Care should be taken to avoid any food contaminated by these cereals or their partial hydrolysates, including beer. Women of childbearing age who experienced amenorrhea due to nutritional deficiencies will probably have a return of regular menstruation and may become pregnant. Men who have had long-standing disease may complain of impotence and infertility. These problems normally resolve within 2 years of starting a gluten-free diet.

• Specific nutritional deficiencies should be treated by replacement: iron, calcium, vitamin B_{12}, folic acid, or magnesium.

Pharmacological treatment

• For most patients, a gluten-free diet is sufficient; extremely ill patients can be given systemic steroids.

Standard dosage	Prednisone, 20–40 mg daily initially, usually rapidly reduced to 5–10 mg daily. Hydrocortisone, 50–100 mg i.v. every 6 h in patients who need i.v. fluid replacement.
Contraindications	Caution in diabetes mellitus, or pregnancy.
Special points	Care should be taken to avoid high-dose (prednisone >10 mg/day), long-term steroid treatment because of side effects.
Main drug interactions	Mild antagonism to thiazide diuretics.
Main side effects	Weight gain, fluid retention, osteoporosis, cushingoid facies, diabetes mellitus.

Treatment aims

To improve general well-being, small intestinal mucosal structure, and associated nutritional deficiencies.

To reduce the risk of development of small intestinal lymphoma.

Prognosis

• With a gluten-free diet, general health is improved within a few weeks.

• Untreated patients are at a 5%–10% risk of developing a small intestinal T-cell lymphoma, the incidence of which probably falls if they maintain a strict diet.

• Failure to improve suggests incorrect initial diagnosis, failure to adhere strictly to a gluten-free diet, or concurrent disorder (*i.e.*, malignancy) [4].

Follow-up and management

• Outpatients must be reassessed 6–8 weeks and 3–4 months after starting a gluten-free diet, when repeat biopsy should be done.

• A further biopsy should be done 1 year after starting treatment, when continued improvement in the structure of the small-intestinal mucosa should be expected.

• Annual hematological screening is recommended to exclude development of specific nutritional deficiencies.

• When the diagnosis is doubtful, a gluten challenge, with 40 g gluten or 4 slices of normal bread daily for 2 weeks (adults) or 6 weeks (children), may be followed by a further jejunal biopsy.

Key references

1. Ciclitira PJ: Coeliac disease and related disorders and the malignant complications of coeliac disease. In *Gastroenterology: Clinical Science and Practice.* Edited by Bouchier I, Hodgson H. London: Baillière Tindall; 1993.
2. Ferguson A, Arranz E, O'Mahony S: Clinical and pathological spectrum of coeliac disease: active, silent, latent, potential. *Gut* 1993, **34**:150–155.
3. Kagnoff MF: Celiac disease: a gastro-intestinal disease with environmental, genetic, and immunologic components. *Gastroenterol Clin North Am* 1992, **21**:405–425.
4. Trier JS: Celiac sprue. *N Engl J Med* 1991, **325**:1709–1719.

Diagnosis

Symptoms

• Symptoms generally include the following, alone or in combination:

Epilepsy: in >50% of patients by presentation; associated focal features may suggest localization of brain tumor; epilepsy of late onset (>25 years) may indicate new brain lesion and should be investigated.

Dysphasia, hemiparesis, intellectual failure, personality change: cranial nerve abnormalities.

Headache, papilledema, visual failure, vomiting: alone or in combination indicate raised intracranial pressure due to intracranial mass lesions.

Signs

Papilledema, impaired visual acuity, visual field defects.

Diplopia: with or without clear III or VI nerve palsy.

Facial weakness.

Dysphasia.

Hemiparesis, hyperreflexia, extensor plantar response, hemisensory loss.

Signs of primary malignancy in secondary brain tumors: *e.g.*, site of previous melanoma excision visible in skin.

Investigations

Neuroradiography: primarily CT and MRI of brain; more invasive procedures (*e.g.*, angiography or positron emission tomography) sometimes needed for further aspects of management.

Chest radiography: important as part of general screening for extracerebral primary or metastatic tumor in lungs.

EEG: possibly needed as secondary investigation to elucidate epileptic manifestations.

Blood tests: possibly needed to clarify differential diagnosis, *e.g.*, blood cultures when metastatic brain abscess suspected.

Lumbar puncture: to identify meningeal spread of malignancy.

Complications

Blindness: papilledema due to progressive raised intracranial pressure leads to blindness if unrelieved.

Herniation: brain shift due to increasing mass of cerebral tumor can lead to central or transtentorial brain herniation, with irreversible ischemic brain damage and fatal apnea due to failure of brain stem function.

Differential diagnosis

Cerebrovascular disease.

Other organic brain disease (*e.g.*, encephalitis or demyelination).

Other extracerebral intracranial tumors (*e.g.*, meningioma).

Cerebral abscess: an important differential diagnosis; often no signs of acute infection in patients, despite relevant history of middle ear disease, bronchiectasis, or valvular heart disease.

Etiology

• The cause of most cerebral tumors remains unknown, although the incidence is increased after exposure to radiation, in patients with neurofibromatosis, and in some rare inherited immunodeficiency diseases.

• Increasing evidence indicates that cerebral astrocytomas are associated with loss of tumor suppressor gene function from chromosomes 17 and 10 and with amplification of epidermal growth factor receptor.

Epidemiology

• Primary cerebral tumors account for ~55% of intracranial tumors in adults and are the tenth most common tumors in men.

• The annual incidence of cerebral tumor is ~10 in 100 000 population.

• The peak incidence is in the fifth decade, with a small male preponderance (55%).

• Secondary brain tumors are common and account for 15%–20% of intracranial tumors in neurological series.

Treatment

Diet and lifestyle

• No special diet is necessary for patients with primary brain tumors.

• Impaired cognitive function and fatigue may limit employment.

Pharmacological treatment

For epilepsy

• Anticonvulsant drug treatment is usually started for supratentorial tumors in both epileptic and nonepileptic patients.

Standard dosage	Phenytoin, 300–400 mg daily, or carbamazepine, 600–1000 mg daily.
Contraindications	Hepatic impairment, severe cytopenia.
Main drug interactions	Analgesics, antibiotics, antidepressants.
Main side effects	Confusion, skin eruptions, gum swelling, diplopia, ataxia.

For raised intracranial pressure and stabilization of brain function

Standard dosage	Dexamethasone, 4 mg every 6 h (adult) initially; up to 20 mg every 6 h may be useful for a few weeks as palliative terminal treatment.
Contraindications	Peptic ulcers.
Special points	When surgical decompression and adjuvant radiotherapy have been completed, steroids may be gradually withdrawn or reduced to a minimum level that keeps the patient asymptomatic. While the patient is taking dexamethasone, the risk of peptic ulcers is increased; H_2 antagonists such as ranitidine, 150 mg twice daily, are usually also prescribed.
Main drug interactions	Hypoglycemia agents, diuretics.
Main side effects	Peptic ulcers, weight gain, demineralization.

For acutely raised intracranial pressure

• In patients who are unconscious as a result of raised intracranial pressure from cerebral tumor or in those who have herniated, with respiratory arrest, artificial ventilation, mannitol as an osmotic diuretic, and i.v. dexamethasone may be needed in an emergency department or intensive care unit setting.

Chemotherapy

• After surgery and adjuvant radiotherapy, antitumor chemotherapy may be indicated for malignant glioma, either as an adjuvant or at the time of relapse.

• Nitrosoureas and procarbazine are the agents chiefly used.

Treatment aims

To relieve symptoms; curing malignant primary or secondary brain tumors is generally not possible.

Other treatments

Surgery: almost always indicated to establish histological diagnosis and grading and, where possible, to reduce tumor bulk.

Radiotherapy: localized to tumor and surrounding area, usually given for malignant primary cerebral tumors; secondary metastatic cerebral tumors treated by whole-brain radiation.

Prognosis

• Prognosis is related to tumor type and histological grade, patient age, and functional performance at the time of treatment.

• The median survival with grade 4 astrocytomas is ~9 months and with grade 2 astrocytomas ~6 years.

Follow-up and management

• Clinical assessment of neurological and performance status, with follow-up brain scanning at intervals of 3–6 months, is used to monitor progress.

• At disease progression, further surgery is considered in 10%–15% of patients, as are novel treatments, *e.g.*, focused radiation or immunotherapy.

• The terminal phase is usually short, from a few days to 6 weeks, and patients may often be managed in the home, although hospice care may sometimes be preferable.

General references

1. Apuzzo MLJ, ed: *Malignant Cerebral Glioma.* Illinois: American Association of Neurological Surgeons, 1990.
2. Mahaley MS: Neuro-oncology index and review (adult primary brain tumors). *J Neurooncol* 1991, **11**:85–147.
3. Thomas DGT, ed: *Neuro-Oncology.* London: Arnold; 1990.

Diagnosis

Symptoms

Pruritis, fatigue: >50% of patients.

Right upper quandrant pain: intermittent.

• Patients may present with symptoms of end-stage liver disease (variceal bleeding, encephalopathy, ascites).

• 25% of patients are asymptomatic; diagnosis is made after discovery of abnormal liver function tests, particularly in patients with ulcerative colitis.

Jaundice: intermittent.

Weight loss.

Fever: unusual unless previous intervention, *e.g.*, endoscopic retrograde cholangiopancreatography, surgery.

Bleeding esophageal varices, edema, ascites: late features.

Signs

• Signs are not always manifest [1].

Right-upper quandrant tenderness, fevers: during episodes of cholangitis.

Hepatomegaly: >50%.

Splenomegaly: ~30%.

Jaundice: in more advanced cases.

Spider nevi, palmar erythema, ascites: late.

Investigations

Liver chemistries: cholestatic pattern with raised alkaline phosphatase, gamma glutamyl transpeptidase, bilirubin (late); low albumin, prolonged prothrombin time (late); antimitochondrial antibody usually negative.

Cholangiography: the diagnostic test; endoscopic retrograde cholangiography first choice, percutaneous route only if endoscopic route fails; bile-duct stricturing interspersed with dilatation (beading); intra- and extrahepatic duct changes in most patients.

Liver biopsy: changes suggestive (portal edema, fibrosis, duct proliferation) rather than diagnostic; biopsy staging: 1, portal changes; 2, periportal extension; 3, septum formation; 4, cirrhosis.

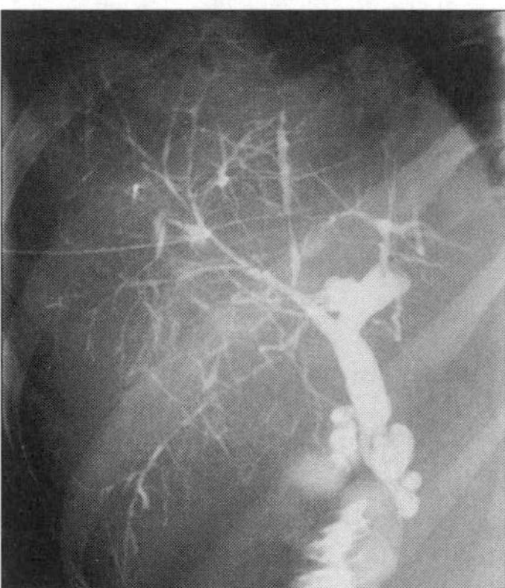

Classic intrahepatic changes of primary sclerosing cholangitis (bleeding and stricturing) on percutaneous cholangiography. The common bile duct is dilated because of involvement of the lower end by primary sclerosing cholangitis. Endoscopic cholangiography was unsuccessful.

Complications

Recurrent cholangitis.

Cholangiocarcinoma: in 10%–15% of patients.

Metabolic bone disease.

Portal hypertension, variceal hemorrhage, edema, ascites, encephalopathy: late.

Differential diagnosis

Bile duct stones.

Cholangiocarcinoma.

Drug-induced cholestasis.

Primary biliary cirrhosis.

Surgical stricture.

Secondary sclerosing cholangitis.

Metastatic tumor.

Granulomatous liver disease (*e.g.*, sarcoid).

AIDS cholangiopathy.

• Distinction of benign primary sclerosing cholangitis stricture from cholangiocarcinoma is very difficult; brush or bile cytology is only 50%–60% sensitive.

Etiology

• Primary sclerosing cholangitis has a known strong association with inflammatory bowel disease (ulcerative colitis) and HLA B8 and DR3.

• The pathogenetic mechanism is unknown.

• The current hypothesis is that infection, or absorption of bacterial products or both occur in predisposed (HLA DR) individuals.

Epidemiology

• 70% of patients with primary sclerosing cholangitis have ulcerative colitis; 4% of patients with ulcerative colitis have primary sclerosing cholangitis.

• The prevalence of primary sclerosing cholangitis is 2–7 in 100 000.

• The male :female ratio is 2 :1.

• The most common age of presentation is 25–45 years.

Treatment

Diet and lifestyle

• Careful attention to adequate nutrition is recommended.

• If steatorrhea is problematic, fat intake may be reduced.

Pharmacological treatment

Symptomatic

• Drugs are indicated to relieve pruritus.

Standard dosage	Cholestyramine, 4–12 g daily.
Contraindications	Complete biliary obstruction.
Special points	May interfere with absorption of fat-soluble vitamins, so supplementation may be needed.
Main drug interactions	Delayed or reduced absorption of digitalis, tetracycline, chlorothiazide, warfarin, thyroxine.
Main side effects	Increased bleeding tendency, constipation, diarrhea.

Prophylactic

• For proven fat-soluble vitamin deficiency or jaundice, the following are indicated:

Vitamin K, 10 mg i.m. monthly.

Vitamin D, 100 000 units i.m. monthly.

Vitamin A, 100 000 units i.m. 3-monthly.

• Adequate calcium intake must be ensured.

Therapeutic

• No medical treatment has been definitively shown to delay progression or reverse changes of primary sclerosing cholangitis [2].

• Ursodeoxycholic acid, 10–15 mg/kg orally daily, improves liver function tests, but benefit for liver histology, cholangiography, or survival has not been established.

• The choice of antibiotics for cholangitis (when no remediable dominant stricture) depends on bile or blood culture; empiric considerations include ciprofloxacin, ampicillin, or a cephalosporin.

Treatment aims

To relieve symptoms.

To prevent recurrence of cholangitis.

Other treatments

Nonsurgical

Endoscopic or radiographic palliation: for symptomatic dominant strictures (cholangitis, itching); endoscopic approach preferable to percutaneous; balloon dilatation possibly with stent.

Surgical

Surgical palliation: appropriate for dominant stricture only if transplantation is not an option and an endoscopic or a percutaneous approach has failed.

Orthotopic liver transplantation: for persistent jaundice, cholangitis, bleeding varices, fluid retention, encephalopathy, malnutrition; ~70% 1-year survival; unexpected cholangiocarcinoma often found (recurs).

Prognosis

• Prognosis varies greatly.

• Factors at presentation related to prognosis (Mayo model) include serum bilirubin concentration, histological stage on liver biopsy, age, and presence of splenomegaly [3,4].

Follow-up and management

• Patients should be monitored clinically for signs and symptoms of cholangitis.

• Patients should be reviewed monthly if they have symptomatic or biochemical deterioration and are approaching transplantation.

Key references

1. Farrant JM, *et al.*: Natural history and prognostic variables in primary sclerosing cholangitis. *Gastroenterology* 1991, **100**:1710–1717.

2. Lindor KD, *et al*: Advances in primary sclerosing cholangitis. *Am J Med* 1990, **89**:73–80.

3. Dickson ER, *et al.*: Primary sclerosing cholangitis: refinement and validation of survival models. *Gastroenterology* 1992, **103**:1893–1901.

4. Wiesner RH, *et al.*: Selection and timing of liver transplantation in primary biliary cirrhosis and primary sclerosing cholangitis. *Hepatology* 1992, **16**:1290–1299.

Chronic fatigue syndrome

Diagnosis

Symptoms

Major

Fatigue: lasting >3–6 months, with 50% reduction in activity; worsened by physical or mental stress; relapsing, with good and bad days.

Prominent disturbance of concentration or short-term memory.

Minor

Initiating viral-like illness, with pyrexia and malaise, common.

Myalgia: especially limb and chest pain; worse after activity.

Joint pain: especially in large joints.

Abdominal pain or bloatedness, nausea, alternating constipation and diarrhea.

Headaches, dizziness, tinnitus, paresthesias.

Sleep disturbance: initially more sleep, followed by disturbed sleep or vivid dreams.

Sensitivity to heat or cold, inappropriate sweating.

Adverse effects of alcohol.

Signs

• Most patients have been previously well; few clinical signs are manifest.

Localized areas of tender muscle: about 1 cm diameter in affected muscle groups.

Enlarged lymph nodes, glands, or inflamed throat: in periods of relapse.

Muscle weakness: in patients who have been ill for many years.

Investigations

• Diagnosis must not be made on the presence of fatigue alone; the two major symptoms and at least four minor items from symptoms, clinical signs, or positive laboratory investigations must be present.

• No diagnostic test exists; investigations are designed to exclude other causes of a similar clinical syndrome.

Initial investigations

• All of the results should be normal, if other illnesses are to be excluded.

Hemoglobin measurement: to exclude anemia.

Leukocyte count: to identify infection or a hematological condition.

Thyroid function tests: to exclude thyroid disease.

Plasma viscosity or ESR and CRP measurement: nonspecific indicator of an underlying disorder.

Further investigations

• Other conditions suggested by the patient's history or examination must be excluded, especially infection, *e.g.*, tick bites (Lyme disease) or consumption of raw meat (toxoplasmosis).

Complications

Psychiatric disorder: especially depression and anxiety.

Irritable bowel syndrome.

Severe disability: patient may become bedridden.

Differential diagnosis

Infections, especially Epstein–Barr virus, Lyme disease, toxoplasmosis, hepatitis A, brucellosis.

Endocrine disease, especially hypothyroidism.

Psychiatric disease, especially if patient has been ill for many years.

Malignancy.

Autoimmune disease, sarcoidosis.

Drugs or toxins.

Etiology

• The cause is unknown; probably several conditions are involved, including continuing infection and immune response to infection.

Epidemiology

• Chronic fatigue syndrome occurs throughout the world.

• ~1.3 in 1000 population are affected.

• Both sexes and all ages are affected; women are more likely to have prolonged illness.

Nomenclature

• Chronic fatigue syndrome is also known as the following:

Postviral fatigue syndrome.

Myalgic encephalomyelitis (ME).

Effort syndrome.

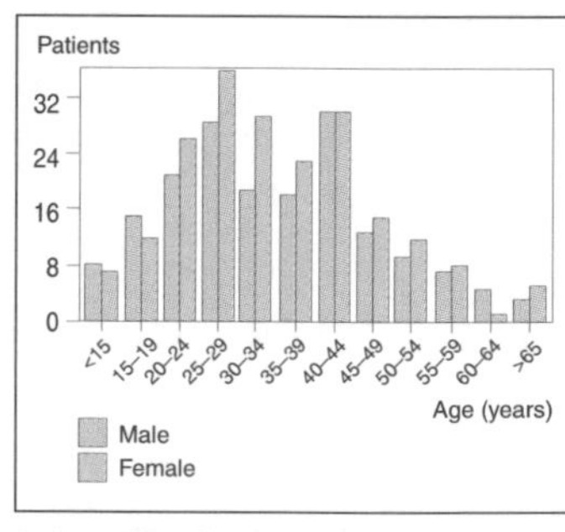

Patients affected by chronic fatigue syndrome, according to age and sex (204 females, 177 males; ratio, 1.2:1.

Treatment

Diet and lifestyle

- If patients have a normal diet, vitamins or mineral supplements are unnecessary.
- Patients should remain within their energy limits; sleep should not be resisted (at least 10 h/day); sleep and relaxation techniques increase energy levels; energy is lost through physical activities and mental exertion (such as concern about jobs, finances, and relationships).

Pharmacological treatment

- Although moderating activity is the best method of controlling symptoms, many patients need additional supportive treatment.
- Several drugs may have to be tried before the most appropriate is found.

Analgesics

- Mild analgesics, *e.g.*, acetaminophen or aspirin, should be tried initially; if they are unsuccessful, dihydrocodeine or ibuprofen may help.

Benzodiazepines

- Because of their hypnotic, sedative, anxiolytic, and muscle-relaxant actions, these drugs are useful in patients who have difficulty sleeping.
- Intermediate-acting compounds are best (temazepam, lormetazepam).

Standard dosage Temazepam, 10 mg orally at night for 3–4 weeks.

Contraindications Respiratory depression, phobic or obsessional states.

Main drug interactions Alcohol.

Main side effects Drowsiness, dizziness.

Antidepressants

- The most useful agents are amitriptyline, doxepin, dothiepin, and fluoxetine.

Standard dosage Amitriptyline, 10 mg orally at night.

Contraindications Heart disease.

Special points Patients should be given low doses initially, with gradual increase if necessary.

Main drug interactions Alcohol.

Main side effects Dry mouth, blurred vision, nausea, constipation.

Treatment aims

To reduce fatigue and prevent relapses.

To relieve other symptoms.

To allow patient to resume normal activity, *e.g.*, to return to work or school.

Prognosis

- Patients may recover after a fluctuating illness, usually in the first 4 years, achieve stability at a lower energy level, or deteriorate and become chronically disabled.

Follow-up and management

- Patients should keep a daily diary, monitoring activities and energy levels.
- Activities may be increased and a return to work or school encouraged when energy levels are 70%–80% of normal.

Causes of treatment failure

Overoptimistic reassurance of recovery.

Patient's inability to change lifestyle.

Too much energy being spent pursuing alternative cures.

General references

1. Ho-Yen DO: *Better Recovery from Viral Illnesses*, edn 3. Inverness: Dodona Books; 1993.
2. Thomas PK: The chronic fatigue syndrome: what do we know? *BMJ* 1993, **306**:1557–1558.
3. Tirelli U, *et al.*: Clinical and immunologic study of 205 patients with chronic fatigue syndrome. *Arch Intern Med* 1993, **153**:116–120.
4. Wessely S: Chronic fatigue syndrome: current issues. *Review of Medical Microbiology* 1992, **3**:211–216.

Diagnosis

Symptoms

Cough: chronic bronchitis is defined as a cough productive of sputum on most days for at least 3 consecutive months in 2 successive years.

Increasing shortness of breath.

Weight loss.

Signs

Barrel-shaped chest, decreased cardiac dullness and reduced breath sounds, palpable liver due to hepatic displacement, signs of hyperexpansion.

Increased respiratory rate, use of accessory muscles of respiration, paradoxical movement of costal margins, "pursed lip" breathing, reduced breath sounds: signs of airflow obstruction.

Cyanosis.

Right ventricular heave, raised jugular venous pressure, peripheral edema: signs of pulmonary hypertension.

Fine inspiratory crackles: frequently found in chronic obstructive airway disease and do not necessarily imply coexistent heart failure.

Investigations

Complete blood count: polycythemia found in a few patients.

ECG: to detect right axis deviation or signs of right-sided strain.

Chest radiography: to detect signs of chronic obstructive pulmonary disease (low flat diaphragms, long thin heart), emphysema (hypodense bullae, large retrosternal airspace on lateral radiography), or pulmonary hypertension (prominent hilum, with reduced peripheral vascular shadows).

Spirometry: to confirm obstructive picture and to show degree of reversibility to therapeutic agents.

Arterial blood gas measurement: to check for hypoxia and carbon dioxide retention; high bicarbonate concentration suggests more chronic carbon dioxide retention.

Complications

Infective exacerbations.

Pulmonary hypertension.

Respiratory failure, death.

Pneumothorax.

Lung cancer: when smoking is cause of chronic obstructive pulmonary disease (COPD).

Differential diagnosis

Shortness of breath

Asthma.

Left ventricular failure.

Large airway obstruction, *e.g.*, proximal tumor.

Recurrent chest infections

Aspiration secondary to esophageal disease.

Immunosuppression.

Etiology

• Causes include the following:

Cigarette smoking.

Atmospheric pollution: much less important than smoking.

Alpha-1 antitrypsin deficiency: rare; homozygous form present in 1 in 5000 people, and not all of these develop chest disease; causes basal emphysema [1].

Intravenous drug abuse.

Epidemiology

• Estimates indicate that about 15 million Americans have COPD.

• Chronic obstructive airway disease is estimated to cause 90 000 deaths per year.

Treatment

Diet and lifestyle

• Stopping smoking reduces the rate of deterioration of lung function to that of non-smokers and, at an early stage, may improve symptoms.

• Loss of weight improves functional capacity.

• Patients' homes can be assessed for the need for aids to daily living.

Pharmacological treatment [2,3]

• Inadequate inhaler technique is one of the main reasons for treatment failure; inhaler technique must always be checked before treatment is initiated or changed.

Inhaled beta-2 agonists (*e.g.*, albuterol, metaproterenol, terbutaline)

Standard dosage Two puffs up to 4 times daily (dosage varies with formulation).

Contraindications Hypersensitivity.

Special points Patient responses vary; clinical improvement may occur but may not be detected on spirometric assessment.

Main drug interactions None.

Main side effects Tremor, hypokalemia after high doses.

Inhaled anticholinergics

Standard dosage Ipratropium bromide inhaler, 20–40 μg 4 times daily.

Contraindications Hypersensitivity; caution in glaucoma (nebulized solutions).

Main drug interactions None.

Main side effects Dry mouth (rare).

Inhaled steroids

• Inhaled steroids are indicated for patients who have shown an objective response.

Standard dosage Beclomethasone dipropionate, 200–1000 μg twice daily.

Contraindications Hypersensitivity.

Special points Systemic absorption can be reduced with a spacer device.

Main drug interactions None.

Main side effects Oral candidiasis.

Oral steroids

• Oral steroids are indicated for exacerbations of chronic obstructive pulmonary disease and for maintenance treatment in severely ill steroid-responsive patients.

Standard dosage Prednisone, 30 mg in the morning for exacerbations; lowest possible dose for maintenance treatment.

Contraindications None.

Special points Steroid responsiveness should be shown by >10% improvement in forced expiratory volume in 1 s after 3 weeks of prednisone, 30 mg.

Main drug interactions None.

Main side effects Osteoporosis, diabetes, steroid psychosis.

Theophyllines

• These have been shown to improve exercise tolerance.

Standard dosage Theophylline, 300–600 mg daily.

Contraindications None.

Special points Plasma concentrations must be monitored; they should be maintained at 10–20 μg/L.

Main drug interactions Cimetidine, erythromycin, ciprofloxacin, and oral contraceptives reduce metabolism; cigarettes, alcohol, phenytoin, and rifampin increase metabolism.

Main side effects Tachycardia, arrythmias.

Treatment aims

To maximize functional capacity.

To reduce decline in lung function.

Other treatments [4]

Long-term oxygen therapy (>16 h daily)

• Indications include the following:

Partial pressure of oxygen <55 mm Hg on two successive occasions when patient is stable.

Forced expiratory volume in 1 s <1.0 L.

Nonsmoking patient.

Failure to show carbon dioxide retention after a trial of oxygen.

At least one episode of peripheral edema.

Nasal intermittent positive pressure ventilation

• This may be suitable in patients who retain carbon dioxide with oxygen therapy.

Smoking cessation.

Prognosis

• The 5-year survival rate after the initial episode of respiratory failure averages 15%–20%.

Follow-up and management

• Forced expiratory volume in 1 s must be monitored.

• Response to treatment must be assessed.

Key references

1. American Thoracic Society: Guidelines for the approach to the patient with severe hereditary alpha 1-antitrypsin deficiency. *Am Rev Respir Dis* 1989, **140**:1494–1497.
2. Isada C, Stoller J: The rational use of antibiotics in chronic bronchitis. *Contemporary Internal Medicine* 1991, 29–40.
3. Skorodin M: Pharmacotherapy for asthma and chronic obstructive pulmonary disease. Current thinking, practices, and controversies. *Arch Intern Med* 1993, **153**:814–828.
4. Ferguson GT, Cherniak RM: Management of chronic obstructive pulmonary disease. *N Engl J Med* 1993, **328**:1017–1022.

Diagnosis

Symptoms

• Disease may be an incidental finding (abnormal liver tests on routine screening for other conditions) or manifest in one of the following ways:

Lethargy and pruritus: in middle-aged women (classic).

Right-sided abdominal pain: uncommon.

Ascites or variceal hemorrhage: indicating portal hypertension.

Signs

Jaundice: in later stages.

Xanthoma and xanthelasma.

Hepatomegaly.

Splenomegaly.

Ascites: may be present in late stage.

Spider nevi: often absent.

Investigations

Full blood count: usually normal, but mean cell volume possibly raised.

Liver tests: show cholestasis; in early stage, raised serum alkaline phosphatase, gamma glutamyl transpeptidase, serum bilirubin concentrations; raised cholesterol concentration.

Immunological tests: raised serum IgM and IgG concentrations (IgG less marked); antimitochondrial antibodies (AMA M_2 subclass) almost diagnostic; other autoantibodies, *e.g.*, antinuclear antibodies, occasionally manifest [1].

Liver histology: shows nonsuppurative destructive cholangitis or hepatitis involving portal tracts, which may also contain granulomas.

Complications

• Complications are the same as for end-stage liver disease.

Variceal hemorrhage.

Ascites.

Osteoporosis: hepatic osteopenia.

Liver failure.

Hepatocellular carcinoma.

Encephalopathy.

Differential diagnosis

Primary sclerosing cholangitis.

Autoimmune hepatitis.

Drug-induced jaundice.

Sarcoidosis.

Chronic viral hepatitis.

Etiology

• The cause is unknown, although the following may have a role:

Infectious agents: bacterial or viral.

Autoimmune disorders.

Drugs: benoxaprofen, chlorpromazine.

Epidemiology

• In the UK, estimates of point prevalence of primary biliary cirrhosis are 2.3–14.4 in 100 000 people.

• The disease is less common in Africa and India.

Associated syndromes

Common

Arthralgia.

Hyperlipidemia.

Osteoporosis

Rare

Thyroid disease.

Sicca syndrome.

Glomerulonephritis.

Pulmonary fibrosis.

Sclerodactyly (CREST syndrome).

SLE.

Addison's disease.

Celiac disease.

Raynaud's phenomenon.

Histology

Stage 1

Florid duct lesions, septal duct damage surrounded by dense inflammatory infiltrate, lymphoid aggregates; granulomas.

Stage 2

Ductular proliferation, fibrosis, fewer ducts.

Stage 3

Scarring (less inflammation), fibrous septa expanding from portal tracts; periportal cholestatis.

Stage 4

True cirrhosis; few or no bile ducts.

Treatment

Diet and lifestyle

• Patients must avoid regular alcohol intake.

• Careful attention must be paid to adequate nutrition.

• Prolonged cholestasis may result in vitamin K deficiency as manifest by a prolonged prothrombin time.

• Calcium and vitamin D supplementation should be considered early.

Pharmacological treatment

Symptomatic

• Drugs are indicated to relieve pruritus.

Standard dosage	Cholestyramine, 4–16 g daily or colestipol.
Contraindications	Complete biliary obstruction.
Special points	May interfere with absorption of fat-soluble vitamins, so supplementation may be needed.
Main drug interactions	Delayed or reduced absorption of digitalis, tetracycline, chlorothiazide, warfarin, thyroxine.
Main side effects	Increased bleeding tendency, constipation, diarrhea.

• Treatment to prevent osteoporosis and supportive treatment for associated symptoms should also be provided.

Definitive

• Treatment should be done under specialist supervision.

• No drug has been shown to arrest disease; anti-inflammatories and antifibrotics (corticosteroids, azathioprine, cyclosporin A, colchicine, methotrexate, penicillamine) have been used with no major clinical benefit [2].

• Ursodeoxycholic acid may help; biochemistry is improved, but data on long-term survival are controversial.

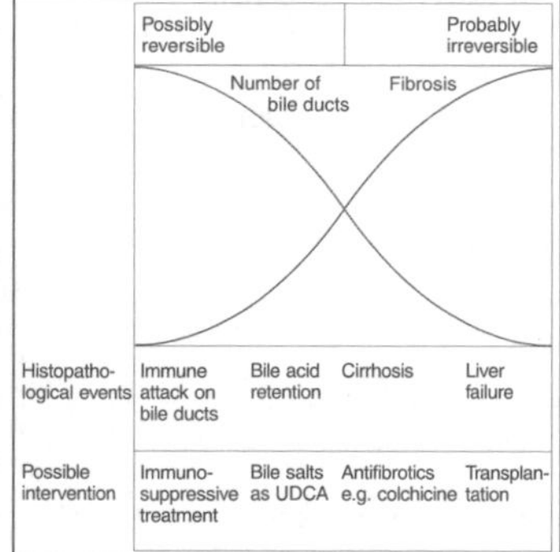

Progression of primary biliary cirrhosis and possible interventions. UDCA, ursodeoxycholic acid.

Treatment aims

To prevent progression.

To reverse symptoms.

Other treatments

Liver transplantation for end-stage disease or intractable symptoms [3].

Prognosis

• Prognosis depends on serum bilirubin concentration: >10 mg/dL implies an 18-month survival.

• The median time from diagnosis to death is 10 years.

Follow-up and management

• Progression must be monitored.

• Complications must be prevented or treated.

Key references

1. Mutchison HC, Bassendine MF: Autoimmune liver disease. *Aliment Pharmacol Ther* 1993, **7**:93–109.
2. Kaplan M: Primary biliary cirrhosis: a first step in prolonging survival. *N Engl J Med* 1994, **330**:1386–1387.
3. Neuberger J, *et al.*: Use of a prognostic index in evaluation of liver transplantation for primary biliary cirrhosis. *Transplantation* 1986, **41**:713–716.

Diagnosis

Symptoms

• Symptoms may be related to primary tumor, metastatic disease, or general effects of malignancies.

Change of bowel habit.

Blood in stools.

Tenesmus: rectal lesions.

Abdominal pain or swelling.

Loss of weight.

Signs

Anemia.

Abdominal mass or distension.

Mass or blood on digital rectal examination.

Peritonitis: perforation.

Mechanical bowel obstruction.

Hepatomegaly: metastatic disease.

Cachexia.

Fecal occult blood.

Investigations

Assessment of primary tumor

• Lesions identified during screening flexible sigmoidoscopy should be biopsied; patients with multiple large adenomas should be referred for colonoscopy.

Colonoscopy: of patients with symptoms or signs of colorectal cancer; any polyps in these patients should be removed for histological examination; malignancy confined to the mucosa or Dukes' stage A (*see* Pathology) do not require surgery or chemotherapy if the lesion can be completely resected via the colonoscope (*i.e.*, the resection margins are free of disease [1].

Assessment of disseminated disease

Liver function tests: metastatic disease often presents with an elevated alkaline phosphatase level.

Chest radiography.

Liver ultrasonography: in absence of CT; inexpensive but lower sensitivity than CT.

Abdominal CT: to assess tumor burden in pelvis and to look for evidence of hepatic disease.

Screening for prevention

Fecal occult blood testing: yearly in asymptomatic patients over age 50 will reduce mortality but requires extensive resources to pursue the large number of false-positive tests [2,3].

Flexible sigmoidoscopy: every 5 years in asymptomatic patients over the age of 50 [4,5].

Colonoscopy: for high-risk groups, *e.g.*, patients with two or more first-degree relatives with colon cancer or one first-degree relative under the age of 50 with colon cancer.

Complications

Obstruction: usually left-sided lesions.

Perforation.

Acute hemorrhage or iron-deficiency anemia.

Fistula formation.

Differential diagnosis

Diverticular disease.
Inflammatory bowel disease.
Irritable bowel syndrome.
Adhesions.
Arterovenous malformations.
Solitary rectal ulcer.

Risk factors

High fat, low fiber diet.
Familial polyposis coli.
Chronic ulcerative colitis.
Genetic: hereditary nonpolyposis colorectal cancer.
Colorectal adenomas.

Epidemiology

• The peak incidence is at 60–69 years.
• It is the second most frequent cause of death due to malignancy in developed countries.

Pathology

Microscopic: adenocarcinoma.
Macroscopic: polypoidal, ulcerative, annular, diffuse, colloidial.

Site

Rectum: 30%.
Cecum and ascending colon: 25%.
Sigmoid colon: 20%.
Descending colon: 15%.
Transverse colon: 10%.

Spread

Direct, lymphatic, venous.

Stage (Dukes' classification)

A: confined to mucosa/submucosa.
B: invasion of muscularis propria.
C: local node involvement.
D: distant metastases.

Treatment

Diet and lifestyle

• For primary prevention, fat intake should be reduced to 30% of energy intake, and dietary unrefined fiber and fruit and vegetable consumption should be increased. Regular aspirin intake has also been associated with a lower risk of colonic adenocarcinoma.

Pharmacological treatment

• Adjuvant chemotherapy (5-fluorouracil and levamisole) is advocated for Dukes' stage B and C lesions; there is no evidence of benefit in disseminated disease [6].

Nonpharmacological treatment

Elective surgery

Curative resection: right hemicolectomy, left hemicolectomy, anterior resection, abdominoperineal excision.

Palliative resection or bypass.

Local treatment for rectal lesions: local transanal resection (open or endoscopic), laser therapy, or intracavity radiation.

Emergency surgery

• 20% of patients present with obstruction, possibly with perforation.

Adjuvant radiotherapy

• For rectal carcinoma, radiotherapy may be used preoperatively to reduce tumor burden.

Management of recurrence

• Management depends on the site, size, and number of metastases.

• Serial carcinoembryonic antigen estimation can predict recurrence and may be followed if the patient is a candidate for aggressive surgical management of extracolonic lesions (*e.g.*, solitary hepatic mestastases).

• Fewer than 20% of patients with recurrence after a "curative" resection are suitable for another resection.

Site of recurrence: local (20%; related to Dukes' stage), hepatic (30%), abdominal (20%), pulmonary (20%), retroperitoneal (10%).

For local disease: 50% amenable to further ablative surgery, with potential cure in 25%; radiotherapy effective palliation for rectal recurrence but limited by myelotoxicity.

For hepatic metastases: <20% (solitary or unilobar) amenable to curative resection; possible short-term benefit from hepatic artery infusion of 5-fluorodeoxyuridine; possible symptomatic relief for capsular distension with fractionated radiotherapy.

Treatment aims

To remove primary tumor and locoregional nodes, including mesorectum for rectal lesions (curative resection).

To remove or bypass the primary lesion with advanced local or metastatic disease, in order to ameliorate symptoms (palliative resection or bypass).

To control local disease in patients unfit for resection.

Prognosis

• 25% of patients have metastases at the time of presentation.

• In-hospital postoperative mortality (5%–7%) is related to intra-abdominal sepsis, obstruction, age, or cardiopulmonary complications.

• Overall 5-year survival rates are 80%–90% for Dukes' stage A, 50%–60% for stage B, 30% for stage C, and 5% for stage D.

Follow up and management

• Patients resected for cure should undergo surveillance colonscopy within 6–12 months of resection to exclude missed lesions, and every 3–5 years in the absence of symptoms.

Key references

1. Bond JH, *et al.*: Polyp guideline: diagnosis, treatment, and surveillance for patients with nonfamilial colorectal polyps. *Ann Intern Med* 1993, **119**:836–843.
2. Ahlquist DA: Accuracy of fecal occult blood screening for colorectal neoplasia. *JAMA* 1993, **269**:1262–1267.
3. Mandel JS, *et al.*: Reducing mortality from colorectal cancer by screening for fecal occult blood. *N Engl J Med* 1993, **328**:1365–1371.
4. Ransohoff DF, *et al.*: Sigmoidoscopic screening in the 1990s. *JAMA* 1993, **269**:1278–1281.
5. Selby JV, *et al.*: A case-control study of screening sigmoidoscopy and mortality from colorectal cancer. *N Engl J Med* 1992 **326**:653–657.
6. Moertal CC: Drug therapy: chemotherapy for colorectal cancer. *N Engl J Med* 1994, **330**:1136–1142.

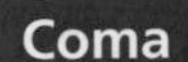

Diagnosis

Definition

• Coma is a state of unresponsiveness to external stimuli in which the patient lies with eyes closed.

• In practice, the condition may usefully be defined as a patient with a Glasgow coma scale of 2:4:2 or less (*see box*).

Symptoms

• Coma is a symptom.

Signs

Fever: indicating infection (meningitis, encephalitis, systemic).
Hypothermia: may be cause or effect.
Neck stiffness, Kernig's sign, papilledema.
Cardiac abnormalities: can indicate subacute bacterial endocarditis or emboli.
Hypertension or hypotension.
Slow, shallow respiration: suggesting drug intoxication.
Rapid respiration: suggesting infection or acidosis.
Anemia, jaundice, rash.
Intoxication, diabetes, hepatic failure.
Organomegaly, polycystic kidneys, subarachnoid hemorrhage.
Meningitis, subarachnoid hemorrhage, raised intracranial pressure.

Investigations

History from a witness: for evolution of coma, circumstances of patient's discovery, trauma, seizure, drugs, previous medical history.

Glasgow coma scale: for level of consciousness [1].

Brain stem function tests: pupillary response, spontaneous eye movements, oculovestibular responses.

Motor function tests: for lateralizing features.

Fundal examination: for papilledema, hemorrhage, emboli.

Blood analysis: for biochemistry, *e.g.*, glucose, electrolytes; hepatic, renal, and thyroid function; toxin exposure; etc.

CT or MRI: for coma with focal signs or if the diagnosis is uncertain.

Lumbar puncture: for coma without focal signs but with stiff neck.

Hematological assays, chest radiography, EEG: for coma without focal signs or stiff neck (raised intracranial pressure must be excluded first).

Cortex
Thalamus
Midbrain reticular formation

The anatomy of consciousness.

Complications

Infections: particularly respiratory or renal, *e.g.*, aspiration pneumonia.
Metabolic abnormalities.
Disseminated intravascular coagulation.
Decubitus ulcers.
Contractures.
Deep venous thromboses.
Corneal abrasion.
Death.

Differential diagnosis

Locked-in syndrome: voluntary response of eye opening and eye closure to command.
Vegetative state: spontaneous eye opening and sleep–wake cycles, but no evidence of cognition.
Psychogenic coma: intact oculovestibular responses and nystagmus to cold water caloric, blepharospasm, intact cranial nerve reflexes.

Etiology

• Causes include the following:
Drug or alcohol overdose.
Trauma.
Space-occupying intracranial lesions.
Infections: encephalitis, meningitis, septicemia.
Intracranial hemorrhage and thrombosis.
Metabolic abnormalities.
Toxins.
Status epilepticus

Epidemiology

• 3% of emergency admissions to hospital are patients in coma.
• 40% of these patients have taken an overdose of sedative drugs.

Glasgow coma scale

Eye opening
1. Nil.
2. To pain.
3. *To speech.*
4. *Spontaneously.*

Motor response
1. Nil.
2 Extensor.
3. Flexor.
4. Withdrawal.
5. *Localizing.*
6. *Voluntary.*

Verbal response
1. Nil.
2. Groans.
3. *Inappropriate.*
4. *Confused.*
5. *Orientated.*

• Italics indicate no coma.

Treatment

Diet and lifestyle

Not relevant.

Pharmacological treatment [2]

• Patients may need treatment for causative or concurrent disorders: antibiotics and antiviral agents, antifungal agents, correction of metabolic abnormalities, removal of toxic substances, treatment of mass lesions, s.c. heparin to prevent thrombotic complications.

• Steroids or mannitol should not be given routinely in comatose patients but may help in specific instances when raised intracranial pressure, due to edema, can be corrected.

Treatment aims

To correct cause.

To maintain hydration and nutrition.

To reverse coma and return normal physiological and psychological function.

Prognosis

• Sedative drugs or alcohol overdoses are not usually lethal, and the prognosis is good if the circulation and respiration are protected.

• The prognosis of other causes of non-traumatic coma depends on the cause (metabolic coma has better prognosis than hypoxic ischemic coma), the depth (the deeper the coma, the worse the prognosis), the duration (the longer the coma, the worse the prognosis), and clinical signs, *e.g.*, brain stem reflexes.

• Overall, only 15% of patients in non-traumatic coma for >6 h make a good or moderate recovery.

Follow-up and management

• The airway must be maintained.

• The patient must be given adequate nutrition.

• Skin, chest, bladder, and bowel must be protected.

• Progress must be monitored.

Key references

1. Plumer F, Posner JB: *Stupor and Coma*, edn 3. Philadelphia: FA Davis; 1982.
2. Bates D: The management of medical coma. *J Neurol Neurosurg Psychiatry* 1993, **56**:589–598.

Diagnosis

Symptoms [1,2]

Headache: present in 75% of patients; at any site, often throbbing, unilateral or asymmetrical, worse at night; scalp soreness and tenderness frequent.

Polymyalgia: proximal limb pain and stiffness in 58%.

Malaise, fatigue, weight loss: in 56%.

Jaw pain and fatigue: masticatory "claudication" in 40%.

Fever: in 35%.

Cough: in 17%.

Amaurosis fugax: in 10%.

Permanent visual loss: in 8%.

Limb claudication: in 8%.

Transient ischemic attack or stroke: in 7%.

Depression or confusional state: in 3%.

Diplopia: in 2%.

Signs

Abnormal temporal artery: tenderness, nodularity, thickening or reduced pulsation in 49% of patients.

Scalp tenderness elsewhere.

Tenderness of common carotid arteries.

Diminished carotid or limb pulses.

Ischemic optic neuropathy: pale, swollen disc in a recently blinded eye [3].

Ophthalmoplegia: due to cranial nerve or brain stem lesion.

Confusional state or encephalopathy.

Investigations

ESR measurement: substantially raised in most patients; mean, 85 ± 32 mm/h (<30 mm/h in 3% of patients).

Full blood count: mild anemia, thrombocytosis, and raised leukocyte count common.

Liver function tests: raised gamma glutamyl transferase, alkaline phosphatase, or aspartate transaminase in 15% of patients.

Lumbar puncture: necessary only if low-grade meningitis or cortical thrombophlebitis considered in differential diagnosis.

Temporal artery biopsy: essential when diagnosis not absolutely clear cut on clinical grounds; at least 2–3 cm length biopsy (longer segment more likely to yield positive result); occipital artery biopsy alternative in selected patients [4].

Angiography: necessary only to exclude arterial dissection or other arteritides in selected patients; may show abnormalities in all major branches of aortic arch in cranial arteritis; lacks sensitivity and specificity as diagnostic test.

Complications

Permanent blindness: in 8% of patients.

Brain stem or carotid territory infarction: in <5%.

Myocardial infarction.

Scalp necrosis.

Limb ischemia.

Aortic rupture.

Differential diagnosis

Raised ESR

Other arteritides (rare in patients >70 years).
Myeloma.
Other skull metastases.
Subacute meningitis.
Infection with venous sinus thrombosis.

Normal ESR

Migraine.
Tension headache.
"Occipital neuralgia."
Cervical spine disease.
Paget's disease of the skull.
Vertebral or carotid dissection.
Temporomandibular joint disease.
Meningioma.

Etiology

• Cranial arteritis is presumed to be an autoimmune disorder, but the antigen is not known (perhaps component of internal elastic lamina).

• Immunoglobulin and complement deposits have been shown at the internal elastic lamina; other histological features suggest that cell-mediated mechanisms are also involved.

Epidemiology [5]

• The incidence is 9.3 in 100 000 population overall and 15–30 in 100 000 aged >50 years.

• The prevalence is 130 in 100 000 aged >50 years.

• Cranial arteritis rarely occurs in people aged <50 years.

• The median age of onset is 75 years (range, 56–92 years in published series).

• The female : male ratio is 3.7 : 1.

Pathology

• Cranial arteritis is an occlusive disease, involving large and medium-sized arteries arising from the aortic arch and sometimes the femoral arteries and aorta itself.

• Biopsy shows arterial luminal stenosis due to intimal proliferation, with disruption of the internal elastic lamina, mononuclear cell infiltration, necrosis of the media, giant cells, and granuloma formation; secondary thrombosis may be present. Involvement is patchy and may be missed by too small a biopsy.

Treatment

Diet and lifestyle

• No special precautions are necessary.

Pharmacological treatment

General principles

• Cranial arteritis requires prompt treatment by corticosteroids to prevent the rare but serious complications, particularly blindness.

• Presenting symptoms are often nonspecific and "atypical" (*e.g.*, pyrexia of unknown origin, weight loss, anemia), so suspicion must be high and treatment initiated as soon as the diagnosis is seriously considered.

• Arterial biopsy is often taken after steroid treatment is started, but it should not be delayed by more than 2–3 days; the yield of positive histology in clinically probable cases falls from 60%–80% with early biopsy to only 10% in patients biopsied 1 week after starting steroid treatment.

• Traditional high doses of prednisolone are justifiable in all patients with visual symptoms or signs and in those with features of cerebral or myocardial ischemia.

• In critical cases (*e.g.*, visual loss in one eye and early symptoms in the other), infusion of high-dose methylprednisolone probably reduces the risk of complete blindness.

• In patients without visual symptoms, prospective trials suggest that most respond to much lower doses (even less needed for polymyalgia without symptomatic arteritis).

• The rate of reduction depends on clinical severity at presentation, starting dose, symptom control, and ESR.

• A maintenance dose of 5–10 mg daily is usually needed for 2–3 years.

• An alternate-day regimen is sometimes possible, when the dose is very low.

• 30%–50% of patients can discontinue treatment after 2 years.

• Some need treatment for several years, and a few apparently need long-term maintenance doses of 2–5 mg daily.

Steroid regimen [6]

Initial dose: prednisolone, 40–80 mg daily;
methylprednisolone, 1 g i.v. daily for 2–5 days in critical cases.

Months 1–2: reduced slowly to 20–40 mg daily.

Months 2–4: reduced slowly to 10–20 mg daily.

Months 4–24: reduced to maintenance dose 5–10 mg daily.

Months 24–36: withdrawal possible in ~50% of patients.

Complications of treatment

Vertebral compression fractures in 26%.

Other symptoms of osteoporosis.

Steroid myopathy in 11%.

Cataracts.

Gastrointestinal symptoms.

Other steroid side effects.

Other drugs

• Azathioprine has a modest steroid-sparing effect but is not of proven efficacy used alone.

• Cyclophosphamide is a possible third option but rarely used.

Treatment aims

To relieve symptoms.

To prevent complications.

To prevent and control steroid side effects.

Prognosis

• Prognosis is excellent with early and adequate steroid treatment, which is usually needed for at least 2–3 years.

• Subsequent morbidity is determined as much by steroid side effects as by the disease itself.

Follow-up and management

• Patients need regular monitoring of clinical symptoms, ESR, and potential steroid effects for at least 2 years, preferably in a specialist clinic (neurology or rheumatology).

Key references

1. Caselli RJ, Hunder GG, Whisnant JP: Neurologic disease in biopsy-proven giant cell (temporal) arteritis. *Neurology* 1988, **38**:352–359.
2. Machado EB, *et al.*: Trends in incidence and clinical presentation of temporal arteritis in Olmstead County, Minnesota, 1950–1985. *Arthritis Rheum* 1988, **31**:745–749.
3. Hayreh SS: Ophthalmic features of giant cell arteritis. *Baillières Clin Rheumatol* 1991, **5**:431–459.
4. Hall S, *et al.*: The therapeutic impact of temporal artery biopsy. *Lancet* 1983, **ii**:1217–1220.
5. Nordborg E, Bengtsson BA: Epidemiology of proven giant cell arteritis (GCA). *Intern Med* 1990, **227**:233–236.
6. Kyle V, Hazleman BL: Treatment of polymyalgia rheumatica and giant cell arteritis. Steroid regimens in the first two months. *Ann Rheum Dis* 1989, **48**:658–661.

Diagnosis

Symptoms

Malaise, anorexia, weight loss.

Diarrhea.

Abdominal pain: due to inflammation, infection, or obstruction.

Tenesmus: with proctitis.

Bloody diarrhea: with Crohn's colitis.

Recurrent perianal abscesses: with local pain.

Growth retardation and failure of normal development: in children.

Signs

Aphthous ulceration in mouth.

Atrophic glossitis: beefy-red tongue, due to vitamin B_{12} malabsorption.

Pallor of mucous membranes: indicating anemia.

Right iliac fossa mass.

Perianal abscesses, fistulas.

Erythema nodosum, pyoderma gangrenosum, clubbing.

Arthritis or tenderness to palpation: *e.g.*, sacroiliac joints.

Growth retardation, weight loss: signs of malabsorption.

Investigations

Full blood count: to check for normochromic anemia of chronic disease, microcytic anemia of iron deficiency, macrocytic anemia (B_{12} and folate deficiency); increased platelets, leukocyte count markers of infection or inflammation.

ESR or CRP measurement: inflammatory markers of disease activity.

Vitamin and mineral measurements: magnesium, vitamin B_{12}, folate, iron, calcium, albumin deficiencies useful markers of absorptive function of small bowel.

Colonoscopy: allows assessment of colonic disease and possibly visualization of terminal ileum and appropriate biopsy; Crohn's is characterized by intermittent disease (*e.g.*, aphthous or serpiginous ulcers) separated by areas of normal mucosa. Although perianal involvement is common, the rectum is often normal; strictures may be evidence of prior inflammation.

Biopsy: reveals crypt distortion and inflammation; classically, granulomas are present, but in practice they often are not seen.

Upper gastrointestinal endoscopy: if relevant symptoms; lesions must be biopsied to confirm that they are due to Crohn's disease.

Radiography: features depend on site of disease; rose-thorn ulceration, string sign, skip lesions, cobblestone mucosa, stricture, fistulous tracts.

Barium imaging: follow-through allows assessment of small-bowel mucosal disease; useful in assessing stricture formation and defining anatomy for surgery; barium enema may complement colonoscopy, particularly in checking for fistulas.

Ultrasonography and CT: useful when checking for extraintestinal blood collections (*e.g.*, abscesses).

Radioisotope-labelled leukocyte scans: may be of use in localizing inflammation and sepsis.

Complications

Intestinal obstruction or perforation, intra-abdominal sepsis.

Fistula formation: to bowel, bladder, vagina, or skin.

Malnutrition, vitamin (*e.g.*, B_{12}) deficiency.

Uveitis, episcleritis.

Amyloid: related to inflammation; rare.

Renal oxalate stones: rare.

Differential diagnosis

Terminal ileal disease

Tuberculosis.

Yersinia spp. infection.

Lymphoma.

Colonic disease

Ulcerative colitis.

Bacterial infections (*Salmonella*, *Shigella*, *Campylobacter* spp.).

Amebic infection.

Pseudomembranous colitis.

Colonic carcinoma.

Etiology

Unknown.

• Crohn's disease is caused by multifocal granulomatous vasculitis.

Possible genetic influences: studies have shown familial clustering, suggesting a genetic predisposition.

Possible viral infections: measles virus identified in vascular endothelium [1].

Epidemiology

• The prevalence of Crohn's disease is 1 in 1000.

• Ethnic clustering has been found.

• Onset may be in childhood.

• The disease most commonly presents in the third decade.

• The male : female ratio is equal.

Histology

Macroscopic

Discontinuous disease with skip lesions.

Transmural inflammation.

Microscopic

Crypt distortion with inflammation.

Noncaseating granuloma.

Lymphocytic infiltrate.

Treatment

Diet and lifestyle

• Nutritional supplementation is needed in patients with severe illness, including total parenteral nutrition in advanced disease.

• Elemental diets may be effective but are poorly tolerated because of unpalatability; remission induced by elemental diets does not continue after diets have been stopped.

Pharmacological treatment

• Disease activity must be monitored using symptoms, signs and occasionally inflammatory markers (ESR).

Corticosteroids

Standard dose Prednisone, 30–60 mg orally (consider i.v. administration in hospitalized patients with poor motility and absorptive function); topical steroids for rectal or perianal disease.

Contraindications Overt sepsis; caution in hypertension and diabetes.

Special points May exacerbate growth retardation by premature fusion of epiphyses.
Hip pain should immediately raise concern about possible aseptic necrosis.
Long-term use should be avoided if possible, especially in young patients.

Main drug interactions Significant immunosuppression with azathioprine: risk of opportunistic infections increased, immunization against varicella should be considered in patients without a history of chicken pox and negative antibody titer.

Main side effects Fluid retention and hypertension, induction of glucose intolerance, osteoporosis, cushingoid features.

5-aminosalicylic acid preparations

• Sulfasalazine, mesalamine, or olsalazine may be of some benefit in extensive ileocolonic disease and in Crohn's colitis [2,3].

Standard dosage Sulfasalazine, 4 g daily; mesalamine, 2.4–4.8 g daily.

Contraindications Salicylate hypersensitivity, sulfonamide sensitivity with sulfasalazine, renal impairment with mesalamine.

Special points Sulfasalazine causes reversible oligospermia, may cause hemolysis; slow-release preparation of mesalamine of particular benefit in small-bowel Crohn's disease.

Main drug interactions None of major clinical importance.

Main side effects Nausea, rashes, occasional diarrhea.

Antibiotics

• Antibiotics are effective in some situations, particularly in perianal disease; they are of some benefit in small bowel disease but mainly of use in colonic disease.

Standard dosage Metronidazole, 500 mg orally 3 times daily.

Contraindications Previous hypersensitivity, peripheral neuropathy.

Special points Patients should avoid using alcohol (Antabuse effect).

Main drug interactions Enhances effects of warfarin; inhibits metabolism of phenytoin.

Main side effects Nausea, metallic taste, risk of neuropathy (long-term use).

Other immunosuppressive drugs

• These are useful as steroid-sparing agents and for additional immunosuppression in resistant disease [4].

Standard dosage Azathioprine, 1.0–1.5 mg/kg once daily.

Contraindications Neutropenia.

Special points Risk of myelotoxicity maximal on starting treatment; whole blood count must be monitored closely, particularly in first few weeks, monthly thereafter.

Main drug interactions Additive immunosuppressive effect with steroids.

Main side effects Rashes, nausea, myelosuppression, increased risk of opportunistic infection, pancreatitis.

Treatment aims

To suppress disease activity.
To restore quality of life.
To prevent complications.
To correct nutritional deficiencies.

Other treatments

• Conservative surgery (limited resection or stricturoplasty when possible to avoid short-bowel syndromes) is indicated for the following:

Acute: acute ileitis with signs of acute abdomen at presentation, fulminating colitis, uncontrolled or severe rectal hemorrhage (rare), intra-abdominal collections (abscesses), refractory to medical management, ruptured viscus with peritonism.

Chronic: subacute intestinal obstruction from fibrosis or scarring, fistulae, chronic debilitating disease unresponsive to medical treatment.

Prognosis

• Modern medical treatment, improved immunosuppressive regimens, and conservative surgery have greatly decreased the incidence of long-term complications.

• The risk of carcinoma is increased slightly in excluded loops.

Follow-up and management

• Close outpatient follow-up, especially during relapse, is recommended.

• Signs and symptoms of a disease flare do not typically require restaging of disease unless medical management fails to arrest the disease or surgery is anticipated.

• Disease activity correlates closely with elevations of the acute-phase reactant, ESR, although this is similarly raised in infective complications.

Key references

1. Podolsky DK: Inflammatory bowel disease (parts I and II). *N Engl J Med* 1991, **325**:928–937.
2. Griffiths A, *et al.*: Slow-release 5-aminosalicylic acid therapy in children with small intestinal Crohn's disease. *J Pediatr Gastroenterol Nutr* 1993, **17**:186–192.
3. Geier DL, *et al.*: New therapeutic agents in the treatment of inflammatory bowel disease. *Am J Med* 1992, **93**:1991–208.
4. Reynolds PD, *et al.*: Pharmacotherapy of inflammatory bowel disease. *Dig Dis* 1993, **11**:334–342.

Diagnosis

Symptoms

Weight gain: face, chest, and abdomen more than arms and legs.

Hirsutism, acne.

Thin skin, easy bruising, stretch marks.

Muscle weakness and aching.

Menstrual disturbance, impotence, loss of libido.

Back pain, loss of height, pain from other osteoporosis-related fractures.

Depression, anxiety, psychiatric disturbance.

Thirst, polyuria, nocturia: sometimes associated with diabetes mellitus.

Signs

Centripetal obesity: may be simply a relative change in fat distribution; many patients with Cushing's syndrome are overweight rather than obese; morbid obesity rare.

"Moon face," hirsutism, facial plethora.

Thin skin relative to age, easy bruising, pigmentation, acne, red abdominal striae (not just stretch marks, which are common in obese patients and after pregnancy).

Proximal myopathy: *e.g.*, difficulty rising from squat without assistance.

Hypertension: incidental finding or with symptoms of cardiovascular complications.

Kyphosis, loss of height.

Lower-limb edema: common.

Androgenic hair loss: occasionally.

Investigations [1]

• All tests may give false-positive and false-negative results, so only the simple screening tests should be done by nonspecialists.

Simple screening tests for Cushing's syndrome

24-h urinary free cortisol measurement: raised concentration in Cushing's syndrome; a simple test when diagnosis is clinically unlikely but must be excluded.

Overnight dexamethasone suppression test: dexamethasone, 1 mg, given orally at 23.00 h. At 08.00 h normal suppression of serum cortisol is to <5 μg/mL; patients with Cushing's syndrome fail to suppress.

Confirmatory investigations for diagnosis of Cushing's syndrome

Low dose dexamethasone suppression: dexamethasone, 0.5 mg orally every 6 h for 2 days. At 08.00 h on day 3 cortisol fails to suppress to <5 μg/mL in Cushing's syndrome.

High dose dexamethasone suppression: dexamethasone, 2 mg orally every 6 h for 2 days. At 08.00 h on day 3 cortisol suppresses to <5μg/mL in patients with Cushing's disease (pituitary tumor) but not in patients with corticotropic hormone (ACTH)–independent Cushing's syndrome (adrenal adenoma).

Differential diagnosis of the cause of proven Cushing's syndrome

Plasma ACTH measurement: undetectable concentration confirms adrenal Cushing's syndrome; values >400 ng/L suggest ectopic tumor.

Plasma potassium measurement: low concentration in most patients with ectopic ACTH.

CT or MRI of adrenals: shows adrenal tumors or macronodular hyperplasia.

MRI or CT of pituitary gland: may show corticotroph adenoma, but false-positives and false-negatives common.

Corticotropin-releasing hormone test: pituitary Cushing's disease frequently shows exaggerated response; other causes do not.

Petrosal sinus sampling catheterization: confirms pituitary ACTH secretion with near certainty. Requires well trained invasive radiologist [2].

Complications

Diabetes, infections, osteoporosis, thromboembolism, ischemic heart disease, cerebrovascular disease, peripheral vascular disease.

Differential diagnosis

Simple obesity.

Polycystic ovarian syndrome.

• Few patients with obesity, hirsutism, bruising, stretch marks, hypertension, or diabetes have Cushing's syndrome.

Etiology [3]

Corticotropic hormone (ACTH)-dependent Cushing's syndrome

• Pituitary Cushing's disease (70% of patients) is usually due to a (basophil) corticotroph microadenoma, but macro-adenoma, corticotroph hyperplasia, and normal tissue structure are found.

• Ectopic ACTH secretion (10%) is usually due to tumors of neuroendocrine origin (carcinoid, metastatic gastrointestinal endocrine tumors).

•Ectopic corticotropin-releasing hormone secretion is rare.

Adrenal Cushing's syndrome

• Causes include adrenal adenoma (10%), adrenal carcinoma (10%), and macro-nodular adrenal hyperplasia (rare).

Iatrogenic Cushing's syndrome

• The most common cause of the clinical syndrome, this is due to steroid or ACTH treatment.

Epidemiology

• Spontaneous Cushing's syndrome is rare.

• Cushing's syndrome and adrenal adenomas occur more often in women.

Ectopic corticotropic hormone (ACTH) syndrome

Occult ectopic ACTH syndrome

• This is usually seen when a neuroendocrine tumor (mostly carcinoid, of bronchial or thymic origin) secretes large amounts of ACTH and mimics a pituitary adenoma.

• The tumor may be only a few millimeters in diameter and only discovered after intensive imaging; diagnosis may prove difficult with conventional tests.

Overt ectopic ACTH secretion

• Many malignant tumors secrete ACTH, most often bronchial small-cell carcinoma; usually the tumor is clinically obvious.

• Patients are rarely cushingoid; they may have no endocrine symptoms or may exhibit pigmentation, myopathy, weight loss, and debility, associated with high cortisol and ACTH concentrations and profound hypokalemic alkalosis.

Treatment

Diet and lifestyle

- Patients must avoid the risk of fractures or skin abrasions.
- Patients should avoid high salt intake when hypertension is present.

Pharmacological treatment

- Medical treatment for Cushing's syndrome is effective in improving the clinical syndrome but is a short-term measure to prepare the patient for surgery, while awaiting the long-term benefit of other treatment, or in patients with inoperable tumors.
- Drugs include metyrapone, ketoconazole, aminoglutethimide, and mitotane; all have significant problems and should be used only under specialist supervision.

Nonpharmacological treatment

For Cushing's disease

Transsphenoidal surgery: treatment of choice for proven pituitary disease, with selective adenomectomy if possible; successful surgery usually results in temporary adrenal insufficiency (due to suppression of normal axis) [4].

Alternatives for surgical failures: pituitary irradiation, bilateral adrenalectomy.

For ectopic corticotropic hormone syndrome

Surgical excision: treatment of choice if technically possible and if tumor secreting hormone can be localized.

Radiotherapy or chemotherapy: for some ectopic tumors.

Alternatives if tumor cannot be localized or removed: longer-term medical treatment, bilateral adrenalectomy.

For adrenal tumors

Excision of adrenal adenomas: usually complete, with cure of clinical syndrome and temporary adrenal insufficiency due to suppression of normal axis.

Excision of adrenal carcinomas: sometimes complete, although these carcinomas are often inoperable and usually recur (in which case, medical treatment is essential).

Treatment aims

To restore a normally functioning hypothalamo–pituitary axis, without damage to other endocrine axes.

Prognosis

- Young patients with mild Cushing's disease cured by transsphenoidal surgery without recurrence should have normal life expectancy.
- Patients with adrenal carcinoma usually suffer recurrence and death within months.
- Before effective treatment was available, 50% of patients with Cushing's syndrome died within 5 years of diagnosis.
- The overall "cure" rate for transsphenoidal surgery is usually 75%–80% but can be as low as 50% (depending on the criteria used to define cure).
- Bilateral adrenalectomy is 100% effective, but patients suffer from life-long hypoadrenalism and are at risk of Nelson's syndrome (pituitary hyperplasia).
- For adrenal adenomas, surgical excision cures most patients.

Follow-up and management

- Follow-up must be life-long because of the risk of recurrence and morbidity.
- Management depends on the individual patient and should be done by specialists.

Key references

1. Trainer PJ, Grossman A: The diagnosis and differential diagnosis of Cushing's syndrome. *Clin Endocrinol* 1991, **34**:317–330.
2. Oldfield EH, *et al.*: Petrosal sinus sampling with and without corticotrophin-releasing hormone for the differential diagnosis of Cushing's syndrome. *N Engl J Med* 1991, **325**:897–905.
3. Howlett TA, Rees LH, Besser GM: Cushing's syndrome. *Clin Endocrinol Metab* 1985, **14**:911–945.
4. Burke CW, *et al.*: Transsphenoidal surgery for Cushing's disease: does what is removed determine endocrine outcome? *Clin Endocrinol* 1990, **33**:525–537.

Diagnosis

Symptoms

Loss of vision, floaters, decrease in visual acuity, unexplained fever: indicating retinitis (asymptomatic at early stage).

Fever, anorexia, weight loss, diarrhea, pain, cramps: indicating gastrointestinal tract infection (esophagitis, gastritis, colitis).

Fever, motor deficit, headaches, seizures, somnolence: indicating polyradiculopathy.

Fever, cough, dyspnea: indicating pneumonitis.

Signs

Fever: in 60%–80% of patients with cytomegalovirus disseminated infection.

Decreased visual acuity: indicating retinitis.

Weight loss, abdominal tenderness, hemorrhages: indicating gastrointestinal tract infections.

Neurological deficit, lethargy, coma: indicating CNS complications.

Increase of respiratory rate, minimal findings at auscultation: indicating pneumonitis.

Investigations

• The disease is caused by recrudescence of a latent infection, so serological tests are of limited value.

Fundoscopy: in retinitis, shows hemorrhagic exudates and necrotic areas.

Endoscopy: in gastrointestinal tract infection, shows submucosal hemorrhages, ulceration; each level of tract may be involved, *e.g.*, esophagus, stomach, duodenum, small intestine, or colon.

Ultrasonography: in cholangitis, shows dilatation of biliary tract.

Biopsy: in cholangitis, shows cytomegalovirus inclusions.

CSF culture: in encephalitis or myelitis, shows increased cells (nonspecific), presence of cytomegalovirus (unusual) in culture or polymerase chain reaction.

CT or MRI: in encephalitis or myelitis, shows ventriculitis or ependymitis, using contrast enhancement.

Transbronchial biopsy: in pneumonitis, shows cytomegalovirus inclusions.

Fundoscopic appearance of cytomegalovirus retinitis.

Complications

Loss of vision, retinal detachment, acute retinal necrosis.

Gastrointestinal tract perforation, hemorrhages.

Respiratory failure.

Coma or death.

Differential diagnosis

Retinitis

Cotton-wool spot.

Toxoplasmosis.

Herpes simplex or varicella–zoster virus.

Acute retinal necrosis.

Syphilis.

Pneumocystis carinii choroiditis.

Gastrointestinal tract

Cryptosporidiosis or microsporidiosis.

Giardia, Entamoeba, Shigella, Salmonella, or *Campylobacter* spp. infection.

Lymphoma.

Kaposi's sarcoma.

Encephalitis or myelitis

HIV encephalopathy or myelopathy.

Progressive multifocal leukoencephalopathy.

Aseptic meningitis.

Herpes virus encephalitis.

Pneumonitis

Pneumocystis carinii infection.

Mycobacteria infection.

Etiology

• Reactivation of latent cytomegalovirus infection due to underlying immune deficiency may be a cause.

• Cytomegalovirus infection is a potential cofactor of HIV disease.

Epidemiology

• >90% of homosexual or bisexual men have latent cytomegalovirus infection.

• Cytomegalovirus disease is found in 20%–40% of AIDS patients.

• End-stage opportunistic infection occurs in 90% of patients with CD4 counts of <50×10^6/L (median, 25×10^6/L).

Treatment

Diet and lifestyle

• No special precautions are necessary.

Pharmacological treatment

Choice of treatment

• Systemic treatment is indicated in acute visceral localization. Ganciclovir and foscarnet have similar efficacy: 90% in retinitis, 80%–95% in gastrointestinal tract disorder, 60%–80% in pneumonitis.

• Maintenance treatment is indicated for retinitis and gastrointestinal tract involvement (non-systematically). Ganciclovir and foscarnet have similar efficacy: 50% relapse within 4 months.

Ganciclovir

• Ganciclovir is more practical than foscarnet.

• It is used for systemic therapy.

• It is active against cytomegalovirus and herpesvirus.

• Disadvantages include hemotoxicity and resistance in some strains of cytomegalovirus.

Standard dosage *Acute:* ganciclovir, 5 mg/kg i.v. twice daily, 20 min infusion for 2–3 weeks.
Maintenance: ganciclovir, 5 mg/kg i.v. once daily long term.

Contraindications Neutropenia, anemia, resistant strains.

Main drug interactions Zidovudine and other hemotoxic drugs.

Main side effects Neutropenia, thrombocytopenia (frequent); rash-convulsion (unusual).

• Recently, oral ganciclovir, 3 g daily, has been shown to reduce progression after i.v. induction. Prophylaxis with this drug for patients with CD4 counts $<100 \times 10^6$/L reduces the rate of subsequent cytomegalovirus disease.

Foscarnet

• Foscarnet is active against all herpesviruses, including cytomegalovirus, and HIV.

• Advantages include absence of hemotoxicity and anti-HIV effect; disadvantages include the long infusion time.

Standard dosage *Acute:* foscarnet, 90 mg/kg in 0.75–1 L saline isotonic solution i.v. twice daily 90 min infusion for 2–3 weeks.
Maintenance: foscarnet, 90 mg/kg 0.75–1 L saline isotonic solution i.v. once daily, 90–120 min infusion.

Contraindications Renal impairment, concomitant nephrotoxic drugs.

Main drug interactions Amphotericin B, i.v. pentamidine.

Main side effects Nephrotoxicity, hypocalcemia, hypophosphatemia, nausea, genital ulcer.

Treatment aims

To prevent replication of cytomegalovirus.

To halt progress of disease.

Prognosis

• The incidence of visceral manifestations of cytomegalovirus is approximately 30%.

• Median survival is 12–18 months.

• With maintenance treatment, retinitis relapse has a high rate (>70%) and occurs approximately 2 months after therapy.

Follow-up and management

• Patients having acute treatment should be followed up every week.

• Patients having maintenance treatment must be followed up every 2–3 weeks.

General references

1. Dieterich D: Cytomegalovirus colitis in AIDS. *J Acquir Immune Defic Syndr* 1991 **Suppl 1**:529–535.
2. Jabs D, SOCA group: Mortality in patients with acquired immunodeficiency syndrome treated with either foscarnet or ganciclovir for cytomegalovirus retinitis. *N Engl J Med* 1992, **326**:213–220.
3. Katlama C, *et al.*: Foscarnet induction therapy from CMV retinitis in AIDS. Comparison of twice daily and three times daily regimens. *J Acquir Immune Defic Syndr* 1992, **5**:518–524.

Diagnosis

Definition

• Dementia is the syndrome of impairment in multiple domains of cognition, which must include memory, with intact consciousness.
• Symptoms, signs, and investigations are used to differentiate potentially treatable causes of dementias from the degenerative dementias.

Symptoms [1]

• Patients may be unaware of deficits and deny symptoms (anosognosia); a history from a caregiver is therefore essential.
Memory loss: the most common presenting symptom.
Psychiatric disturbances: including depression, hallucinations, or behavioral changes.
Dysphasia, dyspraxia, visuospatial dysfunction, behavioral change: usually progressive and may occur in any order.
• Additional symptoms depend on the cause, *e.g.*, the following:
Headache: due to space-occupying lesions or temporal arteritis.
Fatigue: due to systemic disease (*e.g.*, HIV, hypothyroidism).
Weight loss: due to neoplasia.
Peripheral neuropathy: due to vitamin B_{12} deficiency, alcohol.
Seizures: may occur in patients with Alzheimer's disease or may have a focal cause.
Gait disturbances: can be seen in normal pressure hydrocephalus.
Focal neurological symptoms: including hemiparesis can be seen in multi-infarct dementia.

Signs

• The primary degenerative dementias (*e.g.*, Alzheimer's disease) have few signs other than those relating to higher cortical function.
Primitive reflexes (grasp, rooting, sucking), spasticity: late in dementia.
More widespread dysfunction: in dementia plus syndromes, *e.g.*, Huntington's disease (dementia plus chorea), multi-infarct dementia (dementia plus focal motor signs).
Papilledema or focal signs: suggesting a potentially treatable intracranial cause.

Investigations [2]

• Few specific tests are available, and none for the most common cause, Alzheimer's disease.
• Investigations are aimed at excluding secondary causes, *e.g.*, cerebral neoplasms, metabolic disturbances.
Psychometry: to assess pattern and severity of cognitive impairment and influence of the affective components.
Full blood count, ESR measurement, routine biochemistry.
Serum vitamin B_{12} and thyroid function tests.
Treponemal serology.
HIV antibody serology: in some patients.
Chest radiography.
ECG.
EEG: to exclude Creutzfeldt-Jakob disease or concomitant epilepsy.
CT or MRI: to exclude mass lesions, assess vascular changes, and determine regional atrophy.
Positron emission tomography: if available, to assess regional metabolism.
Lumbar puncture: in selected patients with rapidly progressing symptoms to exclude inflammatory changes.
Cerebral biopsy: rarely used; can provide definitive histological diagnosis.

Complications

Bronchopneumonia: due to aspiration.
Parkinsonism or seizures: can be late complications of several degenerative dementias.
Incontinence.

Differential diagnosis

Acute confusional states or delirium with fluctuating impairment of arousal.
Korsakoff's and Wernicke's syndromes secondary to alcohol abuse.
Focal neuropsychological deficits, *e.g.*, dysphasia.
"Pseudodementia" resulting from impairment of cognitive function by anxiety or depression.

Etiology

• Any disease disrupting the function of corticocortical or subcorticocortical connections can cause dementia, *e.g.*, the following:

Causes of degenerative dementia
Alzheimer's disease, frontal-lobe degeneration, Pick's disease, cortical Lewy body disease, Huntington's disease, prion disease.
• Some hereditary dementias are associated with specific genetic markers, *e.g.*, rare families with Alzheimer's disease and amyloid precursor protein (APP) gene mutations, later-onset disease with the apolipoprotein E4 genotype.
• Neuropathologically, dementia of Alzheimer's disease is associated with senile plaques and neurofibrillary tangles in the cerebral cortex.
• ~15% of Alzheimer's disease is familial.

Vascular causes
Multiple cortical or subcortical infarcts, small-vessel disease (Binswanger's disease).

Potentially treatable causes
Neoplasms, normal-pressure hydrocephalus, trauma, subdural and extradural hematomas, drugs or toxins.
Vitamin B_{12} deficiency, hypothyroidism, renal and hepatic dysfunction, inherited metabolic disease.
Multiple sclerosis, temporal arteritis, cerebral vasculitis, sarcoid.
HIV, neurosyphilis, chronic viral encephalitides, chronic meningitides, cerebral Whipple's disease.

Epidemiology

• Dementia is common in elderly patients, occurring in 2%–5% >65 years; 20%–40% >80 years.
• Alzheimer's disease is the most common cause, accounting for 50% of dementia patients and a further 15%–20% in association with vascular disease.

Treatment

Diet and lifestyle

• Patients must avoid fatigue, alcohol, and centrally active medications unless clearly indicated.

• Patients should use cognitive aids, *e.g.*, clear labeling, diary, calendars.

• Medicalert bracelets should be worn.

• Safety issues including driving, using potentially dangerous equipment, and wandering need to be addressed.

Pharmacological treatment [3]

• The treatment of dementia is firstly the treatment of the underlying cause when possible, *e.g.*, removal of meningioma, vitamin B_{12} replacement.

• No drugs are known to alter disease progression of the degenerative dementias.

• The degeneration in Alzheimer's disease particularly affects the glutamatergic cortico-cortical association pyramidal neurones and the subcortico-cortical cholinergic projection neurons; cholinergic enhancement can improve memory in cholinergic-deficit states.

Tacrine may be helpful to slow progression in some early cases [4].

Standard dosage Tetrahydroaminoacridine (tacrine), 40–160 mg daily in divided doses

Contraindications Pregnancy, hepatic disease.

Main drug interactions None.

Main side effects Cholinergic effects, hepatotoxicity.

• Other medications are under investigation.

• Many medications can be useful to manage psychiatric and behavioral problems, including antidepressants and anxiolytics.

Treatment aims

To treat the underlying cause, when possible.

Prognosis

• Prognosis depends on the causative disease.

Follow-up and management

• Management involves many disciplines: neurologists, psychiatrists, and geriatricians.

• Early involvement of social work and community psychiatric services is important.

Social support

Alzheimer's Association, 919 N. Michigan Ave., Suite 1000, Chicago, IL 60611-1676; phone (312) 335-870 or (800) 272-3900.

Legal issues

• Patients should consider referring legal affairs to someone else (power of attorney).

Key references

1. Burns A, Levy R (eds): *Dementia*. London: Chapman Hall, 1994.
2. Cummings JL, Benson DF: *Dementia: A Clinical Approach*, edn 2. Oxford: Butterworth Heinemann; 1992.
3. Rossor MN: Management of neurological disorders: dementia. *J Neurol Neurosurg Psychiatry* 1994, **57**:1451–1456.
4. Knapp MJ, *et al.*: A thirty week randomized controlled trial of high dose tacrine in patients with Alzheimer's disease. *JAMA* 1994, **271**:985–991.

Depression and mania

Diagnosis

Symptoms and signs

• In both mania and major depression, mood-congruent delusions may arise; these may be accompanied by auditory hallucinations.

Mania

Distinct periods of elevated expansion or irritable mood, with three or more of the following:

Hyperactivity.

Pressure of speech.

Flight of ideas.

Subjective self-esteem, euphoria, grandiosity.

Reduced sleep.

Distractability.

Recklessness.

Major depression [1,2]

Distinct periods of dysphoric mood, loss of interest or pleasure in usual activities, with the following:

Change in appetite or weight.

Sleep disturbance.

Psychomotor agitation or retardation.

Anergia.

Difficulty in concentrating or making decisions.

Hopelessness.

Suicidal thoughts or attempts.

Dysthymia

Chronic disturbance with depressed mood, lasting 2 years: similar symptoms to a major depressive episode but less severe.

• A major depressive episode may be imposed on dysthymia ("double depression").

Investigations [1]

• Laboratory investigations are of limited use because of the frequency of false-positive and false-negative results.

• In middle-aged and elderly patients, however, investigations to rule out secondary depression (*e.g.*, associated with occult neoplasm or endocrine disturbance) may be warranted if the patient's symptomatology suggests physical illness.

Assessment of severity of episode: presence of delusions or hallucinations, prominent vegetative symptoms, and large number of symptoms indicate increasing severity; rating scales, *e.g.*, Beck or Hamilton, useful because they give quantitative measurement of severity and can be repeated to produce a serial profile of the episode.

Assessment of probability of suicide: indicated by level of hopelessness, social isolation, presence of delusions, suicide planning or previous attempts, concurrent personality disorder, alcoholism, or drug abuse.

Assessment of impact of episode: on social relationships, work.

Complications

High suicide rate: 15%.

Distress to others in the patient's social network: *e.g.*, spouse, children.

Impairment in occupational function: *e.g.*, reduced productivity, absenteeism, unemployment.

Death due to dehydration and malnutrition: in elderly patients.

Differential diagnosis

Mania or hypomania

Organic affective syndrome: *e.g.*, amphetamines or steroids.
Schizoaffective disorder.
Cyclothymia.

Major depression

Organic affective syndrome: *e.g.*, steroids.
Dementia: in elderly patients.
Schizophrenia, schizoaffective disorder.
Dysthymia, cyclothymia.
Chronic anxiety state.
Uncomplicated bereavement.

Dysthymia

Major depression.
Personality disorder: *e.g.*, dependent, borderline, histrionic.
Normal fluctuation of mood.

Etiology

• Causes include the following:

Biological factors

Genetic: bipolar and major depressive disorders are familial; increased evidence of inheritability for bipolar disorder.
Neurochemical: activity of biogenic amines (*i.e.*, 5-HT, noradrenaline) decreased in depression, increased in mania.

Psychosocial factors

Psychoanalytic: introjection of an ambivalently viewed lost object leads to a rigid superego punishing person for sexual or aggressive impulses.
Cognitive: depression results from habitual maladaptive ways of thinking or from a perceived inability to control events (learned helplessness).
Adverse life event: current adversity (especially loss events) leads to depression by interacting with other vulnerability factors and temperament.

Epidemiology

• The lifetime expectancy of suffering from major depression is 10% in men and 20% in women; for mania, the expectancy is 1% for men and women.

• The female:male ratio is 2:1 for major depression and 1:1 for mania.

Treatment

Diet and lifestyle

• No special precautions are necessary.

Pharmacological treatment

For depression [1]

• Depression is a recurrent disorder; hence the impact of treatment must be evaluated in terms of the following:

Response: reduction of symptoms with treatment.
Remission: resolution of symptoms for a continuous period in an episode.
Recovery: a stable remission lasting at least 4–6 months.
Relapse: symptoms recur during remission.
Recurrence: a new episode after recovery.

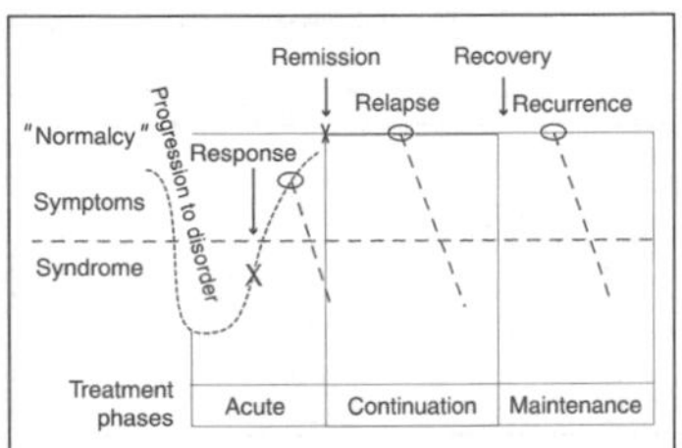

Stages of evaluation for major depression.

Standard dosage	Tricyclic antidepressants, *e.g.*, imipramine, 75 mg, increasing to 150 mg, or specific 5-HT re-uptake inhibitor, *e.g.*, fluoxetine, 20 mg, to obtain remission.
Contraindications	Recent myocardial infarction, heart block.
Special points	Response in ~70% of patients (30% respond to placebo), may take 4–6 weeks; failure may be due to inadequate level of treatment or poor compliance. Medication at full dose or psychotherapy continued for at least 6 months after resolution of symptoms to prevent relapse. The World Health Organization recommends prophylaxis for anyone with more than one severe episode in the preceding 5 years.
Main drug interactions	Hypertensive crises with monoamine oxidase inhibitors.
Main side effects	Anticholinergic effects, sedation, weight gain, sexual dysfunction.

• In patients who do not respond to two successive trials of different medications given for an adequate duration, diagnosis, previous treatment, and compliance must be reviewed.

• Failure to obtain remission is associated with increased duration of symptoms, severity of episode, "double depression," and secondary depression.

• Further interventions include augmentation of the antidepressant regimen with lithium or carbamazepine, simultaneous use of several antidepressants, or electroconvulsive therapy.

For mania or hypomania [3]

Standard dosage	*For acute episode:* combination of major tranquillizer, *e.g.*, haloperidol, 2–10 mg i.m., benzodiazepine, *e.g.*, lorazepam, 2 mg i.m., and lithium to achieve blood concentration 0.8–1.2 mmol/L. *For maintenance treatment:* lithium to achieve blood concentration 0.4–1 mmol/L.
Contraindications	Pregnancy, Addison's disease, renal impairment.
Special points	~50% of patients relapse with monotherapy, so drug may be combined with carbamazepine, clonazepam, or valproic acid; antidepressants (which may cause a relapsing cycle) and antipsychotics generally unhelpful.
Main drug interactions	Thiazide diuretics increase lithium concentration; specific 5-HT reuptake inhibitors increase CNS toxicity.
Main side effects	Gastrointestinal disturbances, fine tremor, polyurea, polydipsia.

• Complications of lithium therapy include hypothyroidism, glomerulonephropathy, and nephrogenic diabetes insipidus.

Treatment aims

To obtain remission and prevent relapse of major depression.

To prevent exacerbation of mania.

Other treatments

Electroconvulsive therapy

• For depressed patients with delusions, catatonic stupor, and severe suicidal tendencies or severely depressed patients in whom pharmacotherapy is not indicated.

• Side effects are cognitive: a transient postictal confusional state, longer-term memory impairment.

Psychotherapy

• Cognitive behavioral therapy or interpersonal psychotherapy are no more effective than pharmacotherapy in obtaining remission but may be more effective in preventing relapse.

• Psychotherapy is less effective when depression is severe.

Prognosis

• 50% of patients with major depression remit by 6 months; 12% fail to remit by 5 years.

• The rate of recurrence of major depression varies widely; some patients need long-term maintenance treatment.

• Patients with bipolar disorders have a poorer prognosis than those with major depression, with recurrence and rehospitalization the norm.

• Only 15% of patients with bipolar disorders remain well.

Follow-up and management

• Bipolar patients and some depressed patients have a chronic disorder needing life-long treatment; specialized mood disorder clinics improve compliance and encourage early intervention and group or peer support.

Key references

1. *Depression in Primary Care*. Rockville: US Department of Health and Human Services, Public Health Agency, Agency for Health Care Policy and Research; 1993. [AHCPR Publication no. 93-055.]
2. Mulrow CD, *et al.*: Case-finding instruments for depression in primary care. *Ann Intern Med* 1995, **122**:913–921.
3. Price LH, Heninger GR: Lithium in the treatment of mood disorders. *N Engl J Med* 1994, **331**:591–598.

Diagnosis

Symptoms

Polyuria, nocturia, excessive thirst (polydipsia).

Enuresis, sleep disturbances, difficulties at school: in children.

• Patients with mild disorder may be asymptomatic.

• During pregnancy, central diabetes insipidus symptoms may worsen because of the placental enzyme, vasopressinase.

Signs

• Central diabetes insipidus has few signs if patients drink enough.

Urine output 3–20 L/24 h.

Hypernatremic dehydration: due to loss of thirst sensation and resulting lack of water intake.

Investigations

Blood glucose and serum sodium, potassium, urea, creatinine, and calcium measurement: to confirm diagnosis of central diabetes insipidus, to identify patients needing specific tests, to exclude other causes of polyuria.

Water deprivation test: cheap and easy to perform but often gives equivocal results; fluid intake during night before test; all fluids withdrawn for up to 8 h (supervision essential); patient weighed hourly (test must be stopped if weight loss >5% of initial body weight); measurement of urine volume and urine and blood osmolality every 1–2 h for 12–16 h; administration of desmopressin, 2 µg i.m.

Infusion of 5% hypertonic saline solution: 2-h infusion, with measurements of plasma osmolality and vasopressin; provides definitive diagnosis of central diabetes insipidus and quick to perform but is expensive and needs facility to measure plasma vasopressin.

Therapeutic trial of desmopressin: 1–2 week trial with close supervision of body weight, urine volume and osmolality, and plasma osmolality differentiates the three major causes of diabetes insipidus (central, nephrogenic, primary polydipsia).

MRI: to identify cause of central diabetes insipidus; shows loss of hyperintense signal in neurohypophysis and presence of tumor.

Serum angiotensin-converting enzyme measurement: to detect sarcoid.

Complications

Bladder distension, hydroureter, hydronephrosis: with bladder outflow obstruction.

Secondary nephrogenic diabetes insipidus: due to renal interstitial solute washout.

Hypernatremic dehydration: if fluid intake inadequate.

Differential diagnosis

Nephrogenic diabetes insipidus.

Primary polydipsia.

Excessive fluid intake (*e.g.*, due to psychogenic polydipsia).

Diabetes mellitus.

Etiology [1]

• Diabetes insipidus is caused by inadequate quantities of osmoregulated vasopressin due to the following:

Familial causes

Dominant inheritance; gene deletions or substitutions.

Diabetes insipidus, diabetes mellitus, optic atrophy, nerve deafness (DIDMOAD).

Acquired causes

Idiopathic: possible infundibular hypophysitis.

Trauma: neurosurgery, head injury.

Tumors: craniopharyngioma, dysgerminoma, metastases.

Granulomas: sarcoidosis, histiocytosis.

Infection: meningitis, encephalitis.

Vascular disorders: Sheehan's syndrome, sickle cell disease.

Epidemiology

• Diabetes insipidus is a rare condition.

• The estimated prevalence is ~1 in 50 000.

• The male : female ratio is 3 : 2.

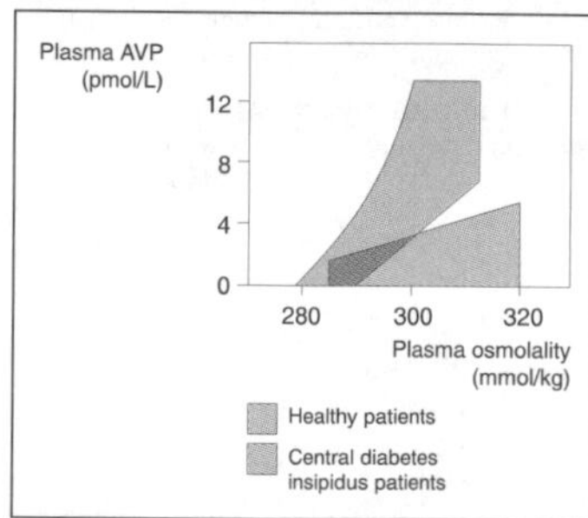

Responses of plasma osmolality and arginine vasopressin (AVP) to hypertonic saline infusion in healthy patients and those with central diabetes insipidus, who have subnormal AVP responses.

Treatment

Diet and lifestyle

• Patients must drink sufficient fluid to quench thirst in order to maintain water balance.

Pharmacological treatment [2,3]

DDAVP (desmopressin)

• DDAVP is a synthetic vasopressin analogue with minimal pressor activity and some resistance to degradation *in vivo;* it is the drug of choice.

Standard dosage	DDAVP, 5–40 μg intranasally daily, divided doses as spray or delivery by rhinal tube; or 0.5–4 μg i.m. or i.v. daily.
Contraindications	Rare hypersensitivity to drug vehicle; caution in renal disease.
Special points	Excessive fluid intake must be avoided. Intranasal preparations less well absorbed when patients have colds or chronic rhinitis. Administration technique must be checked with patients using the rhinal tube.
Main drug interactions	None known.
Main side effects	Hyponatremia (caused by persistent antidiuresis due to DDAVP with continued inappropriate fluid intake).

Pitressin

• This synthetically produced natural human hormone (arginine vasopressin) is not recommended for treatment of central diabetes insipidus because of its pressor activity and very short action.

Other options

• Specific treatment of the cause of central diabetes insipidus may relieve symptoms, *e.g.*, steroids for sarcoidosis (rare).

• Less effective oral preparations include chorpropamide, 250–500 mg daily, (hypoglycemia a major side effect) and carbamazepine, 200–600 mg daily.

Treatment aims

To reduce urine volume to 1–2 L/24 h.

To relieve thirst.

To avoid hyponatremia.

Prognosis

• Prognosis is excellent for treated patients.

• Patients with central diabetes insipidus rarely manage without replacement therapy unless the underlying disease is treated successfully.

Follow-up and management

• Care must be taken to avoid hyponatremia due to overtreatment with vasopressin analogues.

• Serum sodium or plasma osmolality should be measured routinely to ensure normal sodium concentrations.

Key references

1. Baylis PH: Vasopressin: physiology and disorders of hormone secretion. *Med Internat* 1993, **21**:189–196.
2. Robinson AG, Verbalis JG: Diabetes insipidus. *Curr Ther Endocrinol Metab* 1994, **5**:1–6.
3. Buonocore CM, Robinson AG: The diagnosis and management of diabetes insipidus during medical emergencies. *Endocrinol Metab Clin North Am* 1993, **22**:411–423.

Diagnosis

Symptoms

• Symptoms are usually of short duration (days to weeks), often longer in older patients.

Polyuria.

Polydipsia.

Weight loss.

Lethargy.

Diabetic ketoacidosis or coma: if disease undetected or ignored; symptoms more severe, followed by progressive loss of consciousness, with vomiting, abdominal pain, air hunger.

Signs

• Initially no symptoms are manifest.

Mild dehydration, weight loss, ketones on breath.

Shock, severe dehydration, Kussmaul's respiration, reduced level of consciousness: later signs.

Investigations

Laboratory blood glucose measurement: essential for diagnosis; glucose strips, even with meters, not sufficient.

Urinalysis: shows glycosuria and ketonuria.

Arterial blood gas measurement: shows metabolic acidosis.

Electrolyte analysis: wide variation, may show marked hyperkalemia and dehydration.

Complications [1]

• Complications are rare before 5–10 years' duration of diabetes.

Diabetic retinopathy: background affects >75% by 30 years, only affects vision if near macula; proliferative affects fewer but threatens vision by vitreous hemorrhage/fibrosis; treated by laser; most common cause of new adult blindness <65 years.

Diabetic nephropathy: affects up to 40% after 30 years, but rate probably now falling; proteinuria is hallmark, with progressive renal impairment; can be slowed by vigorous antihypertensive treatment, particularly angiotensin-converting enzyme (ACE) inhibitors; end-stage failure can be treated by continuous ambulatory peritoneal dialysis or transplantation.

Diabetic neuropathy: many forms, most common being symmetrical sensory polyneuropathy leading to loss of temperature, vibration, and pain sense, hence easy progression to foot ulceration; also several painful forms.

Large-vessel disease (coronary, cerebrovascular, peripheral): also much more common, especially when patient has nephropathy; possibly more diffuse than nondiabetic large-vessel disease, but otherwise generally similar.

• Other problems include skin disorders, especially necrobiosis, joint disorders, mononeuropathies, and cataracts.

• Intensive treatment and good glycemic control reduce the subsequent incidence of retinopathy, nephropathy, and neuropathy, but at the expense of more frequent hypoglycemia.

Differential diagnosis

• Diagnosis is not usually a problem, after diabetes mellitus has been considered; possible errors include the following:

Drug overdose and other causes of coma.

Pancreatitis or acute abdomen when abdominal pain is prominent.

Anorexia, thyrotoxicosis, malignancy when weight loss is severe.

• Deciding whether the patient is insulin-dependent can be difficult if the diagnosis is made early; in case of doubt, short-term insulin treatment should be given.

Etiology

• Insulin-dependent diabetes mellitus is associated with HLA DR3 and DR4.

• The process occurs via an autoimmune mechanism with antibodies against pancreatic islet-cells, which show insulitis and are progressively destroyed.

• The triggering environmental agent is not known.

Epidemiology

• Insulin-dependent diabetes mellitus can occur at any age, but onset is frequently in juveniles (hence the alternative term "juvenile-onset diabetes mellitus").

• It occurs most often in people of white race, especially in those furthest from the equator (Scandinavia, southern New Zealand); other races differ in genetic susceptibility (*e.g.*, West Indians have similar acute diabetes, but often not truly insulin-dependent or ketosis-prone).

• It affects ~3 in 1000 of the US population.

Treatment

Diet and lifestyle

• Dietetic advice is essential; the diet should be high in unrefined carbohydrate, low in simple sugars, with high fiber and low fat, spread throughout the day, ideally as three meals and three snacks, including one before bedtime.

• Normal activity is advised, except for a few career and driving limitations.

Pharmacological treatment [2]

• After insulin dependency has been established, exogenous insulin is needed.

Types of insulin

• Mainly human biosynthetic insulins are used; pork and beef insulins are still available in some preparations, primarily as Humulin or Novolin.

Short acting: regular or R.

Intermediate-acting (isophane): NPH or N.

Intermediate-acting (zinc): lente or L.

Long-acting: ultralente or U.

Premixed: 70/30.

Types of regimen

Once-daily: suited only for elderly, frail patients and those unable to self-inject.

Twice-daily: minimum for all normal patients, including variable dose self-mixing.

Added bedtime dose: mixture in morning, short-acting before supper, intermediate-acting before bedtime; flexible regimen, especially for patients troubled by overnight hypoglycemia.

Basal-bolus: long-acting overnight, short-acting boluses before meals.

Practical issues

Sites of injection: abdomen, leg or buttock, arm (s.c.)

Timing: usually 30 min before meal.

Exercise needs: extra food or reduced insulin dose.

Insulin infusion (variable rate): best method for ketoacidosis, for unstable diabetes, and during surgery.

Hypoglycemia

• This is the major unwanted effect of insulin treatment and the predominant concern of many patients.

• It is more common with long duration of diabetes, "tight control," and previous severe hypoglycemia.

• It mostly occurs between 10.00 and 13.00 h and overnight.

• Symptoms include sweating, shaking, hunger, palpitation, lack of concentration, confusion, and restlessness, later fits and coma.

• Hypoglycemia should be treated by oral glucose or food, i.v. glucose, or i.m. glucagon.

See Hypoglycemia *for details.*

Treatment aims

To restore normal well-being.

To achieve optimal glycemic control without significant hypoglycemia.

To provide patient education and self-care.

To prevent complications.

Prognosis

• The prognosis is excellent and improving in the short and medium terms, provided that the diagnosis is made and patient and carers are competent; ketoacidosis and hypoglycemia are rare causes of death.

• Longer-term prognosis largely depends on long-term glycemic control and compliance with screening and treatment [3].

• Major causes of death are end-stage renal failure and coronary artery disease.

• Major causes of morbidity include proliferative retinopathy leading to blindness, coronary artery disease and peripheral vascular disease, and neuropathy leading to foot ulceration, claudication, or gangrene.

Follow-up and management

• Long-term follow-up is essential for continued education, checks on control, hemoglobin A_{1c} home capillary blood glucose levels preprandially, and screening for complications (especially eye and foot examination, proteinuria).

• Potentially fertile women must have outstanding control before conception.

• Full patient and family education by specialist nurses and dietitians is essential.

• Most patients should test their own blood glucose and learn to adjust insulin.

Patient support

American Diabetes Association,
1660 Duke Street, Alexandria, VA 22314;
tel 1-800-ADA-DISC.

Key references

1. Day JL: *The Diabetes Handbook: Insulin-Dependent Diabetes*. London: Thorsons, British Diabetic Association; 1992.
2. Tattersall RB, Gale EAM, eds: *Diabetes: Clinical Management*. Edinburgh: Churchill Livingstone; 1990.
3. Diabetes Control and Complications Trial Research Group: The effect of intensive treatment of diabetes on the development and progression of long-term complications in insulin dependent diabetes. *N Engl J Med* 1993, **329**:977–986.

Diabetes mellitus, non–insulin-dependent

Diagnosis

Symptoms

• ~50% of patients are symptomatic, 50% found on routine or accidental screening.

• Common symptoms, often manifest over many months or years, include the following:

Polyuria, polydipsia.

Pruritus vulvae or balanitis.

Weight loss, tiredness, blurred vision.

Hyperglycemic nonketotic coma, with severe dehydration or hyperosmolality: rare manifestation.

Signs

• Generally, no signs are manifest.

• Patients may present with the following:

Obesity.

Foot ulceration or infection.

Diabetic retinopathy or peripheral neuropathy.

Signs of secondary causes of diabetes: *e.g.*, acromegaly, Cushing's disease, thyrotoxicosis.

Investigations

Blood glucose measurement: random capillary/venous blood glucose concentration >200 mg/dL in symptomatic patient is diagnostic; two random values or any fasting value >200 mg/dL is also diagnostic.

Glucose tolerance test: needed when diagnosis in doubt. After a 3-day high carbohydrate (>150 g/day) diet then overnight fast, patient takes 75 g glucose solution. Plasma glucose is measured before glucose administration then every 30 min for 2 h. Plasma glucose interpretation: ≥200 mg/dL at 2 h and any other time diagnostic for diabetes mellitus; ≥200 mg/dL before 2 h but >140 mg/dL and <200 mg/dL at 2 h and <140 mg/dL fasting is defined as impaired glucose tolerance; >200 mg/dL at 1 h but <140 mg/dL at 2 h is inderterminate and may require retesting.

Measurement of hemoglobin A_{1c}: raised concentration.

Measurement of iron and total iron-binding capacity: to rule out hemochromatosis.

Measurement of thyroxine and thyroid-stimulating hormone: to rule out thyrotoxicosis.

• Glycosuria alone and blood strip readings are never diagnostic.

Complications

• Complications are often present at the time of diagnosis (after years of hyperglycemia).

Diabetic retinopathy: may be present at diagnosis, only affects vision if near macula; macular edema frequent with major reduction of visual acuity; proliferative affects fewer but threatens vision by vitreous hemorrhage/fibrosis; both treated by laser.

Diabetic nephropathy: less common than in insulin-dependent diabetes mellitus, except in nonwhite races; proteinuria is marker for high cardiovascular risk, but not necessarily progressive renal impairment; can be slowed by vigorous antihypertensive treatment; end-stage failure can be treated by continuous ambulatory peritoneal dialysis or transplantation.

Diabetic neuropathy: many forms, most common being symmetrical sensory polyneuropathy leading to loss of temperature, vibration, and pain sense, hence easy progression to foot ulceration.

Large-vessel disease (coronary, cerebrovascular, peripheral): much more common especially when patient has nephropathy; possibly more diffuse than nondiabetic large-vessel disease, but otherwise generally similar; these, especially coronary artery disease, are major causes of premature death.

Differential diagnosis

• Diagnosis is not usually a problem, after diabetes mellitus has been thought of; possible errors include the following:

Urinary tract infection.

Prostatic hyperplasia.

Vaginal prolapse.

Primary polydipsia.

Diabetes insipidus.

Etiology [1]

• The cause of non–insulin-dependent diabetes mellitus is unknown; the disorder may be part of a constellation with hypertension and hyperlipidemia (Reaven's syndrome, syndrome X).

• Patients may have a mixture of "relative" insulin deficiency and insulin resistance, contributions of the two varying widely among individuals.

• Very rarely, patients have insulin receptor abnormalities.

• A strong familial component is evident, but the disorder is not directly inherited.

• A marked link with obesity is seen.

Epidemiology

• The prevalence varies widely among races, some populations having a prevalence of >50% by the age of 50 years.

• The US prevalence of diagnosed diabetes is ~3%, although an additional 3% may go undiagnosed.

• The disease is six times more common in Asians, about twice as common in Afro-Carribeans.

• It is probably becoming more common in the developed world.

Treatment

Diet and lifestyle

• The diet should be high in unrefined carbohydrate, low in simple sugars, with high fiber and low fat, spread throughout the day.

• Patients should aim at reducing excess body weight.

• Patients should engage in physical exercise and resume full activities; minimal limitations for those on some drugs include not driving commercial vehicles.

Pharmacological treatment [2]

• Diet alone should be used initially unless the patient is losing too much weight or is seriously symptomatic, in which case diet should be supplemented by pharmacological treatment.

Sulfonylureas

• These increase insulin response to glucose and tend to cause weight gain.

Standard dosage	Glyburide, 2.5–20 mg orally daily, given once or twice each day. Glipizide, 2.5–20 mg orally daily, given once or twice each day.
Contraindications	Breast-feeding, porphyria, pregnancy; caution in elderly patients and those with renal or hepatic failure.
Special points	Used only in conjunction with a diet.
Main drug interactions	Few of major clinical relevance (*see manufacturer's current prescribing information*).
Main side effects	Hypoglycemia is common; otherwise occasional rashes, jaundice, headache.

Biguanide

• Metformin reduces hepatic gluconeogenesis and probably decreases carbohydrate absorption.

Standard dosage	Metformin, 1–2.5 g daily in divided doses.
Contraindications	Hepatic or renal impairment (creatinine >1.4 in men or 1.3 in women), heart failure, pregnancy.
Special points	Does not cause hypoglycemia; may rarely cause lactic acidosis. Should be discontinued 2 days before and 2 days after any radiologic study using i.v. contrast.
Main drug interactions	Alcohol dependence may predispose to lactic acidosis.
Main side effects	Flatulence, anorexia, diarrhea, sometimes transient.

Insulin

• Insulin is indicated for symptomatic or uncontrolled diabetes mellitus despite maximal oral agents, in addition to diet.

• Usually, it is needed only once or twice daily; a longer-acting formulation may be used to control basal hyperglycemia.

See Diabetes mellitus, insulin-dependent *for details.*

Other options

Acarbose, 50 mg 3 times daily (alpha-glucosidase inhibitor): decreases rate of glucose absorption, thereby reducing postprandial glycemia; recent introduction.

Treatment aims

To restore normal well-being.

To achieve optimal glycemic control without significant hypoglycemia.

To provide patient education and self-care.

To prevent complications.

Prognosis

• Mortality is increased as a result of excess cardiovascular disease, myocardial infarction, stroke, and peripheral vascular disease.

• Morbidity is due to the same causes and also to retinopathy, renal disease, and foot ulceration.

• Oral hypoglycemics have not been proved to reduce mortality or morbidity.

Follow-up and management

• Patients need long-term follow-up for treatment aims and screening for development of complications.

• Glycosylated hemoglobin is an objective marker of glycemic control.

Patient support

American Diabetes Association,
1660 Duke Street, Alexandria, VA 22314;
tel 1-800-ADA-DISC.

Key references

1. Day JF: *The Diabetes Handbook: Non Insulin-Dependent Diabetes.* London: Thorsons, British Diabetic Association; 1992.

2. Tattersall RB, Gale EAM, eds: *Diabetes: Clinical Management.* Edinburgh: Churchill Livingstone; 1990.

Diabetic management in children

Diagnosis

Symptoms

• Children may not admit to any symptoms until very late.

Thirst: including unusual forms, *e.g.*, drinking bath water.

Polyuria: bed wetting.

Weight loss.

Decreased appetite.

Vomiting: possibly with abdominal pain.

Confusion: without coma.

Signs

Uncomplicated

Misery, irritability.

Dehydration.

Complicated

Semi-coma.

Deep but rapid respiration: Kussmaul's respiration.

Hypotension.

Infection: in ear, throat, lung, urinary tract.

Investigations

• The urine must always be tested for glucose in a sick child with some of the above symptoms or signs, even if atypical.

Urinalysis: urine should contain 2% glucose, maximum ketones read on text strip, should be cultured to exclude infection.

Blood glucose and plasma sodium, potassium, bicarbonate, and urea measurement: glucose >400 mg/dL; sodium usually within normal range (but is dependent on level of hypoglycemia and dehydration); potassium low, normal, or high (value governs i.v. replacement); bicarbonate low.

Blood pH, oxygen, carbon dioxide, acid–base status analysis: arterial pH <7.3, oxygen normal, carbon dioxide low.

Blood culture: to identify septicemia and responsible organism.

Chest radiography: to identify consolidation due to pneumonia.

Complications

Hypovolemia, circulatory failure, cardiac arrest.

Disequilibrium, with cerebral edema: caused by over-rapid reversal of high hyperglycemia or electrolyte imbalance.

Hypokalemia or hyperkalemia: due to inappropriate i.v. potassium replacement and insulin treatment.

Hypophosphatemia: due to insulin treatment.

Hypoglycemia: due to insulin treatment.

Retinopathy, nephropathy and associated hypertension, neuropathy: long-term complications unusual in childhood.

Differential diagnosis.

Newly diagnosed child

Any condition manifest by nausea and vomiting.

Any condition manifest by polyuria.

Any condition manifest by coma.

Previously diagnosed child

Uncontrolled diabetes mellitus due to intercurrent infection.

Coma due to hypoglycemia.

Etiology

• Causes include the following:

Failure of insulin production and secretion due to lymphocytic infiltration and destruction of beta cells of the islets of Langerhans of the pancreas.

Particular HLA phenotypes (HLA DQ8 and DQ2) and circulating compliment-fixing antibodies to islet tissue and antibodies to insulin itself.

Epidemiology

• ~3 in 1000 US children have insulin-dependent diabetes mellitus.

Treatment

Diet and lifestyle

• Refined carbohydrates must be avoided.

• Diet must be well balanced, with 50% carbohydrates (100 g plus 10 g for each year of childhood life), no high-saturated fats, vegetable oils used for cooking, and high-fiber food (whole-wheat bread, baked beans).

• Meals should be regular, with snacks between main meals and at bedtime.

• No restrictions should be placed on children, but bouts of physical exercise may require additional carbohydrate intake. Hypoglycemia is particularly dangerous during activities in which children are exposed to cold because their thermal regulation fails and hypothermia may occur; this is a major problem, especially in small children.

• Glucose in the form of tablets or gel must be carried by a child or an accompanying adult. Parents should be taught to give glucagon, used when a hypoglycemic child cannot take oral glucose.

Pharmacological treatment [1]

• Oral agents have no place in the management of childhood-onset insulin-dependent diabetes mellitus.

• Insulin is injected before meals, at a frequency and combination meant to achieve maximum glycemic control.

• In small children, this may present a problem because of their sleep patterns. The evening injection can be divided so that the soluble insulin is given before the evening meal and intermediate-acting insulin later in the evening; this can be given while the child is asleep.

• Insulin-containing pens have been produced containing both short- and intermediate-acting insulin.

• Regimens can be altered so that insulin is injected before each meal and intermediate-acting insulin at bedtime, the latter to provide sufficient insulin during the resting period.

Standard dosage	Insulin, 0.5–1 unit/kg daily, adjusted according to blood glucose concentration.
Contraindications	Very rare hypersensitivity (usually due to preservatives in insulin preparation).
Special points	Home blood glucose monitoring essential if hyper- and hypoglycemia are to be avoided.
Main drug interactions	High-dose beta agonists cause severe insulin resistance.
Main side effects	Hyper- or hypoglycemia due to inappropriate dosing.

• Insulin can also be given by continuous infusions (subcutaneous or implanted intraperitoneal) using pumps.

Treatment aims

To return child to health.
To achieve glycemic control.

Prognosis

• Childhood-onset diabetes mellitus is associated with significant complications.

• Life expectancy is reduced by one-third, although this is rapidly improving.

Follow-up and management

• Regular attendance at a combined pediatric and diabetic clinic is vital to monitor growth, provide advice on diet as child gets older, monitor long-term glycemic control, and check for complications [2].

• Management at presentation requires the following:

With hyperglycemia and ketonuria but no vomiting, outpatient management (fluids not needed).
Frequent visits to specialist diabetic unit or frequent visits of staff of the center to the child's home.
Adjustment of dose of insulin on the basis of blood glucose values.
Two or more s.c. insulin injections and change in diet.
With vomiting, hospital admission for i.v. rehydration, insulin treatment, and identification of immediate cause of diabetic ketoacidosis.
Depending on age, education of child about the diabetic process and basic physiology of glucose homeostasis by a skilled member of the diabetic team, usually a specialist nurse.
Education of parents about their child's disease and its control (treatment of hyperglycemia, hypoglycemia, alteration of diet for physical activities, holidays).
Counseling to enable parents to come to terms with their child's life-long disability.

Key references

1. Kostraba JN, *et al.*: Increasing trend of outpatient management of children with newly diagnosed IDDM. *Diabetes Care* 1992, **15**:95–100.
2. Diabetes Control and Complication Trial Group: The effect of intensive treatment of diabetes on the development and progression of longterm complications in insulin dependent diabetes. *N Engl J Med* 1993, **329**:977–986.

Diabetic management in pregnancy

Diagnosis

Symptoms and signs

• Diabetes may already be present or may be manifest for the first time in pregnancy; some patients remain insulin-dependent after pregnancy, whereas in others, the diabetes disappears after pregnancy (gestational diabetes mellitus).

• Patients present with the usual symptoms and signs of pregnancy and possibly of diabetes mellitus; women with gestational diabetes mellitus, however, are usually asymptomatic, the diabetes being detected by screening (most effective at 28 weeks).

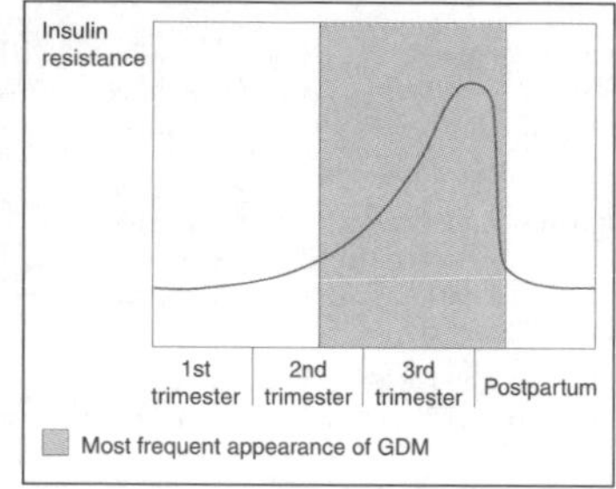

Increase of insulin resistance and the appearance of gestational diabetes mellitus (GDM).

Investigations

• All women with risk factors for gestational diabetes mellitus should be screened at 12 weeks.

• All pregnant women should be screened at 24 to 28 weeks.

• If fasting blood glucose is >90 mg/dL, random blood glucose is >125 mg/dL, or if failed 1-h screening test, a glucose tolerance test should be considered.

Screening test: give 50 g oral glucose solution and measure plasma glucose at 1 h. All women with plasma glucose >140 mg/dL at 1 h should have a 3-h oral glucose tolerance test (GTT).

3-h GTT: in pregnancy, 100 g glucose solution with blood glucose measured at fasting and at 1, 2, and 3 h. Gestational diabetes is diagnosed if two or more values > these parameters: fasting >105 mg/dL; 1 h >190 mg/dL; 2 h >165 mg/dL; 3 h >145 mg/dL.

Blood glucose measurement: 2–6 times daily; targets are 65–90 mg/dL before meals and <120 mg/dL 1 h postprandially.

Electrolytes, blood urea nitrogen, creatinine analysis, full blood count: to assess renal function and anemia.

Urinalysis: for protein, microalbumin; possibly 24-h for measurement of protein and creatinine clearance; hemoglobin A_{1c} should be kept in normal range.

Ultrasonography: at 17–19 weeks for fetal size and to check for malformations; possibly serial ultrasonography of biparietal diameter and abdominal circumference.

Fetal lung maturity measurement: to predict respiratory distress syndrome; lecithin:sphingomyelin ratio may be spuriously high in diabetic patients; low phosphatidyl choline or glycerol concentrations may be better predictors.

• When discrepancies are found between blood monitoring results and hemoglobin A_{1c}, the technique must be checked (meter device more reliable); results checked for falsification; and hemoglobinopathy, splenectomy, and gross anemia considered.

Complications

Maternal

Worsening retinopathy, nephropathy.

Increased pre-eclamptic toxemia.

Hydramnios.

Ketosis, hyperglycemia.

Death.

Fetal

Respiratory distress, jaundice, macrosomia.

Hypoglycemia.

Hypocalcemia.

Polycythemia.

Microcephaly, sacral agenesis.

Congenital malformations.

Congenital heart disease.

Differential diagnosis

Not applicable.

Etiology

Causes of gestational diabetes (increased insulin resistance)

Increased concentrations of progesterone, cortisol, prolactin, and human placental lactogen, which also influence post-receptor metabolism.

Poorly understood immunological processes, which increase insulin need two- to threefold during pregnancy.

Risk factors for gestational diabetes mellitus

Previous gestational diabetes.
First-degree relative with diabetes.
Fasting glycosuria.
Previous unexplained fetal death.
Previous "large for dates" baby.
Previous malformed baby.
Maternal obesity.
Hydramnios, macrosomia.

Epidemiology

• Prevalence of gestational diabetes mellitus in the US is 2%–13%, depending on the diagnostic criteria and population studied.

Pregnancy counseling [2]

• Diabetic women must be advised of the following:

• The risk of death is slightly higher than in nondiabetic women.

• Complications, *e.g.*, retinopathy, nephropathy, and heart disease, may worsen in pregnancy.

• Cesarean section is more probable.

• Numerous antenatal visits and close supervision will be needed.

• Home blood glucose monitoring will be needed several times daily.

• Multiple insulin injections will be needed daily.

• Diet must be adhered to, and smoking and drinking must be stopped.

• The baby will be at increased risk of death, malformations, and serious neonatal complications.

• Risks are, however, minimized by close supervision and cooperation, and maintenance of euglycemia.

Treatment

Diet and lifestyle

• Known diabetic patients should already have consulted a dietitian; those with gestational diabetes must be referred.

• Patients must ensure that 50% of energy intake is carbohydrate and that their diet contains adequate calcium and vitamins.

• Iron and folate supplements are needed.

• Patients should aim to achieve the normal weight gain in pregnancy (average, 10 kg) by appropriate food intake; caloric intake should be restricted to 1500–1800 kcal daily in some overweight pregnant women.

Pharmacological treatment [3]

During pregnancy

• All patients on oral agents should be transferred to insulin, usually given 2–4 times daily, occasionally more often; a mixture of short- and intermediate-acting insulin can be used depending on patient needs, or a late dose of intermediate-acting insulin before bed and short-acting insulin before meals [4].

• Two-thirds of patients with gestational diabetes mellitus may be treated by dietary advice; the remaining one-third need insulin, which can be given as a mixture of short- and intermediate-acting insulin twice daily, with possible supplement of short-acting insulin before lunch.

• Insulin needs increase during pregnancy; >100 units daily may be required; the need may fall at term, dramatically after labor.

During labor and delivery

• 1–4 units of insulin i.v. are needed hourly; insulin is adjusted based on hourly capillary and/or plasma glucose determination.

• Blood glucose must be maintained at near-normal concentrations.

• In prolonged labor or in high-risk patients, an independent energy source, *e.g.*, 10% dextrose, 100 mL i.v. hourly, is needed.

• Insulin should be delivered by an infusion pump (regular insulin, 50 units in 50 mL normal saline solution).

• Beta agonists used for premature labor may cause insulin resistance.

• General anesthesia and cesarean section increase insulin needs.

• After delivery, insulin needs fall dramatically.

• Patients with gestational diabetes mellitus often do not need further insulin treatment but may need medical review.

Treatment aims

To maintain preprandial blood glucose at 65–90 mg/dL, postprandial blood glucose 160 mg/dL, and hemoglobin A_{1c} in normal range.
To achieve a mature fetus, born after 38 weeks by vaginal delivery, with no neonatal or maternal complications.

Prognosis

• Retinopathy and nephropathy can deteriorate during pregnancy but can be minimized by good metabolic control and supervision.
• Perinatal mortality is still increased in diabetic pregnancies; half of the increase is associated with poor control.
• Maternal mortality is slightly higher than in nondiabetic patients.

Follow-up and management

Initial assessment

• Patients are best seen in joint clinic with a diabetologist and an obstetrician.
• Patients should be screened for diabetic complications; visual acuity, fundal examination with dilated pupils, and assessment of renal function are important.
• Blood pressure must be monitored regularly.

Subsequent assessment

• Follow-up should be every 1–4 weeks, depending on the patient's need.
• Patients should be encouraged to change their insulin regimen to attain good metabolic control.
• In gestational diabetes: risk of non–insulin-dependent diabetes mellitus at 5 years is 50%.

Key references

1. Nelson Piercy C, Gale EAM: Do we know how to screen for gestational diabetes? Current practice in one regional health authority. *Diabetic Med* 1994, **11**:493–498.
2. Dornhorst A: Implications of gestational diabetes for the health of the mother. *Br J Obstet Gynaecol* 1994, **101**:286–290.
3. Lowy C: Pregnancy and diabetes mellitus. In *Textbook of Diabetes.* Edited by Pickup J, Williams G. Oxford: Blackwell Scientific Publications; 1991:835–850.
4. Hellmuth E, Damm P, Molsted-Pedersen L: Congenital malformations in offspring of diabetic women treated with oral hypoglycaemic agents during pregnancy. *Diabetic Med* 1994, **11**:471–474.

Diabetic management in surgery

Diagnosis

Symptoms

• Well controlled diabetic patients having an operation have no symptoms.

Thirst and polyuria: indicating poor control in patients with any type of diabetes.

Nausea and abdominal pain: indicating very poor control in insulin-dependent patients.

Signs

Tachycardia, ketosis, dehydration, hypotension: signs of poor diabetic control in insulin-dependent patients; these will most probably develop after the operation if preoperative control of diabetes was poor.

Investigations [1,2]

For elective surgery

Blood glucose profile: 2 days before patient has a major operation; hemoglobin A_{1c} should be within 10% of normal range.

• Other investigations are the same as for nondiabetic patients.

For emergency surgery

Blood glucose measurement: to assess hyperglycemia.

Electrolytes, blood urea nitrogen analysis: to assess renal function and electrolyte balance.

Blood gas analysis: to assess acid-base balance.

Complications

Cardiovascular problems: particularly myocardial infarction; the main perioperative causes of death in diabetic patients.

Infection and poor wound healing: in poorly controlled diabetic patients [3].

Differential diagnosis

• Acute surgical abdominal disorders can be confused with severely decompensated diabetes in insulin-dependent patients: a medical opinion is essential.

Etiology

• The stress response to surgery and anesthesia is characterized by hyperglycemia, suppression of insulin release, and insulin resistance.

• This is due to increases in cortisol, catecholamines, and other counterregulatory hormones.

• The stress response is greater with major surgery.

Epidemiology

• 50% of diabetic patients have operations at some point in their lives.

• Patients with macrovascular disease will probably have several operations.

Treatment

Diet and lifestyle

• Major operations are often followed by a period of relative or absolute starvation: adequate energy intake and insulin must be supplied to diabetic patients because insulin depletion leads to severe catabolic disorders.

• Breakfast and oral agents are omitted if the operation is in the morning.

• If the operation is minor, eating and oral agents can soon be restarted.

Pharmacological treatment [1,2]

• Patients with "brittle" diabetes may need a glucose insulin infusion for 24 h before surgery.

• Regional anesthesia does not produce the same degree of stress response as general anesthesia.

• Infections should be treated aggressively by intravenous antibiotics.

For non–insulin-dependent diabetes: preoperative

• Metformin, which may cause lactic acidosis, and chlorpropamide, because its long action may lead to hypoglycemia, should be avoided.

• Patients should be given shorter-acting sulfonylureas instead, *e.g.*, glyburide, 2.5–20 mg daily, or glipizide, 2.5–20 mg daily.

• Blood glucose concentration must be monitored.

• The main side effect is hypoglycemia.

For non–insulin-dependent diabetes: perioperative

• Intravenous solutions containing glucose should be avoided unless hypoglycemia is a risk.

• If the operation is major, treatment should be the same as for insulin-dependent diabetes until the stress response of surgery is finished [4].

For insulin-dependent diabetes: preoperative

• Preoperative admission for stabilization may be needed to achieve a blood glucose concentration of 100–180 mg/dL.

• If control is good, the insulin regimen need not be changed until the day of surgery; if control is poor before a meal, short-acting insulin achieves rapid metabolic control.

• Blood glucose concentration must be monitored.

• The main side effect is hypoglycemia.

For insulin-dependent diabetes: perioperative

Short-acting insulin, 50 units in 50 mL normal saline solution with an infusion pump; 500 mL 10% dextrose with 10 mEq/L potassium chloride through a separate infusion pump infused 5-hourly.

• Blood glucose concentration must be maintained at 100–180 mg/dL; 1–4 units of insulin may be needed hourly via an infusion pump [4].

Alternatively, glucose–potassium–insulin infusion: 10% dextrose, 500 mL, with potassium chloride, 10 mEq/L, and short-acting insulin, 15 units infused as a mixture 5-hourly.

• Premixed insulins are unsuitable when insulin need changes rapidly.

• If blood glucose is >200 mg/dL, 20 units insulin should be added; if blood glucose is <100 mg/dL, 10 units should be added; other parameters should not be changed.

• The insulin infusion must be continued until the patient's first meal, when s.c. insulin should be started 30 min prior to cessation of insulin infusion; insulin needs will probably be higher than usual.

Treatment aims

To maintain blood glucose at 100–180 mg/dL during the operation.

Prognosis

• Mortality should be similar to that in nondiabetic patients.

Follow-up and management

• Blood glucose should be monitored 3–4 times daily before the operation.

• During and early after an operation, blood glucose should be monitored at least hourly.

• Creatinine and electrolytes should be measured daily, and any deficiencies replaced.

Timing of surgery

• Routine surgery should be postponed in newly diagnosed diabetic patients until good control is attained.

• Acute surgical conditions may lead to ketoacidosis; if possible, surgery should be delayed until metabolic control is achieved.

• Surgery should be done in the morning if possible.

Special situations

Cardiac surgery

• Hypothermic bypass surgery with pump priming and inotropic drugs leads to marked insulin resistance and much higher insulin needs.

• The rapidly changing insulin need makes a separate infusion line for insulin essential.

Pregnancy

• Control of diabetes during cesarean section is critical for mother and fetus.

Key references

1. Clark JDA, Currie J, Hartog M: Management of diabetes in surgery: a survey of current practice by anaesthetists. *Diabetic Med* 1992, **9**:271–274.
2. Gill GV: Surgery and diabetes mellitus. In *Textbook of Diabetes* vol 2. Edited by Pickup J, Williams G. Oxford: Blackwell Scientific Publications; 1991:820–825.
3. Sawyer RG, Pruett TL: Wound infections. *Surg Clin North Am* 1994, **74**:523–524.
4. Smith EA, Kilpatrick ES: Intra-operative blood glucose measurements. *Anaesthesia* 1994, **49**:129–132.

Diagnosis

Indications for dialysis

Acute renal failure: usually part of a multisystem disease, especially with hypovolemia or shock; if the renal failure cannot be reversed rapidly, recovery from the underlying disease is delayed or prevented, possibly resulting in death; early dialysis is needed to reverse acidosis, hyperkalemia, and uremia and to remove fluid from an oliguric patient to allow i.v. treatment and to relieve pulmonary edema.

Chronic renal failure: irreversible, progressive failure is eventually fatal without dialysis; ideally, dialysis should be started before symptoms or signs develop; early dialysis is needed to prevent acidosis, hyperkalemia, uremia, and fluid overload.

Severe heart failure, certain poisonings: rare.

• Treatable causes of renal failure should be excluded before starting dialysis, especially when rapid deterioration in renal function has occurred; these include the following:

Hypovolemia: central venous pressure and lying and standing blood pressure must be checked (postural drop of systolic blood pressure >10 mm Hg suggests up to 10% hypovolemia).

Outflow obstruction: patient must be checked for palpable bladder.

Investigations

Bicarbonate measurement: dialysis indicated in severe renal metabolic acidosis except when renal tubular acidosis occurs (rare).

Potassium measurement: dialysis indicated if concentration >6.5 mEq/L, especially in acute renal failure and if ECG changes are present.

Blood urea nitrogen measurement: difficult to interpret because influenced by generation rate (from protein catabolism); dialysis indicated if concentration >100 mg/dL in well nourished patients or >70 mg/dL in malnourished patients, when uremia present.

Creatinine measurement: generated from muscle protein; dialysis indicated if concentration >10 mg/dL in patients with normal build or >5 mg/dL in patients with low muscle mass (*e.g.*, elderly).

Creatinine clearance tests: most helpful, especially if normalized to patient's surface area; dialysis indicated if clearance rate <10 mL/min/1.75 m^2.

Hepatitis serology: precautions must be taken when dialyzing hepatitis B or C antigen-positive patients.

HIV status: if positive, dialysis not contraindicated, but special precautions are needed.

Complications of dialysis

Acute

Peritonitis: in continuous peritoneal dialysis; usually follows contamination of catheter connections; occurs on average every 1–2 years; rarely fatal; treated by intraperitoneal antibiotics and catheter removal if severe.

Bleeding: due to excessive anticoagulation.

Hypotension: due to excessive fluid removal.

Fever: due to contamination of blood circuit or dialyzer with pyrogens or bacteria.

Disequilibrium: rare; cerebral edema caused by osmotic effects when patient with very high urea concentration is dialyzed excessively rapidly.

Chronic

Amyloidosis: beta-2 microglobulin is poorly cleared by dialysis and accumulates as amyloid; causes a disabling arthropathy and the carpal tunnel syndrome.

Malnutrition: uremia causes anorexia and protein malnutrition unless adequate dialysis is provided; in continuous ambulatory peritoneal dialysis, this is exacerbated by protein losses from the peritoneum and may be masked by obesity caused by excessive uptake of glucose from the dialysis fluid.

Neuropathy: may result from inadequate dialysis or aluminium overload.

Acquired cystic disease: in native kidneys (malignant potential).

• Hypertension, anemia, cardiovascular disease, hyperparathyroidism, and osteomalacia are common in dialysis patients as a result of the uremic state.

Epidemiology (chronic dialysis)

• 600 patients in one million population are on dialysis or have a functioning transplant.

• More than 100 new patients in one million population annually are treated by dialysis.

• The mean age of dialysis patients is 55 years.

• Dialysis costs $35,000 per patient per year.

Patients suitable for dialysis

• Any patient is suitable except those unlikely to survive more than a few months even with normal renal function.

• Dialysis units prefer to decide for themselves if a patient is suitable.

• Many patients on dialysis are elderly or have diabetes, myeloma, or other multisystem disease.

• Patients with severe heart failure need not be refused dialysis; this often improves on dialysis.

Procedures to avoid

Contrast radiography

• Radiography will probably not be helpful and may worsen renal failure.

Cannulation of forearm veins

• Cannulation may destroy the veins needed for dialysis access; hand or antecubital veins should be used.

Urethral catheterization

• In oliguria, catheterization causes urinary tract infection and septicemia and may worsen renal failure.

Blood transfusion

• Transfusion causes fluid overload and hyperkalemia and should be avoided unless performed at the same time as dialysis.

• HLA sensitization may make transplantation difficult.

Treatment

Diet and lifestyle

• Dialysis patients tend to have protein malnutrition and usually need an increased-protein diet or protein supplements; low-protein diets should be avoided.

• Most patients need moderate fluid, potassium, and sodium restriction.

• Supplements of iron and water-soluble vitamins are needed.

Dialysis techniques

Hemodialysis

• The patient's blood is pumped through a dialyzer at 200–500 mL/min.

• Uremic toxins diffuse from the blood through a semi-permeable membrane in the dialyzer into a dialysis fluid.

• Bicarbonate diffuses in the opposite direction to correct the acidosis.

• Up to 140 L of dialysis fluid per treatment is used by the dialysis machine from purified water and an electrolyte concentrate.

• Excess fluid is removed from the patient by ultrafiltration of the blood in the dialyzer, driven by a controlled pressure gradient across the membrane.

• The patient is usually heparinized during treatment.

Hemofiltration (acute renal failure)

• Hemofiltration is similar to hemodialysis but without the dialysate.

• Uremic toxins and excess fluids are removed by ultrafiltration rates up to 150 mL/min across a semi-permeable membrane.

• The ultrafiltrate is then replaced by an i.v. infusion that matches the filtration rate.

• Hemofiltration is more efficient then hemodialysis at removing high-molecular-weight toxins but is more expensive.

• Both hemodialysis and hemofiltration are performed acutely in the intensive care unit. Large volumes of infusate are needed each day and are available ready-prepared in bags, avoiding the need for a dialysis machine.

Continuous ambulatory peritoneal dialysis

• 20% of dialysis patients are now treated by this method.

•. The treatment is done by the patient at home and allows considerable independence.

• Uremic toxins diffuse into 2–3 L of dialysate within the peritoneum.

• Excess fluid is removed by osmosis; the dialysate contains a variable glucose concentration to achieve this.

• The patient aseptically exchanges the dialysate with fresh fluid 4 times daily via a peritoneal catheter.

Home hemodialysis

• Home hemodialysis is suitable for well motivated patients who will probably remain on dialysis for many years.

• It is gradually being replaced by continuous ambulatory peritoneal dialysis in the United States.

Treatment aims

To restore quality of life and prolong life expectancy.

Prognosis

• A typical 60-year-old dialysis patient with coexisting cardiovascular disease has an expected survival of 2–4 years.

• Younger patients with no other disease have a shorter than normal life expectancy.

Follow-up and management

• Dialysis patients are usually followed up at least monthly in the dialysis unit.

• Blood pressure, fluid balance and nutritional status, hemoglobin, calcium, and bicarbonate should be maintained within the normal range.

• Parathyroid hormone (intact or n-terminal assay) should be maintained at about 2–5 times the normal upper limit, and phosphate at <6 mg/dL.

• The amount of dialysis delivered is monitored to ensure adequate dialysis delivery.

Access

Arteriovenous fistula or synthetic graft: created surgically between artery and vein in upper extremity.

Tenckhoff catheter: cuffed, tunneled, silicone catheter implanted into peritoneal cavity for continuous ambulatory peritoneal dialysis.

Long-bore indwelling central venous catheter: can be inserted into right atrium or femoral vein.

General references

1. Nissenson R, Fine R, eds: *Clinical Dialysis*, edn 2. Norwalk: Appleton and Lange; 1990.

Diagnosis

Symptoms

Watery, large-volume diarrhea: >400 mL daily.

Little abdominal pain.

Little vomiting.

Signs

Prominent weight loss and dehydration: possibly.

Investigations

Stool culture: for *Salmonella*, *Campylobacter*, and *Shigella* spp.

Stool staining and microscopy: possibly with concentration of stools; Ziehl–Neelsen stain for cryptosporidia and *Isospora* spp.; trichome or fluorescent stain for microsporidia; microscopy of fresh stool for ameba and cysts of *Giardia* spp.

Small-intestinal biopsy: electron microscopy gold standard for diagnosis of microsporidia, although these are seen by stool staining or light microscopy.

Biopsy: for cytomegalovirus or *Mycobacterium avium* complex colitis, or involvement due to lymphoma or Kaposi's sarcoma.

Tests of malabsorption: protozoan infection associated with partial villus atrophy and malabsorption, particularly of vitamin B_{12} (Schilling test).

Complications

Toxic dilatation: unusual.

Right upper quadrant pain, cholangiographic appearances of "AIDS-related sclerosing cholangitis."

Gross wasting, inanition, death.

Differential diagnosis

Viral diarrhea: cytomegalovirus infection may be bloody and associated with abdominal pain.

Bacterial diarrhea: *Shigella*, *Salmonella*, and *Campylobacter* spp. cause acute diarrhea with systemic symptoms; opportunistic bacterial infection by *Mycobacterium avium intracellulare* causes watery diarrhea in patients with severely reduced CD4 counts (<100×10^6/L).

"Pathogen-negative diarrhea": after complete investigation, large-volume diarrhea with no cause is rare; low-volume irritable-bowel diarrhea is more common in patients with CD4 counts >200×10^6/L.

Etiology

• Causes include the following:

Infectious

Mycobacterium avium.

Cryptosporidia.

Microsporidia (at least two species: *Septata intestinalis* and *Enterocytozoon bienusi*).

Cyclospora spp.

Isospora spp.

Entamoeba spp.

Giardia spp.

Noninfectious

Lymphoma.

Kaposi's sarcoma.

Epidemiology

• Cryptosporidiosis occurs in animal handlers and is associated with sexual transmission; water-borne outbreaks are known.

• Microsporidiosis only occurs in severely immunosuppressed patients (CD4 lymphocyte count <100×10^6/L).

• *Isospora* infection is common in South Americans and Africans; it occasionally occurs in travelers to these continents.

• Infection by *Entamoeba* spp. is common in homosexual men, although these strains are usually not pathogenic.

• *Giardia* infection is common in homosexual men (possible sexual transmission); it is more common in HIV-seropositive men.

Treatment

Diet and lifestyle

• Safe sexual practices reduce sexual transmission.

• Immunosuppressed patients with a CD4 count <200x10^6/L should boil drinking water.

• Care must be taken when gardening or handling pets or domestic animals.

Pharmacological treatment

General treatment

• Patients should be rehydrated, usually with oral rehydration fluids.

• Reduction with antimotility agents (*e.g.*, codeine phosphate, 30–80 mg daily) or stronger opiates may cause toxic megacolon.

• Specific vitamin supplementation should be given for malabsorption.

• Transient stool volume can be reduced during treatment by somatostatin analogues (*e.g.*, octreotide, 50–200 μg 2–3 times daily).

For cryptosporidiosis

• No standard treatment is of proven value.

Standard dosage	Paromomycin, 500 mg 4 times daily (most successful). Alternatively, azithromycin, up to 1.5 g daily.
Contraindications	None.
Special points	*Paromomycin:* stool volumes reduced by 50%, but cryptosporidia not eradicated.
Main drug interactions	None known.
Main side effects	None known.

For microsporidiosis

• No standard treatment is of proven value.

Standard dosage	Albendazole, 400 mg twice daily, or metronidazole, 400 mg 3 times daily.
Contraindications	None.
Special points	*Albendazole:* eradicates *Septata intestinalis*, less effect on *Enterocytozoon bienusi*. *Metronidazole:* may produce symptomatic benefit.
Main drug interactions	*Metronidazole:* alcohol.
Main side effects	*Metronidazole:* nausea.

For *Entamoeba histolytica* infection

• Metronidazole, 400 mg 3 times daily for 1 week is usually given, although the pathogenesis of the organism is often uncertain.

For giardiasis

• Patients can be given metronidazole, 1.2–2 g daily for 3 days; tinidazole, 2 g initially, repeated if necessary; or mepacrine, 100 mg 3 times daily for 5–7 days, repeated after 2 weeks if necessary.

Treatment aims

To resolve diarrhea.

To eradicate organism.

To promote weight gain or prevent weight loss.

Prognosis

Cryptosporidiosis

• In patients with CD4 counts >200x10^6/L, the diarrhea resolves eventually.

• In patients with CD4 counts <200x10^6/L, the diarrhea may be chronic.

• Diarrhea usually continues despite treatment.

• In patients with CD4 counts >200x10^6/L, the prognosis depends on the CD4 count, rather than on the diarrhea.

• In patients with CD4 counts <200x10^6/L, median survival is 1 year.

Microsporidiosis

• Diarrhea usually continues despite treatment.

• Median survival is <1 year.

Other infections

• Diarrhea usually resolves with treatment, but patients may relapse after treatment has stopped.

• The prognosis depends on the underlying CD4 count, rather than on the diarrhea.

Follow-up and management

• Eradication of organism must be checked.

• Continuing diarrhea leads to wasting due to severe anorexia; therefore, the need for supplements, elemental diets, or nasogastric or gastrostomy feeding must be reviewed.

General references

1. Blanchard C, *et al.*: Cryptosporidiosis in HIV-seropositive patients. *Q J Med* 1992, **85**:813–823.

2. Dietrich DT, Rahmin M: Cytomegalovirus colitis in AIDS. *J Acquir Immun Defic Syndr* 1991, **4 (suppl 1)**: S29–S35.

3. Orenstein J, *et al.*: Intestinal microsporidiosis as a cause of diarrhea in human immunodeficiency virus-infected patients. *Hum Pathol* 1991, **21**:475–481.

Diagnosis

Symptoms

• Disseminated intravascular coagulation occurs in a spectrum of guises from a chronic syndrome, diagnosed on laboratory tests, with no symptoms or signs (compensated), to an acute florid clinical bleeding state (uncompensated).

• It is always associated with an underlying disorder.

• The major symptoms are those of the underlying disorder.

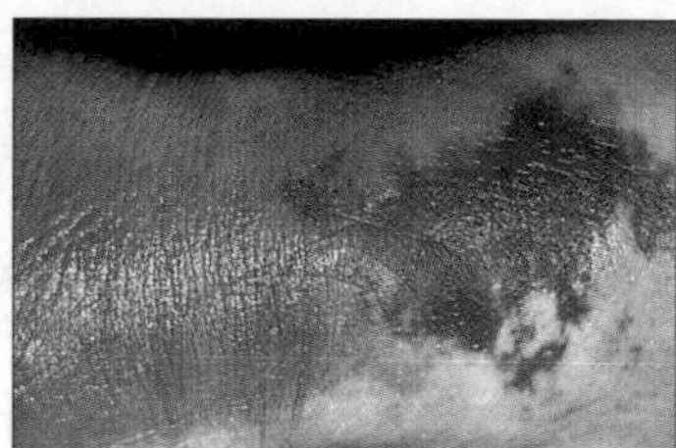

Purpura fulminans, with surrounding extensive subcutaneous hemorrhage.

Generalized bruising: especially over dependent areas.

Bleeding at surgical sites and incisions, around venipuncture sites, indwelling lines, and drainage tubes.

Hematemesis, melena, hemoptysis, hematuria, and vaginal bleeding.

Gangrene of fingers and toes, purpura fulminans, hemorrhagic bullae: microthrombotic lesions in 5%–10% of patients.

Signs

Evidence of bleeding: as detailed under symptoms, when present.

Investigations [1]

• Simple screening tests show reduced levels of clotting factors and platelets.

• Disseminated intravascular coagulation cannot be ruled out by a single set of normal results; serial values may be needed to show consumption.

Measurement of prothrombin time, activated partial thromboplastin time, thrombin time: all times prolonged; prolongation of thrombin time best guide to clinical significance of raised fibrinogen degradation products and low fibrinogen; thrombin time twice normal control value indicates impending overt clinical bleeding.

Fibrinogen measurement: concentration low.

Fibrinogen degradation products and D-dimers measurement: concentrations raised; fibrinogen degradation products sensitive but not specific for disseminated intravascular coagulation; D-dimer specific but not as sensitive.

Platelet count: low.

Blood film: many patients have associated microangiographic hemolytic anemia; erythrocytes fragmented by passing through deposited fibrin strands.

Complications

Uncontrollable hemorrhage.

Microvascular blockage and tissue necrosis of heart, liver, kidney, and brain.

Adult respiratory distress.

Differential diagnosis

• Simple screening tests and the clinical picture are usually diagnostic.

Vitamin K deficiency: normal platelet count.

Liver disease: raised factor VIII concentrations.

Lupus anticoagulant and thrombocytopenia: normal fibrinogen, inhibitor present.

Thrombotic thrombocytopenic purpura: clotting tests usually normal, florid microangiopathic changes on blood film.

Massive transfusion: clinical history.

Etiology

Causes and associated disorders [2]

Infections: meningococcal septicemia, Gram-negative septicemia, malaria, virus (purpura fulminans).

Malignancy: disseminated metastatic carcinomas, myeloid leukemia, promyelocitic leukemia.

Obstetric complications: septic abortion, amniotic fluid embolism, placental abruption, eclampsia, retained dead fetus and placenta.

Tissue injury: severe burns or trauma, extensive surgery, hypo- or hyperthermia, shock.

Immunological phenomena: anaphylaxis, incompatible transfusion, allograft rejection.

Miscellaneous: liver disease and ascitic fluid shunts, extracorporeal circuits, certain snake and insect bites, vascular malformations.

Pathogenesis [2]

• Disseminated intravascular coagulopathy is triggered by inappropriate and continued activation of clotting pathways.

• This leads to excessive thrombin generation, coagulation factor consumption, and platelet aggregation.

• Thrombin also activates protein C and fibrinolytic systems via secondary generation of plasmin.

• Natural inhibitors of the clotting cascade are overwhelmed.

• Coagulation factor consumption, consumptive thrombocytopenia, and hyperfibrinolysis lead to bleeding.

• Uncontrolled fibrin deposition leads to microthrombosis.

Epidemiology

• 60% of clinical cases of disseminated intravascular coagulation are associated with septicemic infection, usually due to gram-negative bacteria.

• Most acute cases are encountered in severely ill patients in intensive care.

Treatment

Diet and lifestyle

• No special precautions are necessary.

Pharmacological treatment

Anticoagulants

• Although controversial, anticoagulants may have a role in acute promyelocytic leukemia (M3), acute intravascular hemolysis (incompatible blood transfusion), and purpura fulminans.

Standard dosage Heparin, 5–10 units/kg/h continuous i.v. infusion.

Contraindications Florid bleeding

Special points Requires antithrombin III for its action, which is often low in patients with disseminated intravascular coagulation; fresh frozen plasma may also be needed to supply antithrombin III to maintain effective heparinization.
Partial thromboplastin time should be kept at 1.5–2 times control.
May increase bleeding tendency; close monitoring and specialist advice needed.

Main drug interactions Other anticoagulants.

Main side effects Bleeding (with overdose).

Fibrinolytic inhibitors

• Because of increased deposition, fibrinolysis is protective against microvascular organ damage in disseminated intravascular coagulation; inhibitors of fibrinolysis are therefore generally contraindicated. In special circumstances of predominant fibrinolysis, however, they may be useful.

• Specialist advice must be sought before use.

Nonpharmacological treatment

See Transfusion medicine *for further details.*

Fresh frozen plasma

• Fresh frozen plasma supplies all clotting factors and naturally occurring inhibitors of coagulation.

• Initially, 10–15 mL/kg should be given.

• It may cause fluid overload.

Cryoprecipitate

• Cryoprecipitate supplies fibrinogen and factor VIII.

• It is used, at a rate of 1 unit/5 kg, when substantial fibrinogen replacement is needed.

Platelet concentrates

• Platelet concentrates are needed when consumptive thrombocytopenia is present.

• They are given, at a rate of 4 units/m^2 body surface area, if the platelet count falls below 50 x 10^9/L and overt bleeding occurs.

Packed erythrocytes

• Packed erythrocytes are needed to treat associated hemolysis or anemia at a rate sufficient to maintain hematocrit >0.3.

• Virus transmission is a risk with any blood product.

• Fluid overload may also be a problem.

Treatment aims

To treat the underlying disorder.

To reverse the coagulopathy (by replacement of clotting factors and platelets or use of pharmacological inhibitors of coagulation).

To provide general supportive care for acutely ill patients.

Prognosis

• The mortality in severe disseminated intravascular coagulation is high and may exceed 80%.

• Death is usually due to progression of the underlying disease; elimination or amelioration of the cause is of utmost importance.

Follow-up and management

• Coagulation screening tests should be repeated to assess the effect of replacement therapy; the aim is a prothrombin time within 3 s of control, partial thromboplastin time within 10 s of control, and fibrinogen >1.0 g/L.

• The need for further replacement should be judged by the results of screening tests and degree of clinical bleeding.

• Laboratory abnormalities correct with successful treatment of the underlying disorder.

Key references

1. Bick R: Disseminated intravascular coagulation and related syndromes: a clinical review. *Semin Thromb Hemost* 1988, **14**:299–307

2. Levi M, *et al.*: Pathogenesis of disseminated intravascular coagulation in sepsis. *JAMA* 1993, **270**:975–979.

Diagnosis

Symptoms

• Diverticulosis is common (*see* Epidemiology) and typically asymptomatic [1].

Symptomatic diverticular disease

Symptomatic diverticular disease may present with the following:

Fever, left lower quadrant pain (diverticulitis).

Maroon stools: from acute lower gastrointestinal bleeding from a diverticula.

Bowel obstruction: from a left-sided stricture caused by recurrent diverticulitis.

Signs

Symptomatic diverticular disease

Fever, tenderness, guarding, palpable inflammatory mass: indicating inflammation due to abscess [2].

Shock, acute abdomen, paralytic ileus: indicating inflammation due to perforation.

Anemia, shock, fresh blood *per rectum*: indicating hemorrhage.

Abdominal distension, obstruction: indicating stricture.

Investigations

• Laboratory tests are usually normal in asymptomatic diverticular disease but can help to exclude other diagnoses.

• Diverticula are easier to identify on barium enema than on colonoscopy.

Full blood count: to identify anemia due to bleeding or elevated leukocytes from inflammation.

Liver function tests: to exclude biliary disease, which can occasionally mimic symptomatic diverticular disease.

Sigmoidoscopy: to exclude colitis or malignancy, which may mimic symptomatic diverticular disease.

Plain abdominal radiography: may show features of ileus or perforation.

Contrast enema: may show obstruction or stricture [3].

Ultrasonography or CT of abdomen and pelvis: may show abscess cavity.

Colonoscopy: may be needed for biopsy of stricture to exclude malignancy.

Tagged red blood cell nuclear scan: to investigate sites of ongoing bleeding.

Complications

Life-threatening gastrointestinal bleeding.

Abscess formation or perforation: leading to subphrenic or pericolic collections.

Intestinal obstruction.

Stricture formation.

Fistula: connection to bladder or vagina.

Differential diagnosis

General

Carcinoma of colon.

Inflammatory bowel disease.

Pseudomembranous colitis.

Abscess or perforation

Pelvic inflammatory disease.

Pyelonephritis.

Perforated peptic ulcer.

Ischemic colitis.

Appendicitis.

Crohn's disease.

Hemorrhage

Polyp in colon.

Angiodysplasia.

Upper gastrointestinal tract bleeding.

Stricture

Radiation damage.

Ischemic colitis.

Endometriosis.

Etiology

• Factors believed to be implicated in the development of diverticula include the following:

Low stool weight, leading to excessive intracolonic pressure.

Dietary fiber deficiency, reducing stool weight and colonic transit time.

Exaggerated colonic pressure due to abnormal colon muscular motility.

Weakness and poor elasticity of colon wall.

Epidemiology

• Colonic diverticula occur in 33% of people >40 years and 50% of people >70 years.

• Diverticulosis appears to be more common in developed countries.

Treatment

Diet and lifestyle

• Increased dietary fiber intake may help some patients, especially those with marked constipation.

• Excessive dietary fiber is contraindicated in patients with excessive narrowing or stricture formation from previous inflammation.

• Regular exercise improves bowel function.

Pharmacological treatment

Diverticulitis

• Antibiotics are administered to patients with acute inflammation, abscess formation, or evidence of systemic toxicity.

• Intravenous antibiotic regimens include cefotetan, 2 g every 12 h, or ciprofloxacin, 400 mg every 12 h, and metronidazole, 500 mg every 6 h.

• Oral antibiotic regimens include metronidazole, 500 mg every 8 h, plus ciprofloxacin, 500 mg every 12 h; trimethoprim, 160 mg/sulfamethoxazole, 800 mg every 12 h; or an oral cephalosporin.

Diverticular bleeding

• Therapy is supportive, with volume expansion and blood products as necessary.

Nonpharmacological treatment

For perforated diverticular disease of the colon: emergency decompression of the colon by colostomy, followed by elective resection of the diseased segment [4].

For life-threatening hemorrhage from diverticular disease: possible surgical control or embolization therapy at the time of selective mesenteric arteriography.

Treatment aims

To relieve acute symptoms.

To improve bowel function.

To reduce incidence of further symptom attacks.

Prognosis

• Most patients with diverticular bleeding have spontaneous cessation and no recurrence.

• Most patients with diverticulitis respond to antibiotic management alone; a small subset will require drainage of an abscess or surgical management of stricutres.

Follow-up and management

• Recurrent symptoms are common, but new or different symptoms need further investigations.

• If symptoms are relieved by fiber supplementation, long-term treatment must be continued.

Key references

1. Cheskin LJ, Bohlman M, Schusler MM: Diverticular disease in the elderly. *Gastroenterol Clin North Am* 1990, **19**:391–403.
2. Jones DJ: Diverticular disease. *BMJ* 1992, **304**:1435–1437.
3. McKee RF, Deignan RW, Krukowski ZH: Radiological investigation in acute diverticulitis. *Br J Surg* 1993, **80**:560–565.
4. Kronberg O: Treatment of perforated sigmoid diverticulitis: a prospective randomized trial. *Br J Surg* 1993, **80**:505–507.

Duodenal ulcer

Diagnosis

Symptoms

Uncomplicated ulcer

Epigastric pain: sometimes described as dull or burning, often occurring 1–4 h after eating and relieved quickly by antacids or food.

Waking at night because of pain.

Complicated ulcer

Hematemesis or melena: indicating bleeding ulcer.

Vomiting: sometimes indicating gastric outflow obstruction.

Severe pain: may indicate pancreatitis or peritonitis, but 50% of patients with fatal complications present without ulcer pain.

Signs

Uncomplicated ulcer

- Few signs are manifest.

Epigastric tenderness: usually midline or to right of midline.

Complicated ulcer

Acute hemorrhage: indicating shock, melena.

Anemia: indicating chronic hemorrhage.

Peritonitis: indicating perforation.

"Succussion splash": indicating gastric outflow obstruction.

Investigations

- Laboratory tests are not diagnostic but can be used to identify complications and exclude other abnormalities.

Full blood count: to identify iron-deficiency anemia.

Serum amylase measurement: raised concentration indicates penetration into pancreas or acute pancreatitis.

Serum gastrin measurement: can be considered in patients with recurrent or multiple ulcers to exclude a gastrinoma.

Fiberoptic endoscopy: allows direct view of ulcer, assessment of scarring or deformity, assessment of *Helicobacter pylori* status (by CLOtest, culture, or histology), photographic documentation, and assessment of coincidental disease; identifies small lesions; treatment of bleeding ulcers possible, particularly ulcers actively bleeding or those with a visible vessel.

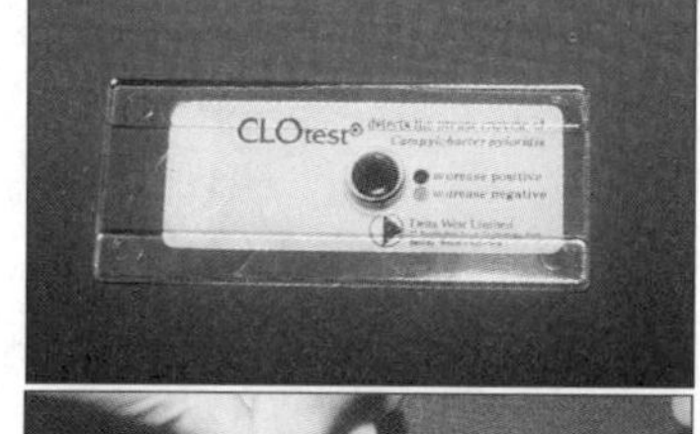

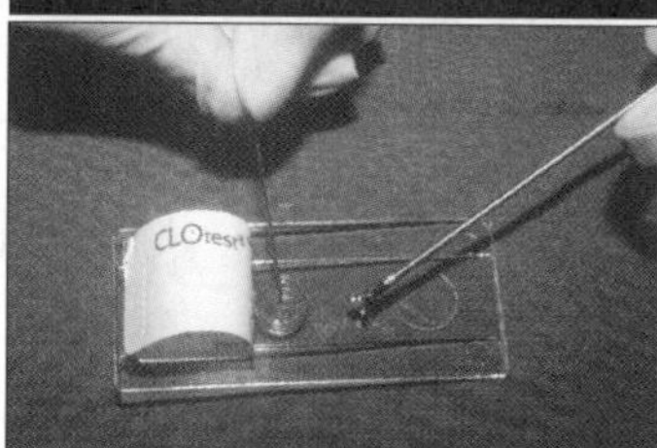

CLOtest detects urease activity in gastric biopsy.

Contrast radiography: less accurate than endoscopy, small lesions may be missed, tissue detection of *H. pylori* not possible, and does not allow tissue diagnosis; relatively cheap, and sedation not needed.

Complications

Acute hemorrhage: in 10% of patients.

Perforation: in 1% (often asymptomatic in elderly or immunosuppressed patients).

Pyloric channel obstruction: may cause weight loss due to vomiting and food aversion.

Differential diagnosis

Chronic pain

Gastroesophageal reflux disease.

Gastric ulcer.

Carcinoma of stomach.

Gallbladder disease.

Chronic pancreatitis.

Irritable bowel syndrome.

Nonulcer dyspepsia.

Acute severe pain

Acute pancreatitis.

Biliary colic.

Aortic dissection.

Acute myocardial infarction.

Aggressive ulceration

Zollinger–Ellison syndrome.

Crohn's disease.

Lymphoma.

Carcinoma.

Cytomegalovirus in imunosuppressed patients.

Ischemia.

Etiology

- Causes include the following:

Helicobacter pylori: in 95% of patients.

Aspirin, NSAIDs (a common etiology).

Increased basal acid secretion: in 30% of patients.

Increased nocturnal acid secretion.

Smoking.

Blood group O association: in nonsecretors.

Genetic: familial clustering.

Epidemiology

- 10% of the population have a duodenal ulcer at some point in their lives.
- Duodenal ulcers occur almost as often in women as in men.

Treatment

Diet and lifestyle

• Bland or milk diets have not been shown to decrease acidity, promote healing, or relieve symptoms.

• Patients should restrict alcohol consumption, eat three balanced meals daily, with no bedtime snacks, avoid aspirin and other NSAIDs, and stop cigarette smoking.

Pharmacological treatment

Antacids

• Antacids are effective for duodenal ulcer, taken 1 and 3 h after meals; some patients may find complying with this regimen difficult.

• Sucralfate, 1 g 4 times daily, is recommended.

H_2-receptor antagonists

• These produce symptomatic relief in days and ulcer healing in 80% of patients at 4 weeks and 95% at 8 weeks; they are also used as maintenance treatment to prevent recurrence at half the usual dose [1].

Standard dosage	Ranitidine, 300 mg; cimetidine, 800 mg; famotidine, 40 mg; or nizatidine, 300 mg in the evening.
Contraindications	Rare hypersensitivity; avoided in pregnancy and lactation.
Main drug interactions	*Cimetidine:* oral anticoagulants, theophylline, phenytoin, warfarin.
Main side effects	Altered bowel habits, headache (both rare). *Cimetidine:* gynecomastia, confusion in elderly.

Proton-pump inhibitors

• Proton-pump inhibitors are associated with faster healing.

• They produce 93% healing after 4 weeks of treatment.

• They are not approved for long-term management.

Standard dosage	Omeprazole, 20 mg daily [2].
Contraindications	Pregnancy and lactation.
Main drug interactions	Diazepam, phenytoin, warfarin.
Main side effects	Diarrhea, headache, rash (all rare); increased risk of enteric infection.

Antibiotic regimens for *Helicobacter pylori* eradication

• Antiobiotic regimens have been shown to decrease the chance of duodenal ulcer relapse, but the optimal regimen remains unclear [3–6].

Alternative regimens	Bismuth subsalicylate, 2 tablets; tetracycline (or amoxicillin), 500 mg; and metronidazole, 250 mg; all taken 4 times daily before food for 2 weeks with omeprazole, 20 mg twice daily; *or* clarithromycin, 250 mg twice daily; metronidazole, 500 mg twice daily; omeprazole, 20 mg daily; all for 1 week.
Contraindications	Pregnancy.
Special points	Patients should avoid alcohol.
Main drug interactions	Warfarin.
Main side effects	Nausea, darkening of stool.

Treatment aims

To relieve pain.

To heal ulcer.

To prevent recurrence and complications.

To eradicate *Helicobacter pylori* infection.

Other treatments

Surgery: for uncontrollable bleeding, second major bleed, perforation or penetration, pyloric stenosis, or antibiotic-resistant *Helicobacter pylori* in young adults.

• Elective surgery is very rarely necessary.

Prognosis

• Untreated, most patients with duodenal ulcers relapse within 1–2 years of initial healing, particularly the elderly, NSAID users, and smokers.

Follow-up and management

• If symptoms continue after 8 weeks of full-dose H_2 blockade, patients should be checked with endoscopy, and the ulcer and antrum should be biopsied.

• Maintenance with half-dose H_2 antagonist should be considered to prevent recurrence for patients with a history of aggressive ulcer (*e.g.*, previous bleeding), the elderly, or those with other illnesses.

Key references

1. Feldman M, Burton ME: Histamine 2-receptor antagonists: standard therapy for acid-peptic diseases. *N Engl J Med* 1991, **323**:1672–1678; 1749–1755.
2. Maton PN: Omeprazole. *N Engl J Med* 1991, **324**:965–975.
3. Peterson WL: *Helicobacter pylori* and peptic ulcer disease. *N Engl J Med* 1991, **324**:1043–1048.
4. Tytgat GNJ: Treatments that impact favourably upon the eradication of *Helicobacter pylori* and ulcer recurrence. *Ailment Pharmacol Ther* 1994, **8**:359–368.
5. Graham DY, *et al*.: *Helicobacter pylori*: current status. *Gastroenterology* 1993, **105**:279–282.
6. Yamada T, *et al*.: *Helicobacter pylori* in peptic ulcer disease. *JAMA* 1994, **272**:65–69.

Diagnosis

Symptoms

Myocardial infarction, angina, claudication, transient ischemic attacks, cerebrovascular accident: indicating accelerated atheroma.

Pancreatitis, confusional states: rare, caused by chylomicronemia.

• Adverse lipid profiles without symptoms are often revealed by well-person screening or through other risk associations, *e.g.*, bad family history.

Signs

• Ectopic lipid deposits should be sought because they suggest the duration of lipidemia (and thus the degree of risk) and alert to asymptomatic lipidemia.

Corneal arcus: traces in 50% of adults by age of 50 years; heavy or early presence can reveal hypercholesterolemia; differential arcus can reveal carotid stenosis.

Xanthomas of tendons: heels, knees, knuckles; indicating long-standing severe hypercholesterolemia, almost always familial.

Xanthomas of soft tissues: elbows, eyelids, palmar creases, rarely elsewhere; typical of mixed lipidemia and triglyceride excess.

Lipidemia retinalis and eruptive xanthomas: indicating chylomicronemia.

Corneal clouding: rare major disorder of high-density lipoprotein.

Carotid bruit, poor or absent peripheral pulses: vascular abnormalities.

Investigations

• The aim of investigations is to clarify the pattern of lipid abnormality and its cause.

• Lipid profiles can be disturbed and difficult to interpret for up to 3 months after myocardial infarction.

Lipid profile: for concentrations of cholesterol, triglycerides, and high-density lipoprotein cholesterol after overnight fasting; random sample adequate for cholesterol.

Secondary lipidemia tests: for thyroid-stimulating hormone concentration, glucose tolerance, alcohol markers; other tests suggested by history or examination.

Second-level tests: apolipoprotein E typing for moderate mixed excess or palmar xanthomas; fibrinogen level, platelet function, lipoprotein (a) concentration also of interest.

Special procedures: for major hypertriglyceridemia, measurement of apolipoprotein CII and lipoprotein lipase; for major high-density lipoprotein deficiency, measurement of lecithin cholesterol acyltransferase activity and apolipoprotein AI and DNA studies.

Family screening: to review suspected genetic problem, notably polygenic or familial hypercholesterolemia.

• Other problems, notably blood pressure, cardiac status, cigarette smoking, and fibrinogen concentration, should be considered in the overall assessment of clinical risk and options for benefit.

Complications

Progressive atheromatous disease.

Graft or angioplasty restenosis.

Attacks of abdominal pain and pancreatitis.

Differential diagnosis

Other causes of premature vascular disease, pancreatitis, corneal clouding.

Etiology

Genetic causes

Monogenic dominant: forms of heterozygous familial hypercholesterolemia (rare homozygotes) and familial combined hypercholesterolemia.

Recessive: most cases of familial dysbetalipoproteinemia (type III).

Polygenic.

Secondary causes

Hypothyroidism in older hypercholesterolemic women.

Alcoholism in executive men.

Diabetes or impaired glucose tolerance in older men or women with mixed lipidemia.

Chronic renal or liver disease.

Etretinate sensitivity.

Unknown causes

Includes diet-dependent effects and possible genetic basis ("common hypercholesterolemia").

Epidemiology

• US cholesterol levels are high by world standards.

• High-density lipoprotein levels are higher and low-density lipoprotein levels lower in women than in men [1,2].

• High-density lipoprotein levels are not affected by age after puberty; low-density lipoprotein levels continue to rise in women and young men.

• Heterozygous familial hypercholesterolemia is present in 0.2% of live births and 6% of patients <50 years admitted to coronary care units.

• Major apolipoprotein E variants are present in 1.7% of live births (type III lipidemia), but only 1% of these have major pulmonary vascular or cardiovascular disease as adults; a secondary problem (*e.g.*, alcohol) is usually needed to provoke clinical expression.

Treatment

Diet and lifestyle

• Reduction in total fat intake (with a greater proportion taken as unsaturates), weight loss, and more steady physical activity should be encouraged.

• Much ingenuity and interpersonal skill is needed to maintain compliance, and committed support by skilled dietitians is invaluable.

• Diet change can also sharpen responses to any subsequent lipid drug treatment.

Pharmacological treatment

• The cause of the abnormal lipid profile must be identified and treated.

• No single drug is universally appropriate; combinations are useful.

Priorities for lipid-lowering treatment in diet-resistant patients

1. Existing coronary heart disease or previous coronary artery bypass grafting, angioplasty, or cardiac transplantation. For such pateints, effective therapy of moderate to severe hypercholesterolemia improves overall survival and freedom from myocardial infarction, revascularization, and cardiac death [4].
2. Several risk factors or major genetic lipid disorder (*e.g.*, familial hypercholesterolemia).
3. Asymptomatic dyslipoproteinemia in men or in postmenopausal women.

Statins

• Statins are powerful cholesterol-lowering agents, alone or with resins.

Standard dosage Statins, 10–40 mg single daily dose, depending on product (*e.g.*, lovastatin, fluvastatin, pravastatin, simvastatin).

Contraindications Liver disease, pregnancy, breast feeding.

Special points Not licensed for children.

Main drug interactions Occasional severe myositis or rhabdomyolysis when used with cyclosporin or fibrates.

Main side effects Rheumatic complaints, severe myositis alone or in combination treatment; reaction time may be delayed.

Resins

• Resins divert bile acids, lower cholesterol, and raise triglycerides; they are first-line treatment in children with familial hypercholesterolemia.

Standard dosage Resins, 1–2 sachets twice daily (up to 4 sachets daily).

Contraindications Biliary obstruction.

Special points Compliance is better with newer formulations.

Main drug interactions May reduce absorption of other medication (should be given before or well after).

Main side effects Gastric irritation, constipation, gas.

Fibrates

• Fibrates are used in patients with mixed lipidemia or low high-density lipoprotein levels; they promote turnover of triglyceride lipoproteins and can generate high-density lipoproteins; some lower fibrinogens, and the level may affect choice.

Standard dosage Depends on product.

Contraindications Severe renal or liver disease, pregnancy.

Special points Some fibrates are licensed for children but rarely so used.

Main drug interactions If used with statins, can affect prothrombin time on oral anticoagulants.

Main side effects Changed bowel habit, rashes, myositis (rare).

Second-line drugs

• Probucol can cause xanthoma regression, but high-density lipoprotein concentrations are reduced.

• Fish oils or polyunsaturates (vegetable or marine) may be antithrombotic.

• Nicotinates can raise high-density lipoproteins and lower lipoprotein (a), but compliance is difficult.

Treatment aims

To improve overall lipid profile in patients with or at risk of coronary heart disease.

To reduce coronary progression [3] and improve outcomes, including death [4].

Prognosis

• Increase in high-density lipoprotein levels is associated with plaque regression.

Follow-up and management

• Dietary support must be reinforced, enthusiastic, and family-based.

• For failing lipid response, compliance and the prospect of a second lipid-related disorder (*e.g.*, hypothyroidism, alcoholism) must be checked.

• Diet or medication changes must be given time to act (*e.g.*, review after 4 months).

Key references

1. Barth JD, Arntzenius HC: Progression and regression of atherosclerosis, what roles for LDL cholesterol and HDL cholesterol. *Eur Heart J* 1991, **12**:952–957.
2. Betteridge DJ *et al.*: Management of hyperlipidaemia: guidelines of the British Hyper- lipidaemia Association. *Postgrad Med J* 1993, **69**:359–369.
3. Brown BG *et al.*: Lipid-lowering and plaque regression: new insights into prevention of plaque disruption and clinical events in coronary disease. *Circulation* 1993, **87**:1781–1791.
4. Scandinavian Simvastatin Survival Study Group: Randomized trial of cholesterol lowering in 4444 patients with coronary heart disease (4S). *Lancet* 1994, **344**:383–389.

Diagnosis

Symptoms

Itching.

Dryness, discoloration, thickening of involved areas; blistering and oozing of skin.

Signs

Xerosis.

Keratosis pilaris.

Dennie-Morgan lines (infraorbital fold of skin).

"Allergic shiners" (infraorbital darkening).

Excoriations.

Lichenification of skin: with predilection for flexural creases.

Follicular prominence: especially in patients with dark skin.

Associated pityriasis alba.

Increased fine line markings of the skin of the palms of bilateral hands.

Secondary impetiginization of excoriated skin.

Investigations

• Atopic eczema is a clinical diagnosis, although family history is helpful.

• Patients often have all or part of the atopic triad (*i.e.*, asthma, allergic rhinitis, atopic eczema).

Skin scrapings: to rule out scabies or dermatophyte infections.

Cultures: to rule out staphylococcal superinfections.

Skin biopsy: rarely performed by experienced clinicians.

Complications

Secondary infection: usually with *Staphylococcus aureus*; Kaposi's varicelliform eruption (eczema herpeticum) occurs when atopic patients get herpes simplex infections that become disseminated over the involved cutaneous surface (may be very severe and life-threatening in young children); molluscum contagiosum not uncommon [1].

Erythroderma (exfoliative erythroderma): possible in severe cases; requires hospital admission with close monitoring to fluid and electrolyte status as well as treatment of any secondary infection that could have triggered the flare.

Differential diagnosis

Scabies.

Tinea.

Psoriasis.

Ichthyosis.

Dermatitis herpetiformis.

Premycosis fungoides (T-cell lymphoma).

Netherton's syndrome (atopic dermatitis is one of the hallmark features).

Wiskott-Aldrich syndrome.

Acrodermatitis enteropathica.

Neurodermatitis.

Contact dermatitis.

HIV infection (especially in children).

Phenylketonuria patients often have atopic eczema during the first year of life.

Etiology

• Although a host of immunological abnormalities have been identified, there is no real consensus as to the cause of atopic dermatitis; it is probable that many factors play a role.

Immunologic abnormalities have included the following:

Elevated serum IgE levels.

Reduced cell-mediated immunity.

Slowed chemotaxis of neutrophils and monocytes.

Relative increase in the number of CD4-positive T-cells that secrete interleukin (IL)-4.

Decrease in CD4-positive T-cells that secrete IL-2 [2].

Epidemiology

Prevalence of atopic dermatitis (atopic eczema) is 7–24 per 1000.

• The highest prevalence is in children.

Onset of disease is in the first year of life in ~50% of patients and before the age of 5 in 85% of patients.

Treatment [3]

Diet and lifestyle

• Rare patients have a definite cutaneous response to certain foods, which obviously should be avoided.

• Children as well as adults should be educated regarding the disease as well as taught how to apply emollients when they "itch" instead of scratching.

• Patients specifically need to know everything that can aggravate their skin condition, *i.e.*, dry ambient environment (especially in households with woodburning stoves), hot baths, harsh soap, wool, fabric softener, dusty environments, stress, scratching, and so forth.

Pharmacological treatment

Topical

• Emollients are the mainstay to prevent dryness.

• Steroids may be used at mild, intermediate, or most potent strength, as follows:

Mild potency: topical steroids, over-the-counter or prescription, 1%–2.5% hydrocortisone; class VI and VII steroids.

Intermediate potency: triamcinolone, flurandrenolide, fluocinolone; Class III–V steroids.

Most potent: desoximetasone, clobetasol, betamethasone; class I and II steroids.

Standard dosage All topical steroids should be applied once or twice a day; intermediate and potent topical steroids should not be used for more than a few days on the face, axillary region, or groin.

Contraindications None.

Special points Potent topical steroids should be tapered off as soon as possible to avoid side effects.

Main drug interactions Atrophy of the skin, steroid folliculitis, systemic absorption (especially in children).

Main side effects Atrophy of the skin, steroid folliculitis, systemic absorption (especially in children).

Systemic therapy

•Systemic treatment is used only in the following situations:

Acyclovir: for secondary infection with herpes.

Antibiotics: for secondary bacterial infection.

Systemic steroids: used only in exceptional cases.

Antihistamines: to relieve pruritis.

Treatment aims

To decrease pruritis.

To prevent secondary infection.

To educate patients so that they can control the disease themselves.

The main objective is to control, not cure, the disease, as it is a chronic skin disease.

Prognosis

Resolves in approximately 40% of patients by adulthood.

The remainder of patients have a chronic course characterized by intermittent flares and remissions.

Follow-up and management

Most patients are treated with topical agents and are followed up until their disease clears.

Some physicians continue to follow-up at 3- to 6-month intervals to educate their patients appropriately.

Key references

1. Bork K, Brauninger W: Increasing incidence of eczema herpeticum: analysis of seventy-five cases. *J Am Acad Dermatol* 1988, **19**:1024–1029.
2. Van der Heijden FL, *et al.*: High frequency of IL-4-producing CD4 positive allergen-specific T-lymphocytes in atopic dermatitis lesional skin. *Invest Dermatol* 1991, **97**:389–394.
3. Hanafin JM: Atopic dermatitis: new therapeutic considerations. *J Am Acad Dermatol* 1991, **24**:1097–1101.

Diagnosis

Definition

Eisenmenger's complex

• Originally described by Eisenmenger, this is defined as pulmonary hypertension at systemic levels due to raised pulmonary vascular resistance, with reversed shunting (*i.e.*, right to left) through a large ventricular septal defect [1].

Eisenmenger's syndrome

• This extension of the term by Wood includes all defects associated with pulmonary hypertension at systemic levels and pulmonary vascular disease; this includes all shunts whether they are atrial, ventricular, or even at the aortopulmonary level [2].

Symptoms

Dyspnea: related to degree of hypoxia; breathlessness least marked in an Eisenmenger patent ductus arteriosus because blue blood is shunted to lower body.

Angina of effort.

Exertional syncope: low cardiac output.

Hemoptysis: pulmonary infarction or capillary rupture.

Ankle swelling: right ventricular failure.

Palpitation: sinus tachycardia, atrial arrhythmias.

Signs

Central cyanosis.

Clubbing: with patent ductus arteriosus, toes clubbed and more cyanosed than hands.

Low-volume pulse, arrhythmias.

Raised venous pressure: with a dominant "a" wave.

Prominent right ventricular impulse with palpable pulmonary second sound.

Right atrial fourth heart sound, pulmonary ejection click, loud pulmonary second sound.

Murmurs: not from defects; low flow across large defects, thus murmurs from effects of pulmonary hypertension; early diastolic murmur due to pulmonary regurgitation, pansystolic murmur of tricuspid regurgitation.

Second sound fixed and split with atrial septal defect, single with ventricular septal defect, normally split with patent ductus.

Ankle edema: with right ventricular failure.

Investigations

ECG: shows P pulmonale (right atrial hypertrophy), right axis deviation, with tall R waves and inverted T waves in right precordial leads (right ventricular hypertrophy).

Chest radiography: shows large main pulmonary artery with narrowed "pruned" peripheral vessels.

Two-dimensional echocardiography: shows anatomy of defect and effects of right ventricular disease (enlarged right ventricle compressing small left ventricle).

Cardiac catheterization: pulmonary pressures at systemic levels, with evidence of shunting on saturation samples.

Complications

Right ventricular failure.

Sudden death.

Polycythemia.

Cerebral abscess.

Hemorrhage.

Paradoxical embolus.

Infective endocarditis.

Hemoptysis.

Hyperuricemia.

Differential diagnosis

Tetralogy of Fallot.

Transposition with pulmonary stenosis.

Primary pulmonary hypertension.

Secondary pulmonary hypertension: *e.g.*, pulmonary vasculitis or pulmonary thromboembolic disease.

• Any of these may coexist with a patent foramen ovale and may confuse the significance of the defect.

Etiology

• Associated defects include the following:

Ventricular septal defect.

Atrial septal defect.

Patent ductus arteriosus.

Aortopulmonary defect.

Double outlet right ventricle.

Truncus arteriosus.

Transposition of great vessels.

Epidemiology

• The incidence of congenital heart disease is ~10 in 1000 live births; only a few of these progress to Eisenmenger's syndrome.

Treatment

Diet and lifestyle

• Pregnancy carries significant mortality and should be avoided.

• Travel to high altitude is extremely poorly tolerated.

• Strenuous exertion and competitive sports must be avoided.

• Oxygen should be given during flights and dehydration avoided.

Pharmacological treatment

Diuretics

• Standard diuretic treatment is appropriate for right ventricular failure, but care must be taken to avoid dehydration.

Digoxin

• Digoxin remains the mainstay for rate control of atrial fibrillation. Role of primary antiarrhythmic agents such as amiodarone has been little studied.

Standard dosage	Digoxin, 0.0625–0.25 mg daily.
Contraindications	Renal failure.
Special points	Hypokalemia must be avoided.
Main drug interactions	None.
Main side effects	Anorexia, nausea, vomiting, arrhythmias.

Antibiotics

• Antibiotics are indicated for invasive procedures and to treat infective endocarditis (*see* Endocarditis *for specific details).*

Anticoagulants

• Anticoagulants are indicated when thromboembolism is clinically evident (*e.g.*, transient ischemic attacks) and for patients with atrial fibrillation.

Standard dosage	Warfarin guided by INR.
Contraindications	Pregnancy, peptic ulcer, severe hypertension.
Main drug interactions	*See manufacturer's current prescribing information.*
Main side effects	Hemorrhage.

Other options

• Nonpharmacological methods of contraception are preferred, but the progesterone-only pill may be used.

• No effective pulmonary vasodilators can be recommended routinely; controlled trials on an individual patient basis may be appropriate.

• Hemoptysis should be treated as a medical emergency; specialist treatment at a cardiac center is recommended.

Treatment aims

To improve symptoms and prolong survival.

Other treatments

• Surgical correction of the anatomical defect is not possible when pulmonary vascular resistance is raised.

• Heart–lung transplantation offers the best chance of survival in severely disabled patients, but they must be free from other disease, *e.g.*, renal failure.

• Phlebotomy should be done, with simultaneous fluid replacement, to avoid symptoms of polycythemia.

Prognosis

• Death occurs most often in the fourth decade, with sudden death being the most common mechanism [3].

• Long-term survival after heart–lung transplantation is possible, but studies are in progress at present.

Follow-up and management

• Patients need careful follow-up.

• Attention must be paid to hematocrit and phlebotomy in polycythemic patients.

• Cardiological input to all aspects of the patient's medical care is essential (*e.g.*, contraception and pregnancy, noncardiac surgery, infections).

Key references

1. Graham TP Jr: The Eisenmenger Syndrome. In *Adult Congenital Heart Disease*. Edited by Roberts WC. Philadelphia: FA Davis; 1987:567–582.
2. Wood P: The Eisenmenger syndrome, or pulmonary hypertension with reversed central shunt. *BMJ* 1958, ii:755–762.
3. Liberthson RR: Congenital Heart Disease: Diagnosis and Management in Children and Adults. Boston: Little Brown; 1989:87–94.

Diagnosis

Symptoms

Headache, behavioral abnormality, fever, photophobia, drowsiness; may progress to confusion, coma, convulsions.

Speech disturbance, limb weakness, incoordination, involuntary movements: indicating focal cerebral involvement.

Seizures.

Signs

Drowsiness, confusion, irritability, coma.

Neck stiffness: due to associated meningeal inflammation (may be absent).

Associated focal cerebral hemisphere signs: *e.g.*, hemiparesis and dysphasia (consider herpes simplex encephalitis).

Ataxia, nystagmus, myoclonus, involuntary movements, extensor plantar responses.

Investigations

CT and MRI of brain: help to exclude other causes and may show brain edema; focal inferior temporal and orbital frontal damage with herpes simplex can take several days to become apparent on plain CT but may be seen earlier on contrast-enhanced CT.

Lumbar puncture and CSF analysis: CSF may be under increased pressure and usually shows lymphocytic pleocytosis, modestly elevated protein, and normal glucose concentration; showing a fourfold rise in specific viral antibody titers is only helpful in retrospect; enzyme-linked immunoassays for viral antigens and gene amplification with polymerase chain reaction are increasingly available to aid early specific diagnosis [2].

EEG: shows widespread slow activity with diffuse brain disorder and may show periodic complexes or focal slowing over temporal region in herpes simplex encephalitis.

Complications

Seizures and status epilepticus: often occur and need vigorous treatment.

Cerebral edema: may cause herniation and calls for measures to reduce intracranial pressure.

Differential diagnosis

Meningitis: bacterial, tuberculous, fungal, or viral.

Acute disseminated encephalomyelitis.

Toxic encephalopathy with systemic infection.

Metabolic encephalopathy: usually no fever, headache, or CSF abnormality.

Cerebral abscess, empyema, subdural hematoma, and other mass lesions.

Meningeal carcinomatosis.

Etiology

• Viral invasion of brain parenchyma causes an inflammatory reaction of varying intensity, associated with perivascular cuffing with lymphocytes and other mononuclear cells and with destruction of nerve cells and glia; hemorrhagic necrosis may occur.

Epidemiology

• Herpes simplex virus is the most common cause of sporadic encephalitis.

• Other herpes viruses, especially herpes zoster, cytomegalovirus, and Epstein-Barr virus, are common causes, particularly when immunity is impaired, as in transplant or AIDS patients.

• Arboviral encephalitis occurs in epidemics in which mosquitoes bite humans.

• Mumps encephalitis and subacute sclerosing encephalitis have declined in incidence with vaccination; the latter is a progressive late complication of measles infection.

• Progressive multifocal leukoencephalopathy, common in AIDS patients, is due to a human polyoma virus (JC) complicating immunodeficiency.

• HIV may cause meningoencephalitis at seroconversion and, later, a slowly progressive dementia.

Treatment

Diet and lifestyle

Not relevant.

Pharmacological treatment

• No effective treatment is available against many of the viruses causing encephalitis; often, the specific causative virus is not identified.

• Seizures need prompt anticonvulsant administration to reduce the deleterious effects of further seizures.

• Full supportive measures are necessary during what is often a self-limiting illness with good recovery.

• Ventilation, mannitol, and dexamethasone can be used acutely to manage edema.

• Intravenous acyclovir started early reduces the morbidity and mortality of herpes simplex encephalitis; treatment should not await the outcome of brain biopsy, which is seldom appropriate [2].

Standard dosage Acyclovir, 10 mg/kg i.v. infusion every 8 h for 10 days (adults), 500 mg/m^2 every 8 h (children aged 3 months to 12 years).

Contraindications Hypersensitivity.

Special points Renal impairment necessitates dose reduction.

Main drug interactions Possible interaction with zidovudine.

• Ganciclovir may be of benefit when cytomegalovirus is the probable cause.

• Improvement of HIV encephalopathy has been reported with zidovudine.

Treatment aims

To treat herpes simplex encephalitis.

To prevent recurrent seizures.

To control raised intracranial pressure.

To provide optimal rehabilitation when necessary.

Prognosis

• The outcome varies with different causative viruses, the age of the patient, and associated underlying disease.

• Death and serious residual disability are frequent with herpes simplex when the diagnosis and treatment are delayed.

Follow-up and management

• Specialized neurological rehabilitation may be important for patients with residual disability in the wake of the illness.

Key references

1. Aurelius E, *et al.*: Rapid diagnosis of herpes simplex encephalitis by nested polymerase chain reaction assay of cerebrospinal fluid. *Lancet* 1991, **337**:189–192.
2. Whitley RJ: Viral encephalitis. *N Engl J Med* 1990, **323**:242–250.

Diagnosis

Definition

• Endocarditis is an infection (usually bacterial) of the lining of the heart (usually the valves); the hallmark is endocardial vegetations consisting of platelet or fibrin thrombi with bacteria and mononuclear cells.

Subacute endocarditis: low-virulence organisms on previously abnormal valves.
Acute endocarditis: high-virulence organisms on previously normal valves.
Culture-negative endocarditis: negative blood cultures may be due to previous partial treatment, infection by an unusual organism (*e.g.*, chlamydiae, rickettsiae, *Brucella* spp, fungi), or noninfective endocarditis.
Noninfective endocarditis: Libman–Sacks endocarditis in SLE; noninfected vegetations occur (mitral more than aortic) with valvular stenosis or regurgitation.
Marasmic endocarditis in terminal illnesses: sterile vegetations, rarely embolizing, often chance post-mortem finding.

Symptoms

Fever, malaise, anorexia, weight loss, rigors: nonspecific symptoms of inflammation.
Progressive heart failure: due to valve destruction (can be dramatic).
Stroke, pulseless limb, renal infarct, pulmonary infarct: due to embolization of vegetations.
Arthralgia, loin pain: due to immune-complex deposition.

Signs

Fever: unless patient is moribund or immunosuppressed.
Murmurs: except in right-sided endocarditis.
Pallor, purpura, petechiae, vasculitis, splinter hemorrhages, erythematous nodules in finger pulps, flat red spots on palms and soles, hemorrhagic retinal infarcts.
Rashes.
Heart failure.
Clubbing, café-au-lait pigmentation, splenomegaly: if disease is chronic.

Investigations

• Diagnosis depends on a high index of suspicion; no single test is "diagnostic."

Blood culture: at least three cultures needed to attempt to identify organism.
Full blood count: shows anemia, raised leukocyte count, hemolysis with paraprosthetic leaks.
Urinalysis: shows microscopic hematuria, proteinuria.
Urea and creatinine analysis: concentrations raised with glomerulonephritis.
CRP, ESR, plasma viscosity analysis: raised as markers of inflammation.
ECG: may reveal conduction disturbances indicative of septal abscess formation (*e.g.*, onset of left bundle branch block may presage heart block or sudden death).
Two-dimensional echocardiography: may reveal vegetations to support diagnosis (absence does not exclude diagnosis); can be used to assess valvular regurgitation or heart chamber size; may detect complications early (*e.g.*, abscess formation).
Transesophageal echocardiography: more sensitive than two-dimensional; indicated if diagnosis in doubt and in patients with prosthetic valves.
Serological tests: *e.g.*, to diagnose infection with *Brucella* spp, chlamydiae, rickettsiae.

Complications

Valve destruction: acute regurgitation, pulmonary edema, heart failure.
Embolism: leading to infarction; in any vascular bed.
Local extension of infection: purulent pericarditis, aortic root abscess (may cause sinus of valsalva fistula), myocardial abscess (conduction disturbance).
Septic emboli to vasa vasorum: may lead to mycotic aneurysms anywhere on vascular tree; most worrying in cerebral vessels, resulting in cerebral hemorrhage.
Distal infection (metastatic): due to septic emboli, *e.g.*, brain abscess, cerebritis.
Candidal endocarditis: may be manifest by fungal endophthalmitis.
Glomerulonephritis.

Differential diagnosis

Pyrexia of unknown origin, tuberculosis, staphylococcal septicemia, paraneoplastic phenomenon (lymphoma, carcinoma).
Systemic vasculitis.
Chordal rupture, aortic dissection, left atrial myxoma.

Etiology

• Damaged valves carry small, short-lived, sterile platelet or fibrin thrombi on their surfaces; these thrombi become infected during transient bacteremia.
• Bacteremia can result from dental manipulations (*Streptococcus viridans*), genitourinary instrumentation or surgery (*Escherichia coli, Strep. faecalis*), mucosal damage due to carcinoma of the colon (*Strep. bovis*), or insertion of intravenous lines or injections (*Staphylococcus aureus* or *epidermidis*).
• Alpha hemolytic streptococci (*Strep. viridans* group) account for 50% of patients.
• Other bacteria include *Strep. pyogenes, Haemophilus parainfluenzae, Neisseria, Pseudomonas,* and *Brucella* spp.
• Nonbacterial organisms include fungi (*e.g., Candida* spp, *Aspergillus* spp), chlamydiae (*e.g., Chlamydia psittaci*), and rickettsiae (*e.g., Coxiella burnetti*).
• Groups at risk include the following:
Patients with previously damaged endocardium (75% of cases: 25% rheumatic heart disease; 25% prosthetic heart valves; 15% bicuspid aortic valve, mitral valve prolapse; 10% congenital heart disease).
Intravenous drug abusers.
Patients with long-standing intravenous lines, *e.g.*, for feeding, chemotherapy, or hemodynamic monitoring: recurrent bacteremia, immunosuppression, and valve trauma caused by the line itself.

Epidemiology

• An average community hospital admits one patient with endocarditis each month.
• An average GP sees one patient with endocarditis every 10 years.

Treatment

Diet and lifestyle

- No special precautions are necessary.

Pharmacological treatment

- The key is accurate, early diagnosis and close cooperation between cardiologist, microbiologist, and cardiac surgeon.
- Patients presenting with fever and suspected endocarditis do not need emergency antibiotic treatment (unless acutely unwell); a delay of 48–72 h allows efforts to make an accurate diagnosis.
- Positive blood cultures allow the initiation of antibiotic treatment based on probable sensitivities, while laboratory confirmation is awaited.
- If the blood culture is negative, appropriate serology for culture-negative organisms should be sent, while "best-bet" antibiotics are given.
- Successful treatment should result in a fall in fever within 10 days and a fall in CRP within 2 weeks.

Standard dosage *For Streptococcus viridans:* penicillin G, 8–24 mU i.v. daily as 6-hourly boluses or continuous infusion.
For Staphylococcus aureus: Nafcillin or oxacillin, 2 gm i.v. every 4 h.
Each with aminoglycoside in synergistic doses (*e.g.*, 60 mg i.v. twice daily), depending on renal function and blood concentrations.
For Strep. faecalis: ampicillin and gentamicin.
For Staph. epidermidis: vancomycin.
For fungi: amphotericin B.

Contraindications Penicillin allergy: vancomycin.

Special points Adequacy of dosing can be checked by using patient's serum to inhibit or kill organisms *in vitro* (back titrations should be >1:8).

Main drug interactions Warfarin dose needs may be altered.
Risk of ototoxicity and nephrotoxicity with combined vancomycin and gentamicin, especially if renal function impaired, also when given with high-dose furosemide.

Main side effects Anaphylaxis, rashes, fever (allergic reactions to initial treatment), oropharyngeal candidiasis, and, rarely, neutropenia (penicillin G), cholestatic jaundice (floxacillin), hepatitis (floxacillin, rifampicin, amphotericin), ototoxicity (vancomycin, gentamicin).

Nonpharmacological treatment

- If the portal of entry was bad teeth, these should be removed.
- After the need for surgery has been identified, treatment must not be delayed.
- Surgery is indicated in the following situations [1]:

Failure of medical treatment to control infective process (possible abscess formation), indicated by continuing fever >10 days, rising CRP concentration, worsening nephritis.

Indications of abscess formation, *e.g.*, conduction abnormalities, cavity on echocardiography, or prosthetic valve dehiscence.

Hemodynamic deterioration, *e.g.*, pulmonary edema or increasing cardiomegaly.

Infection by organisms that are difficult to eradicate, *e.g.*, *Staphylococcus aureus, Candida* spp, *Aspergillus* spp.

Infection on a prosthetic valve.

Recurrent embolization or enlarging, large size vegetations while patient is on effective antimicrobial therapy.

Treatment aims

To eradicate infection and prevent valve damage.

Prognosis

- Despite advances in diagnosis and treatment, mortality remains high at >20%; avoiding delay before diagnosis, isolation of an organism, use of high-dose antibiotics, and appropriate use of cardiac surgery should reduce this figure.
- Some patients have recurrent infection (<10%), and all are at risk of re-infection.

Follow-up and management

- Blood culture, blood count, CRP concentration, and echocardiograph should be checked 3–4 weeks after apparently successful antibiotic treatment has been stopped.
- Removal of the predisposing factor (*e.g.*, ventricular septal defect, patent ductus arteriosus) should be considered.

Prevention

- Patients at risk should maintain good dental hygiene and receive antibiotic prophylaxis for potentially bacteremic maneuvers, *e.g.*, tooth extraction, genitourinary surgery, instrumentation [2].
- This will, however, probably prevent only 10% of cases.

Key references

1. Larbalestier RI, *et al.*: Acute bacterial endocarditis. Optimizing surgical results. *Circulation* 1992, **86 (suppl)**:II68–II74.
2. Working Party of the British Society of Antimicrobial Chemotherapy: Antibiotic prophylaxis of infective endocarditis. *Lancet* 1990, **335**:88–89; 1992, **339**:1292–1293.

Diagnosis

Symptoms

Seizures: usually abrupt onset, transient, stereotyped.

Loss of or altered awareness.

Abnormal posture, tone, movements.

Somatic, visual, auditory, olfactory, gustatory, or visceral sensations.

***Déjà vu, jamais vu*, macropsia, micropsia.**

Signs

• Usually no signs are manifest.

• Patients should be checked for the following:

Mental state and higher mental function.

Focal neurological deficit, head circumference, hemiatrophy.

Evidence of raised intracranial pressure.

Evidence of adverse effects from antiepileptic drugs.

Cardiovascular abnormalities.

Investigations

EEG: routine, with hyperventilation and photic stimulation; if normal and diagnosis in doubt, sleep-deprived and sleep EEG, 24-h ambulatory tape, video-EEG monitoring can be considered (if episodes frequent).

Neuroimaging: MRI superior to CT, necessary for intractable partial seizures or focal deficit, if CT normal or unclear, or if surgical treatment of epilepsy contemplated.

Antiepileptic drug concentration measurement: if prescribed treatment, to check compliance and to assess role of medication levels in symptoms and seizure control.

Blood chemistry: fasting glucose, liver, renal, and complete blood count profiles.

Prolactin measurement: transient rise to 1000 mU/L in serum up to 20 min after tonic–clonic seizures; not raised if attack not epileptic; may rise after complex partial seizure.

Neuropsychology: if cognition or memory causes concern.

Chest radiography, ECG, HIV and syphilis serology: can also be considered.

Complications

Trauma.

Status epilepticus.

Sudden unexpected death, atrial arrythmias.

Psychosocial handicap.

Differential diagnosis

Altered or lost awareness
Syncope, vagal overactivity, breath holding (children), arrhythmia, cardiac outflow obstruction, drug abuse, hypoglycemia, toxic confusional state, narcolepsy or cataplexy, transient global amnesia, psychologically mediated disorders.

Abnormal movements
Paroxysmal movement disorder, oculogyric crisis, tetany from hyperventilation, psychologically mediated disorders.

Neurological deficit
Transient ischemic attack, stroke, migraine, psychologically mediated disorders.

Sleep attacks
Parasomnias, paroxysmal nocturnal dystonia.

Etiology

• Causes include the following:

Cryptogenic.
Idiopathic (often familial).
Hippocampal sclerosis (most frequent cause of refractory temporal-lobe epilepsy).
Cortical dysplasia.
Tumor.
Trauma.
Infection: encephalitis, bacterial meningitis.
Vascular: infarct, hemorrhage.
Hypoxia.
Granuloma: tuberculosis, cystercercosis (in developing countries).

Epidemiology

• 1 person in 40 has a nonfebrile seizure at some time in his or her life.

• The annual incidence in the general population is 1 in 2000.

• The prevalence of active epilepsy (seizure within past 2 years) is 1 in 200 of the general population and 1 in 150 people <15 years.

Classification

• Classification is important for investigation, treatment, and prognosis.

Partial
Simple: aware, responsive, no amnesia.
Complex: impaired awareness, responsiveness, recollection; possible automatisms (orofacial, speech, motor).
Secondary generalized: evolves from partial seizures.

Generalized
Absence, myoclonic, clonic, tonic, tonic–clonic, atonic.

Treatment

Diet and lifestyle

• Patients must avoid excessive fatigue or alcohol excesses.

• Patients are not allowed to drive, swim, or go to heights alone or to operate dangerous tools.

Pharmacological treatment

• Drug interactions are complex.

• The following doses are for adults.

First line

Phenytoin: for all seizure types; may give 20 mg/kg loading dose.

Carbamazepine: for simple, complex, or secondarily generalized partial seizures and for tonic or clonic generalized seizures; 100 mg initially, average maintenance dose 600–2400 mg daily in 3–4 doses.

Clonazepam: for myoclonic seizures (second-line treatment for absences, atonic seizures); 0.5 mg initially, average maintenance dose 0.5–3.0 mg daily in 1–2 doses.

Ethosuximide: for absences; 250 mg initially, average maintenance dose 500–1500 mg daily in 1–2 doses.

Valproate: primarily for generalized or myoclonic seizures; 750 mg initially, average maintenance dose 1000–2500 mg daily in 3 divided doses.

Second line

Gabapentin: for partial seizures; 300 mg initially, average maintenance dose 1800–3600 mg daily in 3 doses.

Lamotrigine: for partial seizures, tonic, clonic, tonic-clonic, or atonic seizures, and absence or atypical absence; 25 mg initially, average maintenance dose 300–500 mg daily in 2 doses; if combined with valproate, initial dosage should be 25 mg increasing on alternate weeks.

Phenobarbitol: for partial seizures, tonic, clonic, tonic-clonic, atonic, or myoclonic seizures, and atypical absences; 60 mg initially, average maintenance dose 60–180 mg daily as single dose.

General adverse effects

Acute, dose-related: sedation, dizziness, nausea, headaches.

Idiosyncratic: skin rash, severe bone-marrow suppression, diplopia, liver failure, behavioral disorder, weight gain, tremor, gingival hyperplasia, soft tissue changes, peripheral neuropathy.

Treatment aims

To control seizures without drug side effects.

Prognosis

• Remission occurs in 70%–80% of patients in 2–5 years; patients have a 30% chance of remission if epilepsy is active for 5 years.
• After the patient is in remission, the overall risk of relapse is 20% in 2 years if the patient remains on medication, and 40% if medication is tapered.
• Risk factors for relapse include juvenile myoclonic epilepsy, generalized spike-wave on EEG, structural brain damage, and difficulty obtaining seizure control.

Follow-up and management

Staged treatment strategy

• This can be followed as far as necessary.

1. Minimizing of epileptogenic stimuli: fever (in children), alcohol, excessive fatigue, epileptogenic drugs, photosensitivity.
2. Initial small dose of first-line drug.
3. Dosage increase if needed, up to maximum tolerated dose.
4. Review of diagnosis, cause, and compliance if no response after treatment.
5. Trial of other first-line drugs alone or combined (80% of patients best treated by monotherapy, 10%–15% by two drugs).
6. Second-line drugs considered.
7. Gradual withdrawal of unhelpful drugs or drugs causing adverse effects.
8. Referral for novel drugs.
9. Referral for possible neurosurgical treatment of partial or secondarily generalized seizures.
10. Gradual drug withdrawal considered in patients free of seizures for 2–3 years.

Essential counseling

• Patients should be advised of the need to take medication regularly, reasonable expectations, driving license regulations, contraception and pregnancy, safe bathing, and safe cooking with a microwave.

General references

1. Wylie E: *The Treatment of Epilepsy.* Philadelphia: Lea and Febiger; 1993.
2. Engel JS: *Seizures and Epilepsy.* Philadelphia: FA Davis; 1989.

Erythema multiforme and Stevens–Johnson syndrome

Diagnosis

Symptoms

• These conditions form a spectrum from the relatively mild erythema multiforme syndrome to the severe and potentially life-threatening Stevens–Johnson syndrome.

Nonspecific upper respiratory tract infection: prodromal syndrome.

Intensely itchy skin rash.

Painful, bullous lesions: involving two or more mucous membranes in Stevens-Johnson syndrome; shallow ulcers result if the bulla ruptures.

Fever, malaise, cough, sore throat, chest pain, vomiting, diarrhea, myalgia, arthralgia: severe systemic reaction in Stevens–Johnson syndrome.

Signs

Erythema multiforme

Classic "target" lesions: develop abruptly and symmetrically, heaviest peripherally; often involve palms and soles.

Urticarial plaques: may develop but do not evolve rapidly as with a true urticaria.

Vesicles and bullae: may develop in pre-existing lesions, usually heralding a more severe form of disease; severe disease with mucosal involvement and constitutional upset indicates Stevens-Johnson syndrome.

Stevens–Johnson syndrome

Bullous lesions on mucous membranes: abrupt appearance 1–14 days after other symptoms; often on oral mucosa, lips, and conjunctivae, often with variable involvement of other mucous surfaces; urethral, vulvo-vaginal, and balanitic involvement may lead to urinary retention.

Pain from oral lesions: possibly severe enough to compromise fluid intake and breathing.

Patchy pulmonary disease, pneumonia, renal failure, diarrhea, paronychia, nail loss, polyarthritis, otitis media, and coma.

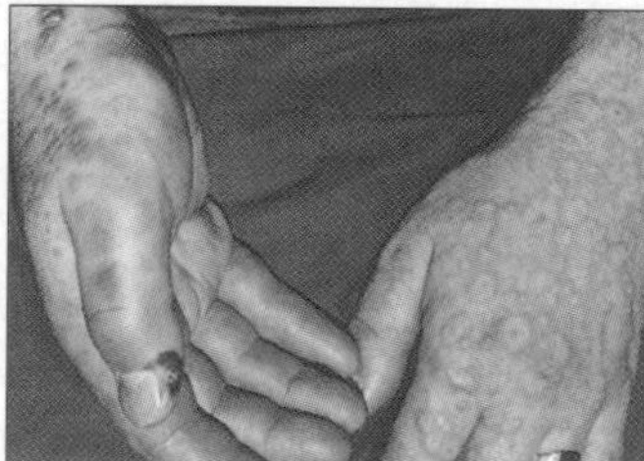

Typical "target" lesions on hands.

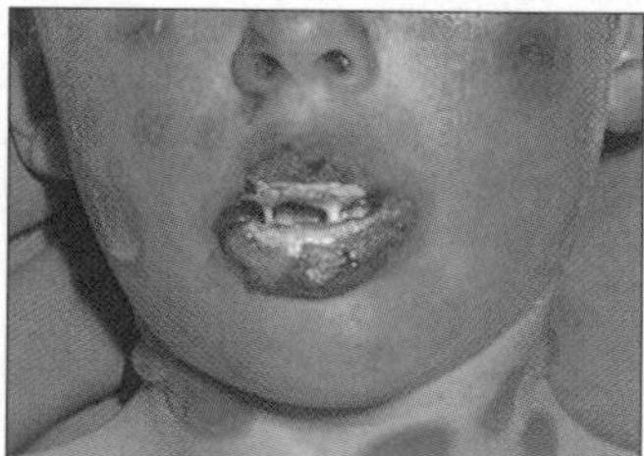

Buccal mucous membrane involvement.

Investigations

History of drug ingestion: very important.

Throat swab: to detect coxsackieviruses, herpes simplex virus, adenoviruses.

Serology: for *Mycoplasma pneumoniae*, coxsackie, herpes simplex virus, adenovirus.

Autoimmune serology: to detect collagen diseases.

Full blood count and ESR measurement: total leukocyte count often raised and may show excess of eosinophils; ESR and CRP usually raised.

U&E and albumin measurement: urea raised because of catabolic state and fluid loss if skin lesions extensive; exudation from lesions may cause hypoalbuminemia.

Skin biopsy: shows characteristic range of changes from mild dermal inflammation to full epidermal necrosis.

Complications

Blindness: caused by corneal involvement.

Recurrence: especially of disease caused by herpes simplex virus or drugs.

Differential diagnosis

• Classic cases with target lesions should prove no problem; atypical cases may resemble any of the following:

Chronic urticaria.

Toxic erythema (drugs or infection).

Collagen diseases.

Secondary syphilis.

Acute HIV seroconversion.

Hemorrhagic fevers.

Kawasaki syndrome.

Toxic epidermal necrolysis.

Chronic meningococcemia.

Etiology

• The condition is produced by a hypersensitivity reaction mediated by immune complexes in dermal blood vessels.

• In ~50% of patients, no cause is identified.

• Common antigenic triggers involve the following:

Infection by virus (especially herpes simplex, enteroviruses), *Mycoplasma pneumoniae*, chlamydiae, histoplasmosis.

Drugs: antibiotics (*e.g.*, penicillins, sulfonamides), anticonvulsants (especially phenytoin), aspirin, corticosteroids, cimetadine.

Neoplasia: leukemia, lymphoma, multiple myeloma, internal (cryptic) malignancy.

Collagen diseases: lupus erythematosis, polyarteritis, rheumatoid arthritis.

Others: sarcoidosis, foods (*e.g.*, emulsifiers in margarine).

Epidemiology

• Erythema multiforme and Stevens–Johnson syndrome account for up to 1% of dermatology outpatient consultations.

• Children <3 years and adults >50 years are rarely affected.

• The incidence peaks in the second and third decades, with 50% of patients <20 years.

• The male : female ratio is 1.5 : 1.

• The illness is most severe in young adults and children, especially boys.

• Seasonal epidemics occur, related to the common provoking agents, *e.g.*, *Mycoplasma* spp., herpesvirus, and adenoviral infections.

Treatment

Diet and lifestyle

• In rare cases of a dietary "trigger," *e.g.*, emulsifiers in margarine, this must be avoided.

• If the oral contraceptive is implicated, obvious lifestyle changes must follow.

Pharmacological treatment

For the underlying "trigger" condition

• Possible drug precipitants should be withdrawn.

• Acyclovir is indicated for herpes simplex virus, and the appropriate antibiotic for *Mycoplasma* infection (macrolide or tetracycline).

Standard dosage	Acyclovir applied directly every 4 h (ointment) or 200 mg 5 times daily. Erythromycin, 500 mg 4 times daily.
Contraindications	*Acyclovir:* renal impairment, severe dehydration. *Erythromycin:* hypersensitivity.
Main drug interactions	*Acyclovir:* other antivirals, *e.g.*, zidovudine (produces lethargy). *Erythromycin:* increase in theophylline concentrations.
Main side effects	*Acyclovir:* rashes, gastrointestinal disturbances. *Erythromycin:* gastrointestinal disturbances, nausea, vomiting, pain, diarrhea.

For skin lesions

• Antihistamines are indicated for pruritus, salicylates or NSAIDs for symptomatic relief (salicylates have been implicated as causative agents), and steroids or icthammol soaks for broken lesions.

Standard dosage	Chlorpheniramine, 4 mg orally every 6–8 h. Naproxen, 250 mg every 6–8 h.
Contraindications	*Naproxen:* active peptic ulceration; to be avoided in children (acetaminophen analgesia instead).
Special points	*Chlorpheniramine:* patients must not drive if drowsiness ensues.
Main drug interactions	*Chlorpheniramine:* alcohol or sedatives. *Naproxen:* oral anticoagulants.
Main side effects	*Chlorpheniramine:* drowsiness, headache, gastrointestinal disturbances. *Naproxen:* gastrointestinal disturbances.

For severe cases (Stevens–Johnson syndrome)

• Withdrawal of any drug precipitant and treatment of infective causes is vital.

• No data from well controlled trials are available, but the dermatological manifestations respond to a short course of high-dose steroids.

• Because of mouth involvement, enteric or parenteral feeding may be needed and should be considered during the first week.

• Intravenous fluid replacement should be instituted early.

Standard dosage	Prednisolone, 80–100 mg daily.
Contraindications	Active peptic ulceration.
Special points	Possible adrenal suppression on withdrawal.
Main drug interactions	NSAIDs, oral anticoagulants.
Main side effects	Cushing's syndrome, growth retardation in children.

Treatment aims

To remove or treat underlying "triggers."

To provide adequate pain relief for mucosal involvement.

To provide symptomatic relief for generalized skin involvement.

To maintain nutrition and fluid replacement in this hypercatabolic state.

Other treatments

• Urethral or renal tract involvement may necessitate catheterization, especially in children.

• Management in a unit used to burns care may be needed for severely ill patients.

• Careful skin nursing is essential to prevent secondary infection.

Prognosis

• The rash heals completely if the precipitant causes are removed or treated.

• Complete recovery is normal, but corneal scarring may occur after *Mycoplasma* infection.

• Untreated Stevens–Johnson syndrome has a 5%–15% mortality.

• Typical erythema multiforme runs a mild course, subsiding to normal after 2–3 weeks.

• Cases related to herpes simplex usually follow a simple course but may recur with further reactivation of herpes simplex; prophylactic acyclovir is then indicated.

• Cases related to *Mycoplasma* infection or drugs often subside more slowly and will more probably progress to Stevens–Johnson syndrome.

Follow-up and management

• Prophylaxis against herpes simplex virus (topical or occasionally systemic acyclovir) is important if the virus precipitates erythema multiforme; this should reduce the incidence of further attacks.

General references

1. Hurwitz S: Erythema multiforme: a review of its characteristics, diagnostic criteria, and management. *Pediatr Rev* 1990, **11**:217–222.
2. Renfro L, *et al.*: Controversy: are systemic steroids indicated in the treatment of erythema multiforme? *Pediatr Dermatol* 1989, **6**:43–50.

Diagnosis

Symptoms

Painful red nodules: on lower legs and occasionally on thighs and forearms; pain worse on weight-bearing; gradual appearance; can become almost confluent; gradual healing (3–6 weeks), with bruising but no scarring.

"Crops" of lesions: occurring at different times, so that lesions manifest at different stages of evolution.

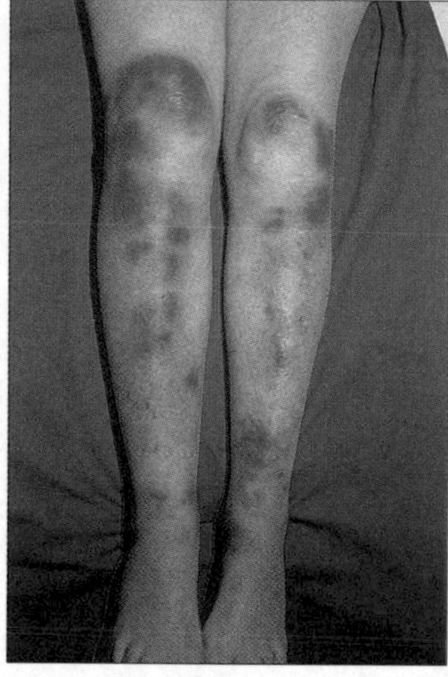

Classic lesions over pretibial region.

Signs

Tender erythematous nodules: 1–5 cm diameter; usually bilateral over pretibial areas; no ulceration or blistering; involution over 3–6 weeks, with yellow–purple bruising.

Fever and systemic reaction: variable but may precede lesions by 1–7 days.

Investigations

• Discovering the cause is important because treatment of this prevents recurrences.

History: for drugs (*e.g.*, oral contraceptive), pregnancy, contact with tuberculosis, inflammatory bowel disease, yersiniosis, histoplasmosis, streptococcal infection.

Full blood count, ESR analysis: acute-phase reactants always raised.

Chest radiography: to detect features of sarcoidosis, tuberculosis, disseminated fungal infection.

Bacteriology: sputum or early morning urine for acid/alcohol-fast bacilli; throat swab or antistreptolysin O titer for evidence of streptococcal infection.

Mantoux test: strongly positive in tuberculosis, negative in sarcoidosis.

Complications

• The skin lesions have no complications.

• Any complications relate to the underlying condition; if this is not controlled, the skin lesion may continue to be manifest (lasting up to 4–5 months).

Differential diagnosis

Erythema nodosum leprosum: in multibacillary leprosy, unrelated acute reactional state to the release of mycobacterial protein during treatment.

Erythematous skin lesions of pretibial area: *e.g.*, pretibial myxedema.

Rheumatoid nodules (usually on elbows, wrists, or palms).

Etiology

• Erythema nodosum is a septal panniculitis in subcutaneous fat due to a hypersensitivity reaction to antigenic or other stimulus.

• Causes include the following:

Drugs: *e.g.*, penicillin, sulfonamides, oral contraceptive pill in 25% of patients.

Infections: *e.g.*, tuberculosis, streptococci, *Yersinia, Salmonella, Campylobacter* spp., deep fungal infection, leprosy.

Inflammatory conditions: *e.g.*, sarcoidosis, inflammatory bowel disease, Behçet's syndrome, pregnancy, thyroid disease.

• 20%–40% of cases are idiopathic.

Epidemiology

• The peak age is 20–30 years, but erythema nodosum can occur at any age.

• The female : male ratio is 3 : 1.

• Patients with tuberculosis-related disease are usually <20 years.

• Patients with disease caused by pregnancy or inflammatory bowel disorders are usually 15–40 years.

• Patients with disease caused by Behçet's syndrome or sarcoidosis are usually 20–40 years.

• Fever and systemic reactions occur more often and for longer in older patients.

Treatment

Diet and lifestyle

• During the acute phase of the inflammation, prolonged weight-bearing should be avoided.

Pharmacological treatment

• Treatment of skin lesions is primarily symptomatic.

• Management of the underlying condition prevents further erythema nodosum.

For pain relief

• NSAIDs should be sufficient.

Standard dosage Naproxen, 250 mg every 6–8 h.

Contraindications Hypersensitivity, active peptic ulceration; caution with concomitant anticoagulation and asthma.

Main drug interactions Warfarin.

Main side effects Gastrointestinal disturbances, discomfort, nausea, ulceration.

Systemic steroids

• Steroids are effective, but extreme caution must be observed; they should be used only if the underlying conditions, *e.g.*, tuberculosis, have been adequately treated.

Standard dosage Prednisolone, 20–40 mg initially, reduced rapidly over 10 days to nil.

Contraindications Active peptic ulceration.

Special points Possible adrenal suppression on sudden withdrawal.

Main drug interactions NSAIDs, oral anticoagulants.

Main side effects Cushing's syndrome, growth retardation in children, glucose intolerance, osteoporosis.

Treatment aims

To provide symptomatic relief of lesion-related pain or discomfort.

To remove or treat underlying cause.

Other treatments

Potassium iodide.

Wet dressings to the lesions for symptomatic relief.

Prognosis

• Lesions usually clear in 3–6 weeks.

• Spontaneous resolution is usual.

Follow-up and management

• The most important aspect of erythema nodosum management is diagnosis of any underlying precipitant.

General references

1. Fox MD, Schwartz RA: Erythema nodosum. *Am Fam Physician* 1992, **46**:818–822.

2. Hannuksela M: Erythema nodosum. *Clin Dermatol* 1986, **4**:88–95.

Diagnosis

Symptoms and signs

• Disease is typically advanced at the time of presentation.

Dysphagia: solids > liquids is the classic presentation.

Inability to swallow saliva: implies high-grade destruction.

Pain: occasionally early symptom; usually manifestation of mediastinal extension.

Weight loss, anemia, cervical lymphadenopathy, hepatomegaly: late symptoms; less specific.

Investigations

Blood count: may reveal iron-deficiency anemia.

Biochemical analysis: may show raised alkaline phosphatase concentration with hepatic or bony metastases; low serum albumin concentration indicates malnutrition.

Barium swallow: shows lesion; endoscopy always needed for confirmation.

Endoscopy: offers direct examination of lesion and provides opportunity to obtain specimens for histology and cytology.

CT, endoscopic ultrasonography: to identify patients with localized tumors for resection.

Complications

Esophageal obstruction.

Malnutrition.

Bleeding.

Fistula to bronchial tree.

Invasion of mediastinum.

Aspiration.

Differential diagnosis

Benign esophageal stricture.

Motility disorders, particularly achalasia.

Extrinsic compression of esophagus: *e.g.*, carcinoma of bronchus.

Schatzki's ring.

Etiology

• Several factors have been identified in association with esophageal cancer, including the following:

Barrett's esophagus [1,2].

More common in lower socioeconomic groups.

Environmental factors poorly characterized (*e.g.*, high-risk regions in Iran, China, and Russia identified).

Increased consumption of tobacco and alcohol.

African-Americans have a 4–5 fold increase compared to whites.

Stasis.

Caustic injury: carcinoma occurs ~40 years later.

Achalasia.

Epidemiology

• Esophageal carcinoma is one of the most common cancers in the world, but wide geographic variations are found.

• It is relatively less frequent in western Europe and North America (incidence, 5 in 100 000).

Histological types

Tumors of upper and middle esophagus: usually squamous cell carcinoma.

Tumors of lower esophagus: mostly adenocarcinoma.

Treatment

Diet and lifestyle

• Adequate nutrition should be ensured, preferably orally.

• The need for a fine-bore enteral feeding tube or percutaneous endoscopic gastrostomy tube should be anticipated, and the tube should be placed prior to high-grade obstruction of the esophagus.

Pharmacological treatment

• Simple analgesics are used for pain control in the early stages, but opiates are needed later.

Standard dosage	Morphine, 5-10 mg every 4 h, titrate as needed.
Contraindications	Raised intracranial pressure.
Special points	Concerns about side effects should not deter use.
Main drug interactions	None significant.
Main side effects	Constipation, nausea, drowsiness.

Nonpharmacological treatment

• Curative surgery or radiotherapy is attempted whenever possible, but most patients are suitable for only palliative treatment [3-5].

Surgical resection: suitable in only about one-third of patients; esophagectomy with primary esophagogastrostomy most frequently chosen.

Endoscopic palliation: to create a wider lumen to allow food and drink to pass; options include simple dilatation (by bougie or balloon), endoscopic intubations (prosthetic stents available), laser therapy, thermal devices (*e.g.*, bipolar coagulation).

Radiotherapy: intracavitary irradiation with cobalt or iridium or external beam irradiation; can be beneficial for pain from mediastinal extension.

Treatment aims

To delay physical deterioration by improving and maintaining swallowing and nutrition.

To diminish pain.

To avoid respiratory complications.

Prognosis

• Most patients die within 4–12 months; in patients with successful surgical resection, the 5-year survival rate is 10%–15%.

• After resection, mortality is 3%–20% and complications are 5%–12%.

• Causes of death from surgery include cardiopulmonary complications and sepsis due to anastomotic leaks; malnutrition is a contributing factor.

Follow-up and management

• Patients who have had curative treatment should be monitored for features of relapse.

• A fistula communicating with the bronchial tree should be considered in patients with progressive disease who develop a cough; stent placement may be beneficial in these patients.

Key references

1. Cameron AJ: Barrett's esophagus and adenocarcinoma. *Gastroenterology* 1993, **102**:1421–1424.
2. Kruse P, *et al.*: Barrett's oesophagus and oesophageal adenocarcinoma. *Scand J Gastroenterol* 1993, **28**:193–196.
3. Cuschieri A: Treatment of carcinoma of the oesophagus. *Ann R Coll Surg Engl* 1991, **73**:1–3.
4. Griffin SM, Robertson CS: Nonsurgical treatment of cancer of the oesophagus. *Br J Surg* 1993, **80**:412–413.
5. Haller DG: Treatments for esophageal cancer. *N Engl J Med* 1992, **326**:1629–1630.

Diagnosis

Symptoms

• Symptoms do not predict the severity of mucosal inflammation.

Heartburn: the most common symptom.

Retrosternal pain: may resemble angina.

Odynophagia (painful swallowing): suggests infectious etiology or pill-induced ulcer.

Regurgitation of food, acid, or bitter juice: may be confused with "vomiting" (but without nausea).

Dysphagia: stricture or motility disorder.

Respiratory symptoms: *e.g.*, nocturnal cough or dyspnea, asthma.

Signs

• Signs are frequently absent.

Pulmonary consolidation or bronchospasm: rarely, if aspiration has occurred as a result of regurgitation.

Investigations

• Blood tests are helpful to exclude other diagnoses, including anemia from ongoing blood loss.

Radiography: not reliable for showing esophagitis (particularly mild forms) or reflux; may be of some use in assessing esophageal motility.

Endoscopy: preferred to radiography because it offers visualization of mucosa and option of obtaining cytology and histology; allows determination of severity of esophagitis.

pH monitoring: for diagnosis of acid reflux without esophagitis; for quantifying reflux to assess effectiveness of treatment or before antireflux surgery.

Manometry: useful to exclude associated motility disorders or before antireflux surgery.

Cardiac tests: to exclude cardiac disease as a source of symptoms.

Complications

Stricture [1].

Barrett's esophagus.

Aspiration, leading to night cough, bronchospasm, pneumonia, asthma, hoarseness.

Bleeding.

Differential diagnosis

Ischemic heart disease.

Esophageal motility disorder.

Peptic ulcer disease.

Gallstone disease.

Esophageal malignancy.

Etiology

• Esophagitis is mucosal damage most commonly caused by gastroesophageal reflux, which occurs when the lower esophageal sphincter is incompetent or esophageal clearance is impaired.

• The damage is caused by prolonged exposure of esophageal mucosa to gastric contents and is more intense if the mucosa is compromised or if gastric emptying is delayed.

• Hiatal hernia is a common condition that rarely causes symptoms; reflux symptoms are often erroneously attributed to hiatal hernia.

Epidemiology

• Two-thirds of the population may suffer from reflux at some time, but only a small proportion seek medical advice.

• Mechanical and hormonal factors make reflux common during pregnancy.

Savary–Miller endoscopic classification

Grade I: nonconfluent mucosal lesions.

Grade II: confluent mucosal lesions.

Grade III: circumferential mucosal lesions.

Grade IV: deep ulcer, stricture, or Barrett's esophagus.

Treatment

Diet and lifestyle

• Reducing weight, stopping smoking, eating small meals, avoiding certain foods (*e.g.*, chocolate, citrus, coffee, mints, alcohol), and sleeping with the head of the bed raised are measures that decrease reflux [2,3].

• Patients should be advised to remain upright for 3–4 hours after a meal.

• NSAIDs, slow-release potassium chloride, nitrates, and calcium blockers (*e.g.*, nifedipine) may also aggravate symptoms.

Pharmacological treatment

Antacids

• Antacids may provide reasonable but short-lasting relief; they have little effect on mucosal inflammation.

Standard dosage 30–60 mL 3–4 times daily.

Contraindications Renal failure (magnesium based).

Main drug interactions Iron, phenytoin, penicillamine, tetracycline.

Main side effects Constipation (aluminum based), diarrhea (magnesium based).

Acid antisecretory agents

• These diminish gastric acid production, thus decreasing exposure of the esophageal mucosa.

• Proton-pump inhibitors (*e.g.*, omeprazole) are more powerful than H_2 antagonists (*e.g.*, ranitidine) and are favored in severe cases.

Standard dosage Ranitidine, 150–300 mg twice daily.
Omeprazole, 20–40 mg daily.
Lansoprazole, 30 mg daily.
Dose can be titrated against symptoms.

Contraindications Known hypersensitivity.

Main drug interactions *Omeprazole, lansoprazole:* warfarin, phenytoin, diazepam.

Main side effects *Ranitidine:* the following side effects are rare and usually not clinically significant: headache, blood disorders, increased liver enzyme levels.
Omeprazole: skin reactions, diarrhea, headache, enteric infections are rarely observed.

Motility-enhancing agents

• These are not widely used, with the exception of cisapride, which is as effective as some H_2 antagonists.

Standard dosage Cisapride, 10–20 mg 3–4 times daily, 30 min before meals.

Contraindications Gastrointestinal hemorrhage or perforation, mechanical bowel obstruction.

Main drug interactions Anticoagulants: effect possibly enhanced; erythromycin.

Main side effects Diarrhea, abdominal discomfort.

Mucosal-protecting agents

• Only sucralfate has proved reasonably effective.

Standard dosage Sucralfate, 1 g 4 times daily.

Contraindications Caution in renal impairment (aluminum toxicity).

Main drug interactions Decreased bioavailability of tetracycline, phenytoin, cimetidine (avoided by separating administration from sucralfate by 2 h).

Main side effects Constipation.

Treatment aims

To control symptoms.

To prevent complications, especially for stricture formation [4].

Other treatments

Antireflux surgery

• Nissen fundoplication and its modifications are the most popular techniques; they are sometimes done laparascopically.

• Surgery is indicated for the following: refractory, debilitating symptoms that are complicated by bleeding, asthma, or severe strictures or that are refractory to aggressive medical management.

Prognosis

• This is a chronic and relapsing condition, but up to 40% of patients remain in remission.

Follow-up and management

• Permanent reflux-reducing measures (particularly weight reduction) must be implemented in order to avoid relapse. Some form of treatment may be necessary to maintain remission. Achievement of esophagitis healing may not be necessary; the simple aim of symptom control may be sufficient.

• Long-term treatment is indicated in patients who have had frequent relapse.

Key references

1. Marks AD, Richter JE: Peptic strictures of the esophagus. *Am J Gastroenterol* 1993, **88**:1160–1173.
2. Pope CE: Acid-reflux disorders. *N Engl J Med* 1994, **331**:656–660.
3. Richter JE: Esophageal chest pain: current controversies in pathogenesis, diagnosis, and therapy. *Ann Intern Med* 1989, **110**:66–78.
4. Sontag SJ: Gastro-oesophageal reflux disease. *Aliment Pharmacol Ther* 1993, **7**:293–312.

Female hypogonadotropic hypogonadism

Diagnosis

Symptoms

Primary or secondary amenorrhea: oligomenorrhea less often.

Delayed puberty: short stature.

Infertility.

Headaches and visual disturbance: indicating pituitary tumors.

Vaginal dryness, thin skin, and scalp hair loss: symptoms of estrogen deficiency.

Eating disorders and weight-loss: often hidden from family and caregivers [1,2].

Signs

• Usually few signs are manifest, particularly shortly after onset of amenorrhea.

Incomplete pubertal maturation: indicating primary amenorrhea.

Low body-mass index: <19 kg/m^2 in eating disorders.

Galactorrhea: in hyperprolactinemia.

Anosmia: Kallmann's syndrome.

Visual impairment: indicating pituitary tumors.

Atrophic vaginal mucosa.

Investigations

For the disorder

Serum follicle-stimulating hormone measurement: concentration not raised (<10 IU/L).

Progestogen challenge test: medroxyprogesterone acetate, 5 mg daily for 5 days, followed by assessment of menstrual response for 7 days; bleeding indicates estrogenization, no bleeding indicates estrogen deficiency.

Ovarian ultrasonography: small inactive or multifollicular ovaries; occasionally, by coincidence, polycystic ovaries are found (pre-existing polycystic ovarian disease overridden by hypothalamo-pituitary failure).

For the underlying cause

Serum prolactin measurement: concentration persistently >50 ng/mL indicates hyperprolactinemia.

Thyroid function tests: primary hypothyroidism is a cause of hyperprolactinemia.

MRI: to define suspected hypothalamic or pituitary tumor.

For complications

Thyroid-stimulating hormone measurement: to screen for panhypopituitarism.

Full pituitary testing: if low thyroid-stimulating hormone, history of pituitary surgery or radiotherapy, or suspicion of pituitary or hypothalamic tumor.

Radiography for bone age: if delayed in girls with primary amenorrhea, low-dose estrogen hormone replacement therapy may be used to try to achieve maximum height potential (ethinyl estradiol, 2 μg daily).

Bone densiometry: no clinical value.

Complications

Anovulatory infertility.

Unwanted pregnancy: resumption of ovulation common in hypothalamic disorders.

Osteoporosis, cardiovascular disease: long-term health risks resulting from estrogen deficiency [3].

Compression of optic chiasma: rare.

Panhypopituitarism: rare.

Differential diagnosis

Uterine malformation (cryptomenorrhea) or atresia.

Asherman's syndrome (uterine synechiae).

Etiology

• Causes include the following:

Hypothalamic

Weight loss, psychological stress, rigorous exercise [1,2].

Tumors (craniopharyngioma).

Kallmann's syndrome (anosmia/isolated gonadotropin-releasing hormone deficiency).

Hyperprolactinemia: anovulation mediated through hypothalamus.

Idiopathic hypothalamic dysfunction.

Pituitary

Prolactin-secreting macroadenomas.

Nonfunctioning pituitary tumors.

Surgery and radiotherapy.

Sheehan's syndrome (postpartum infarction).

Granulomas.

Hyperprolactinemia [4]

Pregnancy and lactation.

Drugs.

Primary hypothyroidism.

Hypothalamic disease.

Pressure on or section of pituitary stalk.

Prolactin-secreting pituitary adenomas.

See Hyperprolactinemia *for further details.*

Epidemiology

• ~40% of cases of anovulation, 55% of amenorrhea, and 6% of oligomenorrhea are due to hypogonadotropic hypogonadism.

Treatment

Diet and lifestyle

• Weight gain (supervised by dietitians and psychologists) is the most appropriate treatment for amenorrhea associated with weight loss; ovulation may be restored.

• Vitamin D and calcium supplementation are needed in patients with anorexia.

• Advice about the risk of atraumatic fractures should be given to women with long-standing untreated amenorrhea.

Pharmacological treatment

For hormone replacement (not hyperprolactinemia)

• Sex-steroid therapy alleviates symptoms of estrogen deficiency and prevents osteoporosis and cardiovascular disease.

• Estrogen is the active agent; progestogens are used to prevent endometrial neoplasia.

• Standard hormone replacement preparations are not contraceptive; women who wish to avoid the small risk of conception should use low-dose combined oral contraceptive (ethinyl estradiol, 20 μg, desogestrel, 150 μg).

Standard dosage Depends on patient's needs.

Contraindications Undiagnosed abnormal menstruation.

Special points *Transdermal estradiol patches:* poor absorption in young women because of thick skin.
Subcutaneous estradiol implants: long duration of estradiol release (up to 36 months); should be avoided in women who may request ovulation induction.
Progestogens: third-generation agent should be used to avoid deleterious effect on lipids.

Main drug interactions Anticonvulsants, warfarin.

Main side effects *Estrogen:* nausea (avoided by slow introduction).
Progestogen: premenstrual symptoms.

For infertility (not hyperprolactinemia)

• Serious causes (*e.g.*, anorexia nervosa) must be treated first.

• Pregnancy must be ruled out before treatment is initiated.

For hypothalamic dysfunction: antiestrogen, pulsatile luteinizing-hormone releasing hormone, exogenous gonadotropins are tried in turn.

For pituitary causes: exogenous gonadotropins.

See Polycystic ovarian disease *for further details.*

For hyperprolactinemia [4]

Associated with primary hypothyroidism: thyroxine.

Associated with prolactinergic drugs: possible removal of drugs.

Associated with prolactinoma: dopamine agonists to reduce tumor size and restore ovulation; surgery and radiotherapy needed rarely for some macroadenomas.

If fertility not required: standard hormone replacement treatment, with low-dose dopamine agonist to prevent tumor expansion.

If fertility required: dopamine agonist to induce ovulation.

See Hyperprolactinemia *for further details.*

Treatment aims

To alleviate underlying causes.

To prevent long-term health risks.

To achieve pregnancy.

Prognosis

• Eating disorders are difficult to control, and patients frequently relapse; sudden death is a risk, perhaps due to arrhythmias.

• Normal conception rates can be achieved for most of the common causes.

• The outcome of pregnancy is poor for underweight women.

Follow-up and management

• Most prolactinomas are <5 mm within 8 weeks of the start of dopamine agonist treatment.

• Prolactin concentration must be measured 6-monthly.

• Previously large prolactinomas may re-expand in pregnancy; visual fields must be checked.

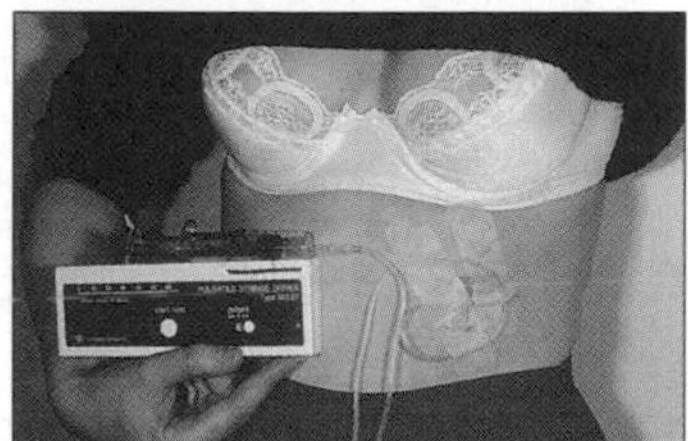

Woman with hypothalamic amenorrhea receiving pulsatile luteinizing hormone–releasing hormone subcutaneously from battery-driven pump.

Key references

1. Abraham S, *et al.*: Should ovulation be induced in women recovering from an eating disorder or who are compulsive exercisers? *Fertil Steril* 1990, **53**:566–568.
2. Patton G, *et al.*: The course of anorexia nervosa. *BMJ* 1989, **299**:139–140.
3. Gulekli B, *et al.*: Effect of treatment on established osteoporosis in young women with amenorrhoea. *Clin Endocrinol* 1994, **41**:275–281.
4. Peillon F: Functional hyperprolactinemia. *Curr Ther Endocrinol Metab* 1994, **5**:37–41.

Diagnosis

Symptoms and signs

Candida infections

White plaques in mouth or tongue, angular cheilitis.
Vulvovaginal discharge, pruritus.
Cutaneous candidiasis, intertrigo, folliculitis, balanitis, perianal or interdigital infection, diaper rash.
Paronychia or onychomycosis.
Cystitis, urethritis.
Disseminated candidiasis involving several organs, intravascular infection, endocarditis, cerebral or hepatic microabscesses.
Pneumonia, allergic wheeze, breathlessness.
Peritonitis, esophagitis.

Aspergillus infections

Wheeze, breathlessness: indicating allergic bronchopulmonary aspergillosis.
Fever, cough, hypoxia, chest discomfort or pleuritic pain, hemoptysis, pneumonia: indicating invasive aspergillosis.
Blocked nose, facial pain, nasal discharge, chronic headache: indicating allergic or saprophytic sinus infection.
Chronic otitis media or externa, meningitis or cerebral microabscesses, endocarditis, endophthalmitis, osteoarticular disorders.

Cryptococcal infections

• Onset is insidious.

Fever, headache, nausea, vomiting, neck stiffness, photophobia: indicating meningitis.
Dyspnea, cough: indicating pneumonia.

Histoplasmosis

Breathlessness, lung infiltrates: indicating pulmonary histoplasmosis.
Pancytopenia, pneumonia, lymphadenopathy, hepatosplenomegaly, oral or gastrointestinal ulcers, adrenal masses: indicating disseminated histoplasmosis.
Enlarged lymph glands: indicating lymphadenopathy.

Agents of mucormycosis (zygomycosis)

Headache, facial pain, orbital cellulitis, lower cranial nerve palsies: indicating rhinocerebral infection.
Pneumonia, disseminated disease.

Investigations

Biopsy of tissue and bone marrow with culture and histology (histoplasmosis only), culture of blood, sputum, fluid (including CSF), and sinuses.
Antigen tests: for cryptococcal infections.
CT for *Aspergillus* infections: of thorax for aspergilloma and invasive infections; of sinuses for allergy, saprophytic, acute invasion; of brain for brain abscess.
Endoscopy, colonoscopy, barium meal, swallow, follow-through: for esophagitis, gastritis, small and large bowel plaques, and ulceration.
Radiography of chest, thorax, and sinuses.
Bronchoscopy: lavage, biopsy, for pulmonary disease and diagnosis.

Complications

Candida infections

Esophageal candidiasis, azole-resistant thrush, endometritis, ascending renal infection in intensive care or surgical patients, prostatitis, multiple organ involvement, hepatosplenic candidiasis in leukemic patients.

Other infections

Pulmonary fibrosis: after 5–10 years; complication of allergic bronchopulmonary aspergillosis.
Hemoptysis: in *Aspergillus* infections and zygomycosis.
Hydrocephalus, impaired mental function, blindness: complications of cryptococcal infections; hydrocephalus usually communicating.

Differential diagnosis

Other infections.
Lymphoma.
Tuberculosis.

Etiology

• Predisposing causes include the following:

Superficial *Candida* infections
Antibiotics, steroids, diabetes mellitus, AIDS immunocompromise, pregnancy, oral contraceptives, macerated skin, occupation, frequent wetting of hands, abnormal T-cell response to *Candida* antigens.

Systemic *Candida* infections
Urinary catheterization, immunosuppression, surgery, burns, premature birth, endocarditis, valvular heart disease, prosthetic valves, peritoneal dialysis, abdominal surgery, bowel perforation, hematological malignancies, CSF shunts.

***Aspergillus* infections**
Asthma, cystic fibrosis, neutropenia, organ transplantation, AIDS, steroids, chronic granulomatous disease, previous pulmonary tuberculosis, sarcoidosis, bronchiectasis, chronic lung disease, diabetes mellitus, alcoholism, previous ear disease, i.v. drug abuse, valve replacement.

Cryptococcal infections
AIDS, lymphoma, steroids, sarcoidosis.

Histoplasmosis
History of exposure, *e.g.*, endemic area, bat caves (acute), emphysema (chronic), AIDS, immunocompromise (disseminated).

Mucormycosis
Acidosis, diabetes mellitus, neutropenia, bone-marrow transplantation, i.v. drug abuse, deferoxamine treatment.

Epidemiology

Environmental saprophytes.

• Vaginal candidiasis affects 70% of all women, and 5% have frequent recurrences.

• Oral thrush affects 90% of AIDS patients and 15%–30% of leukemia patients.

• Invasive aspergillosis affects 5%–40% of immunocompromised patients.

• Cryptococcal meningitis affects 4%–35% of AIDS patients, depending on country.

Treatment

Diet and lifestyle

• No special precautions are necessary.

Pharmacological treatment

Amphotericin B

• Amphotericin B is indicated for the following:

Candida infections (oropharyngeal, urogenital tract, candidemia, endocarditis, pneumonia, visceral, CNS).
Aspergillus infections (invasive or chronic necrotizing aspergillosis, acute invasive sinus, or paranasal granuloma).
Cryptococcal infections (meningitis).
Histoplasmosis (chronic pulmonary, disseminated).
Agents of mucormycosis (rhinocerebral).

Standard dosage	Amphotericin B, 0.5–1.5 mg/kg i.v.
Contraindications	Hypersensitivity.
Special points	Resistant strains include *Candida krusei*, *Fusarium* spp., *Pseudallescheria boydii*, *Trichosporon beigelii*, Mucorales (limited activity).
Main drug interactions	Increased nephrotoxicity with aminoglycosides or cyclosporin.
Main side effects	Infusion-related fever or rigors, nausea, phlebitis, renal toxicity, anemia, electrolyte disturbances.

Azoles

• Fluconazole is indicated for *Candida* infections (oropharyngeal, vulvovaginal, nail infections, chronic mucocutaneous candidiasis, urogenital tract, visceral candidiasis) and for cryptococcal infections (meningitis in AIDS).

• Itraconazole is indicated for *Aspergillus* infections (pulmonary, acute invasive sinus, paranasal granuloma) and for histoplasmosis (severe acute, chronic pulmonary, less seriously ill, disseminated; maintenance in AIDS).

Standard dosage	Fluconazole, 50–400 mg orally or i.v. daily. Itraconazole, 100–200 mg orally daily; 200 mg loading doses 3 times daily initially in severe or life-threatening disease. Ketoconazole, 200–400 mg orally daily.
Contraindications	Azole hypersensitivity.
Special points	*Fluconazole*: resistant strains include *Histoplasma capsulatum*, Mucorales, *Candida krusei* and *glabrata*, *Aspergillus* and *Fusarium* spp. *Itraconazole*: resistant strains include *C. glabrata*, *Fusarium* spp., Mucorales. *Ketoconazole*: resistant strains include *C. glabrata*, *Cryptococcus neoformans*, *Aspergillus* and *Fusarium* spp.
Main drug interactions	Altered azole or drug concentrations with phenytoin, cyclosporin, rifampin, phenobarbital, carbamazepine, warfarin, terfenadine, astemizole, digoxin.
Main side effects	*Fluconazole:* nausea, rash, liver dysfunction (rare). *Itraconazole:* gynecomastia, peripheral edema, hypokalemia, liver dysfunction (rare). *Ketoconazole:* liver dysfunction, nausea, reduced libido, menstrual irregularities, gynecomastia.

Other drugs

Flucytosine, 150 mg/kg orally daily in 4 divided doses only in combination with amphotericin B: for *Candida* infections (candidemia, endocarditis, CNS infections), *Aspergillus* infections (invasive aspergillosis), and cryptococcal infections (meningitis).

Topical nystatin: for mucosal *Candida* infection.

Topical antifungals: for cutaneous *Candida* and dermatophyte infections.

Inhaled steroids, bronchodilators: for allergic pneumonitis.

Oral steroids: for exacerbations of allergic bronchopulmonary aspergillosis.

Treatment aims

To eradicate infection.

To prevent recurrence of infection.

To remove underlying cause.

Other treatments

Removal or replacement of catheter or shunt.

Surgery: for invasive aspergillosis, aspergilloma, allergic sinus infection, fungus ball, paranasal granuloma, rhinocerebral infection (radical clearance).

Removal of CSF in cryptococcal meningitis.

Prognosis

• In patients with candidemia, overall mortality is 55%; in surgical patients with candidal peritonitis, mortality is 37%.

• In patients with invasive aspergillosis, mortality is 30%–90%, depending on the host group: poor prognosis in patients with late-diagnosis and persistent neutropenia, 85%–90% in bone-marrow transplant recipients, 95% in patients with disseminated disease or cerebral aspergillosis.

• In patients with hemoptysis resulting from aspergilloma, mortality is 10%; spontaneous resolution is 10%.

• 50% of leukemia patients with acute invasive *Aspergillus* sinus infection relapse.

• In patients with meningitis, acute mortality is 15%–20%, lower if intracranial hypertension is treated aggressively.

• More than one-third of patients who have had meningitis relapse without prophylaxis.

Follow-up and management

• Patients with life-threatening invasive fungal infections should have specialist treatment and prolonged follow-up.

General references

British Society for Antimicrobial Chemotherapy Working Party: Antifungal chemotherapy in patients with acquired immunodeficiency syndrome. *Lancet* 1992, **340**:648–651.

Denning DW, Stevens DA: Antifungal and surgical treatment of invasive aspergillosis: review of 2121 published cases. *Rev Infect Dis* 1990, **12**:1147–1201.

Warnock DW, Richardson MD, eds: *Fungal Infection in the Immunocompromised Patient*. Chichester: Wiley & Sons; 1991.

Diagnosis

Symptoms

Cosmetic embarrassment.

Mechanical problems: onychodystrophic nails get snagged on clothing; pressure and irritation from footwear.

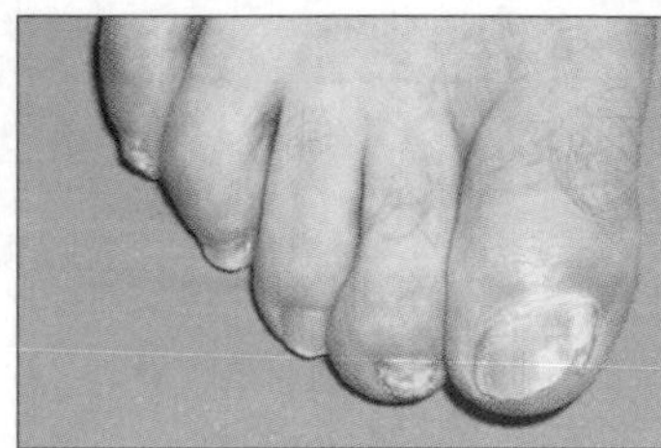

Distal and lateral subungual onychomycosis secondary to dermatophyte infection.

Signs

•Signs can be divided into three varieties of clinical manifestations based on the type of nail infection: (*i.e.*, distal variety, proximal infection, or superficial infection).

Distal infection

Onycholysis: distal or distal-lateral nail separation from nail bed with hyperkeratotic subungual debris and crumbling friable nails; over time extends proximally.

Proximal infection

Discoloration: white to yellow, affecting the proximal ventral nail plate; extends distally and toward the dorsal surface of the nail plate but rarely involves the whole nail (least common type).

Superficial infection

Discoloration: patchy chalk-white, mainly of toenails, known as "superficial white onychomycosis."

Investigations

Microscopic examination: potassium hydroxide preparation of subungual debris (as proximal as possible) will be positive only in 50% of cases.

Culture: positive in only 50% of cases in which microscopy is positive.

Complications

Spread of infection: to other nails or adjacent skin.

Secondary pseudomonas infection (green nail syndrome).

Complete onycholysis: disruption and separation of the entire nail plate from the nail bed.

Differential diagnosis

Psoriasis.

Lichen planus.

Eczema.

Alopecia areata.

Etiology

• With the rare exception of immunosuppressed patients, patients with mucocutaneous candidiasis, and patients with chronic paronychia, most cases are caused by dermatophyte infection.

• *Trichophyton rubrum*, *Trichophyton mentagrophytes*, and *Epidermophyton floccosum* are the most common organisms; *T. mentagrophytes* is usually the cause in superficial white onychomycosis.

• Candida infection is rare and usually occurs when there is candidal chronic paronychia.

Epidemiology

Most likely spreads from skin to nails.

A very common problem, especially in the elderly (extremely rare in children).

Incidence is approximately 20%.

Appears to be more common in men than in women.

Treatment

Diet and lifestyle

•Prophylaxis using antifungal foot powder and prevention of overhydration of feet in occlusive, nonbreathing footwear undoubtedly has merit.

Pharmacological treatment

Topical treatment

• Topical treatment is prophylactic only to control tinea pedis.

• Superficial white onychomycosis can be treated by simply scraping off the superficial fungi from the nail.

Systemic treatment

• Allylamines (terbinafine) and triazoles (itraconazole and fluconazole) are much more effective over a much shorter treatment period than is griseofulvin, which is more effective in fingernail infection than in toenail infection, requires a course of 12–18 months in toenail infections, and has a cure rate of only 10%–50% [1–3].

Standard dosage
Itraconazole (pulse therapy), 200 mg orally twice daily for the first 7 days of months 1, 2, 3, and 4.
Itraconazole, 400 mg orally daily for 1 week, then repeated at monthly intervals for 4 months.
Fluconazole, 150 mg orally every week for up to 9 months.

Contraindications
Pregnancy.

Main drug interactions
Terbinafine: rifampin or phenobarbital will result in decreased serum levels of terbinafine.
Cimetidine will increase terbinafine levels.
Itraconazole: minimal risk of drug interactions because of the lack of significant inhibitory or inducing effect on hepatic microsomal enzymes; otherwise, same as terbinafine.
Fluconazole: primary route of excretion is renal not hepatic; high specificity for fungal cytochrome P-450, otherwise similar to itraconazole and terbinafine.

Main side effects
Terbinafine: gastrointestinal upset, skin reactions (drug rash).
Itraconazole: nausea, gastrointestinal upset, elevated liver function tests (0.3%–5% of patients).
Fluconazole: gastrointestinal upset, elevated liver function tests (especially patients who are HIV-positive).

Treatment aims

To eradicate the infection.

To prevent recurrence.

Other treatments

Nail avulsion combined with systemic therapy.

Prognosis

Better for fingernail involvement (approximately 50% cure rate).

High relapse rate.

Follow-up and management

• It is very important to monitor liver function tests because of the possibility of hepatotoxicity (as with ketoconazole).

• The systemic drugs are relatively new agents that should be used cautiously and monitored carefully.

Key references

1. Roberts DT: Oral therapeutic agents in fungal nail disease. *J Am Acad Dermatol* 1994, **31**:578–581.
2. Raza A: Ecology and epidemiology of dermatophyte infections. *J Am Acad Dermatol* 1994, **31**:521–525.
3. Cohen PR, Scher RK: Geriatric nail disorders: diagnosis and treatment. *J Am Acad Dermatol* 1992, **26**:521–531.

Diagnosis

Symptoms

• Up to 70% of patients are asymptomatic or have nonspecific dyspeptic symptoms.

Uncomplicated

Biliary colic: sudden-onset severe epigastric or upper right quadrant abdominal pain, lasting for several hours, usually radiating to back, sometimes associated with nausea and vomiting.

Complicated

Fever, persistent abdominal pain, nausea and vomiting: indicating acute cholecystitis.

Fever, pain, jaundice: indicating acute cholangitis.

Abdominal pain radiating to the back, vomiting: indicating acute pancreatitis.

Signs

Uncomplicated

• Few signs are manifest.

Tenderness in right upper quadrant: usually during or after episodes of biliary colic.

Complicated

Jaundice: indicating stone impaction in common bile duct.

Murphy's sign (a halt in deep inspiration when deep palpation in the right upper quadrant results in pain)**: indicating acute cholecystitis.**

Hypotension: indicating acute pancreatitis or sepsis from cholangitis.

Investigations

• Gallstones are frequently found incidentally by ultrasonography or abdominal radiography (if calcified).

• Laboratory tests are not diagnostic but are useful for identifying complications and excluding other abnormalities.

Serum alkaline phosphatase and bilirubin measurement: elevation suggests biliary tract disease.

Leukocyte count: frequently elevated with inflammation of the biliary tract.

Serum amylase measurement: >100 IU/dL suggests acute pancreatitis.

Antimitochondrial antibody tests: in atypical cases (*e.g.*, pruritis, painless jaundice) to exclude primary biliary cirrhosis.

Ultrasonography: first choice test to identify stones; may also detect small stones and biliary sludge; no exposure to radiation; detects dilated bile ducts and can identify disease in other organs.

Plain abdominal radiography: identifies ~20% of stones that are calcified.

Oral cholecystography: identifies radiolucent stones, good for determining gallbladder contraction and cystic duct patency and for identifying anatomical abnormalities in gallbladder; not sensitive for detecting small stones and invalid in case of nonopacifying gallbladder.

CT: less sensitive than ultrasonography for detecting gallbladder stones or bile duct dilatation.

Cholescintigraphy: using ^{99m}Tc-HIDA (hepatic iminodiacetic acid) helpful in suspected acute cholecystitis (*i.e.*, gallbladder does not fill); parenchymal liver disease or significant cholestasis may lead to false-positive results.

Complications

Acute cholecystitis.
Acute cholangitis.
Acute pancreatitis.
Hydrops, empyema of gallbladder.
Malignancy of gallbladder.
Perforation.
Internal and external biliary fistulas.
Gallstone ileus.
Hemobilia.
Choledocholithiasis.

Differential diagnosis

• Few patients with gallstones have typical biliary colic (<10%).

Obstructive jaundice

Pancreatic neoplasm.

Bile-duct stricture.

Cholestatic hepatitis

Biliary colic

Pancreatitis.

Esophagitis.

Peptic ulcer.

Irritable bowel syndrome.

Etiology

• No unifying cause has been found, but the following may have a role:

Pathogenesis

Cholesterol supersaturation of bile.

Impaired gallbladder emptying.

Rapid cholesterol nucleation.

Predisposing factors

Obesity.

High fat diet.

Disease: cirrhosis of liver, ileal dysfunction.

Drugs: *e.g.*, octreotide, oral contraceptives.

Epidemiology

• 10%–15% of the adult population have cholesterol gallstones.

• The incidence is 0.6% of the population.

• Gallstones occur more often in women, and their occurrence increases with age.

Treatment

Diet and lifestyle

• No evidence suggests that diet high in fiber and low in cholesterol dissolves stones or prevents their recurrence.

• Patients at risk of gallstones should avoid obesity and not miss meals.

• Rapid weight reduction should also be avoided.

• Diets high in polyunsaturated fat should be avoided.

Pharmacological treatment

• Drugs are indicated for patients with other major medical problems that are contraindications for nonpharmacological treatment and in those with infrequent or mild symptoms, radiolucent stones, and functioning gallbladder [1,2].

• Bile-acid treatment is used for patients with small stones (<15 mm diameter); bile acids dissolve cholesterol gallstones by micellar solubilization or liquid crystal formation; they also reduce cholesterol absorption by intestine or secretion by liver.

Standard dosage	Ursodeoxycholic acid (UDCA), 10 mg/kg daily. Chenodeoxycholic acid (CDCA), 15 mg/kg daily. UDCA and CDCA, 5 mg/kg each daily. All as single bedtime dose for up to 2 years.
Contraindications	Pregnancy and lactation. *CDCA:* chronic liver disease or diarrhea. *UDCA:* active peptic ulcers.
Special points	Dissolution of stones requires 12 months or more of treatment, and recurrence is common when the medication is discontinued; UDCA or combination better than CDCA alone.
Main drug interactions	Sex hormones, oral contraceptives, blood cholesterol-lowering agents.
Main side effects	*CDCA:* diarrhea, hypertransaminasemia (reversible and dose-dependent). *UDCA:* gallstone calcification resulting in treatment failure.

Nonpharmacological treatment

Surgery

• Surgery is the preferred management for almost all patients with symptomatic gallstones.

• Open cholecystectomy is the traditional treatment.

• Laparoscopic cholecystectomy is rapidly becoming the procedure of choice.

Endoscopic retrograde cholangiography with sphincterotomy and stone extraction

For patients with choledocholithiasis.

Often performed in conjunction with laparoscopic cholecystectomy [3].

Extracorporeal shock-wave lithotripsy

• Lithotripsy is possible for 1-3 stones <30 mm in diameter; however, surgical management or dissolution therapy is the preferred approach.

• Expensive equipment is needed.

• The incidence of biliary colic and hematuria hematobilia is higher than with other approaches.

• It is contraindicated in hemolytic disorders.

Contact dissolution with methyl tert-butyl ether (MTBE)

• MTBE is a powerful cholesterol solvent (dissolves stones in a few hours).

• The procedure is invasive (percutaneous, transhepatic gallbladder cannulation) and is performed only in a few specialized centers; it is rarely used since the advent of laparoscopic cholecystectomy.

• Leakage causes drowsiness, nausea, and duodenitis.

• The risk of recurrence is higher because of undissolved debris.

• It is contraindicated in hemolytic disorders.

Treatment aims

To dissolve stones, with consequent relief of symptoms and prevention of complications [4,5].

Prognosis

• Gallstones recur after dissolution therapy in 50% of patients within 5 years.

• If recurrent stones are detected early and treated, >80% of patients remain gallstone-free in the long term.

Follow-up and management

• Regular ultrasonography is needed every 6–12 months after dissolution to detect early recurrence.

• Bile acid treatment (full dose) is needed for recurrent stones.

Causes of pharmacological treatment failure

Patients' noncompliance with treatment.

Presence of radiolucent pigment stones or subradiographic calcification of stones.

Development of nonfunctioning gallbladder.

Inadequate dose (especially in obese patients).

Key references

1. Jonston DE, Kaplan MM: Pathogenesis and treatment of gallstones. *N Engl J Med* 1993, **328**:412–421.
2. Jazrawi RP, *et al.*: Optimum bile acid therapy for rapid gallstone dissolution. *Gut* 1992, **33**:381–386.
3. Cuschieri A, *et al.*: The European experience with laparoscopic cholecystectomy. *Am J Surg* 1991, **161**:385–387.
4. Sauerbruch T, Paumgartner G: Gallbladder stones: management. *Lancet* 1991, **338**:1121–1124.
5. Ransohoft DF, *et al.*: Treatment of gallstones. *Ann Intern Med* 1993, **119**:606–619.

Diagnosis

Symptoms

Epigastric pain, "ulcer-like dyspepsia."

Dyspepsia: lasting more than a few weeks, in middle-aged or older patients.

Rapid satiety, fullness.

Dysphagia: with adeocarcinoma of the cardia or distal esopohagus.

Vomiting.

Hematemesis or melena.

Weight loss.

Malaise.

Signs

• Often no signs are manifest.

Pallor: due to anemia.

Koilonychia: iron deficiency (rare).

Abdominal epigastric mass: palpable gastric tumor.

Nodular, hard enlarged liver: with metastatic disease.

Succussion splash: due to pyloric stenosis.

Ascites.

Pleural effusion.

Hard fixed supraclavicular node: sentinel node of Virchow; in left supraclavicular fossa.

Left anterior axillary node.

Mass: rectal shelf of Blumer; on rectal examination.

Infiltration of the umbilicus: Sister Joseph's nodule.

Investigations

• Laboratory tests are not diagnostic but may suggest bleeding or liver metastases.

Full blood count: to identify iron-deficiency anemia.

Liver function tests: raised alkaline phosphatase may suggest metastases.

Fiberoptic endoscopy: allows direct view of cancer and assessment of extent of cancer; allows biopsy (a minimum of eight tissue samples should be obtained, especially from the edge) and cytology; infiltrating cancer (linitis plastica) and lymphoma may need deep or large biopsy at repeat endoscopy to make diagnosis; allows assessment of obstruction to cardia or pylorus; superficial cancers may be difficult to recognize [1].

Double-contrast barium meal: blunting, fusion, clubbing, or tapering of mucosal folds suggests cancer; less accurate than endoscopy.

Ultrasonography: conventional abdominal ultrasonography to assess liver metastases; endoscopic ultrasonography superior but not yet widely available.

CT: to assess extent of disease, metastases.

Complications

Tumor spread: lymphatic, hematogenous (liver, lungs, bone, adrenals), local dissemination into esophagus, invasion of adjacent organs (pancreas, mesocolon, liver).

Differential diagnosis

Ulcer or nonulcer dyspepsia.

Reflux esophagitis.

Anemia of other causes.

Depression.

Etiology

• Risk factors include the following:

Smoked foods, salt fish, pickled foods, high salt and starch intake (inverse association with refrigeration, vitamin C, fresh fruit and vegetable intake).

Genetic factors: including blood group A, family history, and Lynch syndrome II.

Helicobacter pylori infection (an important cause of gastritis).

Epidemiology

• In the US, the annual incidence is 10 cases per 100 000 population.

• The male to female ratio is 1.5:1.0.

• There has been a considerable decline in the incidence of gastric cancer over the past 30 years.

• Patients with early gastric cancer are, on average, 8 years younger than those with advanced disease [2].

Pathology

Malignant neoplasm of stomach

90% adenocarcinoma; 5% lymphoma; 5% others (carcinoid, leiomyosarcoma, adeno-acanthoma, squamous, hepatoid, liposarcoma).

• Advanced cancer may be polypoidal or fungating, ulcerating with a raised border, or diffusely infiltrating (linitis plastica).

Early gastric cancer

Confined to gastric mucosa or submucosa, irrespective of lymph-node invasion.

Three types: protruded (type I), superficial (type II, most common), excavated (type III).

Associated conditions

Chronic atrophic gastritis/achlorhydria.

Dysplasia.

Adenomatous polyps.

Pernicious anemia: 8% may develop gastric tumors (cancers and carcinoids).

Hypertrophic gastropathy (Menetrier's disease): 10% may develop gastric cancer.

Previous gastrectomy (especially 10–20 years after Billroth II with gastrojejunostomy).

Treatment

Diet and lifestyle

• After gastrectomy, patients are at risk for dumping syndrome.

• Liquids should be taken prior to a meal but not during or immediately after ingestion of solid food.

• Patients should be advised to ingest frequent, small meals.

• Lying down immediately after a meal may be helpful.

• Patients with dysphagia should have a semi-liquid diet, with enteral feeding supplements.

• Patients should be encouraged to lead a normal lifestyle.

Pharmacological treatment

• Chemotherapy has not been shown in trials to produce increased survival; it can produce effective reduction in tumor size and has been used for palliation.

• Symptoms may respond to treatment, as follows:

Ulcer-type pain: H_2 blockers.

Thrush or odynophagia pain: nystatin or ketoconazole if candidal infection is present.

Infiltrative pain: opiate analgesics.

Constipation: laxatives.

Vomiting (infiltrative: incompetence of gastroesophageal sphincter): metoclopramide or cisapride (rarely responds).

Nonpharmacological treatment

Curative resection: for the 30%–50% of patients without evidence of distant metastases [3,4].

Total gastrectomy: if tumor is extensive or close to cardioesophageal junction; higher mortality and morbidity than partial gastrectomy; side effects include small reservoir or bilious vomiting, diarrhea, and malabsorption.

Partial gastrectomy: for early gastric cancer or infiltrative advanced cancer with 5 cm distance clear of cancer from the cardia; side effects include weight loss and altered eating ability.

Dissection of lymph glands draining stomach: important even in early gastric cancer.

Palliation of symptoms, as follows:
For obstructive pain or obstructive vomiting due to pyloric stenosis: bypass surgery.
For dysphagia: laser treatment or repeat dilation.
For bleeding: surgery, endoscopic laser or electrocautery treatment.
For depression, anxiety, or anger: careful discussion, enlistment of family, and palliative care team support.

• Palliative surgery for locally advanced disease involving adjacent organs may benefit patients with bleeding or pyloric obstruction even with metastatic spread.

• Complications after surgery include anastomotic leakage and small gastric residue.

Treatment aims

To provide curative resection when still possible.

To provide effective symptomatic palliation when cure not possible [5].

Prognosis

• In patients having an "open and close" laparotomy confirming unresectability, mean survival is 4–12 months, with almost no 5-year survivors.

• In patients having apparent curative resection, mean survival is 28 months, and the 5-year survival rate is 40%.

• The 5-year survival rate is 15% overall, 50% in patients without lymph-gland involvement, and 30% in those with lymph-gland involvement.

• The prognosis of early gastric cancer is much better, with a 5-year survival rate of 80%, compared with 20% for advanced gastric cancer after resection (types I and II better prognosis than type III) [6,7].

Follow-up and management

• Gastrectomy patients may need iron and vitamin B_{12} or D supplements.

• Some total gastrectomy patients need careful nutritional support.

• Endoscopy, ultrasonography, or CT may be needed during follow-up to diagnose local or distant recurrence.

Key references

1. Takemoto T, *et al.*: Impact of staging on treatment of gastric carcinoma. *Endoscopy* 1993, **25**:46–50.
2. Lechago J, Correa P: Prolonged achlorhydria and gastric neoplasia: is there a causal relationship? *Gastroenterology* 1993, **104**:1554–1557.
3. Cushieri A: Gastrectomy for gastric cancer: definitions and objectives. *Br J Surg* 1986, **73**:513–514.
4. Gouzi JL, *et al.*: Total versus subtotal gastrectomy for adenocarcinoma of the gastric antrum. *Ann Surg* 1989, **2**:162–166.
5. Valen B, *et al.*: Treatment of stomach cancer. A national experience. *Br J Surg* 1988, **75**:708–710.
6. Thompson GB, van Heerden JA, Sarr MG: Adenocarcinoma of the stomach: are we making progress? *Lancet* 1993, **342**:713–718.
7. Green PHR, *et al.*: Increasing incidence and excellent survival of patients with early gastric cancer. *Am J Med* 1988, **85**:658–661.

Gastric ulceration

Diagnosis

Symptoms

Uncomplicated disease

• This is often clinically indistinguishable from duodenal ulcer.

Epigastric pain: described as dull, burning discomfort; variably affected by food; relieved by antacids.

Nocturnal pain.

Complicated disease

Hematemesis or melena.

Severe abdominal pain: when perforation occurs.

Nausea or vomiting and upper abdominal distension: with gastric outflow obstruction.

Marked anorexia, weight loss: suggesting malignant gastric ulceration.

Signs

Uncomplicated disease

Epigastric tenderness.

Complicated disease

Signs of hemodynamic compromise: in acute hemorrhage.

Local or generalized peritonitis: if ulcer has perforated.

Upper abdominal distension, succussion splash, visible peristalsis: with gastric outflow obstruction.

Investigations

Full blood count: to detect iron-deficiency anemia or decreased hemoglobin in acute bleeds.

Serum gastrin measurement: in recurrent or multiple ulceration, for Zollinger–Ellison syndrome [1].

Chest radiography: plain film may show subdiaphragmatic gas in perforation.

Contrast radiography: barium studies may identify an ulcer crater within the gastric mucosa.

Fiberoptic endoscopy: investigation of choice (biopsy and cytology essential to exclude malignancy); allows direct visualization of ulcer; may help to diagnose small lesions or mucosal abnormalities; allows histological confirmation of diagnosis; allows assessment of *Helicobacter pylori* status.

Complications

Perforation.

Hemorrhage.

Gastric outflow obstruction.

Differential diagnosis

Chronic pain

Duodenal ulceration.

Chronic gastritis.

Gastric carcinoma.

Chronic pancreatitis.

Irritable bowel syndrome.

Gastroesophageal reflux disease.

Acute pain

Acute pancreatitis.

Myocardial infarction.

Aortic dissection.

Biliary colic.

• Pain due to peptic ulceration is usually not severe enough to suggest the above diagnoses.

Etiology

• Causes include the following:

NSAIDs inhibiting protective prostaglandin synthesis.

Basal and peak acid secretion usually within normal range; mucosal defenses impaired, with subsequent back-diffusion of acid into mucosa.

Helicobacter pylori infection in 70% of patients.

Epidemiology

• The incidence of gastric ulceration increases with age.

• The male : female ratio is equal.

• Gastric ulceration is more prevalent in low socioeconomic groups.

Treatment

Diet and lifestyle

• In addition to specific pharmacological treatment, avoiding aspirin and other NSAIDs and alcohol excess is useful.

• Patients should eat regular meals and avoid smoking.

• Smoking and NSAIDs are also associated with delayed healing and early relapse.

Pharmacological treatment

• If *Helicobacter pylori* is present, most clinicians would attempt eradication [2] (*see* Duodenal ulcer *for further details*).

Antacids

• These may give temporary symptomatic relief if taken 1 and 3 h after meals.

H_2-receptor antagonists

• The mainstay of treatment, these produce symptomatic relief within days and have ulcer healing rates of 80% at 4 weeks and 90% at 8 weeks [3].

Standard dosage Ranitidine, 300 mg; cimetidine, 800 mg; famotidine, 40 mg; all given as single dose at night.

Contraindications Known hypersensitivity (rare), pregnancy and lactation.

Main drug interactions *Cimetidine:* oral anticoagulants, theophylline, phenytoin.

Main side effects *Cimetidine:* headache, constipation or diarrhea, gynecomastia (all unusual).

Prostaglandins

• Prostaglandins are probably most useful with continuing predisposing factors, *e.g.*, concomitant NSAID treatment. Healing rates are inferior to those of H_2 antagonists [4].

Standard dosage Misoprostol, 400 µg in 4 divided doses.

Contraindications Pregnancy or planned pregnancy.

Special points Small doses of synthetic prostaglandins have been shown to exhibit a cytoprotective effect and to inhibit gastric acid secretion.

Main drug interactions None known.

Main side effects Diarrhea, abdominal pain, flushing, menorrhagia.

Proton-pump inhibitors

• The primary role is management of resistant ulceration or treatment of Zollinger–Ellison syndrome; however, faster healing has been noted when compared with other agents.

Standard dosage Omeprazole, 20 mg daily for 8 weeks [5].

Contraindications Known hypersensitivity.

Special points Long-term treatment not indicated.

Main drug interactions Diazepam, phenytoin, warfarin.

Main side effects Headache, diarrhea, nausea, skin rashes (all unusual).

Treatment aims

To relieve symptoms.

To heal ulcer.

Other treatments

• Surgery is indicated for uncontrolled ulcer-related hemorrhage (early operation important in elderly patients), second major bleed, perforation, or malignant ulceration or delayed healing.

Prognosis

• After completion of a healing course of H_2 antagonists, the chance of recurrence in 1 year is 50%.

Follow-up and management

• Endoscopic confirmation of mucosal healing at 8–12 weeks is essential, with repeated biopsy and further endoscopy if ulcer healing has not occurred.

• After ulcer healing, treatment is usually discontinued unless an obvious and continuing predisposing factor is present.

• Recurrence of symptoms must be reassessed with further endoscopy.

• Recurrent ulceration is managed by maintenance treatment with half-dose H_2 blockade.

Key references

1. Soll H: Pathogenesis of peptic ulcer and implications for therapy. *N Engl J Med* 1990, **322**:909–916.
2. Peterson WL: *Helicobacter pylori* and peptic ulcer disease. *N Engl J Med* 1991, **324**:1043–1048.
3. Feldman M, Burton ME: Histamine 2-receptor antagonists: standard therapy for acid peptic disease. *N Engl J Med* 1991, **323**:1672; 1749–1755.
4. Walt RP: Misoprostol for the treatment of peptic ulcer and antiinflammatory-drug-induced gastroduodenal ulceration. *N Engl J Med* 1992, **327**:1575–1580.
5. Maton PN: Omeprazole. *N Engl J Med* 1991, **324**:965–975.

Diagnosis

Symptoms

Hematemesis: fresh red blood or darker altered blood that may resemble ground coffee.

Melena: passage of black, sticky, foul-smelling stool; fresh blood takes ~14 h to be altered to hematin.

Rectal bleeding (hematochezia): passage of fresh red blood or darker red "maroon" from rectum; may be unaltered blood, blood mixed into the stool, blood clots, or bloody diarrhea.

Collapse, loss of consciousness, angina, shortness of breath, malaise, headache: symptoms of hypotension or anemia.

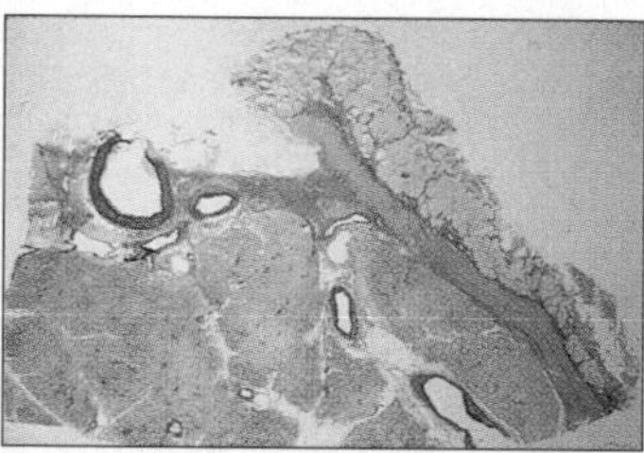

Large hole in an artery in the large duodenal ulcer in a patient who died.

Signs

Tachycardia: earliest sign of shock.

Hypotension: especially postural.

Splenomegaly, spider nevi, palmar erythema: stigmata of chronic liver disease (varices should be considered).

Abdominal tenderness: unusual.

Mass, hepatomegaly, lymph-gland enlargement, Kaposi's sarcoma: signs of cancer.

Findings of telangiectasia: Osler-Weber-Rendu syndrome, or liver disease.

Lax skin: pseudoxanthoma elasticum.

Lax joints: Ehler-Danlos syndrome.

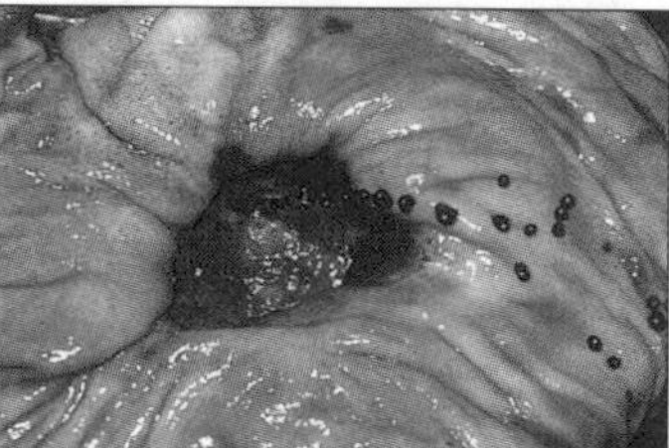

Bleeding gastric ulcer.

Investigations

Hemoglobin and hematocrit analysis: time needed for hemodilution, so initial hemoglobin may not reflect severity of bleeding.

Mean cell volume measurement: raised volume with alcohol-related disorders or may indicate a raised reticulocyte count.

Platelet count: raised with recent bleeding or iron deficiency, may be low in liver or HIV-related disease.

Prothrombin time, partial thromboplastin time: elevated in patients with liver disease or easy bruising.

Urea (BUN) measurement: concentration often elevated with bleeding and may rise further in hypotensive patients.

Fiberoptic endoscopy: stigmata of hemorrhage in peptic ulcers allow prediction of further bleeding (absence of stigmata suggests low chance of further bleeding); visible vessel in peptic ulcer indicates 50% chance of further hemorrhage and increased risk of death; large varices and cherry-red spots may predict increased risk of further bleeding; endoscopy superior to barium studies in making diagnosis in most situations.

Angiography: occasionally useful for severe recurrent bleeding (needs bleeding rate of >5 mL/min); presence of barium may compromise angiography.

^{99m}Tc-labeled erythrocyte scanning: may detect bleeding rate of 1 mL/min and is used to locate site of bleeding distal to the ligament of Treitz.

Tc pertechnate scanning: useful for Meckel's diverticulum because isotope taken up by ectopic gastric mucosa in diverticulum.

Complications

Recurrent or continued bleeding.

Exsanguination.

Aspiration (upper gastrointestial bleeding).

Differential diagnosis

Hematemesis

Nose bleeds and hemoptysis, with subsequently swallowed blood.

Melena

Ingestion of iron, bismuth-containing preparations, producing black stool.

Etiology

History of previous bleeding, ulcer, or gastrointestinal disease (in <50% of patients).
Alcohol, NSAID, or anticoagulant intake.
Hematemesis preceded by retching (suggesting Mallory–Weiss tear).
Liver disease, coagulopathy, amyloidosis.
Family history of bleeding.
Previous surgery for peptic ulcer or arterial bypass grafts.

Causes of upper gastrointestinal bleeding

Gastric erosions, duodenal ulcer, gastric ulcer, varices, esophagitis, erosive duodenitis, Mallory–Weiss tear, neoplasm, esophageal ulcer, stomal ulcer.
Osler–Weber–Rendu syndrome (autosomal dominant), pseudoxanthoma elasticum, Ehler–Danlos syndrome (autosomal dominant and recessive types).
Reflux esophagitis and hiatal hernia.
Helicobacter pylori and AIDS-related disease [1].

Causes of lower gastrointestinal bleeding

Hemorrhoids, polyps, cancer, inflammatory bowel disease, angiodysplasia, diverticular disease, radiation enteritis, ischemic colitis, drug-induced ulcer or solitary rectal ulcer.
Meckel's diverticulum, leiomyoma, adenocarcinoma, lymphoma, aortoenteric fistula (especially in the distal duodenum), mesenteric ischemia.

- Hemorrhoids are the most usual cause of lower gastrointestinal bleeding. Bright blood unmixed with stool often seen only on toilet paper; this is rarely a cause of major bleeding. Blood from hemorrhoids can reflux to splenic flexure. 25% of patients with prolapsing hemorrhoids have another cause of rectal bleeding.

Epidemiology

- The incidence of upper gastrointestinal bleeding is 50–150 hospital episodes in 100 000 population.

Treatment

Diet and lifestyle

• Patients should be warned not to take aspirin or other NSAIDs and should be advised not to smoke.

• Alcoholic patients, especially those with liver disease, should be advised to stop drinking alcohol and should be given medical, family, and nonmedical support.

• Patients must not eat just before endoscopy or surgery; at other times, no evidence suggests that starving or feeding patients confers benefit.

Pharmacological treatment

For peptic ulcer

• Little evidence indicates that drug treatment affects outcome from bleeding peptic ulcer; administration of omeprazole (bleeding peptic ulcers) or octreotide (bleeding varices) may reduce the risk of recurrent bleeding when added to endoscopic management [2].

• Treatment by long-term H_2 blockade or eradication of *Helicobacter pylori* may reduce the incidence of readmission with peptic ulcer bleeding.

For bleeding varices

• Drug treatments are probably ineffective in the treatment of bleeding varices. Some clinicians claim that a somatostatin analogue (octreotide) or propanolol may improve outcome.

Nonpharmacological treatment

Transfusion

Whole blood or packed cells; not for patients with minor bleeding or who are at low risk for further bleeding.

For peptic ulcer

Endoscopic treatment (laser, monopolar, bipolar, heater probe, and injection of adrenaline alone, adrenaline and a sclerosant, or alcohol): can reduce rebleeding rate, need for surgery, and mortality; repeat endoscopic treatment may be preferable to surgery in elderly patients [3-5].

Surgery: in patients with continued or recurrent bleeding in hospital; if surgery necessary, best done before repeated episodes of hypotension have impaired chances of recovery.

For bleeding varices

Endoscopic variceal injection sclerotherapy, using sclerosants such as monoethanolamine, alcohol, sodium tetradecyl sulfate, or sodium morrhuate: has been shown to reduce the incidence of further bleeding and to reduce mortality in patients with recent bleeding from esophageal varices, and it can stop bleeding from varices.

Endoscopic variceal band ligation: less invasive than surgery, has lower complication rate than endoscopic sclerotherapy.

Balloon tamponade: stops bleeding in 85% of patients, but bleeding recurs in 21%–60% and survival not improved; complications include esophageal rupture and aspiration pneumonia, with lethal complications of 10%.

Percutaneous transhepatic cannulation of portal vein: with injection of sclerosant or obliterative substance, *e.g.*, Gelfoam, thrombin, cyanoacrylate.

Transjugular intrahepatic portacaval shunt: for patients who have recurrent variceal bleeding despite sclerotherapy or ligation therapy.

Surgery: for the few patients who do not respond to endoscopic treatment; options include portosystemic shunt, esophageal transection, devascularization, or hepatic transplantation [6].

Complications of treatment

After surgery: pneumonia, renal or cardiac failure, further bleeding.

With endoscopy for bleeding peptic ulcer: precipitation of acute bleeding, perforation, infarction of stomach or duodenum (with injection).

With endoscopy for bleeding varices: esophageal ulceration, perforation, septicemia, distant thrombosis, pleural effusion, aspiration.

Treatment aims

To reduce mortality, need for urgent surgery, and rebleeding rate.

Prognosis

• For peptic ulcer bleeding, the risk of rebleeding in hospital is 15%–30%, of needing urgent surgery 15%–20%, and of death 5%–10%.

• The risk of death after admission with first variceal bleeding is 30%.

• 70% of patients with bleeding varices die within 1–4 years.

• Bleeding due to Mallory–Weiss tear, esophagitis, gastritis, and duodenitis has excellent prognosis.

• Most patients with bleeding upper gastrointestinal cancer die within 1 year.

Follow-up and management

• Ulcer patients with major bleeding should have follow-up endoscopy to check healing and eradication of *Helicobacter pylori*.

• Patients with second major bleed should be considered for surgery.

• Patients with bleeding varices need repeat endoscopy and sclerotherapy until varices are eradicated.

Key references

1. Laine L: Upper gastrointestinal bleeding. *Alimentary Pharmacol Ther* 1993, **7**:207–232.
2. Laine L, Peterson WL: Medical progress: bleeding peptic ulcer. *N Engl J Med* 1994, **331**:717–727.
3. Consensus Development Panel, National Institutes of Health 1990: Consensus statement on therapeutic endoscopy and bleeding ulcers. *Gastrointest Endosc* 1990, **36**:S62–S63.
4. Cook DJ, *et al.*: Endoscopic therapy for acute nonvariceal upper gastrointestinal hemorrhage: a meta-analysis. *Gastroenterology* 1992, **102**:139–148.
5. Fleischer D: Endoscopic hemostasis in non-variceal bleeding. *Endoscopy* 1992, **24**:58–63.
6. Wheatley KE, Dykes PW: Upper gastrointestinal bleeding: when to operate. *Postgrad Med J* 1990, **45**:926–936.

Diagnosis

Definition

• Glomerulonephritis is an immunologically mediated glomerular inflammation, often with associated tubulointerstitial lesions and is sometimes part of a multisystem vasculitis.

• In different patients, the same cause can produce different histological lesions; similarly, different histological appearances can be caused by similar insults in different patients.

• The following classification is based on that of the World Health Organization (terms are purely descriptive and are not necessarily specific disease entities):

Nonproliferative

Minimal-change glomerulonephritis: normal on light microscopy.

Membranous glomerulonephritis: thick-basement membranes, subepithelial immune complexes.

Focal segmental glomerulosclerosis: mesangial and capillary loop scarring.

Proliferative: endocapillary

Diffuse proliferative glomerulonephritis: overcellular glomeruli.

Focal segmental proliferative glomerulonephritis: overcellular glomeruli.

Mesangial IgA disease: large deposits of IgA in mesangium.

Mesangiocapillary glomerulonephritis: thick capillary loops with expanded overcellular mesangium; also called *membranoproliferative glomerulonephritis*.

Focal necrotizing glomerulonephritis: segment of necrosis in peripheral capillary loop.

Proliferative: extracapillary

Crescentic glomerulonephritis: sheaves of macrophages and other cells filling all or part of Bowman's space with variable underlying glomerular lesions.

Symptoms and signs

• Glomerulonephritis is often silent, manifesting as chronic renal failure after insidious deterioration in renal function.

Proteinuria: asymptomatic (usually <2 g/24 h); nephrotic (>3 g/24 h).

Hematuria: microscopic (detected by stick test); macroscopic (smoky urine).

Acute nephritic illness.

Acute renal failure.

Chronic renal failure.

Investigations

Urine microscopy (phase contrast): dysmorphic erythrocytes and casts imply glomerular inflammation.

24-h urinalysis: for creatinine clearance and urine protein.

Blood urea nitrogen and creatinine measurement.

Albumin and lipid measurement.

Tests for lupus and vasculitis: *e.g.*, anti-double-stranded DNA antibody, anti-neutrophil cytoplasmic antibody (ANCA).

Antiglomerular basement membrane antibody measurement.

Investigation for appropriate associated infections.

Complement studies: CH50, C3, C4.

Plain abdominal radiography and ultrasonography or intravenous pyelography.

Renal biopsy: light, electron, and immunofluorescent microscopy all needed.

Complications

Hypertension: can be severe.

Acute or chronic renal failure.

Nephrotic syndrome: venous and arterial thromboses, pleural effusions, ascites, intravascular volume depletion, infection, accelerated atherosclerosis.

Differential diagnosis

Nephritic syndrome

Severe hypertension.

Scleroderma renal crisis.

Thrombotic microangiopathies (*e.g.*, hemolytic uremic syndrome).

Acute interstitial nephritis.

Nephrotic syndrome

Pre-eclampsia.

Amyloidosis.

Diabetes mellitus.

Congestive cardiac failure.

Cirrhosis with edema and ascites.

NSAID use.

Other

Orthostatic proteinuria.

Other causes of hypertension or acute or chronic renal failure.

Etiology

Immunopathogenesis

Immune complex: in-situ formation (built up within glomerulus) or, less commonly, deposition of preformed immune complexes from circulation.

Direct antibody-mediated injury: antiglomerular basement membrane antibody (Goodpasture's syndrome); this is rare.

Unknown, but possibly cell-mediated; probably important in many forms of glomerulonephritis.

Associated diseases

Primary: no known association (idiopathic).

Secondary: postinfectious, *e.g.*, viruses, (hepatitis B, HIV), bacterial (poststreptococcal), protozoal (malarial);
drug-induced, *e.g.*, gold or penicillamine;
associated with vasculitis;
associated with neoplasia.

Epidemiology

• Glomerulonephritis is the most common cause of chronic renal failure (~20%–25%).

• Minimal-change glomerulonephritis is the most common cause of nephrotic syndrome in children.

• Mesangial IgA disease is the most common cause of recurrent episodes of macroscopic hematuria in young adults.

Treatment

Diet and lifestyle

- Patients must not have added salt if they have edema or hypertension.
- Nephrotic patients should have a normal protein intake.
- Renal failure patients should have a low protein intake (0.5 g/kg daily).
- Oral intake of fluids should be restricted if the patient is edematous.
- Pregnant patients are at increased risk of pre-eclampsia (high risk if creatinine raised).
- Occasionally, pregnant patients experience deterioration of renal function.

Pharmacological treatment

Immunosuppression

- Patients are chosen on the basis of clinical syndrome and histology.
- Aggressive treatment is indicated for heavy proteinuria or falling glomerular filtration rate.
- Histology is most helpful for choosing treatment.

For minimal-change glomerulonephritis:
remission induction: high-dose steroids, cyclosporin A;
maintenance: low-dose steroids or cyclosporin A;
prevention of relapse: cyclophosphamide.

For membranous glomerulonephritis: trial of steroids, possibly with chlorambucil or cyclophosphamide in selected patients.

For focal segmental glomerulosclerosis: high-dose steroids or cyclosporin A, or both (prolonged treatment needed).

For mesangial IgA disease: fish oil (eicosapentaenoic acid).

For postinfectious diffuse proliferative glomerulonephritis: treat infection.

For mesangiocapillary glomerulonephritis: no treatment effective; trial of immunosuppression in selected patients.

For focal necrotizing or crescentic glomerulonephritis: steroids with cyclophosphamide (pulse i.v. methylprednisolone for 3 days may help); additional plasma exchange in selected patients (immediate plasma exchange mandatory in Goodpasture's syndrome).

Supportive

Control of fluid balance: diuretics (combinations may be needed).

Control of blood pressure: angiotensin-converting enzyme inhibitors if possible; calcium antagonists should be avoided (edema).

Aggressive treatment of intercurrent infections (cellulitis, pneumonia, spontaneous bacterial peritonitis).

Anticoagulation: should be considered for nephrotic patients, especially if they are immobile.

Treatment aims

To suppress glomerular inflammation.

To prevent progressive glomerular scarring and progression to chronic renal failure.

To minimize proteinuria.

To control hypertension and fluid balance.

To avoid overimmunosuppression, particularly of burnt-out glomerulonephritis with intrarenal scarring.

Prognosis

- A poor prognosis is associated with severe hypertension, heavy persistent proteinuria, and raised creatinine when first seen.
- Prognosis is closely related to histology:

Minimal-change glomerulonephritis: excellent, eventually resolves despite relapses.
Focal segmental proliferative glomerulonephritis: <10% of patients progress to chronic renal failure (CRF).
Membranous glomerulonephritis: 30% resolve, 30% remain static, 30% progress to CRF
Mesangial IgA disease: 25% progress to CRF.
Postinfectious diffuse proliferative glomerulonephritis: >90% resolve.
Mesangiocapillary glomerulonephritis: >75% progress to CRF.
Focal necrotizing and crescentic glomerulonephritis: <30% progress to CRF if given early aggressive treatment.

Follow-up and management

- Follow-up should be for life if the patient has raised creatinine, persistent hematuria, proteinuria, or hypertension.
- Strict control of blood pressure is needed, using angiotensin-converting enzyme inhibitors whenever possible because this class of drug reduces glomerular blood pressure and proteinuria and may protect the kidney.
- Immunosuppressive drugs must be titrated to disease activity.
- Lipids must be controlled.

General references

D'Amico G: Influence of clinical and histological features on actuarial renal survival in adult patients with idiopathic IgA nephropathy, membranous nephropathy and membranoproliferative glomerulonephritis. *Am J Kidney Dis* 1992, **20**:315–323.

Mason PD, Pusey CD: Glomerulonephritis: diagnosis and treatment. *BMJ* 1994, **309**:1557–1563.

Diagnosis

Symptoms

Acute pain in a single joint: usually base of great toe; often starting at night; self-limiting but tendency to recur.

Mild systemic disturbance, with irritability and low-grade fever.

Polyarticular attacks: in 5%–10% of patients (50% of elderly patients).

Chronic asymmetrical polyarthritis: after repeated acute attacks.

Signs

Exquisite tenderness.

Swollen, shiny, red, tender joints.

Desquamation: as attack subsides.

Tophi in helix of ear, elbow, and over small joints of hands and feet: in severe cases.

Olecranon bursitis: "boozer's elbow"; common.

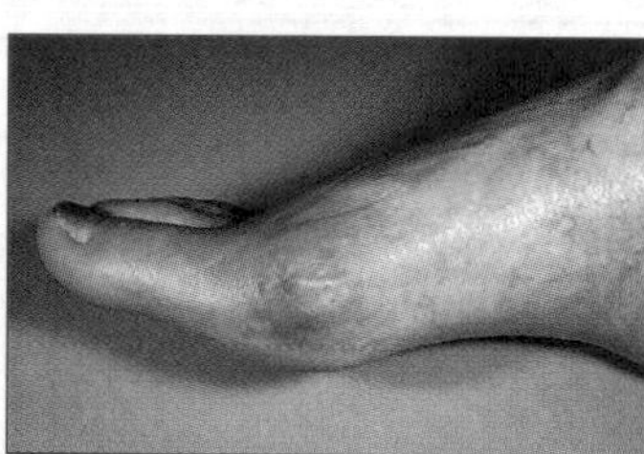

Acute gout in big toe.

Investigations

Polarized light microscopy: needle-shaped, negatively birefringent crystals in synovial fluid from the affected joint are diagnostic.

Serum uric acid measurement: concentration usually raised but may fall to normal during acute attack.

Full blood count: to exclude secondary cause, *e.g.*, lymphoproliferative disorder.

ESR measurement: may be raised during acute attack.

Creatinine measurement: renal failure may result from or be caused by hyperuricemia.

Fasting lipids measurement: hyperlipidemia common.

Urinary urate excretion measurement: differentiates overproducers from underexcretors (while on low-purine diet).

Radiography: may show characteristic juxta-articular punched-out erosions without accompanying osteoporosis around joints ("overhanging edges") in patients with chronic arthritic gout.

Complications

Prolongation of acute attack: by incorrect use of allopurinol.

Gastrointestinal bleeding: due to high-dose NSAIDs.

Renal impairment: due to drug interference with renal cortical blood flow.

Differential diagnosis

Acute gout

Septic arthritis.

Cellulitis.

Pyrophosphate arthritis ("pseudogout").

Chronic tophaceous gout

Rheumatoid arthritis.

Septic arthritis.

Hyperlipidemia with xanthomata.

Nongout

Painful bunion with asymptomatic hyperuricemia.

Etiology

- Gout is often precipitated by alcohol overindulgence, surgery, or intercurrent illness.
- Primary gout may be caused by a genetic predisposition to overproduction or underexcretion of urate or failure to inhibit crystallization in tissues.
- Secondary gout may be caused by diuretics (particularly in older women), renal impairment, diet (high purine intake coupled with obesity), high cell turnover (malignant disease), alcohol excess, or heavy-metal poisoning, especially lead (saturnine gout).

Epidemiology

- Gout is particularly prevalent in middle-aged men, postmenopausal women, and patients with renal failure.

Treatment

Diet and lifestyle

• Patients with associated obesity may benefit from caloric restriction.

• Alcohol intake should be moderated because alcohol inhibits urate excretion by the kidney and is often associated with acute attacks [1].

• Consumption of high purine foods (*e.g.*, shellfish) should be restricted because they may provoke acute attacks; a purine-free diet is impractical.

Pharmacological treatment

For acute attack

Standard dosage Rapidly acting NSAID, *e.g.*, indomethacin, 25–50 mg initially, followed by 25–50 mg 3 times daily until attack starts to subside, then reduced dose [1,2].
Colchicine, 0.5 mg hourly to a maximum of 12 mg in first 24 h; do not repeat dose for 7 days.

Contraindications *Indomethacin:* peptic ulcer, anticoagulants, renal impairment.
Colchicine: hypersensitivity.

Special points *Colchicine:* can be used to prevent recurrence at 0.5 g once or twice daily.
Alternatives for resistant or difficult cases include intra-articular or oral steroids.

Main drug interactions *Indomethacin:* warfarin.

Main side effects *Indomethacin, diclofenac:* indigestion, gastric bleeding, headache, nausea, dizziness (worse with indomethacin).
Colchicine: nausea, diarrhea.

For hyperuricemia

• Treatment can be considered between attacks if the serum urate concentration remains raised [1,2].

• Allopurinol is indicated for recurrent attacks of gout, chronic tophaceous gout, renal impairment due to hyperuricemia, induction of chemotherapy, and asymptomatic hyperuricemia (>12 mg/dL) or for any gouty patient with a history of renal stones.

Standard dosage Allopurinol, 300 mg initially; reduce dosage for renal insufficiency.

Contraindications Acute gout, hypersensitivity.

Special points Lower dose in renal failure to prevent build up of metabolites; additional prophylactic NSAID or colchicine for first 3 months to prevent multiple attacks of gout.

Main drug interactions Azathioprine.

Main side effects Rash.

Treatment aims

To control inflammation during acute attack.

To prevent recurrent acute attacks and chronic gouty arthritis by lowering serum urate concentrations.

Prognosis

• The prognosis is excellent; with modern hypouricemic treatment, most patients are effectively cured.

Follow-up and management

• Patients are usually followed up by the primary care physician, who should monitor serum urate concentrations to adjust the dose of hypouricemic treatment and to ensure compliance.

• Referral to a specialist is indicated if the diagnosis is in doubt, response to treatment is poor, or drug sensitivity develops.

Key references

1. Star VL, Hockberg MC: Prevention and management of gout. *Drugs* 1993, **45**:212–222.

2. Tan N, Lertratanakul W, Barr WG: Acute gouty arthritis: modern approaches to an ancient disease. *Postgrad Med* 1993, **94**:73–75; 78; 83–84.

Diagnosis

Symptoms

Sweats, chills, or rigors.

Cough, possibly with sputum, pleuritic chest pain, breathlessness.

Dysuria, urinary frequency.

Abdominal pain, nausea, vomiting, diarrhea.

Headache, neck stiffness, confusion.

Signs

• Focal clinical signs, if present, may help to localize the site of infection.

Tachycardia: >90 beats/min.

Tachypnea: >20 breaths/min.

Temperature >38°C or <35.6°C: hypothermia associated with worse prognosis.

Hypotension: systolic blood pressure <90 mm Hg or fall of 40 mm Hg from baseline.

Oliguria: <20 mL/h.

Petechial or purpuric skin rash: suggesting meningococcal septicemia; ecthyma gangrenosum associated with *Pseudomonas* infection in neutropenic patients.

Investigations

• Investigations are directed towards ascertaining the microbiology, site of infection, severity, and complications of gram-negative sepsis.

• Ideally, culture specimens should be taken before antimicrobial treatment, but treatment should not be unduly delayed in seriously ill patients.

Blood cultures: at least two, preferably three.

Urine and sputum microscopy and culture.

Gram-stain and culture of available pus or body fluids: may provide rapid diagnosis.

Chest radiography, further radiography directed by clinical picture.

Hemoglobin count: to detect severe anemia (may need to be corrected).

Leukocyte count: to detect neutrophil leukocytosis or toxic granulation; leukopenia associated with poor prognosis.

Platelet count and coagulation studies: for evidence of disseminated intravascular coagulation.

Arterial blood gas analysis: shows respiratory alkalosis early and metabolic acidosis later; possibly hypoxia.

Liver function tests: abnormal results in 40%–60% of patients.

Complications

Renal failure: acute tubular necrosis, usually reversible.

Disseminated intravascular coagulation.

Adult respiratory distress syndrome: in 15%–40% of patients.

Hepatic failure.

Differential diagnosis

• More than one factor may contribute to shock in an individual patient.

Other causes of shock: cardiogenic, hypovolemic, redistribution of fluid (*e.g.*, burns, pancreatitis, anaphylaxis), toxins.

Other infections: *e.g.*, Gram-positive bacteria, fungi, malaria, or viral infections, staphylococcal or streptococcal toxic shock syndrome.

Etiology

• Gram-negative septicemia is usually associated with *Escherichia coli, Klebsiella, Enterobacter, Serratia, Proteus,* and *Pseudomonas* spp., and *Neisseria meningitidis;* enteric gram-negative bacteria account for most cases.

• The most common sources are intra-abdominal or urinary tract infections and pneumonia.

• Host risk factors include the following:

Surgery (especially gastrointestinal, genitourinary, hepatobiliary).

Abnormalities of genitourinary tract.

Intravenous lines.

Hospitalization.

Cancer.

Neutropenia.

Immunosuppression.

Epidemiology

• Gram-negative septicemia and shock have been increasing over the past 30 years.

• Bacteremia is found in ~7 in 1000 hospital admissions.

• Septic shock complicates 20% of bacteremias.

Pathogenesis of gram-negative shock

• Bacterial endotoxin (lipopolysaccharide) and other bacterial products initiate the release of inflammatory mediators from monocyte/macrophages, endothelial cells, and polymorphonuclear leukocytes.

• The interaction of these mediators leads to an "inflammatory cascade" of reactions, leading to widespread endothelial damage, hypotension, refractory shock, multiorgan failure, and death.

Treatment

Diet and lifestyle

• No special precautions are necessary.

Pharmacological treatment

Indications

• Antibiotic treatment depends on the site of the infection and host and environmental factors.

Urinary tract (community-acquired): quinolone.

Urinary tract or pneumonia (hospital-acquired): ceftazidime, or piperacillin with gentamicin.

Intra-abdominal: cefotaxime with metronidazole, or piperacillin with gentamicin.

Biliary tract: piperacillin with gentamicin.

Cefotaxime or ceftazidime

Standard dosage	Ceftriaxone, 1–2 g daily, or ceftazidime, 1–2 g 8-hourly.
Contraindications	Previous cephalosporin hypersensitivity.
Special points	Dose adjusted in moderate to severe renal failure.
Main drug interactions	None.
Main side effects	Rashes, diarrhea, hemolysis, or raised transaminases (rare).

Amoxicillin and clavulanate

Standard dosage	Amoxicillin/clavulanate, 1.2 g 8-hourly.
Contraindications	Penicillin hypersensitivity.
Special points	Dose adjusted in moderate to severe renal failure.
Main drug interactions	None.
Main side effects	Pseudomembranous colitis, hypersensitivity.

Gentamicin

Standard dosage	Gentamicin, 4 mg/kg daily (normal renal function).
Contraindications	Myasthenia gravis, pre-existing renal failure.
Special points	Concentrations must be monitored before and after dose.
Main drug interactions	Loop diuretics, curare-type anesthetic agents.
Main side effects	Nephrotoxicity, ototoxicity.

Quinolones

Standard dosage	Ciprofloxacin, 500 mg twice daily.
Contraindications	Pregnancy, childhood.
Special points	Dose adjusted in severe renal failure.
Main drug interactions	None.
Main side effects	Diarrhea, renal failure.

Piperacillin

Standard dosage	Piperacillin, 2 g 6-hourly.
Contraindications	Penicillin hypersensitivity.
Special points	Dose adjusted in moderate to severe renal failure.
Main drug interactions	Inactivates aminoglycosides if mixed in solution.
Main side effects	Hypersensitivity, hepatotoxicity in 3% of patients, platelet dysfunction.

Treatment aims

To control infection.
To maintain organ perfusion and tissue oxygen delivery.
To minimize complications

Other treatments

Drainage of infected collections of pus.
Surgical debridement of dead or infected material.

Prognosis

• Mortality is 10%–20% in patients with bacteremia, 40%–60% in those with shock, and >90% in those with multiorgan failure.

Follow-up and management

• Patients need careful management in the convalescent stage, which may be prolonged after acute septic shock; they may relapse if the predisposing condition remains.

Management of gram-negative bacterial shock

• Monitoring of the following is needed:
Systolic blood pressure (must be kept >90 mm Hg or high enough to maintain renal perfusion).
Central venous pressure or postcapillary wedge pressure (to exclude hypovolemia).
Cardiac output.
Systemic vascular resistance (normal, >1000; in septic shock, generally <1000).
Catheterization (for urine measurement).
Oxygen saturation (arterial pressure falls, venous pressure rises because of failure in tissue oxygenation).

• Treatment includes the following:
Colloid to restore intravascular volume (blood for severe anemia).
Pressor or inotropic agents, if necessary.
Renal dopamine 2–4 μg/min to maintain renal perfusion.
Inspired oxygen at minimum to maintain arterial oxygenation.
Nutritional support.

General references

Edwards JD: Management of septic shock. *BMJ* 1993, **306**:1661–1664.

Parillo JE: Pathogenetic mechanisms of septic shock. *N Engl J Med* 1993, **328**:1471–1477.

Rietschel ET, Brade H: Bacterial endotoxins. *Sci Am* 1992, **267**:26–31.

Diagnosis

Symptoms

• Symptoms are often nonspecific, with a wide variety of manifestations.

Initial or indolent phase

Cough, dyspnea.

Nasal and ocular symptoms: in Wegener's granulomatosis.

Wheeze or asthma, abdominal pain: in Churg–Strauss syndrome.

Active or aggressive phase

Fever, malaise, anorexia, weight loss.

Cough, dyspnea, hemoptysis, chest pain.

Skin rash, arthralgia.

Signs

• Manifestations are widely varied.

Chest signs: often little, compared with extent of radiographic changes.

Wheeze: feature of Churg–Strauss syndrome and bronchocentric granulomatosis.

Nasal inflammation and granulation: in Wegener's and lymphomatoid granulomatoses.

Ocular inflammation or proptosis: in Wegener's granulomatosis.

Vasculitic or nonspecific skin rash.

Peripheral or cranial neuropathy.

Investigations

Full blood count: anemia common; eosinophilia >1.5 × 10^9/L in Churg–Strauss syndrome.

ESR and plasma viscosity measurement: usually raised values.

Renal function test: abnormalities frequent in Wegener's granulomatosis.

Chest radiography: varied appearances; can show mass lesion, consolidation, or diffuse shadowing; cavitating nodules typical of Wegener's granulomatosis.

Anti-neutrophil cytoplasmic antibodies (ANCA): cANCA present in 90% of patients with active Wegener's granulomatosis, pANCA present in some Churg–Strauss, lymphomatoid, or Wegener's sufferers; other serology usually negative.

Biopsy: ideally open lung biopsy; bronchoscopic or renal biopsy may give specific histology; nasal and skin biopsy usually nonspecific.

Complications

General

Pulmonary hemorrhage: uncommon.

Infection: common.

Peripheral or cranial neuropathy, mononeuritis multiplex.

Wegener's granulomatosis

Renal impairment: in 40% of patients.

Deafness: in 30%.

Churg–Strauss syndrome [1]

Cardiac involvement: in 50% (most common cause of death).

Differential diagnosis

General

Collagen-vascular diseases.

Other systemic vasculitides, subacute bacterial endocarditis, atrial myxoma.

Pulmonary disease alone

Sarcoid, tuberculosis, neoplasm, infection.

Pulmonary and renal disease

Goodpasture's syndrome, SLE.

Eosinophilic disease

Eosinophilic pneumonia, bronchopulmonary aspergillosis, hypereosinophilic syndrome, drug reaction.

Etiology

• The cause is unknown but may be a granulomatous or vasculitic response to infection or neoplasm.

• Bronchocentric granulomatosis is associated with aspergillus infection.

• Lymphomatoid granulomatosis may be a form of lymphoma.

Epidemiology

• Granulomatoses are rare conditions, of which Wegener's is by far the most common.

• They occur at all ages but mainly in people aged 35–55 years.

Diagnostic pointers

• Histology is often unavailable or inconclusive; diagnosis therefore rests on a combination of clinical features, investigations, and histology.

Wegener's granulomatosis [2]

Necrotizing, granulomatous vasculitis, involving upper and lower respiratory tract and kidneys; c-anti-neutrophil cytoplasmic antibody positive.

Churg–Strauss syndrome [1]

Asthma, eosinophilia, and vasculitis; p-anti-neutrophil cytoplasmic antibody often positive.

Lymphomatoid granulomatosis [3]

Nonnecrotizing, involving upper and lower respiratory tract; rare.

Necrotizing sarcoid or bronchocentric granulomatosis

Lung shadows without extrapulmonary features.

Treatment

Diet and lifestyle

• Stopping smoking should be encouraged in view of the risk of chest infection from disease and treatment.

Pharmacological treatment [4]

Prednisone

• Prednisone is important in all initial treatment and in maintenance for Churg-Strauss syndrome, necrotizing sarcoid granulomatosis, and bronchocentric granulomatosis.

Standard dosage Prednisone, 60–80 mg orally daily initially.
Optional initial pulse methylprednisolone 1 g i.v. on 3 successive days.
Steady dose reduction and alternate-day use after 1 month.
Wegener's patients should be weaned off drug entirely after remission.

Contraindications Caution in diabetes mellitus, hypertension, or peptic ulceration.

Special points Patients must be given a steroid-warning card; blood glucose and blood pressure must be checked.

Main drug interactions Rifampin, carbamazepine, phenytoin, phenobarbital.

Main side effects Fluid retention, hypertension, proximal myopathy, mental disturbance, osteoporosis, skin fragility, increased risk of infection.

Cyclophosphamide

• Cyclophosphamide is essential in Wegener's granulomatosis, advised in lymphomatoid granulomatosis, and sometimes needed in Churg–Strauss syndrome.

Standard dosage Cyclophosphamide, 2 mg/kg orally daily.
Optional initial pulse cyclophosphamide, 0.5 g i.v., followed by 0.5–1 g i.v. monthly, according to leukocyte count.

Contraindications Porphyria, pregnancy.

Special points Dose reduced in patients with renal impairment; should be adjusted according to regular leukocyte counts and side effects; usually continued for 1 year after remission has been induced.

Main drug interactions Allopurinol, succinylcholine.

Main side effects Bone-marrow suppression, nausea and vomiting, hair loss, cystitis, sterility, bladder cancer, lymphoma.

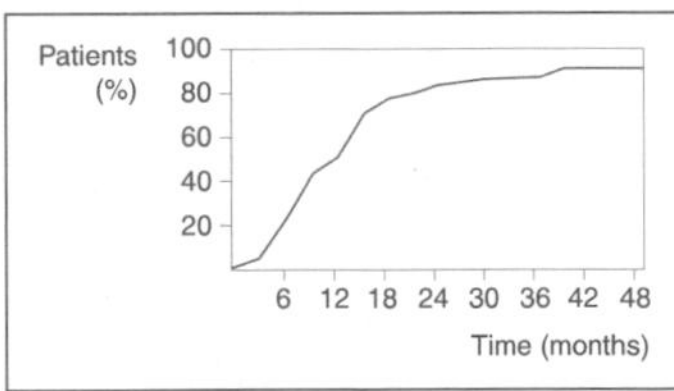

Cumulative remission rate on standard treatment for Wegener's granulomatosis (in the 75% of patients who achieve complete remission).

Treatment aims

To achieve remission and prevent relapse.

Prognosis

Wegener's granulomatosis

• Long-term survival is >80%, but relapse is common, and >80% of patients suffer permanent morbidity.

Churg–Strauss syndrome

• Long-term survival is high, but cardiac complications are the main cause of death.

Lymphomatoid granulomatosis

• The 5-year survival rate is 50%, less if lymphoma is present.

Necrotizing sarcoid or bronchocentric granulomatosis

• The prognosis and response to steroids are good.

Follow-up and management

• Long-term monitoring is required; ESR and chest radiography are guides of disease activity.

• Antineutrophil cytoplasmic antibody titers are helpful guides in Wegener's granulomatosis; they do not rise in infective episodes but may rise some time before relapse occurs.

• Renal function in Wegener's granulomatosis should be monitored.

Key references

1. Lanham JG: Churg–Strauss syndrome. *Br J Hosp Med* 1992, **47**:667–673.
2. Hoffman GS, *et al.*: Wegener's granulomatosis: an analysis of 158 patients. *Ann Intern Med* 1992, **116**:488–498.
3. Pisani RJ, DeRemee RA: Clinical implications of the histopathologic diagnosis of pulmonary lymphomatoid granulomatosis. *Mayo Clin Proc* 1990, **65**:151–163.
4. Fauci A, *et al.*: Wegener's granulomatosis: prospective clinical and therapeutic experience in 85 patients for 21 years. *Ann Intern Med* 1983, **98**:76–85.

Diagnosis

Symptoms

• Patients present with short stature at all ages.

Height less than the third height centile or short for family.

Delayed puberty: in patients short for a reason.

Signs

• Signs are not always manifest.

• Features of hypothyroidism with goiter may be seen.

Disproportionate growth: *e.g.*, short legs.

Dysmorphic features: *e.g.*, in Turner's syndrome, intrauterine growth retardation.

Investigations [1,2]

Anthropometry: height of child should be recorded on two occasions separated by at least 3 months to calculate annual growth rate; assessments of nutrition (weight, skinfold thickness) helpful; Tanner stages of puberty must be elicited; heights of parents should be measured; short person growing at normal rate for age and stage of puberty may need explanation of how shortness arose (*e.g.*, low birth weight).

Radiography: to assess skeletal maturity (bone age) as guide to long-term outlook; skeletal survey needed for disproportionate short stature and for children with height prediction small for family, who may have occult skeletal dysplasia.

Hematology: to identify anemia (vitamin B_{12}, folate, ferritin malabsorption).

ESR measurement: to exclude inflammatory disease.

Chemical pathology: electrolyte and creatinine analysis, measurement of calcium to exclude metabolic disease; measurement of thyroxine, gonadotropins, gonadal steroids, and prolactin in short children of pubertal age showing no or few signs of puberty; measurement of growth hormone secretion for short children growing slowly for otherwise unexplained reasons.

Karyotyping: XO in Turner's syndrome.

Complications

Premature fusion of epiphyses: through injudicious treatment.

Differential diagnosis

Not applicable.

Etiology [1,2]

• All disease in childhood causes a decrease in growth velocity that ultimately becomes manifest as short stature.

• The following may play a role:

Nutritional disorders: in infants.

Diminished growth hormone secretion: in the absence of physical signs in children.

Functional or organic failure of the hypothalamo–pituitary–gonadal axis: at 14 years.

Endocrine condition: in short, fat patients with low growth velocity.

Disease in any body system: in thin patients.

Epidemiology

• Boys with delayed puberty (and its consequent short stature) outnumber girls by 20 to 1.

• Most other conditions have a roughly equal gender distribution.

Treatment

Diet and lifestyle

• In infants, adequate nutrition must be promoted, including correction of malabsorption.

Pharmacological treatment [1,2]

• In childhood, growth hormone is appropriately prescribed to correct insufficiency; at puberty, sex steroids are appropriate first-line treatment.

• Long-term alleviation of short stature is achievable only when an abnormal growth velocity can be corrected; the height of a normal child cannot be increased.

Growth hormone: depends on pretreatment growth rate, condition being treated, and response required; hypopituitary children need 15 units/m^2 s.c. weekly as daily divided injections; 20 units/m^2 weekly needed to increase normal pretreatment rate; 30–40 units/m^2 weekly for children with abnormal skeletons (*e.g.*, in Turner's syndrome).

Thyroxine: 100 µg/m^2 orally as single daily dose.

Ethinyl estradiol: initially 2 µg daily, increased to 5, 10, 15, 20, and 30 µg daily at 6 monthly intervals; progestogen added when dose of 15 µg achieved or if breakthrough bleeding occurs earlier; contraindicated if family history of thrombotic disorder.

Testosterone: initially 50 mg testosterone esters at 4-weekly intervals, increased to 100 mg every 4 weeks after 6 months; increased to 3-weekly intervals over a further 6 months and then to 2-weekly intervals; causes accelerated fusion of epiphyses.

Treatment aims

To redress abnormal growth.

Prognosis

• The prognosis is not good in patients who are well developed at puberty.

• Treatment of disease promotes catch-up growth, but ultimate stature is determined by the deficit at presentation (height for bone age).

• Pre-existing deficits (low birth weight) or those caused by delay in diagnosis cannot be corrected.

Follow-up and management

• 6-monthly anthropometry is needed to record effects on growth and to readjust doses for increase in size.

Key references

1. Brook CGD: *A Guide to the Practice of Paediatric Endocrinology.* Cambridge: Cambridge University Press; 1993.
2. Brook CGD, ed: *Clinical Paediatric Endocrinology* edn 3. Oxford: Blackwell Scientific Publications; 1995.

Diagnosis

Symptoms

• Symptoms are usually minimal.

Clumsiness or accident-proneness: *e.g.*, because furniture is too small.

Aggression: patients stronger than their peers.

Behavior disorder: patients trying to show that they are not as old as they seem.

Symptoms of hyperthyroidism: rarely.

Signs

• Tall children usually look normal.

Dysmorphic features.

Signs of early puberty or thyrotoxicosis.

Isolated signs of virilization: pubic hair, acne, cliteromegaly; probably due to adrenal androgen secretion, the cause of which should be investigated.

Joint hypermobility, arachnodactyly, iridonodesis, high arch palate: signs of Marfan syndrome.

Investigations [1]

• Tall stature associated with precocious puberty must be fully investigated in boys; girls with no neurological signs and consonance of pubertal signs with pelvic ultrasonographic findings do not need invasive procedures.

Anthropometry: height of child and both parents should be measured; Tanner stages of puberty should be recorded; measurement of sitting height to determine leg length more helpful than measurement of span.

Radiography: assessment of skeletal maturity enables height prediction; radiographic appearance of iliac apophyses helps to asses potential for spinal growth; skull radiography (at least) for pituitary fossa.

Special tests: measurement of thyroxine and thyroid-stimulating hormone may reveal thyrotoxicosis; low basal concentration of growth hormone excludes gigantism, but proof of this diagnosis requires demonstration of measurable concentrations of growth hormone throughout 24 h, which leads to raised concentration of insulin-like growth factor 1.

Complications

Scoliosis.

Lens dislocation.

Cardiovascular problems.

Osteoarthritis.

Differential diagnosis

Not applicable.

Etiology [1]

• Causes include the following:

Normal growth rate and appearance

Tall parents.

Obesity of infantile onset.

Marfan, Klinefelter's, or Sotos' syndrome.

Excessive growth rate

Early puberty.

Androgen secretion (congenital adrenal hyperplasia, adrenal neoplasm, adrenarche).

Thyrotoxicosis.

Growth hormone excess.

Epidemiology

• 1% of the population is tall.

Treatment

Diet and lifestyle

• No special precautions are necessary.

Pharmacological treatment [1]

• Treatment of children for limitation of tall adult stature after puberty has begun is probably a waste of time because insufficient time for maneuver is available; tall children should be referred before the age of 8 years.

• Precocious puberty and adrenal, thyroid, and pituitary conditions need appropriate treatment.

• Patients with Klinefelter's syndrome and inadequate puberty need androgens to prevent gynecomastia.

• If excessive height in adulthood is predicted, height can be lost by (early) induction of puberty at a height 30 cm less than that desired.

• If the age at which puberty induction would be needed to limit final stature is extremely low (*i.e.*, the patient is and will be extremely tall), growth hormone secretion can be reduced using somatostatin analogues.

Ethinyl estradiol: initially 2 µg daily, increased to 5, 10, 15, 20, and 30 µg daily at 6 monthly intervals; progestogen added when dose of 15 µg achieved or if breakthrough bleeding occurs earlier; contraindicated if family history of thrombotic disorder.

Testosterone: initially 50 mg testosterone esters at 4-weekly intervals, increased to 100 mg every 4 weeks after 6 months; increased to 3-weekly intervals over a further 6 months and then to 2-weekly intervals; causes accelerated fusion of epiphyses.

Treatment aims

To reduce adult stature.

Prognosis

• The prognosis depends on the diagnosis.

Follow-up and management

• Children with Marfan syndrome need ophthalmological and cardiac opinions.

Key reference

1. Brook CGD, ed: *Clinical Paediatric Endocrinology*, edn. 3. Oxford: Blackwell Scientific Publications; 1995.

Diagnosis

Symptoms

Ascending, symmetrical weakness in all limbs: legs usually affected first, with patient initially noticing difficulty climbing stairs, rising from sitting, and, eventually, walking and standing.

Paresthesias of extremities, with distal sensory loss: in 95% of patients.

Neck, shoulder, back, and sciatic pain: may be severe.

Diplopia, drooling, nasal regurgitation of food or drink, slurred speech, weak cough: indicating cranial nerve involvement.

Dyspnea: late symptom, reflecting intercostal and diaphragmatic weakness.

Fatigue: possibly profound and often persisting after return of muscle strength.

Hesitancy and urinary retention: usually when weakness more advanced (vs. acute myelopathy, in which sphincter symptoms appear early).

Signs

Weakness in limbs: flaccid, usually symmetrical, arms usually less severely affected.

Cranial nerve palsies: facial nerve most often affected, followed by bulbar muscles.

Hyporeflexia, areflexia: early.

Sensory deficit: may be absent or minor despite prominent symptoms.

Profound sensory loss: in some patients.

Ataxia, ophthalmoplegia, areflexia, with little or no weakness: Miller-Fisher syndrome; rare.

Investigations

Initial

Lumbar puncture: classically, raised protein concentration associated with normal cell count (albuminocytological dissociation); protein possibly normal within first week.

Serum potassium measurement: to exclude hypo- or hyperkalemic paralysis.

Antinuclear antibodies analysis: positive in rare cases associated with SLE.

Liver function tests: often abnormal.

Heavy metal screening: only if clinically indicated.

Porphyrin screening: positive in acute intermittent porphyria, which may manifest like Guillain-Barré syndrome.

Lyme titers.

Specialist

Nerve conduction studies: to identify multifocal conduction block and slowed conduction, confirming demyelinating neuropathy; studies early in disease may be only mildly abnormal, *e.g.*, delayed or absent F waves; axonal degeneration may also occur [1].

Electromyography: in patients without sensory involvement, to help to rule out neuromuscular conduction block or muscle disease and to document axonal degeneration.

Antiganglioside antibody analysis: anti-GM_1 antibodies present in 20%–30% of patients and are associated with poor prognosis; anti-GQ1b antibodies associated with Miller-Fisher syndrome.

Complications

Death: if airway not adequately protected.

Atelectasis, pneumonia, deep-vein thrombosis, pulmonary embolism, joint contractures, pressure sores, anxiety and depression, pain [2].

Cardiac arrhythmias, including bradycardic and asystolic episodes, labile blood pressure: due to autonomic instability.

Differential diagnosis

Brain stem encephalitis or infarct.

Acute myelopathy.

Poliomyelitis.

Other neuropathies: porphyria, vasculitis, critical-illness neuropathy, drug-induced neuropathy, toxins (*e.g.*, heavy metals, organophosphates), Lyme disease, or HIV.

Neuromuscular conduction block: myasthenia gravis, botulism.

Muscle disease: hypokalemia (with or without periodic paralysis), polymyositis, acute rhabdomyolysis.

Functional disease: hysteria, malingering.

Etiology

• The cause of Guillain–Barré syndrome is unknown, but, in 60%–70% of patients, it is associated with antecedent infection.

• Inflammatory demyelination with variable axonal degeneration in the peripheral nervous system due to autoimmune mechanisms is triggered by many different agents, including the following:

Viruses: cytomegalovirus, Epstein–Barr virus, HIV (usually around seroconversion).

Bacteria: *Mycoplasma pneumoniae, Campylobacter jejuni.*

Vaccines against rabies or swine influenza.

Surgery.

Epidemiology

• Guillain–Barré syndrome has become the most frequent cause of acute generalized neuromuscular paralysis in developed countries since the virtual eradication of poliomyelitis.

• The incidence is 1–2 in 100 000 population.

• More men than women are affected.

• The disease occurs more often in young women and elderly patients.

• It is not contagious.

• No seasonal variation is evident.

Treatment

Diet and lifestyle

• No special precautions are necessary.

Pharmacological treatment

General measures

Frequent measurement of vital capacity and continuous ECG monitoring during progressive phase.

Admission to intensive care unit if vital capacity falling rapidly or patient unable to swallow saliva.

Regular turning, mouth and eye care, aspiration of secretions.

Heparin, 5000 units s.c. twice daily.

Nasogastric feeding if patient has bulbar palsy or is too weak to eat.

Plasma exchange

• Plasma, 50 ml/kg, exchanged five times over 5–10 days is indicated for any patient unable to walk unaided.

• Treatment should be initiated as soon as the diagnosis is made because it is more effective in early disease.

Immunoglobulin [3]

Standard dosage	Immunoglobulin, 0.4 g/kg i.v. daily for 5 days or 1 g/kg daily for 2 days.
Contraindications	IgA deficiency due to circulating anti-IgA antibodies.
Special points	May cause aseptic meningitis and acute or chronic renal failure.
Main side effects	Fever, hypersensitivity reactions, fluid overload.

Treatment aims

To prevent respiratory failure.

To relieve pain.

To prevent complications of immobility.

To optimize functional recovery.

Other treatments

Early tracheostomy: to assist tracheal toilet and increase patient comfort.

Ventilatory assistance: if vital capacity 20 mL/kg or falling rapidly (oxygen saturation best monitored by pulse oximetry) or patient unable to protect airway.

Endocardial pacemaker: for episodes of bradycardia or sinus arrest.

Prognosis

• ~5% of patients relapse; 80% make a good recovery (median time to full independence, 9 months); 20% have permanent disability; 5% die.

• Poor prognostic indicators include age >40 years, rapid onset of weakness, ventilation, high titers of IgG anti-ganglioside GM_1 antibodies, and previous diarrheal illness.

Follow-up and management

• A high level of vigilance must be maintained until recovery has started and the tracheostomy has been closed.

• The patient should be reassured that recovery is probable and is nearly complete in most cases.

• Rehabilitation, *e.g.*, physical therapy, must be continued after discharge.

• Immunization injections must be avoided, especially tetanus toxoid, which has been associated with relapse.

Key references

1. Albers JW: Acquired inflammatory demyelinating polyneuropathies: clinical and electrodiagnostic features. *Muscle Nerve* 1989, **12**:435–451.
2. Hughes RAC, Bihari D: Acute neuromuscular respiratory paralysis. *J Neurol Neurosurg Psychiatry* 1993, **56**:334–343.
3. van der Meché FGA, Schmitz PIM, the Dutch Guillain–Barré Study Group: A randomized trial comparing intravenous immune globulin and plasma exchange in Guillain–Barré syndrome. *N Engl J Med* 1992, **326**:1123–1129.

Diagnosis

Definition

• Heart block is a disturbance of conduction of the electrical impulse from atrium to ventricle.

• Failure of the sinus impulse to penetrate the atrium (sinoatrial block) and bundle branch block are not considered here.

First-degree atrioventricular block: delayed conduction of impulses from atrium to ventricle, with a prolonged PR interval, but all impulses are conducted.

Second-degree atrioventricular block: intermittent complete failure of conduction of atrial impulse to ventricle, with dropped (nonconducted) P waves on ECG.
Mobitz type I (Wenckebach): progressive lengthening of PR interval until conduction completely fails; atrioventricular conduction recovers after dropped beat, and sequence is repeated.
Mobitz type II: occasional or repetitive failure of conduction without previous lengthening of PR interval; may be every second (2 : 1) or third (3 : 1) beat or occasional random dropped P waves [1].

Third-degree (complete) atrioventricular block: complete failure of conduction of all atrial impulses to ventricles; escape rhythm is either narrow complex (if level of block is in atrioventricular node, escape pacemaker arises in bundle of His) or broad complex (if block is infranodal).

Symptoms

First-degree and Mobitz type I

• Patients are usually asymptomatic but may progress to higher-grade atrioventricular block.

Mobitz type II and complete heart block

Syncope (Adams–Stokes attack): loss of consciousness is abrupt, without warning, and the patient appears pale; rare in Mobitz type II.

Presyncope and dizzy spells, fatigue, dyspnea, sudden death.

Signs

First-degree

• No signs are manifest.

Mobitz type I

Irregular pulse with dropped beats.

Mobitz type II

Occasional dropped beats: irregular pulse.
2 : 1/3 : 1 block, etc.: bradycardia, edema, raised venous pressure.

Complete heart block

Bradycardia, large-volume pulse, raised venous pressure with occasional cannon waves, variable intensity of first heart sound, peripheral edema.

Investigations

Resting ECG: usually diagnostic.

24-h Holter monitoring: if heart block is intermittent or continuous "event recorder" if symptoms are infrequent.

Complications

Injury: from syncope.

"Heart failure": underlying ventricular function may be normal, but low cardiac output due to bradycardia and loss of atrioventricular synchrony may mimic ventricular disease.

Ventricular tachycardia and fibrillation: leading to sudden death, may complicate complete heart block.

Differential diagnosis

• ECG diagnosis is usually definitive; the only differential should be in etiology.

Etiology

• Causes include the following:

Idiopathic fibrosis: increasing frequency with age.

Ischemic heart disease, particularly acute myocardial infarction.

Calcific aortic stenosis: involvement of ring close to atrioventricular node.

Drug toxicity: many antiarrhythmic agents, including digoxin and calcium channel blockers.

Postoperative: especially aortic valve replacement.

Congenital complete heart block.

Complex congenital heart disease.

Infection: aortic valve endocarditis with root abscess, diphtheria, Lyme disease, rheumatic fever.

Multisystem disease: sarcoidosis, amyloidosis, ankylosing spondylitis, Reiter's syndrome, rheumatoid arthritis, scleroderma, SLE.

Muscular dystrophy, myotic dystrophy, Refsum's disease.

Epidemiology

• >200 000 permanent pacemakers are implanted world wide each year; most of these are for heart block.

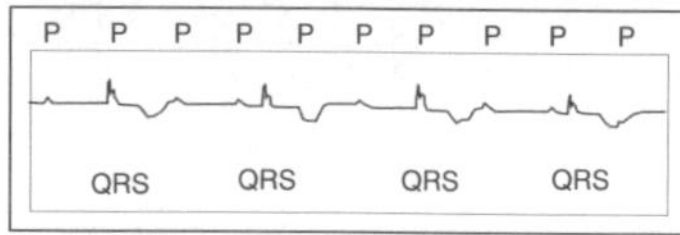

Rhythm strip of ECG for complete heart block demonstrating complete dissociation between P waves and QRS complexes and slow ventricular escape rhythm of 32 beats/min.

Treatment

Diet and lifestyle

• Patients should lead a normal life after heart block has been treated.

• Permanent pacemaker implantation places certain restrictions on patients, *e.g.*, avoidance of contact sports, which might damage the device or lead.

Pharmacological treatment

• Atropine (0.5–1 mg i.v. bolus) and isoproterenol (200 μg i.v. bolus or 0.5–10 μg/min infusion) may be used as temporary measures before temporary or permanent pacemaker implantation or when heart block needs treatment during resuscitation, although external temporary pacing should also be considered in such circumstances.

Nonpharmacological treatment

• Implantation of a permanent pacemaker in a patient with complete heart block is one of the most cost-effective interventions in modern medicine.

Indications for permanent pacemaker implantation

Second-degree Mobitz type II heart block.

Complete heart block.

Indications for temporary pacing

Symptomatic second-degree Mobitz type II and complete heart block, pending implantation of a permanent pacemaker.

Acute myocardial infarction: complete heart block, second-degree Mobitz type II, development of alternating bundle branch block, development of right bundle branch block with left axis deviation, especially when in combination with first-degree or second-degree heart block.

Treatment aims

To return patient to a full and active life.

Prognosis

• Implantation of a permanent pacemaker dramatically improves the prognosis of patients with complete heart block.

Follow-up and management

• Patients with first-degree or second-degree Mobitz type I heart block should be followed carefully to check for development of higher-grade atrioventricular block.

• Patients with a permanent pacemaker need regular follow-up in a pacemaker clinic to ensure continued normal function of the device.

• Permanent pacemakers must be changed every 7–10 years.

Key reference

1. Rowlands DJ: Conduction Disturbances. In *Understanding the Electrocardiogram: Rhythm Abnormalities*. Macclesfield: ICI; 1987:483–507.

Diagnosis

Definition

• Hemolytic uremic syndrome (HUS) is a syndrome, not a disease; it is defined by the following:

Acute renal insufficiency.

Microangiopathic hemolytic anemia.

Thrombocytopenia.

• Thrombotic thrombocytopenic purpura (TTP) is closely related and often indistinguishable from HUS; the term should be reserved for the following:

A relapsing form of HUS.

Associated fever and fluctuating CNS signs.

• Both HUS and TTP are associated with normal clotting times. Thrombocytopenia and a microangiopathic hemolytic anemia with prolonged clotting times indicate septicemia and disseminated intravascular coagulation.

Symptoms

Malaise, nausea, tiredness: nonspecific symptoms of renal insufficiency.

Oliguria, discolored urine, difficulty concentrating, other subtle CNS changes.

Abdominal cramps; watery diarrhea, then bloody diarrhea; fever <38°C: indicating infection by *Escherichia coli*.

Signs

Pallor: from anemia.

Yellow tinge: occasionally, from the hemolysis.

Bruising or prolonged bleeding: if thrombocytopenia is severe.

Investigations

Full blood count: shows thrombocytopenia; fragmented erythrocytes seen on film.

Clotting times: prothrombin time and partial thromboplastin time should be normal.

Biochemistry: shows raised urea, creatinine, and urate concentrations, hyponatremia, hypoalbuminemia in severely ill patients, raised lactate dehydrogenase (an index of erythrocyte hemolysis).

Renal biopsy: usually not needed in children; contraindicated during severe thrombocytopenia; typically shows glomerular and arteriolar thrombosis and acute tubular necrosis in patients with diarrhea, and severe intimal proliferation of preglomerular arterioles and small arteries, with varying degrees of glomerular endothelial injury, in patients without diarrhea.

Stool culture for *Escherichia coli* 0157:H7 and isolation of verotoxin: can confirm diagnosis in patients with associated diarrhea.

Serology: for neutralizing antibodies to *E. coli* 0157:H7.

Complications [3]

Bloody diarrhea, gut infarction, rectal prolapse: in patients with associated diarrhea.

Severe malignant hypertension, cardiomyopathy: in patients without diarrhea.

Irritability, restlessness, twitching, generalized or focal seizures, transient visual disturbance, drowsiness, cerebellar ataxia, reduced level of consciousness, decerebrate spasms, coma.

Skin petechiae or purpura: rare unless platelets are $\leq 20 \times 10^9$/L.

Differential diagnosis [1,2]

Septicemia associated with disseminated intravascular coagulation

Gram-negative bacilli.

Infection by *Staphylococcus aureus, Pneumococcus* spp., or *Meningococcus* spp.

Psittacosis.

Mycoplasma.

Viral and other diseases: thrombocytopenia without hemolysis

Hantavirus.

Dengue hemorrhagic fever.

Malaria.

Leptospirosis.

Snake bite.

Associated with pregnancy (associated with disseminated intravascular coagulation)

Septic abortion.

Amniotic fluid embolus.

Prolonged intrauterine fetal death.

Antepartum hemorrhage.

Etiology

Infectious causes [1]

Escherichia coli associated with diarrhea (in most patients): infection acquired from contaminated beef or dairy products.

Shigella spp.

HIV.

Sporadic, noninfectious causes [1]

Idiopathic or familial disorders, drugs (mitomycin, cyclosporin A), tumors, pregnancy, SLE, transplantation, scleroderma, malignant or accelerated hypertension.

Superimposed on glomerulonephritis.

Epidemiology

• Patients with diarrhea-associated hemolytic uremic syndrome are usually aged <5 years or >65 years.

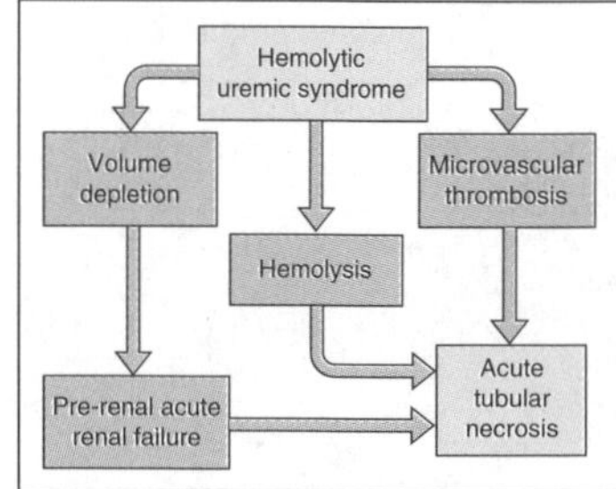

Pathogenesis of acute tubular necrosis from hemolytic uremic syndrome.

Treatment

Diet and lifestyle

• No special precautions are necessary.

Pharmacological treatment

Intravenous saline solution and furosemide: to correct circulating volume and reverse prerenal failure and to establish diuresis.

Antiplatelet drugs (*e.g.*, aspirin, dipyridamole): have a logic but no proven benefit.

Prostacyclin infusions: of theoretical value and useful to control hypertension.

Nonpharmacological treatment [4]

Erythrocyte transfusion: for anemia.

Platelet transfusion: if count $<50\times10^9$/L and some surgical intervention needed.

Hemodialysis: when indicated, *i.e.*, for volume overload, hyperkalemia, "uremia," acidosis.

Infusions of fresh frozen plasma: may induce remission; amount necessary not known but probably 1-2 L daily; mechanism of benefit not known but may include neutralizing toxins, restoring antioxidant activity, and inducing prostacyclin synthesis; infusions should be continued until erythrocyte fragmentation ceases and platelet count rises $\sim100\times10^9$/L.

Plasma exchange: may be needed to create intravascular space for repeated infusions of fresh frozen plasma.

Treatment aims

To establish diuresis if possible.

To provide dialysis if necessary.

To control blood pressure.

To try to induce hematological remission.

To prevent seizures.

Prognosis

• The natural history of hemolytic uremic syndrome, when preceded by a diarrheal illness and associated with glomerular thrombi, is one of spontaneous recovery, although patients may have some residual injury; most children are in this category.

• Idiopathic patients, particularly adults, often have major preglomerular vascular disease and irreversible renal failure.

• 3%–10% of patients die during the acute illness (usually from CNS involvement); 10%–20% remain dependent on dialysis; 10% have long-term neurological sequelae; 70% recover with no residual evidence of renal disease.

Follow-up and management

• Recovery of renal function and disappearance of proteinuria must be established.

• If this is not possible, long-term follow-up is needed.

• Blood pressure should be controlled by angiotensin-converting enzyme inhibitors, which may help to limit occlusive arteriopathy.

Key references

1. Milford DV, Taylor CM: New insights into the hemolytic uremic syndromes. *Arch Dis Child* 1990, **65**:713–715.
2. Neild GH: Hemolytic uremic syndrome: clinical practice. *Lancet* 1994, **343**:398–401.
3. Neild GH: Hemolytic uremic syndrome (including disseminated intravascular coagulation and thrombotic purpura). In *Oxford Textbook of Clinical Nephrology*. Edited by Cameron JS, *et al.* Oxford: Oxford University Press; 1992:1041–1060.
4. Rock GA, *et al.*: Comparison of plasma exchange with plasma infusion in the treatment of thrombotic thrombocytopenic purpura. *N Engl J Med* 1991, **325**:393–397.

Diagnosis

Symptoms

Hemophilia

Episodic spontaneous hemorrhage: into joints and muscles.

Deep-tissue hematoma: particularly after trauma or surgery.

Von Willebrand's disease

Bruising.

Epistaxis and melena.

Excessive bleeding after dental extraction or surgery.

Postpartum bleeding, rarely hemarthroses and muscle hematomas.

Signs

Hemophilia

Hot, swollen, painful joint; unexpected bleeding after surgery: acute.

Crippling joint deformity: chronic.

Investigations

Hemophilia

Activated partial thromboplastin time measurement: prolonged.

Hemophilia A, factor VIII:C; hemophilia B, factor IX; and hemophilia C, factor XI assays: all three show low values.

Coagulation factor activity measurement: correlated with disease severity in hemophilia A and B (normal range, 50–150 units/dL):
<2 units/dL indicates severe disease, manifest as frequent spontaneous bleeding episodes, joint deformity, and crippling;
2–5 units/dL indicates moderate disease, manifest as posttraumatic bleeding, occasional spontaneous episodes;
5–20 units/dL indicates mild disease, manifest as posttraumatic bleeding.

Von Willebrand's disease

Bleeding time measurement: prolonged.

Factor VIII clotting activity, von Willebrand factor antigen and activity measurement: low values.

Platelet function tests: reduced aggregation of platelets with ristocetin.

• Von Willebrand's disease is classified on the basis of the type of protein abnormality; this is important for deciding treatment.

Complications

Transfusion-transmitted disease [1]

Hepatitis A: has been a problem with a solvent detergent sterilized product; all patients with bleeding disorders should be vaccinated.

Hepatitis B: although all blood donors are tested for this, sterilization processes for clotting factor concentrate cannot be regarded as 100% safe; vaccination mandatory in patients with bleeding disorders [2].

Hepatitis C: all patients treated by unsterilized clotting factor concentrates have been infected (sterilization introduced in 1985); some patients progress to chronic liver disease; treatment by interferon may normalize transaminases; HIV co-infection results in faster progression of hepatitis C liver disease [2].

HIV infection: occurred in patients receiving concentrates between 1979 and 1985 [3,4].

Inhibitors

Neutralizing antibodies: occurring after infusion of concentrates.

Chronic arthropathy

Chronic disabling arthritis: caused by recurrent hemarthroses.

Differential diagnosis

Other clotting factor deficiencies or platelet function disorders.

Etiology

Causes of hemophilia

Quantitative deficiency of clotting factors.

Factor VIII: hemophilia A (most common).

Factor IX: hemophilia B.

Factor XI: hemophilia C.

Causes of von Willebrand's disease

Quantitative or qualitative deficiency of von Willebrand factor, important in primary platelet hemostasis, acting as an adhesive protein and a carrier protein for factor VIII.

Genetics

Hemophilia A and B: X-linked (men affected, but some women carriers may need concentrate for surgery or trauma).

Von Willebrand's disease: autosomal-dominant.

Hemophilia C (severe disease): autosomal-recessive or compound heterozygote.

Epidemiology

• 1 in 5000 men is affected by hemophilia A or B; 1 in 6 patients with hemophilia has hemophilia B.

• Hemophilia C is common in Ashkenazi Jews; it may occur in any ethnic group.

• Von Willebrand's disease is the most common inherited bleeding disorder if all grades of severity are considered; clinically significant disease occurs in ~125 in one million population.

Carrier detection and antenatal diagnosis

• Carrier status and presence of the disorders in fetuses can be detected by the following:

Restriction fragment length polymorphisms.

Variable-number repeat sequences.

Direct mutational analysis (research).

Chorionic villus sampling before 10 weeks (for carriers with a molecular marker).

Fetal sexing and choriocentesis (for carriers without a molecular marker).

Treatment

Diet and lifestyle

• Patients should avoid contact sports, but regular exercise, *e.g.*, swimming, should be encouraged.

Pharmacological treatment

• Intramuscular injections must be avoided in patients with bleeding disorders.

• Aspirin or NSAIDs that impair platelet function must also be avoided.

Indications

For hemophilia A: factor VIII concentrate or DDAVP (desmopressin).

For hemophilia B: factor IX concentrate.

For hemophilia C: factor XI concentrate [5].

For von Willebrand's disease: factor VIII concentrate rich in von Willebrand's factor or DDAVP.

Clotting factor preparations [6]

Recombinant: Recombinate (VIII), Kogenate (VIII).

Extracted by immunoaffinity chromatography: Hemofil M (VIII), Antihemophilic Factor (American Red Cross) Monoclate P (VIII), Mononine (IX), Humate P (von Willebrand's factor).

Extracted by conventional separation: *very high purity (>100 units/mg):* Alphanine (IX) SD; *intermediate purity (<50 units/mg):* Humate P (von Willebrand's factor), (IX).

• The units of clotting factor needed, x, can be calculated by the following equation:
$x = [\text{rise in clotting factor required (\%)} \times \text{weight (kg)}] \div K$
where K = 1.5 for factor VIII, 1 for factor IX, and 2 for factor XI.

• Approximate levels for hemostasis are as follows:

15–20 units clotting factor/dL plasma for minor spontaneous hemarthroses and hematomas.

20–40 units clotting factor/dL plasma for severe hemarthroses and muscle hematomas, minor surgery.

80–100 units clotting factor/dL plasma for major surgery.

DDAVP

• DDAVP releases factor VIII:C and von Willebrand's factor from endothelial cells.

• It is used to cover minor procedures in patients with mild hemophilia and von Willebrand's disease.

• It is not indicated for severe hemophilia or severe and variant types of von Willebrand's disease.

Standard dosage	DDAVP, 0.3 µg/kg in 100 mL normal saline solution i.v. infusion over 20 min.
Contraindications	Vascular disease.
Special points	Response should be monitored using factor assays.
Main drug interactions	None.
Main side effects	Hyponatremia and seizures (in children <2 years), coronary occlusion (in patients >60 years).

Tranexamic acid and aminocaproic acid

• Tranexamic acid, an inhibitor of fibrinolysis, reduces blood loss, particularly in mucosal bleeding, *e.g.*, oral surgery, epistaxis, and tonsillectomy.

Standard dosage	Tranexamic acid, 1 g orally or i.v. 3–4 times daily; in children, 25 mg/kg 3 times daily. Aminocaproic acid, 5–30 g in divided doses every 3–6 h for 5–7 days.
Contraindications	*Tranexamic acid and aminocaproic acid:* hematuria, risk of "clot colic."
Special points	*Tranexamic acid and aminocaproic acid:* dose should be reduced in patients with renal impairment.
Main drug interactions	None.
Main side effects	*Tranexamic acid and aminocaproic acid:* nausea, dizziness.

Treatment aims

To prevent spontaneous bleeds and to make surgery safe.

Prognosis

• With the advent of virally safe blood products and home-treatment programs, many severely hemophilic patients can lead a relatively normal life.

• Mild disease, whether hemophilia or von Willebrand's disease, may impinge little unless an injury occurs or surgery is planned.

Follow-up and management

• All patients with bleeding disorders should be registered and regularly reviewed at a designated hemophilia center; regular review and access to treatment are of paramount importance for the successful long-term management of these patients.

Key references

1. Vermylen J, Briet E: Factor VIII preparations: need for prospective pharmacovigilance. *Lancet* **342**:693–694.
2. Lee CA, Dusheiko G: Hepatitis and hemophilia. In *Viral Hepatitis.* Edited by Zuckerman AJ, Thomas HC, 1993.
3. Goerdert JJ, *et al.*: A prospective study of human immunodeficiency virus type I infection and the development of AIDS in subjects with hemophilia. *N Engl J Med* 1989, **321**:1141–1148.
4. Lee CA, *et al.*: Progression of HIV disease in a hemophilic cohort followed for 11 years and the effect of treatment. *BMJ* 1991, **303**:1093–1094.
5. Bolton-Maggs PHB, *et al.*: Production and therapeutic use of a factor XI concentrate from plasma. *Thromb Haemostas* 1992, **67**:314–319.
6. Mannucci PM: Modern treatment of hemophilia: from shadows towards light. *Thromb Haemostas* 1993, **70**:17–23.

Diagnosis

Symptoms

• In most patients, symptoms occur 24–48 h after infection (usually upper respiratory tract infection) or drug ingestion (antibiotics).

• ~50% of adults develop only the characteristic rash and malaise.

Florid palpable purpuric skin rash: predominantly on lower legs but also on buttocks and arms (cardinal symptom).

Cramping abdominal pains: in 60%–70% of patients

Joint pains: in 60%–70%.

Blood in urine or stool: in 20%–30%.

Symptoms of intestinal obstruction: due to intussusception, in young children.

Fever and toxicity: if severe.

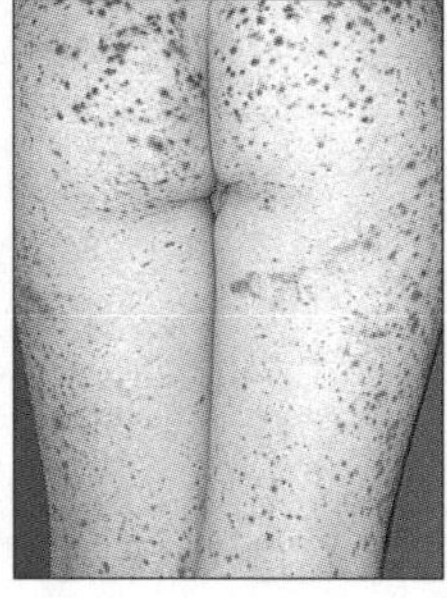

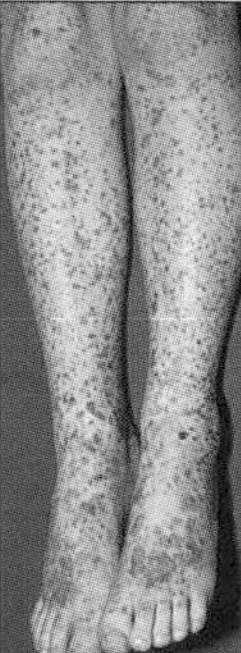

Typical purpuric lesions on buttocks (left) and pretibial areas and lower legs (right).

Signs

Rash: "papular purpura" lesions that do not blanch on pressure, some forming a necrotic center that may vesiculate, usually on buttocks, natal cleft, and extremities; usually painless; in adults, may persist or recur for up to 2 months.

Joint involvement: mild to moderate symmetrical arthropathy in 60%–70%; some periarticular swelling; a few patients also have angioedema of hands and feet.

Gut involvement: cramping abdominal pain, and some rebound tenderness in 25%; frank blood in stool in 10%–20%; obstructive symptoms (intussusception) or perforation.

Renal involvement: ~30% of patients develop nephritis.

Investigations

Skin biopsy: may show cutaneous necrotizing venulitis but does not indicate cause.

History: may be positive for recent infective episodes or drug ingestion (antibiotic).

Full blood count: may show mild polymorphonuclear leukocytosis.

Serology: for recent viral or streptococcal infection.

Stool and urine analysis: regularly during and after rash, with formal microscopy if positive; 30% of patients show evidence of erythrocytes, raised protein concentration, and casts on urinalysis.

Formal renal investigations, including biopsy: if findings indicate renal disease.

Complications

• In children, this condition is often thought of as "harmless."

Secondary infection of vasculitic lesions.

Glomerulonephritis, IgA nephropathy: in ~30% of patients; 15%–20% of these progress to renal failure in 6 months (adults).

Renal failure: in 5%–10% of all patients.

Gastrointestinal or surgical problems: *e.g.*, intussusception or perforation in young children; of the 60%–70% of patients with gastrointestinal complications, a few develop intramural hematomata, associated with intussusception, infarction, or gut perforation; protein-losing enteropathy.

Renal problems: *e.g.*, immunoglobulin nephropathy in older children and adults.

Differential diagnosis

Other forms of vasculitic or purpuric rash (*e.g.*, meningococcal septicemia).

Embolic phenomena from acute or subacute bacterial endocarditis.

Systemic gram-negative sepsis.

Collagen vascular disease, especially polyarteritis nodosa.

Etiology

• Henoch–Schönlein purpura is essentially idiopathic.

• Triggers include the following:

Nonspecific upper respiratory infection (in ~33% of patients).

Sulfonamide or penicillin treatment.

Streptococcal infection.

Streptokinase treatment for myocardial infarction.

Epidemiology

• Henoch–Schönlein purpura can occur at any age, but it predominantly affects children.

• It has a seasonal variation, occurring most often in winter months in temperate climates.

Treatment

Diet and lifestyle

• Other than bed rest during the acute phase, no special precautions are necessary.

Pharmacological treatment

• Treatment is symptomatic and does not alter the course or outcome of the condition or its complications.

• Local treatment of the rash, if needed, should be designed to prevent secondary infection, *e.g.*, potassium permanganate soaks.

• Steroids have no effect on renal abnormalities and are associated with a significant incidence of gastrointestinal side effects.

For pain relief

Standard dosage NSAIDs, *e.g.*, naproxen, 250 mg every 6–8 h (adults).

Contraindications Active peptic ulceration.

Special points Asthma may be exacerbated.

Main drug interactions Oral anticoagulants.

Main side effects Gastrointestinal disturbances, discomfort, nausea, or ulceration.

For joint abnormalities

Standard dosage Corticosteroids, *e.g.*, prednisolone, 40–60 mg daily.

Contraindications Active peptic ulceration.

Special points Possible adrenal suppression on sudden withdrawal.

Main drug interactions NSAIDs, oral anticoagulants.

Main side effects Cushing's syndrome, growth retardation in children, osteoporosis.

Treatment aims

To prevent secondary infection in vasculitic skin lesions.

To relieve symptoms of joint or abdominal pain.

Other treatments

• Renal replacement therapy may be needed in the 5%–10% of patients who develop renal failure or nephrotic syndrome.

Prognosis

• The prognosis of the rash alone is good.

• Crops of lesions may recur within 4–8 weeks, especially in adults.

• Spontaneous remission is the norm.

• Relapses of the rash alone often occur in adults.

• 15%–20% of adults with IgA nephropathy progress to renal failure in 6 months.

• Generally, 5%–10% of patients develop renal failure; this is most probable in adults or adolescents.

Follow-up and management

• Renal function or urinary sediment must be monitored for evidence of renal involvement.

• If renal involvement is detected, full renal investigation, including biopsy is needed.

General references

Fogazzi GB, *et al.*: Long term outcome of Schönlein Henoch nephritis in the adult. *Clin Nephrol* 1989, **31**:60–66.

Ford EG, Jennings LM, Andrassay RJ: Management of Henoch–Schönlein purpura and polyarteritis nodosum. *Tex Med* 1987, **83**:54–58.

Schreiner DT: Purpura. *Dermatol Clin* 1989, **7**:481–490.

Diagnosis

Definition

• Hepatic encephalopathy is a reversible neuropsychiatric syndrome that is a complication of fulminant or chronic liver disease [1].

• Hepatic encephalopathy may also be present in the rare cases of urea-cycle enzyme defects and portosystemic shunting in the absence of liver disease.

• Latent encephalopathy is a subclinical form occurring in chronic liver disease, only detected by psychometric testing.

Symptoms

• Wide differences are seen in presentation and evolution (*see* Classification).

Inversion of normal sleep pattern.

Deterioration of intellectual function.

Slurred speech.

Tremor: absent at rest.

Personality changes: features of frontal-lobe syndrome.

Coma.

Symptoms of precipitating causes: *e.g.*, infection or gastrointestinal bleeding.

Signs

• Patients with impaired consciousness have intact pupillary reflexes.

Asterixis.

Fetor hepaticus.

Constructional apraxia: Reitan trail test.

Brisk tendon reflexes: except in coma.

Increased muscle tone and rigidity.

Hyperventilation in deep coma.

Signs of precipitating causes: *e.g.*, spontaneous bacterial peritonitis.

Investigations

• No single parameter confirms the diagnosis.

• The underlying liver disease or its complications must be identified.

• A precipitant cause must always be sought.

• A careful evaluation for infection is warranted including paracentesis if ascites is present.

Psychometric testing: essential to detect subclinical encephalopathy; number connection test (Reitan trail) and drawing a clock face easiest to perform.

EEG: slowing of normal frequency to severe slowing; characteristic triphasic waves; changes appearing first in frontal regions.

CT of head: to exclude subdural hematomas and other intracranial diseases; some atrophy of brain usually manifest, particularly in chronic encephalopathy.

Blood ammonia measurement: concentration usually raised, but false-positive and false-negative results may occur.

Complications

Increase in intracranial pressure: in patients with fulminant liver failure; due to cerebral edema, which can lead to brain death.

Complications of coma: *e.g.*, aspiration in patients with encephalopathy.

Structural neuronal damage: with demyelination and a spastic paraplegia, in patients with chronic encephalopathy (rare); chronic cerebellar or basal ganglia signs may also be present with Parkinsonian features.

Focal seizures: rare, other causes must be sought.

Differential diagnosis

Alcoholic brain damage.

Alcohol withdrawal syndrome.

Wernicke's encephalopathy.

Chronic subdural hematoma or other space-occupying lesion.

Other causes of metabolic coma.

Postictal state.

Meningitis, encephalitis.

Etiology

• Precipitant causes include the following:

Constipation.

Gastrointestinal bleeding (occult or apparent).

Infection.

Overdiuresis.

Hypovolemia.

Sedative and opiate drugs.

Diarrhea and vomiting.

Dietary indiscretion.

Protein excess.

Acute worsening of chronic liver disease.

Urea and electrolyte abnormalities.

Uncontrolled diabetes.

Hypoglycemia.

Surgery.

Epidemiology

• Chronic liver disease is usually progressive, so that most patients develop hepatic encephalopathy at some time, particularly secondary to a precipitant cause.

• Intermittent encephalopathy is the most common pattern.

• Subclinical or latent encephalopathy is present in most patients, but its clinical significance is unclear.

• Fulminant liver failure is a rare disorder that warrants immediate referral to a liver transplant center.

Classification

Grade 1: confusion, altered behavior, psychometric abnormalities.

Grade 2: drowsiness, altered behavior.

Grade 3: stupor, obedience to simple commands, great confusion.

Grade 4: coma responsive to painful stimuli.

Grade 5: coma unresponsive to painful stimuli.

Treatment

Diet and lifestyle

• Careful attention must be paid to adequate nutrition, and this should take priority over protein restriction which is required (*e.g.*, <30 g/day), only in a subset of patients with encephalopathy that is difficult to control pharmacologically.

• The possible manifestations of encephalopathy must be explained to patients and their families so that early medical opinion can be obtained.

Pharmacological treatment

• Encephalopathy typically resolves when the precipitating cause is corrected [2].

For acute encephalopathy in chronic liver disease

Lactose or sorbitol administered by nasogastric tube or enema.

Correction of electrolyte abnormalities.

Intravenous thiamine in alcoholics.

Long-term treatment

Standard dosage	Lactulose or sorbitol, 30 mL 4 times daily initially and titrated to produce two soft bowel movements daily.
Contraindications	Known hypersensitivity.
Special points	Demyelination, electrolyte abnormalities should be watched for.
Main drug interactions	None known.
Main side effects	Abdominal bloating, flatulence.

Encephalopathy of fulminant liver failure

Correction of hypoglycemia: 20% dextrose i.v.

Correction of electrolyte abnormalities.

Bowel decontamination: oral antibacterial agents.

Early treatment of infection.

Other options

Flumazenil, a benzodiazepine receptor antagonist, may temporarily reverse symptoms.

Treatment aims

To correct or remove precipitating cause.

To prevent recurrence.

Other treatments

Refashioning, embolization, or ligation of surgical shunt.

• Oral, nonabsorbable antibiotics (*e.g.*, neomycin) may be considered for patients refractory to treatment with lactulose or sorbitol.

Liver transplantation: for recurrent acute or chronic encephalopathy, and fulminant liver failure with adverse prognostic factors.

Prognosis

• Prognosis is determined by the underlying liver disease and avoidance of precipitating factors.

Follow-up and management

• Follow-up depends on the severity of the underlying liver disease, but clinic visits every 1–3 months are common; patients usually should keep a 3-monthly diary and stool chart.

Key references

1. Fraser CL: Hepatic encephalopathy. *N Engl J Med* 1985, **313**:865–873.
2. Butterworth RF: Pathogenesis and treatment of portal-systemic encephalopathy. *Dig Dis Sci* 1992, **37**:321–327.

Diagnosis

Symptoms

• Acute hepatitis is often asymptomatic.

Constitutional symptoms

Malaise, headache, myalgias, arthralgias, anorexia, nausea, right upper quadrant discomfort, and fevers.

Later symptoms

Jaundice, pruritis, acholic (pale) stools, dark urine.

Signs

• Signs may be absent.

Jaundice.

Tender hepatomegaly.

Splenomegaly: uncommon.

Stigmata of chronic liver disease: absent in uncomplicated acute hepatitis.

Fetor hepaticus, hepatic encephalopathy, or asterixis: signs of severe disease.

Vasculitis: rare.

Investigations

Biochemical assays: should confirm hepatitis, with elevated serum transaminases, mild increase in alkaline phosphatase, variable increase in bilirubin; as disease progresses, cholestatic picture may evolve before recovery.

Full blood count or blood film: not usually helpful; features consistent with hypersplenism, however, suggest underlying chronic liver disease.

Prothrombin time: If elevated, fulminant hepatic failure should be watched for; underlying chronic liver disease should be considered.

Virology tests: used with thought and precision on basis of probable cause, as follows:
Hepatitis A: check for IgM antibody (indicates acute infection; IgG antibody present for life and suggests previous infection) [1].
Hepatitis B: check for IgM anticore antibody (develops early in illness) and surface antigen (present in most symptomatic patients but may be eliminated quickly) [2].
Hepatitis C: antibody may take several months to convert, although most patients become positive within 3 months (viral assay using polymerase chain reaction is positive early) [3].
Hepatitis D: sought by detection of antibody; superinfection with hepatitis D virus in a chronic hepatitis B virus carrier (IgM anticore negative) may be differentiated from coinfection by hepatitis B (IgM anticore to hepatitis B positive).
Hepatitis E: can be sought by enzyme-linked immunosorbent assay (very rare) [4].
Cytomegalovirus and Epstein-Barr virus: should be sought when viral cause suspected and other serological tests negative.

Liver biopsy: may be indicated in rare circumstances when diagnostic confusion exists or when underlying liver damage is suspected.

Complications

Fulminant liver failure: in 1%–5% of cases.

Progression to chronic hepatitis: may occur with hepatitis B (~10%), hepatitis C (30%–50%).

Anemia.

Aplastic anemia, vasculitis, cryoglobulinemia: rarely, in cases of hepatitis B or C.

Differential diagnosis

Acute manifestation of chronic liver disease: *e.g.*, acute onset of autoimmune disease with rapid progression, Wilm's tumor.

Acute disease in a patient with underlying chronic liver disease: *e.g.*, episode of acute alcoholic liver damage.

Etiology and epidemiology

Hepatitis A virus: transmitted by fecal–oral route; infection associated with foreign travel, consumption of shellfish, and some sexual practices; often, no source identified.

Hepatitis B virus: often transmitted sexually; vertical transmission also important; i.v. drug users at risk; no identifiable risk factors in 50%.

Hepatitis C virus: associated with i.v. drug use and transfusion; less effectively transmitted vertically or sexually compared to hepatitis B; no identifiable risk factor in 50%.

Hepatitis D virus: hepatitis D transmitted predominantly by i.v. drug use, occurs only in patients with concomitant hepatitis B infection.

Hepatitis E virus: transmitted by fecal–oral route in developing countries (in epidemics, pregnant women most vulnerable).

Epstein–Barr virus.

Cytomegalovirus (particularly in immunosuppressed patients).

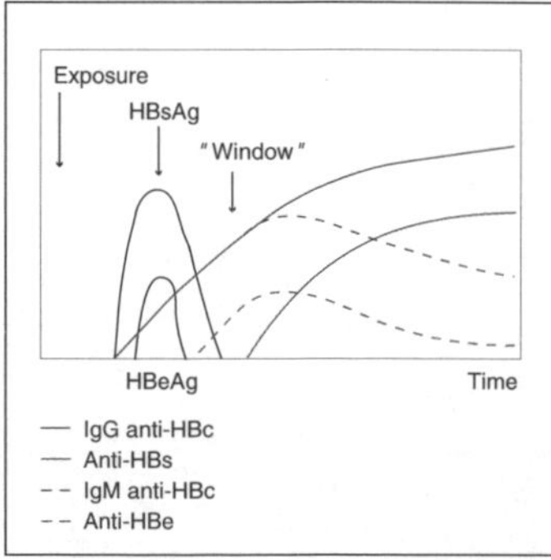

Serological diagnosis of acute hepatitis B (HB) infection. HBeAg, HBe antigen; HBsAg, HB surface antigen.

Treatment

Diet and lifestyle

• Abstinence from alcohol until recovery should be recommended.

• Rest is recommended; many patients are unable to return to work for weeks or months and, even after return, may need time before normal function fully returns.

• Patients must understand the routes by which the hepatitis infection has been acquired and may therefore be transmitted; this may place certain restrictions on professional or sexual activities in the short term.

Pharmacological treatment

• The onset of jaundice is often associated with loss or significant reduction of infectivity in patients with hepatitis A and B; no specific treatment is available for acute viral hepatitis.

• Symptomatic improvement may be obtained in patients with prolonged cholestasis using ursodeoxycholic acid, 600 mg at night.

• For hepatitis A virus, an effective vaccine is available for protective immunization; immunoglobulin has a well defined role in short-term prophylaxis and for household contacts of patients with acute hepatitis.

• For hepatitis B virus, an effective vaccine is available; vaccination soon after exposure may still be effective; hepatitis B immunoglobulin no longer has less of a role in this setting but is given with vaccination to infants born of mothers who are hepatitis B surface antigen–positive.

Treatment aims

To palliate symptoms.

To prevent infection.

To observe for progression to fulminant hepatic failure.

Prognosis

• Acute hepatitis is often a debilitating illness, but recovery is usual, although patients may experience fatigue for several months before full recovery.

• Over 40% of patients infected by hepatitis C virus and ~10% infected by hepatitis B become carriers; for the latter, chronic infection is less common after a severe, acute illness.

• The immediate prognosis for patients with hepatitis C who become carriers is excellent; chronic liver disease often develops, however.

Follow-up and management

• Patients with acute hepatitis A, B, or E should be followed until the liver function tests have returned to normal and the patient has made a full symptomatic recovery.

• Patients with hepatitis B should also be followed until hepatitis B surface antigen is eliminated; persistence of hepatitis Be antigen beyond 6 weeks suggests that a carrier state may be evolving.

• For hepatitis D, the prognosis depends ultimately on the outcome of the hepatitis B infection; a patient who remains hepatitis B surface antigen–positive may well develop chronic liver disease; follow-up should therefore be for life.

• In the present state of uncertainty about the prognosis of patients with hepatitis C, they should be followed every 6–12 months unless evidence for persistent hepatitis C is lacking, *i.e.*, disappearance of hepatitis C virus antibody or RNA.

Key references

1. Ross BL, *et al.*: Hepatitis A virus and hepatitis A infection. *Ad Virus Res* 1991, **39**:209–257.
2. Brown JL, *et al.*: The hepatitis B virus. *Baillières Clin Gastroenterol* 1990, **4**:721–747.
3. Bradley DW: Virology, molecular biology and serology of hepatitis C virus. *Transfus Med Rev* 1992, **6**:93–102.
4. Krawczynski K: Hepatitis E. *Hepatology* 1993, **17**:932–941.

Diagnosis

Symptoms

• Patients may present with symptoms of gastrointestinal bleeding from varices, encephalopathy, or ascites.

Malaise, anorexia: most common symptoms, although many patients are asymptomatic.

Signs

• Signs of advanced disease include the following:

Muscle wasting.
Palmar erythema, spider telangiectasias.
Jaundice: unusual in mild disease.
Testicular atrophy, gynecomastia: in men.
Ascites.
Caput medusae.
Splenomegaly.

Investigations

Liver function tests: show chronic hepatocellular disease; ALT and AST typically elevated to a greater degree than alkaline phosphatase; elevation in bilirubin variable.

Coagulation screening: impaired hepatic synthetic function causes prolonged prothrombin time and low albumin.

Full blood count: hypersplenism may result in leukopenia and thrombocytopenia.

Serum protein electrophoresis: loss of alpha spike in alpha-1 antitrypsin, immunoglobulins elevated in chronic liver disease but particularly prominent in autoimmune hepatitis (especially IgG).

Autoantibody analysis: antinuclear antibody, double-stranded DNA, and smooth-muscle antibody often positive in autoimmune disease.

Serum ferritin: elevated in hemochromatosis.

Hepatitis B serology: interpreted as follows:
Immune, postvaccination: sAb+, sAg–, cAb–, eAg–, eAb–, DNA–.
Immune, past exposure to hepatitis B virus: sAb+, sAg–, cAb+, eAg–, eAb+, DNA–.
Infected, carrier: sAb–, sAg+, cAb+, eAg–, eAb+, DNA–.
Infected, high risk of transmission: sAb–, sAg+, cAb+, eAg+, eAb–, DNA+.

Hepatitis C serology: interpreted as follows:
Positive, active disease: ELISA+, RIBA+ (2–4 bands), ALT increased, RNA+.
False-positive: ELISA+, RIBA– or indeterminate (1 band), ALT normal, RNA–.

Ceruloplasmin: decreased and 24-h urine copper increased in Wilson's disease.

Liver ultrasonography or CT: often normal but may show small liver with splenomegaly.

Liver biopsy for histology: shows the following:
Hepatitis B/D virus: inflammatory cells spreading into parenchyma from enlarged portal tracts; hepatitis B sAg on immunohistochemistry; hepatitis D infection increases severity and can be detected by immunohistochemistry.
Hepatitis C virus: usually mild chronic hepatitis with lobular component, prominent lymphoid follicles in portal tracts, acidophil body formation, focal hepatocellular necrosis; no immunohistochemical staining currently available.
Autoimmune disease: periportal inflammatory infiltrate and piecemeal necrosis; negative to hepatitis B/D staining on immunohistochemistry.

Complications

Cirrhosis: in 20%–50% of patients.

Variceal bleeding, PSE, ascites: due to portal hypertension.

Hepatocellular carcinoma: increased incidence in patients with cirrhosis.

Differential diagnosis

Primary biliary cirrhosis.
Primary sclerosing cholangitis.
Granulomatous hepatitis: multiple granulomata (on liver biopsy), sarcoid, tuberculosis, histoplasmosis, Q fever, brucella, lymphoma.
Alcoholic liver disease.
Hemochromatosis.

Etiology

• Causes include the following:

Viral infection: hepatitis B, C, or D (B/D in 20% of patients, C in 40%) [1].
Autoimmune disorder (in 20%).
Drugs: methyldopa, isoniazid, oxyphenisatin.
Genetic: Wilson's disease, alpha-1 antitrypsin deficiency.
Steatohepatitis

Definition

Hepatic dysfunction (*i.e.*, abnormal liver enzyme levels, often with progression to abnormal synthetic function) of at least six months' duration secondary to inflammation of the hepatic parenchyma.

Abbreviations

ALT	alanine aminotransferase
AST	aspartate aminotransferase
cAb	Hepatitis B core antibody
eAb	Hepatitis B e antibody
eAg	Hepatitis B e antigen
ELISA	enzyme-linked immunosorbent assay
PSE	portosystemic encephalopathy
RIBA	recombinant immunoblot assay
sAb	Hepatitis B surface antibody
sAg	Hepatitis B surface antigen

Treatment

Diet and lifestyle

• Alcohol must be avoided.

• Patients infected by hepatitis B virus should be advised on barrier methods of contraception unless the partner is vaccinated; sexual transmission of hepatitis C occurs, but at a much lower frequency.

Pharmacological treatment

• Treatment should be given under specialist supervision.

For hepatitis B virus infection

• Treatment is indicated for patients who have histological evidence of chronic hepatitis and are positive for hepatitis B e antigen or virus DNA.

• Meaningful remission can be achieved in 40%–50% of patients with hepatitis B virus.

Standard dosage Interferon-α, 10 MU s.c. three times a week for 4–6 months [2]. Alternative regimens also available.

Contraindications Hypersensitivity.

Main drug interactions None.

Main side effects *Induction:* low-grade fever, malaise, arthralgia, myalgia, headache, anorexia, nausea, vomiting, diarrhea.
Maintenance: fatigue, anorexia, weight loss, alopecia, depression, neutropenia, thrombocytopenia, exacerbation of autoimmune disease, induction of thyroid disease, myalgia.

• Steroid pretreatment may cause rebound immune stimulation; available data do not indicate that combination is superior to interferon alone.

For hepatitis C virus infection

• Treatment is indicated for patients with histological evidence of hepatitis or who are positive for recombinant immunoblot assay (2–4 bands) or virus RNA.

• Remission persists in only 25% of patients after treatment is stopped.

Standard dosage Interferon-α, 3 MU s.c. 3 times weekly for 4–12 months [3].

Contraindications hypersensitivity.

Main drug interactions None.

Main side effects As above.

For hepatitis D virus infection

• Patients may respond to interferon-α, but remission does not usually persist after treatment is discontinued.

For autoimmune disease

• Treatment is indicated for patients with raised transaminase and IgG, histological evidence of chronic hepatitis, and serologic test results consistent with autoimmune hepatitis (*e.g.*, ANA, SMA, LKM antibodies) [4].

Standard dosage Prednisone, 20–40 mg initially, reduced gradually (depending on clinical response); 5–10 mg daily maintenance dose may be needed.
Azathioprine, 50–70 mg orally daily as adjunct.

Contraindications Systemic infection; previous serious reaction to corticosteroids (*e.g.*, psychosis).

Main drug interactions None.

Main side effects *Steroids:* osteoporosis, proximal myopathy, skin thinning, cataracts, diabetes mellitus, weight gain, amenorrhea, depression, hypertension.
Azathioprine: pancreatitis, bone marrow suppression.

Vaccination

Hepatitis B: surface antigen suspension, 20 μg i.m. injection at 0, 1, and 6 months; surface antibody must be >100 IU after third dose to ensure adequate seroconversion (if inadequate, a fourth dose should be given).

Hepatitis C: no vaccine available.

Hepatitis D: protection provided by preventing hepatitis B infection.

Treatment aims

To induce remission and thus prevent progression to cirrhosis.

To eliminate active replication of viruses.

Other treatments

• Orthotopic liver transplantation is the treatment of choice for end-stage liver disease in chronic hepatitis [5].

• The 5-year survival rate is 50%–70%, depending on the cause; however, reinfection is frequent in patients with hepatitis B and is often accompanied by chronic liver disease.

Follow-up and management

• During interferon-α treatment, patients must be monitored closely for leukopenia and thrombocytopenia.

• Thyroid function must be checked because autoimmune disease can be exacerbated.

• Patients on long-term corticosteroid treatment should be monitored for steroid side effects and should have annual bone densitometry to check for osteoporosis.

• Patients who have progressed to cirrhosis are at risk of hepatocellular carcinoma; some investigators advocate surveillance with alpha fetoprotein and ultrasound evaluations every 6 months.

Key references

1. Scheuer PJ: Classification of chronic viral hepatitis: a need for reassessment. *J Hepatol* 1991, **13**:372–374.
2. Perillo RP: Interferon in the management of chronic hepatitis B. *Dig Dis Sci* 1993, **38**:577–593.
3. Davis GL, *et al.*: Treatment of chronic hepatitis C with recombinant interferon alpha. *N Engl J Med* 1989, **321**:1501–1506.
4. Johnson RL, *et al.*: The natural course and heterogeneity of autoimmune chronic active hepatitis. *Semin Liver Dis* 1991, **11**:187–196.
5. Lake JR, Wright TL: Liver transplantation for patients with hepatitis B: what have we learned from our results? *Hepatology* 1992, **13**:796–799.

Hepatocellular carcinoma

Diagnosis

Symptoms

• Small hepatocellular carcinomas (<2 cm diameter) are usually asymptomatic; symptoms have insidious onset and usually consist of the following:

Upper abdominal pain: right hypochondrial or epigastric.

Weight loss, weakness, anorexia.

Abdominal swelling: may be due to ascites or enlarged liver.

Low-grade pyrexia.

Features of cirrhosis.

Metastatic symptoms: *e.g.*, bone pain.

Signs

• The liver is typically enlarged and tender.

Arterial bruit: heard in 20% of patients.

Ascites.

Splenomegaly: in 20–30%.

Wasting: with more advanced disease.

Jaundice: in later stages of illness.

Stigmata of chronic liver disease.

Investigations

Biochemistry: elevation of alkaline phosphatase common; aspartate aminotransferase and alanine aminotransferase elevations often mild.

Hematology: may show evidence of pancytopenia (hypersplenism) or erythrocytosis.

Alpha-fetoprotein: combined with ultrasonography for early detection; alpha fetoprotein possibly normal in small hepatocellular carcinoma.

Chest radiography: may show raised right hemidiaphragm or metastases.

CT: useful to stage tumor.

Ultrasonography: may be useful for screening patients with cirrhosis for small hepatocellular carcinoma; 1-cm lesions can be detected, often as hypoechoic lesions.

Celiac axis angiography: tumors usually hypervascular; useful for staging disease that does not appear confined or in distinguishing benign nodules from malignant lesions.

Lipiodol CT: sensitive method for detecting small hepatocellular carcinoma; lipiodol, an oil contrast medium, cleared by hepatocytes but not by hepatocellular carcinoma; CT done 2 weeks after intra-arterial injection.

Liver biopsy: directed biopsy usually indicated; aspiration biopsy can be performed but is less diagnostic.

Complications

Acute intraperitoneal hemorrhage: often the terminal event.

Intravascular and intraductal growth.

Portal vein, inferior vena cava, and right atrial involvement.

Metastases: lung, bone, skin, brain, adrenal, and lymphogenous.

Hypoglycemia, hypercalcemia, polycythemia, hyperlipidemia.

Hepatic failure.

Variceal bleeding.

Differential diagnosis

Cystic lesions, hepatic metastatic carcinoma from other sites, abscess, adenoma, focal nodular hyperplasia.

Benign hemangioma.

Etiology

• Most cases of hepatocellular carcinoma develop in the setting of cirrhosis, including disease caused by the following [1]:

Chronic hepatitis B or C virus infection.

Alcoholic liver disease.

Autoimmune hepatitis or primary biliary cirrhosis.

Hemochromatosis.

Other inherited disorders of metabolism.

Tyrosinosis, alpha-1-antitrypsin deficiency.

Environmental carcinogens: aflatoxin is a potent chemical carcinogen, produced by *Aspergillus flavus*, which contaminates food in high-incidence areas; genetic changes have been documented.

Membranous inferior vena cava obstruction.

Androgenic anabolic steroids.

Contraceptives (controversial).

Epidemiology

• Areas of high, intermediate, and low incidence correspond crudely to prevalence of hepatitis B and C infection; low-incidence areas include northern Europe and North America.

• Hepatocellular carcinoma is more frequent in immigrants from high- and intermediate-prevalence countries (sub-Saharan Africa, China, southern and eastern Europe, Middle East).

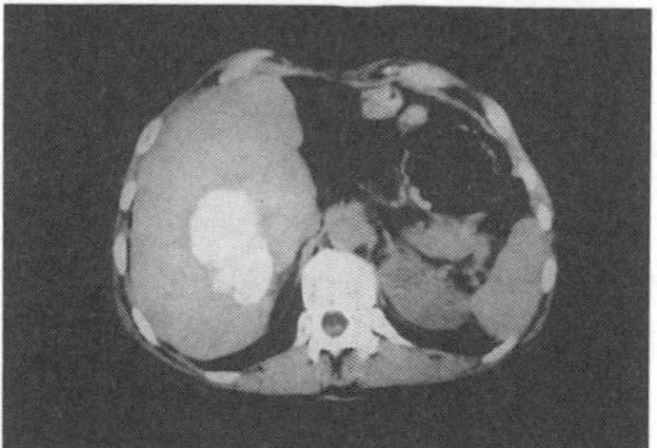

Retention of lipiodol within a hepatocellular carcinoma.

Treatment

Diet and lifestyle

• No special precautions are necessary.

Surgical treatment

• Surgical management is reserved for lesions that are confined to the liver and that do not involve the hepatic capsule [2].

• In patients who are candidates for surgery, liver transplantation may be required for those with chronic liver disease who would not tolerate partial hepatic resection [3].

Pharmacological treatment

Chemotherapy for palliation

• Treatment should be given under specialist supervision.

Standard dosage	Doxorubicin, epirubicin, cisplatin, mitoxantrone every 3–4 weeks.
Contraindications	*All:* hypersensitivity. *Doxorubicin:* bone-marrow suppression, buccal ulcerations (after first dose). *Cisplatin:* pre-existing renal impairment, hearing disorders, bone-marrow suppression.
Special points	Other adjunctive agents, *e.g.*, tamoxifen, interferon, and interleukin 2, may be used. *Doxorubicin:* ECG, ejection fraction, and echocardiogram must be monitored. *Cisplatin:* hydration must be maintained; blood count, serum creatinine, and blood-urea-nitrogen must be monitored; audiometry needed.
Main drug interactions	*Cisplatin:* use with aminoglycoside or cephalosporins may cause increased ototoxicity or nephrotoxicity.
Main side effects	*Doxorubicin:* mucositis, bone-marrow suppression, alopecia, nausea, vomiting, diarrhea, cardiotoxicity. *Cisplatin:* nephrotoxicity, myelosuppression, neurotoxicity, ototoxicity, immunosuppression, nausea, vomiting. *Mitoxantrone:* leukopenia, thrombocytopenia, anemia, nausea, vomiting, alopecia, diarrhea, mucositis, cardiovascular effects (rare), blue-green discoloration of urine.

Treatment aims

To cure disease or prolong survival without recurrence.

To alleviate symptoms.

Other treatments

Transcatheter arterial embolization: for unresectable carcinoma, not for portal-vein thrombosis or Child's C cirrhosis; side effects include abdominal pain and fever; can be used with lipiodol-targeted chemotherapy.

• Target injection of tumor using alcohol or lipiodol (*e.g.*, alcohol, 10–20 mL intratumoral injection 3 times weekly for twelve treatments) may be palliative.

Prognosis

• <25% of patients have partial responses to current chemotherapeutic regimens.

• 60% 5-year survival rates have been reported after intratumoral injection of alcohol for small tumors, but injection is without benefit in other series.

• 1-year survival rates as high as 78% after transcatheter arterial embolization have been reported.

• The 5-year survival rate after surgery is 25%; patients with encapsulated tumors, negative resection margins, no intracapsular or intravascular invasion of tumor cells, and Child's class A have better prognosis for surgical management [4].

Follow-up and management

• Serial imaging of the liver, lung, and bones is suggested to detect recurrence.

• Serial alpha-fetoprotein concentrations should be measured if initially high.

Key references

1. Simonetti RG, *et al.*: Hepatocellular carcinoma: a worldwide problem and the major risk factors. *Dig Dis Sci* 1991, **36**:962–972.
2. Dusheiko GM, *et al.*: Treatment of small hepatocellular carcinomas. *Lancet* 1992, **340**:285–288.
3. Di Bisceglie AM, *et al.*: Hepatocellular carcinoma. *Ann Intern Med* 1988, **108**:390–401.
4. Okuda K: Hepatocellular carcinoma: recent progress. *Hepatology* 1992, **15**:948–963.

Diagnosis

Symptoms

Pain, burning, itching, tingling lasting 6–12 h, vesicles (generally ulcerating or crusting within 48 h): recurrent orolabial herpes (cold sores).
Fever, malaise, headache, altered personality, confusion, convulsions, paresis, paralysis, or coma: herpes encephalitis.
Fever, malaise, headache, nausea, vomiting, photophobia, neck stiffness: herpes meningitis.
Pain, photophobia, edema of the eyelid, lacrimation, blurring of vision: ocular herpes (spectrum ranges from superficial infections to stromal keratitis and iridocyclitis affecting inner eye).
Fever, sore mouth, swelling of gums, vesicles, ulceration in anterior half of mouth, tender anterior cervical lymph nodes: primary gingivostomatitis (frequently asymptomatic).
Pain, burning, itching, tingling, vesicles followed by ulcers and crusts in perineum, vaginal discharge, dyspareunia: genital herpes; symptoms vary in severity, extent, and duration, depending on whether the infection is primary (usually most severe) or recurrent; may be asymptomatic.
Vesicles, ulcers, crusts, malaise, fever, lymphadenopathy: eczema herpeticum.
Pruritis, severe localized pain, vesicles, ulcers, crusts, fever, lymphadenopathy: other cutaneous herpes infections (herpes whitlow or gladiatorum, herpetic nipple).

Signs

Erythema progressing to vesicles, ulcers, and crusts: cutaneous lesions.
Altered personality, fluctuating levels of consciousness, focal or generalized convulsions, focal neurological findings, drowsiness, stupor, coma: herpes encephalitis.
Neck stiffness, positive Kernig's test: herpes meningitis.
Small blister or predendritic ulcers on cornea: ocular herpes; dendritic ulcers have serpentine branching appearance on fluoroscopy after fluorescein instillation.

Investigations

Cutaneous lesions

• Laboratory tests are usually not needed because symptoms and signs are diagnostic.

Tzanck test: may show multinucleated giant cells.
Immunofluorescence: can show viral antigens in cell smears.
Virus culture: from vesicle fluid or ulcers.

Herpes encephalitis

CT, MRI, EEG: show temporal lobe localization; EEG shows temporal spike and slow wave activity in 80% of patients.
CSF analysis: shows pleocytosis, usually 50–500 cells/mm^3, with lymphocyte predominance; erythrocytes often present, specimen may be xanthochromic; protein or red erythrocyte count may be raised, sugar usually normal; CSF can be examined for virus DNA (polymerase chain reaction) or viral antigens (immunology), but treatment should not await results.

Herpes meningitis

Lumbar puncture: to show CSF abnormalities of aseptic meningitis; herpes meningitis assumed when findings accompany mucocutaneous herpes, usually primary genital.
EEG: localized abnormalities in temporal lobe.

Ocular herpes

Ophthalmic examination and fluorescein: show presence of dendritic ulceration.
Abrasion of corneal cells: shows viral antigens; can be used for virus isolation.

Complications

Erythema multiforme, aseptic meningitis, urethritis, urinary retention, myelitis: due to mucocutaneous herpes.
Death, severe neurological sequelae: due to herpes encephalitis.
Visual loss, rupture of the globe (rare): due to recurrent ocular herpes.

Differential diagnosis

Mucocutaneous lesions
Causes of gingivitis and stomatitis.
Aphthous ulceration.
Coxsackievirus infection (hand, foot, and mouth).
Behçets syndrome.
Inflammatory bowel disease.
Varicella–zoster virus.
Sexually transmitted disease.

Herpes encephalitis
Other encephalitides.
Space-occupying lesions (*e.g.*, abscess, tumor, tuberculoma).

Herpes meningitis
Other causes of meningitis (*e.g.*, viruses, bacteria, fungi).

Ocular herpes
Ocular infections.

Etiology

Herpes simplex virus types 1 and 2: enveloped DNA viruses.
Exposure to strong sunlight, ultraviolet light, pneumonia, meningitis and malaria: cause reactivation (cold sores).
Fever, stressful events, depression, menstruation, sexual activity: causes of recurrences of genital herpes.
Immunosuppression: cause of mucocutaneous herpes.
Inoculation of virus into a finger or direct contact: cause of herpetic whitlow and herpes gladiatorum.
Bites and other traumatic forms of viral inoculation (*e.g.*, from needles, razors, contaminated finger nails): causes of herpetic nipple.

Epidemiology

• Seroepidemiological studies show that 30%–50% of patients in higher socioeconomic groups and 100% of those in lower groups are infected with herpes simplex virus 1 by puberty.
• The prevalence of antibodies to herpes simplex virus 2 varies from 3% in nuns to ~70% in prostitutes.
• The prevalence of herpes encephalitis is 0.1–0.4 in 100 000 people.

Treatment

Diet and lifestyle

- Parents or grandparents with cold sores should not kiss young children.
- Laboratory tests have shown latex condoms to be effective mechanical barriers to herpes simplex virus.

Pharmacological treatment

- Acyclovir is of proven clinical value in some infections.
- It is not recommended for orolabial herpes or treatment of recurrent genital herpes.
- No other licensed compound has the combined safety and efficacy of acyclovir.
- Famcyclovir is now available and quite effective.

Standard dosage
For initial genital herpes: acyclovir, 200 mg 5 times daily for 10 days.
For recurrent genital herpes (prophylaxis): acyclovir, 400–800 mg daily in 2–4 divided doses (continuous suppressive therapy).
For mucocutaneous herpes in immunocompromised patients: acyclovir, i.v. or oral.
For herpes encephalitis: acyclovir, 10 mg/kg i.v. 3 times daily for 10 days.
For ocular herpes simplex: acyclovir, 400 mg 5 times daily, more effective than 3% ointment.

Contraindications
Hypersensitivity.

Special points
Limited experience in pregnancy and lactation so should be used only when potential benefits outweigh risks
Bioavailability of drug possibly reduced in patients being treated for malignancy so i.v. route advised.

Main drug interactions
Probenecid increases acyclovir half-life.
No detrimental interactions recognized.

Main side effects
Raised urea and creatinine concentrations due to deposition of acyclovir crystals in tubules after rapid bolus doses, occasional nausea and vomiting, inflammation and ulceration at site of infusion if extravasation of drug occurs.

Treatment aims

To accelerate healing.

To reduce virus replication and dissemination.

To prevent recurrence, death and neurological complications, and blindness.

Prognosis

- Treatment of mucocutaneous herpes results in accelerated healing and reduced viral shedding.
- Treatment of herpes encephalitis results in reduced mortality and morbidity, especially in young patients with high Glasgow Coma Scale scores who are treated early.
- Treatment of ocular herpes has varying outcomes, depending on previous inflammation and scarring.
- Prophylactic treatment reduces the incidence and severity of recurrences in patients with recurrent genital herpes and viral shedding in immunocompromised patients.

Follow-up and management

- Pregnant women should inform their obstetrician of a past history of genital herpes.

General reference

Prober CG, *et al.*: The management of pregnancies complicated by genital infections with herpes simplex virus. *Clin Infect Dis* 1992, **15**:1031–1038.

Herpes zoster and varicella

Diagnosis

Symptoms

Chickenpox (varicella)

Fever and malaise: in prodromal phase, variable.

Headache, myalgia.

Vesicular rash: frequently itchy.

Shingles (herpes zoster)

Pain in affected dermatome: may precede rash by a few days.

Mental confusion, depression: common in elderly patients.

• Symptoms often continue for weeks or months.

Signs

Chickenpox

Vesicular rash: maximal on face and trunk; rapidly evolving from macules and papules to vesicles and crusts; crops of new vesicles continuing to appear for 3–4 days; drying up in 7–10 days; possibly involving conjunctivae, oropharynx, vulva, vagina; larger lesions and slow evolution suggest underlying immune deficiency.

Shingles

Unilateral, segmental skin rash: lesions similar to chickenpox but often confluent; possibly ulcerating; often a few scattered lesions elsewhere; severe multiple dermatome or recurrent disease suggests underlying immune deficiency, including HIV infection.

Investigations

• Virological investigations are needed only when the clinical diagnosis is uncertain.

Tzanck smear: of material from vesicular skin lesions for rapid confirmation of herpes virus infection.

Tissue culture: to distinguish varicella-zoster virus from herpes simplex virus.

Complications

Chickenpox

Secondary bacterial infection of skin: usually *Staphylococcus aureus* or *Streptococcus pyogenes*.

Chickenpox pneumonia: particularly in adults and pregnant women.

Systemic spread: to liver, brain, lung of immunocompromised patients.

Hemorrhagic rash: in immunocompromised patients.

Encephalitis, polyneuritis, transverse myelitis: rare.

Reye's syndrome: in children, rare.

Hemolytic anemia, coagulopathy with hemorrhagic rash: rare.

Shingles

Uveitis, keratitis: in patients with ophthalmic herpes zoster.

Lower motor neuron paralysis.

Ramsey Hunt syndrome: herpes zoster of geniculate ganglion, with facial palsy, loss of taste, ipsilateal oral ulcers and skin lesions in pinna of ear.

Bowel and bladder dysfunction: in patients with sacral herpes zoster infection.

Encephalitis: rare.

Cerebral vasculopathy: trigeminal herpes zoster virus infection, with delayed cerebral infarction and hemiplegia; rare.

Differential diagnosis

Herpes simplex virus.

Other vesicular rashes, especially erythema multiforme.

Etiology

• Chickenpox is caused by direct contact or airborne transmission of varicella–zoster virus from either chickenpox or shingles.

• After primary infection, the virus probably incorporates its DNA into the satellite cells of dorsal-root or cranial-nerve ganglion cells.

• Later reactivation causes shingles.

Epidemiology

•2% of cases of chickenpox but 25% of deaths due to the disease occur in people aged >20 years.

• The prevalence of shingles rises steadily with age, 1 in 100 people >80 years being affected.

• Shingles in infants and young children probably is caused by a reactivation of intrauterine infection.

• Both chickenpox and shingles are cross-infection hazards in hospitals.

Infection in pregnancy

• Chickenpox in pregnant women may be severe and complicated by varicella pneumonia; patients should be monitored closely.

• Intrauterine infection may damage the fetus and cause limb scarring and hypoplasia, microcephaly or hydrocephalus, and eye abnormalities.

• This fetal varicella syndrome has an incidence of 1%–3% in the first trimester (much lower risk in subsequent trimesters).

• Termination of pregnancy on the grounds of maternal chickenpox is not indicated, because the risk to the fetus is small and unpredictable.

• Maternal herpes zoster infection is not a risk to the fetus.

Infectivity

Incubation period (chickenpox): 17 days.

Infectivity: from 2 days before onset of rash until lesions have dried.

Increased infectivity and susceptibility with immunodeficiency or immunosuppression.

Treatment

Diet and lifestyle

• Patients should avoid contact with susceptible individuals (*e.g.*, immunocompromised) until their skin lesions have dried.

Pharmacological treatment

Acyclovir

• Acyclovir is a highly selective antiviral agent that inhibits viral DNA polymerase and causes premature DNA chain termination.

Standard dosage — *For chickenpox and shingles in immunocompromised patients, chickenpox pneumonia:* acyclovir, 10 mg/kg i.v. 8-hourly.
For cutaneous shingles: acyclovir, 800 mg orally 5 times daily for 7 days (started within 72 h of rash onset).
For ophthalmic shingles: acyclovir orally as above for 10 days.
For severe maternal or neonatal chickenpox: acyclovir i.v.

Contraindications — Hypersensitivity.

Special points — High cost; no effect on latency or recurrence; not licensed for uncomplicated chickenpox.

Main drug interactions — Extreme lethargy has been reported on administration of zidovudine with i.v. acyclovir.

Main side effects — Rashes and gastrointestinal disturbances (occasionally), alterations in biochemical and hematological indices (more rarely), headaches and neurological reactions, particularly with i.v. administration, some risk of crystalluria and renal impairment at high dose (maximum oral dose in renal failure, 800 mg 3 times daily).

Varicella–zoster immune globulin

• This is distributed by the Public Health Laboratory Service (in short supply).

• It is used for highly susceptible contacts of chickenpox or shingles, including the following:

Bone-marrow transplant recipients (despite history of previous chickenpox).
Patients with debilitating disease (despite history of previous chickenpox).
HIV-positive patients with symptoms but no known varicella–zoster virus antibody.
Pregnant women without antibody (patients without a definite history of previous chickenpox must be screened for antibody).
Immunosuppressed patients who have been treated by high-dose steroids within the 3 months before contact (screened first).
Neonates up to 4 weeks old whose mothers develop chickenpox between 1 week before and 1 month after delivery or those in contact with chickenpox or shingles whose mothers have no history of previous varicella–zoster infection or no antibody.
Premature babies <30 weeks gestation or weighing <1 kg at birth in contact with chickenpox.

Standard dosage — Varicella–zoster immune globulin, depending on age: *0–5 years,* 250 mg; *6–10 years,* 500 mg; *11–14 years,* 750 mg; *≥15 years,* 1000 mg.

Contraindications — Hypersensitivity to human immunoglobulin.

Special points — Must be given as soon as possible and not more than 10 days after exposure.

Main drug interactions — None.

Main side effects — Hypersensitivity reactions (rare).

• Live attenuated varicella vaccine is available, on a named-patient basis, for immunocompromised patients, especially children with leukemia.

Treatment aims

Chickenpox

To relieve symptoms in previously healthy patients.

To contain infection and reduce morbidity and mortality in immunocompromised patients or those with chickenpox pneumonia or maternal or neonatal infection.

Shingles

To accelerate healing and curtail pain.

To prevent complications in patients with ophthalmic herpes zoster.

To prevent progressive disease in immunocompromised patients.

Prognosis

• Mortality from chickenpox is increased in patients aged >20 years.

• Morbidity and mortality are reduced by acyclovir treatment in immunocompromised patients.

Follow-up and management

• Patients must be monitored for the development of complications.

• Pain continuing at the site of herpes zoster infection 30 days or more after an acute attack indicates postherpetic neuralgia, which should be treated by amitriptyline or sodium valproate. *See* Neuralgia, postherpetic *for details.*

General references

Anonymous: Acyclovir in general practice. *Drug Ther Bull* 1992, **30**:101–104.

Anonymous: Varicella/herpes zoster. In *Immunisation Against Infectious Diseases.* London: HMSO; 1992.

Bowsher D: Neurogenic pain syndromes and their management. *Br Med Bull* 1991, **47**:644–666.

Gilbert GL: Chickenpox during pregnancy. *BMJ* 1993, **306**:1079–1080.

Wallace MR, *et al.*: Treatment of adult varicella with oral acyclovir. A randomized, placebo-controlled trial. *Ann Intern Med* 1992, **117**:358–363.

Diagnosis

Symptoms

- The usual presentation is a lymph-node mass noticed by the patient.
- Fluctuation in size is not unusual.
- ~25% of patients have other symptoms.

"B" symptoms: unexplained fever >38°C, loss of >10% body weight in 6 months, night sweats.

Pruritis: may lead to extensive excoriation from scratching.

Alcohol-induced nodal pain: rare and nonspecific.

Anorexia, lethargy.

Signs

Palpable lymphadenopathy: usually; careful examination of all node-bearing areas essential.

Extranodal involvement: *e.g.*, bone-marrow, liver, CNS; in 10%–20% of patients.

Investigations

- Initially, a good biopsy specimen must be carefully examined to make the diagnosis. Reed–Sternberg cells are the hallmark of Hodgkin's disease and the putative malignant cell.
- Investigation is then systematic to "stage" the disease.

Full blood count: possible neutrophilia, eosinophilia, lymphopenia, leukoerythroblastic picture if bone-marrow is involved.

ESR measurement: rate sometimes raised; can be useful disease marker and prognostic feature.

Liver function tests: abnormalities raise possibility of liver involvement.

Lactate dehydrogenase measurement: useful disease marker and prognostic feature.

Chest radiography: to look for nodal and pulmonary disease.

CT of chest and abdomen: to detect nodes; poor at detecting hepatic and splenic disease.

Lymphangiography: in centers with expertise, better than CT for assessing retroperitoneal nodes.

Bone-marrow examination: with trephine; rarely reveals unsuspected bone-marrow involvement.

Staging laparotomy: controversial now; in theory, might detect unsuspected splenic disease and change treatment plan.

Complications

Infection related to underlying defect in cell-mediated immunity: herpes zoster seen in 20%, and tuberculosis not unusual.

Differential diagnosis

Non-Hodgkin's lymphoma.

Infections, *e.g.*, Epstein-Barr virus, toxoplasma, cytomegalovirus.

Angioimmunoblastic lymphadenopathy.

Etiology [1]

- The origin of the Reed–Sternberg cell, the putative malignant cell, is still debated; cell surface marker CD15 is usually expressed; T- or B-lymphocyte markers are also sometimes expressed.
- Recent evidence implicates Epstein–Barr virus (EBV) in the cause of some cases of Hodgkin's disease; the EBV genome has been found incorporated into DNA in Reed–Sternberg cells, and serological evidence links EBV with Hodgkin's disease.

Epidemiology [1]

- Hodgkin's disease has a bimodal distribution, with a first peak at 15–40 years, then increasing incidence with increasing age.
- Male patients are more frequently affected than female patients.
- The incidence is higher in whites.

Classification

Based on the Rye system:

1. Nodular sclerosing (>80% of patients): dense bands of collagen with nodules of tumor.
2. Lymphocyte predominant: infiltrate of small lymphocytes.
3. Mixed cellularity: pleomorphic infiltrate.
4. Lymphocyte depleted: few Reed–Sternberg cells seen.

Staging

- Hodgkin's disease appears to start unifocally and to spread to adjacent lymph nodes in an orderly fashion. Staging (based on the Ann Arbor Scheme) is important for rational planning of treatment.

Stage I: involvement of single lymph-node region.

Stage II: two or more lymph-node regions on same side of diaphragm.

Stage III: lymph-node involvement on both sides of diaphragm, including spleen.

Stage IV: diffuse involvement of extranodal sites.

Suffix A: no systemic symptoms.

Suffix B: "B" symptoms as described earlier.

Treatment

Diet and lifestyle

• Some patients continue a normal lifestyle during chemotherapy; others feel quite unwell.

Pharmacological treatment

• Hodgkin's disease is a chemo- and radiosensitive disease.

• Treatment decision depends on accurate staging and should also take into account current clinical trials.

Radiotherapy [2]

• Patients with stage I and IIA disease and no other adverse prognostic features can be cured by radiotherapy alone.

• This is usually given to an extended field beyond the area of overt nodal disease over 1 month.

• Initial treatment with combined chemo- and radiotherapy provides no survival advantage in early-stage disease and may lead to increased toxicity.

Chemotherapy [3]

• For more advanced disease, several standard four-drug combinations are used, *e.g.*, MOPP (mechlorethamine, vincristine, procarbazine, prednisone), LOPP (chlorambucil, vincristine, procarbazine, prednisone), ABVD (doxorubicin, bleomycin, vinblastine, dacarbazine), or EVAP (etoposide, vincristine, doxorubicin, prednisone).

• Precise details of treatment should always be decided by an experienced hematologist or oncologist.

• Good intravenous access is needed because some drugs, particularly vinca alkaloids and anthracyclines, are vesicant.

• Admission to the hospital is not usually required for treatment, although treatment should commence as soon as practical after initial diagnosis and staging.

Treatment after relapse

• Relapse after initial treatment may still be compatible with long-term survival.

• Patients who relapse after radiotherapy can be "salvaged" with chemotherapy with similar overall survival to those who were initially treated with both modalities; the converse is rarely true.

• The longer the duration of first remission, the greater is the chance of obtaining a second remission on standard treatment.

• Increasing dose intensity of treatment is of benefit in Hodgkin's disease; ~50% of patients resistant to standard treatment can still achieve long-term survival with high dose chemotherapy regimens such as BEAM (BCNU [carmustine], etoposide, cytarabine, melphalan) and autologous hematopoietic stem cell support [4].

Complications of treatment

Skin reactions and pneumonitis after radiotherapy.

Myelosuppression, emesis, hair loss, and neurotoxicity after chemotherapy.

Second malignancy: lung cancer; acute myeloid leukemia (~ 1%), peak incidence 4–11 years after initial treatment.

Impaired fertility after chemotherapy.

Pulmonary fibrosis.

Treatment aims

To cure the disease with minimal toxicity from the treatment.

Prognosis

• The overall survival at 10 years is ~60%.

• Poor prognostic features include the following:

Older age.

Presence of B symptoms.

Mixed cellularity/lymphocyte-depleted histology.

Stage III or IV disease at presentation.

ESR >40 mm/h.

Lactic dehydrogenase >normal.

Mass >10 cm.

Failure to obtain complete remission after adequate first-line treatment.

Follow-up and management

• Regular review during treatment is essential to detect complications and assess response.

• Full blood count is mandatory before administration of each cycle of treatment.

• After treatment is finished, full restaging is needed.

• Follow-up interval may gradually lengthen but should be continued indefinitely to detect late complications of treatment or relapse.

Key references

1. Collins RH Jr: The pathogenesis of Hodgkin's disease. *Blood Rev* 1990, **4**:61–68.
2. Horwich A: The management of early Hodgkin's disease. *Blood Rev* 1990, **4**:181–186.
3. DeVita VT Jr, Hubbard SM: Drug treatment: Hodgkin's disease. *N Engl J Med* 1993, **328**:560–565.
4. Linch DC, *et al.*: Dose intensification with autologous bone marrow transplantation in relapsed and resistant Hodgkin's disease: results of a BNLI randomised trial. *Lancet* 1993, **341**:1051–1054.

Diagnosis

Symptoms

• Hypercalcemia causes either no symptoms or nonspecific symptoms, *e.g.*, the following:

Tiredness and lethargy.

Nausea and vomiting.

Constipation.

Polydipsia and polyuria.

Muscle weakness.

Impaired mental function and occasional loss of consciousness: in severe cases.

Signs

• Specific signs of hypercalcemia are rare.

Corneal and soft-tissue calcification.

Signs of dehydration: caused by moderate to severe hypercalcemia.

Investigations

Serum calcium measurement: total serum calcium influenced by serum protein concentration, especially albumin.

Parathyroid hormone measurement: high concentration indicates probable hyperparathyroidism.

Tests for anemia, liver function tests, alkaline phosphatase and ESR measurement: malignancy more probable if concentrations are abnormal or raised.

Chest and skeletal radiography: indicated if malignancy probable.

• Specific investigations of other causes of hypercalcemia are indicated when the more common causes have been excluded.

Complications [1]

Dehydration: common and, unless corrected, causes worsening of hypercalcemia.

Kidney stones: may complicate hyperparathyroidism.

Bone pain: common in malignancy, rare in hyperparathyroidism.

Pancreatitis: rare complication of chronic hypercalcemia.

Differential diagnosis

Not applicable.

Etiology

• 97% of cases of hypercalcemia in general medical practice are due either to primary hyperparathyroidism or to malignancy, which is usually disseminated.

• Other causes include the following:

Severe thyrotoxicosis.

Vitamin D excess.

Vitamin A excess.

Calcium treatment to bind phosphate in chronic renal failure.

Sarcoidosis.

Familial benign or hypocalciuric hypercalcemia.

Diuretic phase of acute renal failure.

Milk-alkali syndrome.

Addison's disease.

Epidemiology

• Primary hyperparathyroidism increases markedly after middle age and is three times more common in women than in men.

• Hyperparathyroidism may be a feature of multiple endocrine neoplasia type I or II.

• Many malignancies can be complicated by hypercalcemia.

• Sarcoidosis is complicated by hypercalcemia in <1% of patients.

Treatment

Diet and lifestyle

• A low-calcium diet is of no value in treating hypercalcemia, although high calcium intake exacerbates the disorder.

• Patients with hyperparathyroidism treated conservatively should be advised to maintain an adequate fluid intake, especially when they are unwell.

Pharmacological treatment [2]

For hyperparathyroidism [3]

• The only effective treatment of primary hyperparathyroidism is surgical.

For malignancy [3]

• Intravenous rehydration is mandatory.

• The bisphosphonate drugs are the initial treatment of choice for severe hypercalcemia.

Standard dosage	*For severe hypercalcemia:* pamidronate, 60–90 mg i.v. by continuous infusion. *For mild hypercalcemia:* etidronate, 5–10 mg daily.
Contraindications	Caution in renal failure.
Special points	Serum calcium falls to or towards normal within 3–5 days. Oral bisphosphonates must be taken on an empty stomach; they are much less effective than i.v. preparations. Newer, more potent and effective oral biphosphonates are now becoming available, *e.g.*, alendronate.
Main drug interactions	Absorption of oral drug reduced by antacids, iron, and calcium.
Main side effects	Gastrointestinal upset.

For sarcoidosis

• Hypercalcemia responds rapidly to steroids.

Standard dosage	Prednisone, 20 mg daily, reduced to lowest dose that controls hypercalcemia.
Contraindications	Systemic infections; caution in peptic ulceration or diabetes.
Main drug interactions	None.
Main side effects	Cushingoid appearance (with maintained high doses), dyspepsia.

Adjunctive therapy

• Calcitonin may be used early as an adjunct to treat hypercalcemia.

Standard dosage	Calcitonin, 4 IU/kg s.c. or i.m. every 12 h; dose may be increased to 8 IU/kg every 12 or every 6 h if necessary.
Contraindications	Allergy to synthetic salmon calcitonin.
Main drug interactions	Effective within 12 h but effectiveness greatly diminished by 72–96 h.
Main side effects	Hypocalcemia.

Nonpharmacological treatment

For hyperparathyroidism

• Surgery should be reserved for all younger patients and those with complications of the disease (*e.g.*, renal stones).

• Elderly asymptomatic patients can be followed conservatively [4].

• Surgery must be done by an experienced parathyroid surgeon.

• After successful surgery, serum calcium is usually normal within 24 h.

• Transient hypocalcemia may occur; rarely, permanent hypoparathyroidism may follow.

For malignancy

• Surgical cure is rare because the disease is usually disseminated.

Treatment aims

Hyperparathyroidism

To cure disease by surgery.

To monitor asymptomatic patients.

Malignancy

To alleviate symptoms.

Prognosis

Hyperparathyroidism

• Effective surgical treatment of hyperparathyroidism is associated with a normal life expectancy.

• After a patient has been cured, a recurrence of hypercalcemia is unusual, except when hyperplastic glands are present.

• In hypercalcemia of malignancy, unless curative chemotherapy can be offered, the prognosis is poor, most patients dying within 6 months.

Malignancy

• Hypercalcemia frequently recurs unless the malignancy is well controlled.

Follow-up and management

• Follow-up of the malignant disease is essential, to check for recurrence of hypercalcemia if the malignancy has not been cured.

Key references

1. Larsson K, *et al.*: The risk of hip fractures in patients with primary hyperparathyroidism: a population based cohort study with a follow-up of 19 years. *J Int Med* 1993, **234**:585–593.
2. Bilezikian JP: Management of hypercalcaemia. *J Clin Endocrinol Metab* 1993, **77**:1445–1449.
3. Heath DA: The treatment of hypercalcaemia of malignancy. *Clin Endocrinol* 1991, **34**:155–157.
4. Proceedings of the NIH Consensus Development Conference on diagnosis and management of asymptomatic primary hyperparathyroidism. Bethesda, Maryland, October 29–31, 1990. *J Bone Miner Res* 1991, **6 (suppl 2)**:81–166.

Hyperglycemic emergencies

Diagnosis

Symptoms

Hyperglycemia

Polyuria, thirst, polydipsia.

Weight loss.

Tiredness, lassitude, general malaise.

Decreasing level of consciousness.

Ketoacidosis

Nausea, vomiting, abdominal pain.

Dyspnea.

Precipitating cause

Symptoms of infection, myocardial infarction, or other illness.

Signs

General

Dehydration: particularly marked in hyperosmolar coma.

Hypotension.

Variable level of consciousness.

Signs of precipitating cause.

Ketoacidosis

Kussmaul's respiration, ketones on breath.

Peripheral vasodilatation, warm skin, tachycardia, generalized abdominal tenderness.

Investigations [1,2]

To establish diagnosis

Capillary blood glucose analysis.

Urinalysis: for glucose, ketones.

To confirm diagnosis

Laboratory blood glucose analysis.

Serum sodium, potassium, bicarbonate, and creatinine measurement.

Measurement of arterial or capillary pH, partial oxygen and carbon dioxide pressure, and base excess: if serum bicarbonate <20 mmol/L or ketonuria; shows acidosis, high oxygen pressure, low carbon dioxide pressure.

To identify precipitating cause

Chest radiography: may show infection or pulmonary edema.

ECG: may show acute myocardial infarction or signs of electrolyte disturbance.

Blood, urine, and throat cultures.

Abdominal ultrasonography or paracentesis: to exclude acute abdominal disease if abdominal signs do not resolve quickly.

Complete blood count: to look for anemia or leukocytosis.

Complications

Cardiac arrest.

Thromboembolism: particularly if patient is hyperosmolar.

Inhalation pneumonia.

Renal failure.

Rhabdomyolysis: rare.

Differential diagnosis

Ketotic

Hyperventilation, chest infection, lactic acidosis.

Acute abdominal disease.

Nonketotic

Hypercalcemia.

Cerebrovascular disease.

Thyrotoxicosis.

Etiology [2]

- Causes include the following:

Diabetes (initial presentation).

Other physical stress, precipitating rise in counter-regulatory hormones and relative deficiency of insulin (*e.g.*, infection, myocardial infarction, stroke).

Omission of insulin.

Epidemiology

- The incidence is not declining, despite advances in diabetes education.
- 3–8 episodes occur in 1000 diabetic patients each year.

Treatment

Diet and lifestyle

• No special precautions are necessary.

Pharmacological treatment [3]

• Rehydration and correction of electrolyte imbalance must begin immediately.

• A central venous pressure measurement may be a useful guide to fluid replacement in elderly patients or those with cardiac or renal disease.

• If the patient is comatose, a nasogastric tube should be passed.

• Urinary catheterization may be needed to allow accurate monitoring of urinary output.

Rehydration

0.9% saline solution, 1L in first hour to restore circulating volume, raise blood pressure, and open renal circulation; then 1 L in 2 h, 1 L in 4 h, 1 L in 6 h, 1 L 8-hourly thereafter as needed.

• The infusion rates should be adjusted as clinically indicated.

• 0.45% saline solution should be used if serum sodium is >155 mEq/L.

• Colloid solution can be given if the patient remains hypotensive.

Insulin

By continuous i.v. infusion: *if ketotic*: 6 units/h by pump; *if nonketotic*: 3–4 units/h.

• Adjust based on patient's usual daily insulin requirement.

By intermittent intramuscular injection: *if ketotic*: 20 units initially, then 10 units/h; *if nonketotic*: 10 units initially, then 6 units/h.

• Treatment is continued until blood glucose is 250 mg/dL; then the dose of insulin should be halved, and i.v. infusion of 10% dextrose commenced at 80 mL/h.

• Patients should be told not to stop insulin treatment if intercurrent illness supervenes associated with anorexia or vomiting; insulin needs increase in these circumstances.

Potassium

• The total body deficit of potassium is ~1000 mEq.

• Infusion should be started when serum potassium is <5.0 mEq/L.

• Potassium chloride, 20–80 mEq/h, well diluted in rehydration fluid, should be given.

• Treatment should be monitored by serum potassium measurement and ECG.

Sodium bicarbonate

• This is indicated only if the pH is <6.9.

• Sodium bicarbonate, 100 mL 8.4% in 30 min, with 20 mEq potassium chloride, should be given.

• The pH should be checked after 30 min, and treatment should be repeated if necessary until the pH is >6.9.

Other options

Anticoagulation: low-dose s.c. heparin for all; full-dose i.v. heparin if serum osmolality >360 mOsmol/kg.

Antibiotics: broad spectrum if any suspicion of infection.

• Replacement of other electrolytes (magnesium, phosphate) is rarely indicated.

Complications of treatment

• Most complications are avoidable with meticulous care and attention to detail.

Hypo- or hyperkalemia.

Hypoglycemia.

Fluid overload, especially in elderly patients.

Cerebral edema.

Adult respiratory distress syndrome.

Treatment aims

To save the patient's life.
To rehydrate the patient.
To restore acid-base and electrolyte balance to normal.
To achieve euglycemia in 24–48 h.

Prognosis

• Mortality remains at 5%–15% in diabetic ketoacidosis and 30%–50% in hyperosmolar coma, even in experienced units.
• In elderly patients, the cause of death is often the underlying precipitating disorder rather than the metabolic upset.

Follow-up and management

Response to treatment

• Response should be monitored at the bedside (pulse, blood pressure, respiratory rate every 30–60 min, capillary glucose hourly) and in the laboratory (glucose, sodium, potassium, bicarbonate, creatinine, pH on admission and at 2, 5, and 12 h of treatment, or more often if clinically indicated).

Later management

• Patients should be given fluids or a light diet when able to eat, but i.v. or i.m. insulin should be continued.
• When patients can tolerate oral intake, they should be transferred to s.c. insulin: quick-acting before each of the three main meals and intermediate-acting before bed.
• A 30-min overlap must be allowed before i.v. insulin is discontinued, to allow time for s.c. absorption.

Follow-up

• The events leading to admission should be reviewed in an effort to educate the patient and prevent further admissions; all patients should be taught "sick-day" rules, including advice on seeking professional help early.
• Patients presenting in hyperosmolar coma may not need long-term insulin, but continuing it for a few weeks is probably safer, before stopping under close supervision.

Key references

1. Walker M, Marshall SM, Alberti KGMM: Clinical aspects of diabetic ketoacidosis. *Diabetes Metab Rev* 1989, **5**:651–663.
2. Marshall SM: Hyperglycaemic emergencies. *Care of the Critically Ill*, 1993, **9**:220–223.
3. Berger W, Keller U: Treatment of diabetic ketoacidosis and non-ketotic hyperosmolar coma. *Clin Endocrinol Metab* 1991, **6**:1–22.

Hyperkalemia and hypokalemia

Diagnosis

Symptoms

• Often no symptoms are manifest.

Hyperkalemia

Skeletal muscle weakness: causing collapse, paralysis.

Diarrhea.

Hypokalemia

Muscle weakness and fatigue.

Polyuria and polydipsia.

Palpitations.

Signs

Hyperkalemia

Skeletal muscle weakness.

Irregular pulse.

Ileus.

Bradycardia, heart block, cardiac arrest (asystolic).

Hypokalemia

Postural hypotension.

Ileus.

Skeletal muscle weakness: quadriplegia, respiratory distress.

Cardiac arrhythmias: atrial and ventricular premature beats, atrial or ventricular tachycardia.

Investigations

• Estimation must be repeated urgently with optimal venipuncture technique and rapid transfer to laboratory.

Renal function tests: blood urea nitrogen (BUN), creatinine.

ECG.

Acid–base analysis.

Urinary potassium and pH measurement.

Plasma magnesium measurement.

Creatine kinase measurement.

Plasma phosphate measurement.

Plasma glucose measurement.

Complications

Hyperkalemia

Sudden death: asystole.

Hypokalemia

Rhabdomyolysis on vigorous exertion (acute).

Growth retardation in children.

Nephrogenic diabetes insipidus.

Negative nitrogen balance.

Interstitial nephritis: renal impairment.

Glucose intolerance.

Myocardial fibrosis.

Differential diagnosis

Artifact of sampling technique (hyperkalemia).

Etiology

Hyperkalemia

• The most common cause is a combination of renal impairment with the following:

Excessive potassium intake: due to diet, salt substitutes, potassium penicillins, transfusion of stored blood.

Redistribution: due to acidosis, exercise, hyperkalemic familial periodic paralysis, hormonal deficiencies (insulin, aldosterone, cortisol), drugs (beta blockers, alpha antagonists), release from damaged tissues, hyperosmolality.

Impaired renal excretion: due to acute or chronic renal failure, potassium-conserving diuretics, inadequate mineralocorticosteroid hormones, angiotensin-converting enzyme inhibitors, NSAIDs, cyclosporin A, pentamidine, type IV renal tubular acidosis.

Impaired gut excretion: due to colectomy in patients with pre-existing renal failure.

Hypokalemia

• The most common cause is a combination of gut loss with the following:

Inadequate intake: due to diet.

Redistribution: due to anabolic states, correction of severe anemia, transfusion of washed or frozen erythrocytes, metabolic alkalosis, some myeloproliferative disorders, beta agonists, correction of hyperglycemia, hypokalemic periodic paralysis, barium intoxication.

Gut losses: due to vomiting or nasogastric aspiration, diarrhea, purgative abuse.

Urinary losses: due to diuretics, hyperaldosteronism, Bartter's syndrome, Cushing's syndrome, licorice abuse, excess adrenocorticotropic hormone, renal tubular acidosis, tubular toxins (*e.g.*, cisplatin, amphotericin, aminoglycosides), urinary diversion into gut, magnesium depletion.

Epidemiology

• Hyperkalemia rarely occurs without renal impairment.

• Hypokalemia is more common, being associated with the use of common drugs (diuretics and purgatives) and as a common complication of diarrheal states.

Treatment

Diet and lifestyle

• Hyperkalemic patients with underlying chronic renal failure need dietary advice to restrict the daily potassium intake to 40–60 mEq/day; high-potassium foods include fruits, chocolate, nuts, and instant coffee.

• Hypokalemia can rarely be corrected by dietary means.

Pharmacological treatment

For hyperkalemia: moderate

• For moderate hyperkalemia with an acute rise in potassium to <6.5 mEq/L and a normal ECG, the following measures should be taken:

Intake of potassium decreased.

Offending drug removed.

Good urinary output ensured.

Plasma potassium concentration measured every 6 h to ensure falling values.

For hyperkalemia: severe

• An acute rise in potassium to >6.5 mEq/L and abnormal ECG or chronically raised potassium >8 mEq/L is a medical emergency.

• ECG monitoring is needed.

• Rapid correction is vital.

• Emergency dialysis is needed if the patient is oliguric and volume overloaded.

Standard dosage 10% calcium gluconate solution, 10 mL i.v. slowly.
50% glucose solution 50 mL, containing insulin, 10 units, i.v. 4-hourly.
8.4% sodium bicarbonate solution, 50 mL i.v. only if acidotic.
Sodium polystyrene sulfonate, 15 g, and lactulose, 10 mL orally 6-hourly or sodium polystyrene sulfonate by rectal retention enema if no ileus present.
Furosemide or bumetanide i.v. every 4–6 h to achieve urine flow rate >50 mL/h, *e.g.*, bumetanide 1 mg initially, increased to 5 mg.
Beta-adrenergic agonist can be given via inhaled route.

Contraindications None.

Special points Patient must be checked for hypoglycemia after i.v. glucose and insulin.
Calcium gluconate: a cardioprotective agent, does not lower plasma potassium concentration.

Main drug interactions None.

Main side effects None.

For hypokalemia

Standard dosage Effervescent potassium chloride, 80–200 mEq orally daily.
Potassium chloride, 60–120 mEq i.v. over 24 h.

Contraindications None.

Special points Potassium as chloride must be used with alkalosis to avoid continued urinary losses of potassium.
Oral supplements should be used whenever possible.
Intravenous repletion is potentially dangerous: 10 mEq/h is usually safe; higher rates may be used, but ECG monitoring is essential.

Main drug interactions Hypokalemia exacerbates digoxin toxicity.

Main side effects Late hyperkalemia due to delayed gastrointestinal absorption after oral potassium supplements.

Treatment aims

To restore acid–base balance and plasma potassium slowly over 24–72 h.

Prognosis

• Prognosis depends on the underlying condition.

Follow-up and management

• If deviations are gross, frequent and repeated measurements of plasma potassium are essential for several days.

General references

Androgue HJ, Wesson DE: Potassium. In *Blackwell's Basics of Medicine*. Oxford: Blackwell Scientific Publications; 1994.

Jacobsen HR, Rector FC, eds: Renal regulation of extracellular fluid composition. *Kidney Int* 1990, **38**:569–743.

Schrier RW, ed: *Renal and Electrolyte Disorders*, edn 4. Boston: Little Brown & Co; 1992.

Tannen RL: Potassium metabolism. In *Current Nephrology*, vol 15. Edited by Gonick HC. St Louis: Mosby Year Book; 1992:109–148.

Hypernatremia and hyponatremia

Diagnosis

Symptoms

Hypernatremia

Restlessness.

Irritability.

Lethargy.

Muscle twitches.

Hyponatremia

Lethargy.

Confusion and disorientation.

Agitation.

Anorexia.

Nausea.

Muscle cramps.

Signs

Hypernatremia

Increased reflexes.

Increased muscle tone.

Depressed consciousness.

Convulsions.

Coma.

Hyponatremia

Decreased reflexes.

Hypothermia.

Pseudobulbar palsy.

Convulsions.

Cheyne–Stokes respiration.

Coma.

Altered consciousness.

Investigations

- Most sodium is extracellular, so changes in sodium balance are reflected in changes in extracellular fluid volume (ECFV).
- Changes in serum sodium concentration reflect alterations in the sodium : water ratio in the extracellular fluid and can occur with increased, normal, or decreased ECFV (increased, normal, or reduced total body sodium).

Detection of edema, estimation of jugular venous pressure, tissue turgor, erect and supine pulse and blood pressure, peripheral perfusion, auscultation of lung bases, and patient weighing: vital for accurate documentation of state of ECFV; edema always indicates raised total body sodium (water, being freely diffusable, does not accumulate as edema).

Renal function tests, chest radiography, ECG, liver function tests, albumin and glucose measurement, urine and plasma osmolality, endocrine tests (thyroid and adrenal), echocardiography if cardiac disease suspected.

Complications

Hypernatremia

Shrinkage of brain cells.

Rupture of cerebral veins.

Cerebral venous (sinus) thrombosis.

Intracranial hemorrhage.

Hyponatremia

Cerebral edema.

Raised intracranial pressure.

Herniation of brain stem.

Central pontine myelinolysis: related to over-rapid correction; causes permanent residual neurological deficits.

Differential diagnosis

Hyperlipidemia or hyperproteinemia: may cause pseudohyponatremia; reduced water volume of plasma reduces apparent sodium concentration/mL whole plasma.

Etiology

Causes of hypernatremia

Normal (slightly reduced) extracellular fluid volume (ECFV): diabetes insipidus, dry ventilation, hypodipsia, sweating.

Increased ECFV (edema): excessive sodium intake, excessive adrenocortical hormones.

Decreased ECFV (without free access to water): excessive loss of sodium in urine, excessive loss of gastrointestinal secretions, burns, sweating.

Causes of hyponatremia

Normal (slightly expanded) ECFV: excessive water intake, syndrome of inappropriate antidiuretic hormone secretion (drug-induced).

Increased ECFV (edema): acute or chronic renal failure, cardiac failure, cirrhosis with ascites, nephrotic syndrome, pregnancy.

Decreased ECFV (with free access to water): excessive loss of sodium in urine, excessive loss of gastrointestinal secretions, burns, sweating.

Epidemiology

- Hypernatremia is common in elderly patients (hypodipsia) and in immobile or unconscious patients.
- Hyponatremia is common in hospitals because of inappropriate fluid replacement, usually with dextrose saline solution or over-diuresis of patients with cardiac failure.

Treatment

Diet and lifestyle

• Hypernatremia and hyponatremia usually develop in hospitals; the primary underlying disease dominates the clinical picture.

• Alterations in sodium intake are needed for patients with changes in their extracellular fluid volume, *e.g.*, sodium restriction for those with edema.

• Compulsive water drinkers and drug abusers may need psychiatric counseling.

Pharmacological treatment

Hypernatremia

• Extracellular fluid volume must first be defined and corrected; a decrease should be corrected by normal saline solution, an increase by diuretics or dialysis.

• Then the hypernatremia can be corrected *slowly* by 0.5% dextrose or dextrose saline or 0.9% saline solution, replacing about half of the calculated replacement over the first 24 h.

• Central venous pressure monitoring and urethral catheterization for monitoring urine output may be needed.

Hyponatremia

• For mild to moderate chronic dilutional hyponatremia, restriction of water intake alone may be sufficient.

• For edematous states, diuretics should be given, with human albumin if the patient is nephrotic or cirrhotic.

• Patients with true sodium depletion should be given 0.9% saline or 5% hypertonic saline solution infused slowly, with diuretics to correct serum sodium concentrations—over-rapid correction may cause brain damage (hyponatremia should be corrected by 1.5–2 mEq/h if acute onset or ≤ 1 mEq/h if chronic).

• Administration of sodium to edematous patients may precipitate cardiac failure; diuretics may be needed to normalize intravascular volume.

• Restoring plasma oncotic pressure with albumin solutions may be needed, but their sodium content can be high (160 mEq/L); serum sodium must be measured every 4–6 h, with treatment adjusted to achieve desired correction rate.

• In severe cases, central venous pressure monitoring and urethral catheterization to monitor urine output are needed.

Treatment aims

To correct extracellular fluid volume.

To correct serum sodium concentration.

Prognosis

• Prognosis depends on the underlying condition.

• Acute changes in onset or correction are more dangerous than slow changes.

• Very old or very young patients are most vulnerable.

• Permanent neurological deficits are common, especially if correction is over-rapid.

Follow-up and management

• Follow-up depends on the underlying condition.

General references

Adrogue HJ, Wesson DE: Salt and water. In *Blackwell's Basics of Medicine*. Oxford: Blackwell Scientific Publications; 1994.

Richardson RMA: Water metabolism. In *Current Nephrology* vol 15. Edited by Gonick HC. St Louis: Mosby Year Book; 1992:149–206.

Schrier RW: Body fluid volume regulation in health and disease: a unifying hypothesis. *Ann Intern Med* 1990, **113**:155–159.

Sterns RH: Central nervous system complications of hyponatremia. In *International Year Book of Nephrology*. Edited by Andreucci VE, Fine LG. Berlin: Springer-Verlag; 1992:55–74.

Diagnosis

Symptoms

• Symptoms can be subdivided into those directly related to hyperprolactinemia and those due to the mass effect of a pituitary macroadenoma.

Hyperprolactinemia

Galactorrhea.

Amenorrhea, oligomenorrhea: in women.

Impotence: in men.

Infertility.

Reduced libido.

Macroadenoma

Headache: frontal.

Visual field defect: bitemporal hemianopia.

Diplopia.

Convulsions: temporal-lobe epilepsy due to local extension of tumor.

Cerebrovascular accident.

Signs

Macroadenoma

Hypopituitarism.

Optic atrophy: if tumor compressing optic nerve.

Loss of secondary sexual characteristics, postural hypotension, hypothyroidism, delayed or arrested puberty: signs of hypopituitarism.

Investigations [1,2]

Detailed drug history.

Serum prolactin measurement: thyroid-releasing hormone and other dynamic stimulation tests are of no value.

Thyroid function tests: hypothyroidism is a cause of raised serum prolactin.

Gonadotropin and gonadal steroids measurement: to diagnose polycystic ovary syndrome, a cause of hyperprolactinemia.

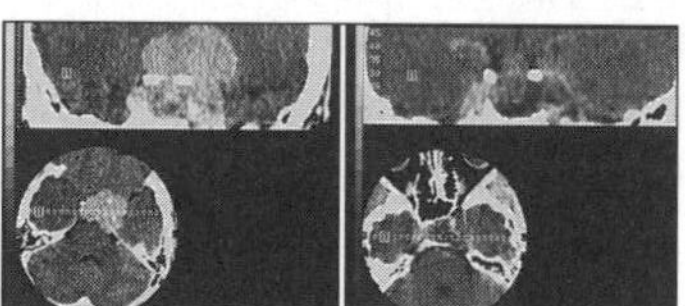

Axial and coronal view of large prolactinoma (left). Repeat scan (right) showing virtual disappearance of tumor on treatment by bromocriptine.

Corticotropic hormone and cortisol measurement.

Dynamic pituitary function testing: consider doing if necessary.

Skull radiography, pituitary MRI or CT: to identify tumor.

Complications

Hyperprolactinemia

Infertility, impotence.

Osteoporosis.

Polycystic ovarian disease: in 25% of patients with a prolactinoma.

Macroadenoma

Hydrocephalus.

Blindness.

Hypopituitarism.

Cranial nerve palsy.

Differential diagnosis

Prolactinoma.

Pseudoprolactinoma (prolactin usually <150 ng/mL).

Hypothyroidism.

Medication (prolactin usually <150 ng/mL): substituted benzamides (metoclopropamide, sulpiride), phenothiazines, butyrophenones, reserpine, methyldopa.

Stress: *e.g.*, venipuncture, epilepsy.

Polycystic ovarian disease (prolactin usually <50 ng/mL): hyperprolactinemia can be secondary to polycystic ovarian disease; alternatively, polycystic ovarian disease occurs in 25% of patients with a prolactinoma.

Possible breast stimulation.

Chest wall processes (tumor, herpes zoster).

Etiology [1,2]

• Prolactinomas are monoclonal tumors that secrete prolactin.

• Pseudoprolactinomas are tumors of any type that interrupt the tonic inhibition, by hypothalamic dopamine, of prolactin secretion, *i.e.*, the prolactin is secreted from the healthy pituitary.

• Estrogens are not causative but can encourage prolactinoma growth, particularly the combined oral contraceptive pill and pregnancy.

Epidemiology

• Prolactinomas occur much more often in women than in men.

Treatment

Diet and lifestyle

• Estrogens, *e.g.*, the combined oral contraceptive, are contraindicated unless taken with dopamine agonists.

• Pregnancy and breast feeding can encourage tumor growth and must be undertaken with caution.

Pharmacological treatment [1–4]

Standard dosage Bromocriptine, 1.25 mg initially, in the middle of a snack last thing at night; dose must be titrated against serum prolactin, median being 7.5 mg; ultimately, once-daily dose in the middle of a meal.

Contraindications Toxemia of pregnancy, sensitivity to ergot alkaloid, history of psychosis.

Special points An alternative dopamine agonist in cases of bromocriptine intolerance or resistance is pergolide [5].

Main drug interactions None.

Main side effects Gastrointestinal disturbance, particularly nausea; postural hypotension; first-dose hypotension (effect negated by drugs that raise prolactin concentration).

Treatment aims

To normalize serum prolactin concentration.

To retain normal pituitary function.

Other treatments [1–3]

Transsphenoidal microadenectomy: for dopamine agonist intolerance or resistance, infertility, pseudoprolactinoma.

Pituitary radiotherapy: for failed transsphenoidal hypophysectomy, macroprolactinoma (possibly before pregnancy to avoid expansion during pregnancy), dopamine agonist intolerance or resistance.

Prognosis

• 15%–20% of microprolactinomas resolve during long-term dopamine agonist treatment.

• 40% of patients with macroadenomas have normal serum prolactinomas after transsphenoidal hypophysectomy.

Follow-up and management

• Patients must be maintained on the minimum dose of bromocriptine necessary to normalize serum prolactin concentrations.

• Bromocriptine should be stopped every 2 years and serum prolactin concentration checked.

• Long-term follow-up is necessary.

Key references

1. Levy A, Lightman SL: Diagnosis and management of pituitary tumours. *BMJ* 1994, **308**:1087–1091.
2. Serri O, Beauregard H, Somma M: Prolactinoma. *Curr Ther Endocrinol Metab* 1994, **5**:41–43.
3. Cunnah D, Besser GM: Management of prolactinomas. *Clin Endocrinol* 1991, **34**:231–235.
4. Faglia G: Should dopamine agonist treatment for prolactinomas be life-long? *Clin Endocrinol* 1991, **34**:173 174.
5. Webster J, *et al.*: A comparison of cabergoline and bromocriptine in the treatment of hyperprolactinemic amenorrhea. Cabergoline Comparative Study Group. *N Engl J Med* 1994, **331**:904–909.

Diagnosis

Symptoms

• Patients are usually symptomless; hypertension is discovered at opportunistic or organized screening visits or detected after a hypertensive complication has intervened (myocardial infarction, cardiovascular accident, peripheral vascular disease, heart failure).

• Patients should be asked about symptoms of underlying causes of hypertension, *e.g.*, flushing and palpitations with pheochromocytoma, also other endocrine causes.

Headaches: occasionally.

Poor vision, shortness of breath, angina: rare.

Signs

Uncomplicated mild hypertension

• No signs other than raised blood pressure are manifest.

Moderate to severe hypertension

Displaced forceful apex beat, fourth heart sound, left atrial lift: signs of cardiac hypertrophy.

Silver wire arterioles, arteriovenous nipping, hemorrhages, exudates, papilledema.

Hypertensive complications

Signs of heart failure, renal failure, peripheral vascular disease, strokes.

Underlying causes (much less common than essential hypertension)

Signs of Cushing's syndrome, renal artery stenosis, aortic coarctation, pheochromocytoma, acromegaly.

Investigations

Blood pressure measurement: to confirm diagnosis; repeated over several visits or by ambulatory monitoring.

Chest radiography: for coarctation, *e.g.*, rib-notching and double aortic shadow.

Renal function and electrolyte analysis: to check for renal failure, low potassium in Conn's syndrome.

Urine microscopy: for hematuria, casts, proteinuria in nephritis.

24-h urinary catecholamines, metanephrines, vanillylmandelic acid analysis: for pheochromocytoma.

Ultrasonography of kidneys: show small scarred kidneys of pyelonephritis or end-stage renovascular disease; obstructive nephropathy.

Nuclear renography or renal angiography: for renal artery stenosis.

Endocrine tests: for Cushing's syndrome, acromegaly, thyroid disease.

ECG or echocardiography: for left ventricular hypertrophy in patients with moderate to severe hypertension.

Microalbuminuria measurement: for kidney damage in patients with moderate to severe hypertension.

Complications

Atrial fibrillation, ischemic heart disease, heart failure.

Peripheral vascular disease.

Nephrosclerosis, renovascular disease, renal failure.

Transient ischemic attacks, cardiovascular accidents, encephalopathy.

Hemorrhage, infarction, papilledema, blindness.

Differential diagnosis

"White-coat" hypertension.

Pseudohypertension.

Etiology

• In most patients, no cause is found (essential hypertension).

• Underlying causes include the following.

Renal artery stenosis, nephritis, obstructive uropathy.

Coarctation.

Pheochromocytoma, Cushing's syndrome, Conn's syndrome, acromegaly, thyroid disease.

Cyclosporin, steroids, NSAIDs.

Pre-eclampsia, occasional autonomic neuropathy.

Epidemiology

• The frequency of hypertension depends on diagnostic cut-off levels of blood pressure: 10%–15% of the adult population have hypertension, increasing with age.

• Incidence and associations differ in non-white populations: *e.g.*, with insulin resistance in Asians, low-renin hypertension in Afro-Caribbeans.

Treatment

Diet and lifestyle

• Patients should be encouraged to lose weight, increase physical exercise, reduce salt intake, moderate alcohol intake, stop smoking, and consider other risk factors, *e.g.*, hyperlipidemia.

Pharmacological treatment

Angiotensin converting enzyme inhibitors

Standard dosage Depends on choice of agent (*see manufacturer's current prescribing information*).

Contraindications Angioedema, renal artery stenosis, pregnancy.

Main drug interactions Hyperkalemia, synergistic with potassium-sparing diuretics.

Main side effects Cough, renal impairment, angioedema (rare).

Calcium antagonists

Standard dosage Depends on choice of agent (*see manufacturer's current prescribing information*).

Contraindications Heart failure (relative).

Special points Useful in black patients.

Main drug interactions Bradycardia with diltiazem or verapamil and beta blockers.

Main side effects Edema, flushing.

Beta blockers

Standard dosage Depends on choice of agent (*see manufacturer's current prescribing information*).

Contraindications Asthma, heart failure, heart block.

Special points Less effective in elderly patients.

Main drug interactions Bradycardia with diltiazem or verapamil.

Main side effects Lethargy, fatigue, impotence.

Thiazide diuretics

Standard dosage Low doses, depending on choice of agent (*see manufacturer's current prescribing information*).

Contraindications Diabetes (relative).

Special points Particularly beneficial in elderly patients [2,3,5,6].

Main drug interactions Other diuretics.

Main side effects Hypokalemia, glucose intolerance.

Alpha blockers

Standard dosage Depends on choice of agent (*see manufacturer's current prescribing information*).

Contraindications Known hypersensitivity.

Special points First-dose hypotension and tolerance may occur.

Main drug interactions Few specific interactions.

Main side effects Flushing, occasionally lupus-like syndrome.

Combination therapy

• Logical and synergistic combinations should be chosen, such as thiazides and angiotensin converting enzyme inhibitors; fixed-dose combinations are a disadvantage.

Treatment aims

To reduce blood pressure to <140/90 mm Hg and to improve other cardiovascular risk factors.

Prognosis

• Prognosis is excellent if blood pressure is controlled (almost always possible).

Follow-up and management

• Follow-up must be for life.

Key references

1. Collins R, *et al.*: Blood pressure, stroke, and coronary heart disease: part II. Short-term reductions in blood pressure: overview of randomised drug trials in their epidemiologic context. *Lancet* 1990, **335**:827–838.
2. Dahlöf B, *et al.*: Morbidity and mortality in the Swedish Trial in Old Patients with Hypertension (STOP-Hypertension). *Lancet* 1991, **338**:1281–1285.
3. MRC Working Party: Medical Research Council trial of treatment in older adults: principal results. *BMJ* 1992, **304**:405–412.
4. Sever P, *et al.*: Management guidelines in essential hypertension: report of the second working party of the British Hypertension Society. *BMJ* 1993, **306**:983–987.
5. Mulrow CD, *et al.*: Hypertension in the elderly. *JAMA* 1994, **272**:1932–1938.
6. SHEP Co-operative Research Group: Prevention of stroke by antihypertensive drug treatment in older persons with isolated systolic hypertension. *JAMA* 1991, **265**:3255–3264.

Diagnosis

Symptoms

Weight loss, fatigue, sweating, heat intolerance, neck swelling.

Palpitations, shortness of breath.

Tremor, weakness, nervousness.

Increased frequency of bowel movements.

Staring, gritty eyes, swelling around eyes.

• Classic symptoms and signs may be absent in elderly patients.

Signs

Sinus tachycardia, atrial fibrillation, cardiac failure.

Fine tremor, proximal myopathy.

Goiter: diffuse, with or without bruit, nodular, solitary nodule.

Lid retraction, lid lag, periorbital puffiness, chemosis, proptosis, corneal ulceration, ophthalmoplegia.

Pretibial myxedema, palmar erythema, acropachy (finger clubbing).

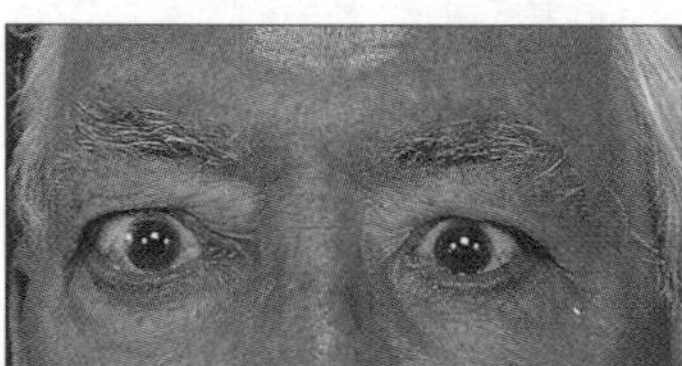

Periorbital edema, mild lid retraction and chemosis in a patient with Graves' ophthalmopathy.

Investigations

Serum thyroid hormone measurement: total or free thyroxine (T_4) to indicate severity of hyperthyroidism; total or free triiodothyronine (T_3) to indicate severity and diagnose T_3 toxicosis if T_4 normal but thyroid-stimulating hormone (TSH) low.

Serum TSH measurement: undetectable in hyperthyroidism; normal value excludes primary hyperthyroidism (use of a sensitive assay obviates need for thyrotrophin-releasing hormone testing); in pituitary-driven hyperthyroidism (rare), TSH is detectable.

Autoantibody tests: antithyroid peroxidase and antithyroglobulin antibodies often positive in Graves' disease; anti-TSH receptor antibodies often positive in Graves' disease but not measured routinely.

Radioisotope scanning and uptake measurements: not routinely indicated; ^{99m}Tc scintigraphy distinguishes Graves' disease from toxic nodular goiter; increased uptake of ^{131}I confirms hyperthyroidism; uptake low in thyroiditis.

Complications

Cardiac disease: especially atrial fibrillation and congestive cardiac failure (more common in elderly patients).

Reduced bone density and increased risk of osteoporotic fractures.

Graves' ophthalmopathy: may be progressive and occasionally sight-threatening because of corneal ulceration or optic nerve compression [1].

Differential diagnosis

Psychiatric disorders: *e.g.*, anxiety.

Anemia.

Malignancy.

Pheochromocytoma.

Alcohol withdrawal.

Excess caffeine intake.

Etiology [2]

Common causes (95% of patients)

Graves' disease.

Autoimmune cause associated with antibodies to thyroid-stimulating hormone (TSH) receptor on thyroid cell.

Toxic nodular goiter: multinodular, single toxic adenoma.

Thyroiditis: subacute, silent, postpartum.

Uncommon causes

Exogenous iodide: kelp ingestion, amiodarone, radiographic contrast agents.

Factitious: ingestion of thyroid hormones.

Inappropriate secretion of TSH by pituitary: TSH-secreting tumor, thyroid hormone resistance syndromes.

Neonatal hyperthyroidism: baby born to mother with history of Graves' disease.

Epidemiology

• The prevalence of hyperthyroidism is ~20 in 1000 females and ~2 in 1000 males.

• Toxic nodular goiter is part of a spectrum of endemic or sporadic goiter, often found in patients with a long history of goiter; the peak incidence is at ~60 years.

Treatment

Diet and lifestyle

• Increased iodine intake may precipitate hyperthyroidism in patients with euthyroid goiter.
• Cigarette smoking significantly increases the risk of ophthalmopathy in Graves' disease.

Pharmacological treatment [2]

Thionamides [3]

• Thionamides are first-line treatment in patients <40 years with Graves' hyperthyroidism; they are short-term treatment in older patients and those with relapsed hyperthyroidism before radioiodine treatment.
• They produce biochemical improvement and symptomatic relief within 2 months in most patients; a full course of 18 months is important to allow remission of disease.

Standard dosage Methimazole, 30 mg single daily dose at diagnosis, reduced to maintenance dose of 5–10 mg.
Propylthiouracil, 100 mg 3 times daily at diagnosis, reduced to maintenance dose of 50 mg 1–2 times daily.

Contraindications Thionamide-induced agranulocytosis or other serious side effects.

Main drug interactions No major interactions.

Main side effects Agranulocytosis (rare; patients must be warned to stop treatment and seek an urgent blood test if they develop a sore throat or other infection), hepatitis, cholestatic jaundice and lupus-like syndromes (rare but serious), skin rashes and arthralgia (common but not serious).

Beta-adrenergic blockers

• Beta-andergenic blockers are recommended for patients with moderate or severe symptoms until serum thyroid hormones have returned to normal; often they are the only treatment needed for thyroiditis.
• They provide quick symptomatic relief of tremor and palpitations that resemble sympathetic overactivity.

Standard dosage Propranolol, 20–80 mg 3 times daily (higher dose may be needed because of increased first-pass metabolism).
Atenolol, 50–100 mg daily.

Contraindications Asthma, obstructive pulmonary disease; caution in heart failure, even if induced by hyperthyroidism.

Main drug interactions *See manufacturer's current prescribing information.*

Main side effects *See manufacturer's current prescribing information.*

Radioiodine

• Radioiodine treatment must be done under specialist supervision.
• It is increasingly used as first-line treatment in patients with the first episode of hyperthyroidism; it is the treatment of choice in patients aged >40 years at presentation and in those with relapse after drug treatment or surgery.

Standard dosage Radioiodine single dose initially; second dose after 6 months if hyperthyroidism not cured (one-third of patients); larger initial doses for elderly patients or those with severe disease to produce rapid effect and induce hypothyroidism.

Contraindications Pregnancy (must be avoided for 6 months after treatment), breast feeding, hyperthyroidism secondary to thyroiditis; caution in patients with active ophthalmopathy.

Special points Thionamides should be withdrawn at least 4 days before and avoided for 4 days after treatment.
Can exacerbate hyperthyroidism and rarely induce "thyroid storm."

Main drug interactions None.

Main side effects Hypothyroidism (within 25 years of treatment), may be intended outcome if larger dose of radioiodine used for thyroid ablation and thyroxine replacement.

Treatment aims

To relieve symptoms.
To restore thyroxine and triiodothyronine values to normal range.
To obtain long-term euthyroidism.

Other treatments

Partial thyroidectomy: for Graves' disease in patients with large goiter and relapse after thionamide treatment or with large toxic nodular goiter.
• Patients must be rendered euthyroid before surgery by thionamide or beta blocker with potassium iodide.

Prognosis

• Only 30% of patients with Graves' hyperthyroidism remain euthyroid in the long term after a course of thionamide; 15% become hypothyroid even without treatment.
• Medium-dosed radioiodine treatment and partial thyroidectomy are each associated with a 50% risk of permanent hypothyroidism; larger doses ablate the thyroid.

Follow-up and management

• Serum thyroxine and thyroid-stimulating hormone concentration should be monitored every 4–6 weeks in patients on high-dose thionamides and every 3 months in those on maintenance doses.
• Thyroid function should be checked annually (continuing risk of hypothyroidism).

Management of hyperthyroidism in pregnancy

• Thionamides are the most appropriate agents; propylthiouracil is preferred (crosses placenta less than methimazole, excreted less in breast milk).
• Dosage must be adjusted to maintain serum thyroxine at the upper end of normal range (these drugs cause fetal goiter and hypothyroidism in high dose).
• Low doses are needed in Graves' hyperthyroidism (usually remits in pregnancy).
• Relapse is frequent after delivery.

Key references

1. Fells P: Thyroid-associated eye disease: clinical management. *Lancet* 1991, **338**:29–32.
2. Franklyn JA: The management of hyperthyroidism. *N Engl J Med* 1994, **330**:1731–1738.
3. Reinwein D, *et al.*: A prospective randomised trial of antithyroid drug dose in Graves' disease therapy. *J Clin Endocrinol Metab* 1993, **76**:1516–1521.

Diagnosis

Symptoms

• Patients may be asymptomatic.

Severe cardiac failure: in infants.

Premature unexpected death: may be presenting symptom in children or young adults [1].

Dyspnea on exertion: in ~50% of patients.

Chest pain: in ~50%; may be exertional or occur at rest.

Syncope: in 15–25%.

Dizziness, palpitations.

Signs

• In patients without outflow tract gradient, abnormalities may be subtle.

Rapid upstroke arterial pulse: best felt in carotid area.

Forceful left ventricular impulse: best appreciated on full held expiration in left lateral position.

Ejection systolic murmur: best heard at left sternal border; radiating towards aortic and mitral areas but not into neck.

Palpable atrial beat: reflecting forceful atrial systolic contraction.

Investigations

Two-dimensional echocardiography: important for assessing left ventricle structure and function, gradients, valvular regurgitation, and atrial dimensions.

ECG: may be normal in <5% of patients or show abnormalities reflecting left ventricular hypertrophy, atrial fibrillation, left axis deviation, right bundle branch block, and myocardial disarray (*e.g.*, ST- and T-wave changes, intraventricular conduction defects, abnormal Q waves); bizarre or abnormal findings in young patients should raise suspicion of hypertrophic cardiomyopathy, especially if a family member also affected.

Chest radiography: may be normal or show evidence of left or right atrial or left ventricular enlargement.

Treadmill exercise test with maximum oxygen ventilatory capacity: simple and noninvasive; provides useful functional information; maximum oxygen ventilatory capacity often moderately reduced; one-third of patients have abnormal blood pressure response, with drops of 25–150 mm Hg from peak systolic recordings (probably of prognostic significance); ST segment changes of >2 mm documented in 25%, associated with symptoms of angina.

48-h Holter monitoring: arrhythmias common during ECG monitoring; established atrial fibrillation in ~10% of patients, paroxysmal supraventricular arrhythmias in 30%, nonsustained ventricular tachycardia in 25%; ventricular tachycardia invariably asymptomatic during Holter monitoring, but most useful marker of risk of sudden death in adults; sustained supraventricular arrhythmias often symptomatic and predispose to thromboembolic complications.

Thallium scintigraphy: fixed and reversible perfusion defects common, useful in assessment of ischemia, particularly when resting ECG grossly abnormal and exercise changes uninterpretable.

Cardiac catheterization and left ventriculography: invasive evaluation not needed for diagnosis, but coronary arteriography often necessary in older patients with angina to exclude coronary artery disease; endomyocardial biopsy possibly necessary to exclude specific heart muscle disorder (amyloid, sarcoid) but has no other role in diagnosis because of patchy nature of myofiber disarray.

Complications

Atrial fibrillation.

Systemic embolism.

Infective endocarditis.

Sudden death.

Differential diagnosis

Aortic valve disease.

Systemic hypertension.

Etiology

• Hypertrophic cardiomyopathy is an autosomal dominant heart muscle disorder.

• Mutations in the gene encoding contractile proteins cause disease in 50–60% of patients [2].

Pathology

Macroscopic: hypertrophied myocardium; thickened anterior leaflet of mitral valve; contact lesion upper anterior septum.

Histological: interstitial fibrosis; myofiber disorganization and whorling; myocyte hypertrophy.

Pathophysiology

Systolic: hyperdynamic contraction; left ventricular outflow tract gradient (30%; associated mitral regurgitation).

Diastolic: impaired relaxation; impaired filling; decreased compliance.

Epidemiology

• The male:female ratio is equal, although the disease tends to affect younger men and older women.

• In children and adolescents, myocardial hypertrophy often occurs during growth spurts; a negative diagnosis made before adolescent growth has been completed must be tempered by the proviso of subsequent reassessment.

• Myocardial hypertrophy does not ordinarily progress after adolescent growth is completed.

• The annual mortality from sudden death is 2.5% in adults and at least 6% in children and young adults.

• First-degree relatives of affected patients have a 50% chance of carrying the disease gene; they should be investigated by ECG and two-dimensional echocardiography.

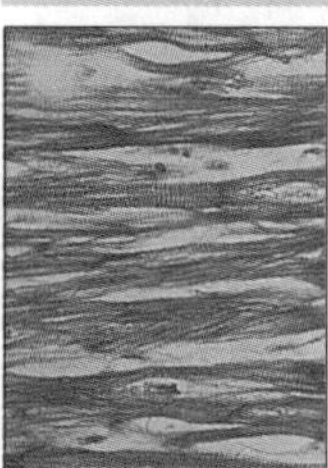
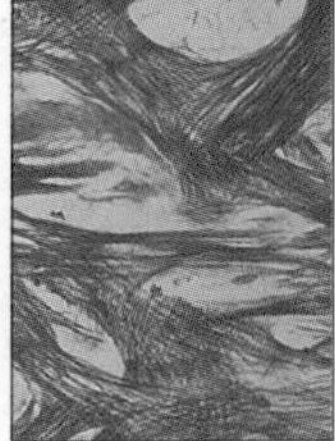

Myofibrillar stain from a normal person (*left*) and one with myocardial disarray (*right*).

Treatment

Diet and lifestyle

• Competitive exercise is not recommended, especially in high-risk patients.

Pharmacological treatment

Beta blockers

• Beta blockers may reduce symptoms and increase exercise capacity, but they do not reduce the incidence of ventricular arrhythmia or risk of sudden death.

Standard dosage	Propranolol, 80–320 mg daily. Atenolol, 50 mg daily.
Contraindications	Conduction disease.
Main drug interactions	Other drugs that suppress impulse formation.
Main side effects	Other unwanted adrenergic blocking effects.

Calcium antagonists

• Calcium antagonism can improve hemodynamics and relieve symptoms but gives no reduction in risk of sudden death.

Standard dosage	Verapamil, 120–480 mg daily.
Contraindications	Outflow-tract gradient.
Special points	Verapamil fails to abolish ventricular arrhythmia.
Main drug interactions	Digoxin.
Main side effects	High-grade conduction block, negative inotropic effect.

Antiarrhythmics

• Antiarrhythmics are effective in short-term and long-term control of supraventricular and ventricular arrhythmias and can improve survival in adults with nonsustained ventricular tachycardia (low dose).

Standard dosage	Amiodarone, 100–200 mg daily.
Contraindications	Hyperthyroidism.
Special points	Plasma concentration should be maintained <1.5 mg/L.
Main drug interactions	Anticoagulants, digoxin.
Main side effects	Photosensitivity, sleep disturbance.

Other options

Anticoagulation: important in patients with paroxysmal or established atrial fibrillation.

Endocarditis prophylaxis: for patients with obstruction and valvular regurgitation (*see* Endocarditis *for details*).

Treatment aims

To improve symptoms.

To prevent complications.

To prevent sudden death.

Other treatments

Surgical myectomy [3]

• In patients with left ventricle outflow tract obstruction, this provides symptomatic and hemodynamic improvement.

• Perioperative mortality is high, at 5–10%.

Dual-chamber permanent pacing

• Recently proposed for treatment of obstructions [4], this provides a reduction in outflow gradient and improvement in symptoms.

• Further assessment is needed.

Cardiac transplantation

• Transplantation is limited to patients who develop severe systolic impairment.

Prognosis

• Nonsustained ventricular tachycardia is the best marker of high risk in adults.

• Other patients at high risk are children and adolescents who have had recurrent syncope and patients with two or more siblings with hypertrophic cardiomyopathy who have died suddenly.

Follow-up and management

• Patients must be monitored for disease progression and risk of complications.

Key references

1. Maron BJ, *et al.*: Hypertrophic cardiomyopathy. *N Engl J Med* 1987, **316**:780–789.
2. Rosenzweig A, *et al.*: Preclinical diagnosis of familial hypertrophic cardiomyopathy by genetic analysis of blood lymphocytes. *N Engl J Med* 1991, **325**:1753–1760.
3. Seiler C, *et al.*: Long-term follow-up of medical vs. surgical therapy for hypertrophic cardiomyopathy. *J Am Coll Cardiol* 1991, **17**:634–642.
4. Fananapazir L, *et al.*: Impact of dual chamber permanent pacing in patients with obstructive hypertrophic cardiomyopathy with symptoms refractory to verapamil and beta-blocker therapy. *Circulation* 1992, **85**:2149–2156.

Diagnosis

Symptoms

Paresthesia: especially around face, hands, and feet.

Tetany: causing painful cramps culminating in hands going into tetanic spasm position.

Epilepsy.

Bone pain: common in vitamin D deficiency.

Signs

• Mild hypocalcemia may be asymptomatic; signs are due to neuromuscular irritability.

Twitching of local facial muscles: after tapping over facial nerve in front of and below ear; Chvostek's sign (positive in some normal people, rarely in those with hypokalemia).

Development of tetanic spasm (Trousseau's sign): after inflation of a sphygmomanometer cuff on arm (a painful procedure and not recommended).

Proximal myopathy: common in vitamin D deficiency.

Obesity, "moon" face, shortened metacarpals and metatarsals: signs of pseudohypoparathyroidism.

Investigations [1]

Serum calcium measurement: low concentration.

Serum phosphorus measurement: low concentration in vitamin D deficiency, high in hypoparathyroidism, pseudohypoparathyroidism, and renal failure.

Serum creatinine measurement: raised concentration in renal failure.

Serum alkaline phosphatase measurement: often raised concentration in vitamin D deficiency.

Serum magnesium measurement: low concentration can cause hypocalcemia.

Serum parathyroid hormone measurement: raised concentration in vitamin D deficiency, pseudohypoparathyroidism, and renal failure.

Radiography: of wrists and knees in suspected rickets, chest and pelvis in suspected osteomalacia.

Complications

Epilepsy.

Cataracts and basal ganglia calcification: in longstanding hypocalcemia.

Differential diagnosis

Previous neck surgery.

Hypomagnesemia, especially if patient is an alcoholic, has extensive small-bowel disease or resection, or is on aminoglycoside drugs or cisplatinum.

Etiology [2]

• Causes include the following:

Low plasma proteins (not true hypocalcemia).

Acute or chronic renal failure.

Vitamin D deficiency.

Hypoparathyroidism: rarely idiopathic, usually after neck surgery.

Pseudohypoparathyroidism.

Hypomagnesemia.

Severe acute pancreatitis.

Malabsorption.

Epidemiology

• Vitamin D deficiency is more common in Asians who are vegetarians.

• Hypocalcemia is manifest most often at times of increased calcium shifts (*i.e.*, neonatal period, growth spurt, and pregnancy).

Treatment

Diet and lifestyle

• Patients should have an adequate calcium intake (800–2000 mg daily).

• Low-dose vitamin D supplementation should be considered if exposure to sunlight is inadequate.

Pharmacological treatment [1]

For acute symptomatic hypocalcemia

Standard dosage	10% calcium gluconate, 10 mL i.v. slowly, followed by 50–100 mL i.v. in 1 L saline solution over 24 h at a rate to relieve symptoms.
Contraindications	None.
Main drug interactions	None.
Main side effects	Tissue necrosis (if extravasation outside vein).

For hypoparathyroidism

Standard dosage	Calcitriol, 0.5–1.0 μg orally daily.
Contraindications	None.
Special points	Regular serum calcium monitoring.
Main drug interactions	None.
Main side effects	Hypercalcemia.

For vitamin D deficiency

Standard dosage	Calciferol, 500–1000 units orally daily.
Contraindications	None.
Main drug interactions	None.
Main side effects	None at this dose range.

For renal failure

Standard dosage	Calcitriol, 0.5–1.0 μg orally daily.
Contraindications	None.
Special points	Hyperphosphatemia should be controlled.
Main drug interactions	None.
Main side effects	Hypercalcemia.

For hypomagnesemic hypocalcemia

• Patients with severe, symptomatic hypomagnesemia are best treated initially by an intravenous preparation: magnesium sulfate, 5–10 mg 50% solution in 1 L 5% dextrose over 3–4 h.

• Daily infusions may be needed until serum magnesium is maintained within the normal range.

• If magnesium losses continue (*e.g.*, short bowel syndrome), this can be treated by intermittent infusions or oral therapy. Various oral preparations are available, all of which may cause gastrointestinal problems.

Treatment aims

To correct hypocalcemia.

Prognosis

• Hypoparathyroidism usually needs life-long treatment.

• For vitamin D deficiency, treatment is needed throughout the period of increased vitamin D requirement.

Follow-up and management

• All patients on high doses of vitamin D need regular serum calcium measurements to prevent the occurrence of hypercalcemia.

Key references

1. Tohme JF, Bilezikian JP: Hypocalcemic emergencies. *Endocrinol Metab Clin North Am* 1993, **22**:363–375.
2. Ledger GA: Hypocalcemia and hypoparathyroidism. *Curr Ther Endocrinol Metab* 1994, **5**:508–510.

Diagnosis

Symptoms

Sweating, shaking, anxiety, feeling hot, nausea, palpitations, tingling lips: due to sympathetic and adrenergic response to low blood glucose concentration (autonomic).
Dizziness, tiredness, confusion, difficulty speaking, inability to concentrate, headache: due to impaired cerebral cortical function resulting from low blood glucose level.
Hunger, weakness, blurred vision.
Headache, malaise, confusion: posthypoglycemic.

• Patients with recurrent hypoglycemic attacks often present with symptoms of decreased cognitive function or conscious level for which they have no subjective awareness.

Signs

Pallor, diaphoresis, tremor, tachycardia or occasionally bradycardia, increased pulse pressure, dilated pupils: autonomic.
Altered behavior, irrational speech or behavior, slurred speech, irritability, decreased level of consciousness, seizure, coma: neuroglycopenic.
Transient focal neurological defects: posthypoglycemic.

Investigations [1]

For all cases

Blood glucose measurement: confirmed by laboratory measurement, although treatment may be started after bedside capillary blood glucose strip testing; concentration <40 mg/dL, in treated diabetic patients ≤60 mg/dL.

For recurrent or unexplained episodes

Plasma insulin and c-peptide analysis.
Blood and urine screening: for sulfonylureas.
Blood urea nitrogen, creatinine, liver function, insulin antibody tests.
Thyroid and adrenal function tests, gastric emptying studies, growth hormone measurement: to investigate recurrence in treated diabetic patients.

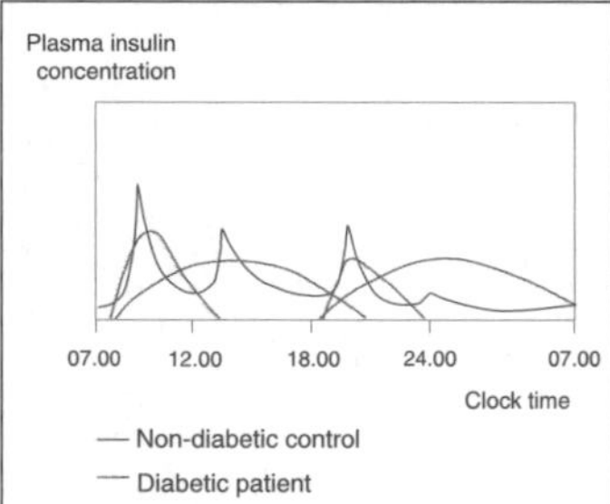

Plasma insulin concentrations over 24 h from a patient on twice-daily injections of mixed exogenous insulins and an approximation of the plasma insulin profile of a nondiabetic person eating 3 meals daily, showing times of risk of hypoglycemia.

For suspected insulinoma

Fasting glucose, insulin, c-peptide, and pro-insulin measurement: repeated during 72-h fast or until hypoglycemia documented; care needed in children, in whom other metabolites should be measured; high c-peptide and insulin suggest insulinoma, sulfonylureas, or insulin autoantibodies (rare); high insulin with low c-peptide indicates exogenous insulin.
CT, celiac axis or mesenteric angiography, endoscopic pancreatic ultrasonography, laparotomy, and perioperative ultrasonography: to localize insulinoma.

For noninsulinoma, nondiabetes related hypoglycemia

09.00 h cortisol and cosyntropin test, growth hormone profile, insulin-like growth factors analysis, liver function tests.

For suspected "reactive" hypoglycemia

Home blood glucose testing: patients must be taught to collect capillary blood samples at home during episodes for later laboratory estimates of blood glucose concentration.

Complications

Trauma: while patient is hypoglycemic.
Seizure.
Loss of subjective awareness of subsequent episodes.
Permanent neurological sequelae: usually only with large insulin overdosage.
Death.

Differential diagnosis

Acute

Other causes of coma or confusion, including the following:
Ketoacidosis, nonketotic hyperosmolar coma, intoxication or poisoning, uremia, epilepsy, stroke, intracranial hemorrhage, meningitis, head injury.

Recurrent

Epilepsy, arrhythmias, psychiatric disorder, pheochromocytoma.

Etiology [2]

• Causes include the following:

Excess insulin action in diabetic patients [3]

Missed, small, or late meals, error in time or dose, exercise (effect may last 18 h), alcohol (delayed effect), hypothyroidism, renal failure, gastroparesis: with pharmacological treatment of diabetes mellitus (insulin, sulfonylureas, rarely metformin).
Vigorous insulin response to rapidly absorbed glucose or gastric surgery: in "reactive or postprandial" hypoglycemia.
Insulinoma, nesidioblastosis.

Excess insulin action in nondiabetic patients

Tumors secreting insulin-like growth factor.
Surreptitious or malicious administration of insulin or sulfonylurea.

Increased insulin sensitivity

Cortisol deficiency.
Growth hormone deficiency.
Hypopituitarism and adrenal insufficiency (especially in children).

Defects of hepatic glucose production

Liver disease.
Alcohol toxicity.
Glycogen storage diseases.
Ketotic hypoglycemia of childhood.
Prematurity.
Defective fatty acid oxidation.

Epidemiology

• 3% of the US population have diabetes mellitus; 10% of these have the insulin-dependent form; 4%–40% experience severe hypoglycemia.
• 10% of insulinomas are multiple, 10% are malignant, 9% with multiple endocrine neoplasia.

Treatment

Diet and lifestyle

• In "reactive hypoglycemia," patients should eat small, regular meals with high complex carbohydrates and should avoid simple sugars.

• In childhood disorders of metabolism, frequent high-carbohydrate, low-fat meals should be eaten.

• In patients with diabetes, regular meals and snacks are essential, with patient-led dosage adjustments for certain situations, *e.g.*, excessive exercise.

Pharmacological treatment [1]

For conscious patients

Rapidly absorbed carbohydrates (20 g, *e.g.*, 4 glucose tablets or ½ glass orange juice), then snack.

Contraindicated for loss of gag reflex or severely impaired level of consciousness.

For confused patients

Oral glucose gel.

Contraindicated for loss of gag reflex or severely impaired level of consciousness.

For unconscious patients

50% glucose, 50 mL, or 20% glucose, 100–150 mL i.v.

In children: 20% dextrose, 2.5 mL/kg.

In infants: 10% dextrose, 2.5 mL/kg.

Alternatively, glucagon, 1 mg i.m., followed by 30 g complex carbohydrate orally on recovery.

• Extravasation of glucose must be avoided.

• If hypoglycemia is due to sulfonylurea treatment, massive insulin overdose, or unknown cause, the patient should be admitted to hospital for observation and i.v. glucose infusion considered.

• Glucagon may not be effective in very undernourished or very alcohol-intoxicated patients.

Treatment aims

To achieve recovery from acute event.

To prevent further episodes.

Other treatments

Surgery for insulinomas, tumors secreting insulin-like growth factor, nesidioblastosis.

Prognosis

• For diabetes, the prognosis is that of the underlying disease, but the patient may be prone to further attacks.

• For tumors secreting insulin-like growth factor, prognosis is poor.

Follow-up and management

Prevention of further episodes

• The diabetes regimen should be adjusted.

• Diazoxide can be given for insulinoma, after the diagnosis is established, pending definitive surgical management.

• Diet regimens should be followed for metabolic defects.

Key references

1. Service FJ: Hypoglycemic disorders. *N Engl J Med* 1995, **332**:1144–1152.
2. Amiel SA: Glucose counterregulation in health and disease: current concepts in hypoglycaemia recognition and response. *Q J Med* 1991, **293**:707–727.
3. Amiel SA: Hypoglycaemia in diabetes mellitus. *Med Int* 1993, **21**:279–280.

Diagnosis

Symptoms

• Symptoms may be due to an underlying cause or to hormone deficiencies, which usually have a gradual onset if secondary to an expanding pituitary lesion and tend to occur in a sequential order: growth hormone, luteinizing or follicle-stimulating hormone, thyroid-stimulating hormone, corticotropic hormone.

Impotence or amenorrhea, decreased libido: due to deficiency of gonadotropins.
Poor growth and development: in children, due to deficiency of growth hormone.
Cold intolerance, weight gain, tiredness, lethargy: due to deficiency of thyroid-stimulating hormone.
Dizziness, nausea, vomiting: due to deficiency of corticotropic hormone.
Urinary frequency, nocturia: due to deficiency of vasopressin.
Headache or visual disturbance: due to macroadenoma.
Galactorrhea: due to prolactinoma or pituitary stalk compression by lesion.

Signs

Small soft testes, loss of pubic and axillary hair: due to deficiency of gonadotropins.
Short stature: in children, due to deficiency of growth hormone.
Cool skin, absent or slow reflexes: due to deficiency of thyroid-stimulating hormone.
Postural hypotension, shock: due to deficiency of corticotropic hormone.
Visual field defect, diplopia or cranial nerve palsies, papilledema, CSF rhinorrhea, excessive hormone production or galactorrhea: indicating macroadenoma.
Signs of acromegaly.

Investigations

Cortisol measurement for adrenal axis: if 09.00 h cortisol >20 μg/dL, significant deficiency improbable; if <2 μg/dL, corticotropic hormone (ACTH) deficiency very probable unless patient is taking steroids; intermediate values need insulin tolerance test to assess ACTH reserve.
Thyroid tests: thyroxine, free thyroxine (T_4), triiodothyronine (T_3), thyroid-stimulating hormone (TSH); secondary hypothyroidism suggested by low T_4 or free T_4 index unaccompanied by raised TSH.
Sex hormone measurement for gonadal axis: *in men:* 09.00 h testosterone, sex hormone-binding globulin (high level can give rise to high total bound testosterone, while free level remains low), luteinizing hormone (LH) or follicle-stimulating hormone (FSH); gonadotropin deficiency suggested by low basal testosterone and no rise of LH/FSH; *in women:* estradiol, sex hormone-binding globulin, LH/FSH, progesterone on day 21 (normal concentration implies normal gonadal axis).
Prolactin test: on 2–3 occasions; hyperprolactinemia may suppress pulsatile gonadotropin secretion in either sex in absence of absolute deficiency.
Growth hormone (GH) measurement: basal values usually undetectable and therefore unhelpful; insulin tolerance or glucagon test necessary to assess GH reserve [1].
Plasma and urine osmolality measurement for posterior pituitary: plasma osmolality >295 mOsm/L and urine : plasma osmolality ratio of <2 : 1 suggest diabetes insipidus.
Insulin tolerance test: to assess ACTH and GH reserve; must be done in a specialized unit; contraindicated in patients with ischemic heart disease, epilepsy, or unexplained blackouts; particular caution in children and elderly patients [2].
Releasing hormone tests: thyrotropin-releasing and gonadotropin-releasing hormone tests only assess only "readily releasable" pool of anterior pituitary hormones and cannot be used to diagnose normality of physiological secretion of the hormone.
Radiography: may show double floor of pituitary fossa due to pituitary enlargement.
MRI or CT of pituitary gland: to visualize macroadenomas and most microadenomas.

Complications

Cardiovascular collapse: resulting from adrenocortical insufficiency.
Expanding pituitary mass: with optic chiasm compression and local invasion of brain.
Hydrocephalus: with third ventricular compression by tumor.
Temporal-lobe epilepsy: with temporal extension of tumor.

Differential diagnosis

Primary adrenal or thyroid insufficiency.
Anorexia nervosa.

Etiology

• Causes include the following:
Pituitary tumors: most common.
Iatrogenic disorders: previous surgery or radiotherapy [3].
Secondary deposits: especially breast, lung.
Infectious disease: *e.g.*, tuberculosis.
Vascular disease: *e.g.*, Sheehan's syndrome, postpartum necrosis.
Severe exercise or malnutrition: may cause reversible loss of gonadotropin-releasing hormone release.

Epidemiology

• The incidence of panhypopituitarism is difficult to determine, but ~1 in 10 000 patients each year develops a pituitary tumor.

Treatment

Diet and lifestyle

• Patients need a steroid card, Medicalert bracelet or necklace, and emergency pack of parenteral hydrocortisone (for deficiencies of pituitary–adrenal axis).

Pharmacological treatment

For deficiencies of pituitary–adrenal axis

Standard dosage Hydrocortisone, 15 mg on waking, 10 mg with evening meal (variable).

Contraindications None.

Special points Response monitored by clinical assessment and hydrocortisone day curve.
For mild cold or sore throat, no change in dosage; with moderate illness manifested primarily with fever, double hydrocortisone dose; with severe illness, especially vomiting or diarrhea, or for perioperative cover, parenteral treatment is needed (hydrocortisone, 100 mg i.m. every 6 h).

Main drug interactions Estrogens increase cortisol-binding globulin and thus hydrocortisone concentration.

Main side effects Iatrogenic Cushing's syndrome due to over-replacement.

For thyroid deficiencies

Standard dosage Thyroxine, 100–150 μg daily.

Contraindications None.

Special points Response monitored by clinical assessment and serum thyroxine and triiodothyronine measurement (if patient taking the latter); 09.00 h cortisol must be >100 4 μg/dL before replacement; can precipitate angina during replacement in patients with ischemic heart disease.

Main drug interactions Estrogens increase thyroid-binding globulin and raise total thyroxine; free thyroxine should be used for monitoring.

Main side effects None.

For growth hormone deficiencies [1]

• Children should be given growth hormone, 2–4 units s.c. daily (0.5 units/kg/week).

• Growth hormone is likely to be of benefit in adults because it improves psychological well-being and muscle strength and decreases adiposity, although expense is an issue.

For deficiencies of pituitary–gonadal axis

Standard dosage *Men:* testosterone enanthate or cypionate, 200 mg i.m. every 2 weeks or 300 mg every 3 weeks; transdermal testosterone patch daily.
Women: ethinyl estradiol, 30 μg daily, and medroxyprogesterone acetate, 5–10 mg on days 1–14 of calendar month.

Contraindications Prostatic cancer, breast cancer.

Special points Response monitored by potency and serum testosterone, menses, and symptoms of estrogen deficiency.

Main drug interactions Estrogen increases many binding globulins and thus total hormone concentrations.

Main side effects Aggression due to over-replacement of testosterone.

For posterior pituitary deficiencies

Standard dosage Desmopressin, 10–20 μg at night by intranasal spray; dose may also be needed in morning.

Contraindications None.

Special points Response monitored by plasma and urine osmolality.

Main drug interactions None.

Main side effects Dilutional hyponatremia due to over-replacement.

Treatment aims

To achieve patient's clinical well-being.

To achieve normal target gland hormone concentrations.

To remove underlying cause.

Other treatments

• Surgery is indicated for the following.

Pituitary tumors.

Visual field defects.

Cranial nerve palsies.

CSF rhinorrhea.

Prognosis

• Accurate and careful hormone replacement restores a normal life expectancy.

Follow-up and management

• Initial close supervision is necessary to ensure the correct dosage.

• Thereafter, patients should be reviewed every 6–12 months.

Key references

1. Cuneo RC, *et al.*: The growth hormone deficiency syndrome in adults. *Clin Endocrinol* 1992, **37**:387–397.
2. Jones SL, *et al.*: An audit of the insulin tolerance test in adult subjects in an acute investigation unit over one year. *Clin Endocrinol* 1994, **41**:123–128.
3. Littley MD, *et al.*: Hypopituitarism following external radiotherapy for pituitary tumors in adults. *Q J Med* 1989, **70**:145–160.

Hypothyroidism

Diagnosis

Symptoms [1]

Weight gain, fatigue, cold intolerance, neck swelling, hoarseness.

Angina, shortness of breath.

Aches and pains, depression, carpal tunnel syndrome.

Dry skin.

Menorrhagia, infertility, galactorrhea secondary to hyperprolactinemia.

Constipation.

Poor growth, mental retardation, delayed puberty: in children.

Signs

Bradycardia, pericardial effusion (rare), cardiac failure.

Hoarseness, deafness, cerebellar ataxia, delayed relaxation of tendon reflexes, psychosis ("myxedema madness").

Anemia: iron-deficiency, normochromic, normocytic, macrocytic, pernicious.

Goiter: small firm diffuse (Hashimoto's thyroiditis), nodular or diffuse (iodine deficiency).

Dry skin, myxedema, vitiligo, erythema *ab igne*.

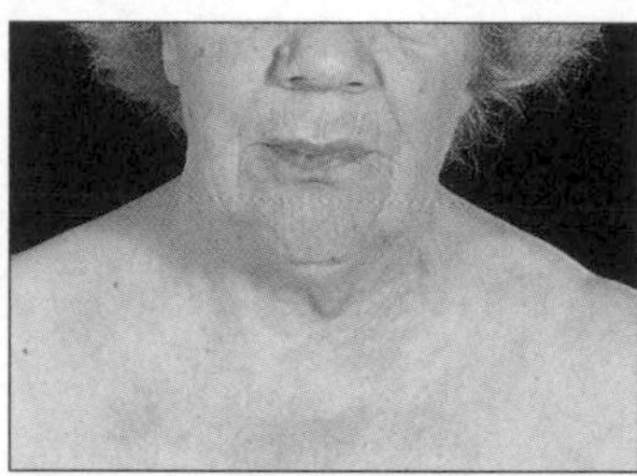

Hypothyroid appearances of an elderly patient with severe untreated Hashimoto's thyroiditis.

Investigations [2]

Serum thyroid hormone measurement: reduction in free or total thyroxine indicates severity of hypothyroidism; serum triiodothyronine usually normal except in severely ill patients, so measurement not helpful.

Serum thyroid-stimulating hormone (TSH) measurement: elevation indicates primary thyroid failure; raised TSH with normal thyroxine is termed "subclinical" hypothyroidism; TSH within or below normal range, with low serum thyroxine, suggests secondary hypothyroidism (hypothalamic/pituitary; same picture seen in "nonthyroidal" illness and treatment by certain drugs, *e.g.*, glucocorticoids).

Autoantibody measurement: antithyroid peroxidase and antithyroglobulin antibodies often present in high titer in Hashimoto's thyroiditis.

Complications

Hypothermia and coma: in severely ill patients, typically in the elderly in cold weather

Hyperlipidemia and ischemic heart disease: associated with longstanding hypothyroidism.

Differential diagnosis

• Middle-aged, overweight, depressed women often appear mildly hypothyroid and should always be screened.

Neurasthenia.
Menstrual disorders.
Weight change.
Anemia.
Unexplained heart failure (unresponsive to digoxin).
Hyperlipidemia.
Unexplained ascites.
Primary amyloidosis.
Depression, primary psychosis, cerebral disorders (arteriosclerosis, tumor).

Etiology [2]

Causes of primary thyroid failure

Autoimmune thyroiditis: Hashimoto's thyroiditis.
Previous treatment by radioiodine or thyroidectomy.
Idiopathic atrophy.
Iodine deficiency.
Antithyroid drugs or excess iodine.
Subacute and silent thyroiditis.
Poor compliance with thyroxine replacement.
Dyshormonogenesis, agenesis, infiltrative disease (uncommon).

Causes of secondary thyroid failure

Disease of pituitary or hypothalamus.

Epidemiology

• The prevalence of hypothyroidism is 5–15 in 1000 females, ~1 in 1000 males.

• In the US, >90% of cases are due to autoimmune thyroiditis, idiopathic atrophy, or previous treatment for hyperthyroidism.

Congenital hypothyroidism

Prevalence: 1 in 5000 infants in US.
Detection: routine screening of all infants.
Possible causes: thyroid agenesis, ectopic or hypoplastic thyroid tissue, inherited disorders or hormonogenesis, transplacental passage of thyroid-stimulating hormone receptor blocking antibodies (such cases resolve spontaneously within 2 months).

Iodine-deficient hypothyroidism

• Iodine deficiency is the major cause of hypothyroidism worldwide. It is typically found in mountainous regions.

• Iodine supplementation programs are effective in abolishing symptoms.

Treatment

Diet and lifestyle

• Long-term ingestion of iodine-containing compounds, *e.g.*, kelp preparations or expectorants, can result in hypothyroidism in adults.

Pharmacological treatment [3–5]

• Thyroxine for patients with symptomatic hypothyroidism; triiodothyronine is used occasionally in patients with myxedema coma to produce more rapid effect.

• Symptoms begin to resolve within 2–3 weeks of the beginning of treatment, but treatment at full dose for 8 weeks may be needed to restore serum thyroid-stimulating hormone to normal.

Standard dosage	Thyroxine, 100–150 μg daily as single dose. Triiodothyronine, 20 μg orally 2–3 times daily.
Contraindications	Caution in severe ischemic heart disease (patient should be admitted to hospital).
Main drug interactions	None.
Main side effects	Generally none; exacerbation of ischemic heart disease may follow initiation of treatment; can precipitate acute adrenal failure in patients with subclinical adrenal disease.

Treatment aims

To relieve symptoms.

To restore serum thyroid-stimulating hormone and thyroxine to normal values.

Prognosis

• Life expectancy is not adversely affected by long-term thyroxine treatment.

• Thyroxine treatment (in doses that reduce serum thyroid-stimulating hormone to below normal) may reduce bone density and may increase risk of osteoporotic fractures.

• Up to 25% of patients in the community prescribed thyroxine have biochemical evidence of undertreatment that may be associated with hyperlipidemia and increased risk of ischemic heart disease.

Follow-up and management

• Serum thyroid-stimulating hormone should be measured 8 weeks after starting treatment to check whether the dose needs to be increased and should be measured annually in patients on established treatment to ensure continuing compliance.

• Treatment is for life, except in mild cases occurring within the first 6 months after radioiodine treatment, pregnancy, or partial thyroidectomy (possibly temporary) and in patients who are hypothyroid secondary to subacute or silent thyroiditis.

Key references

1. Anonymous: Hypothyroidism? *Lancet* 1990, **335**:1316.
2. Lazarus JH, Hall R, eds: Hypothyroidism and goitre. *Ballières Clin Endocrinol Metab* 1988, **2**.
3. Toft AD: Thyroxine therapy. *N Engl J Med* 1994, **331**:174–180.
4. Utiger RD: Therapy of hypothyroidism. When are changes needed? *N Engl J Med* 1990, **323**:126–127.
5. Singer PA, *et al.*: Treatment guidelines for patients with hyperthyroidism and hypothyroidism. Standards of Care Committee, American Thyroid Association. *JAMA* 1995, **273**:808–812.

Infections in hematological malignancy

Diagnosis

Definition

• Infections in hematological malignancy are opportunistic infections that arise during the treatment of hematological malignancy due to the development of neutropenia. Patients are particularly vulnerable when the neutrophil count falls below 0.5×10^9/L.

Symptoms and signs

Fever: the only consistent indication of established infection.

Investigations

• Full examination should always be made, including mouth, pharynx, genitalia, perianal region, and central line sites.

• Surveillance cultures can be predictive of infection, *e.g.*, with *Pseudomonas aeruginosa,* allowing planning of empirical treatment for individual patients and monitoring of prophylaxis, as well as facilitating infection control.

• Stool should be screened, *e.g.*, for parasites, if patient comes from a high-risk area.

Blood cultures: from central line and peripheral vein, for bacteria and fungi.

Hickman swab: if inflamed or cutaneous discharge.

Specimens from clinically suspicious sites.

Urinalysis and culture.

Chest radiography.

CT of thorax: invaluable in invasive aspergillosis.

Bronchoalveolar lavage: especially in bone-marrow transplant patients with dry cough or chest radiography lesions early on.

Skin lesion aspiration: valuable in diagnosis of disseminated fungal infection.

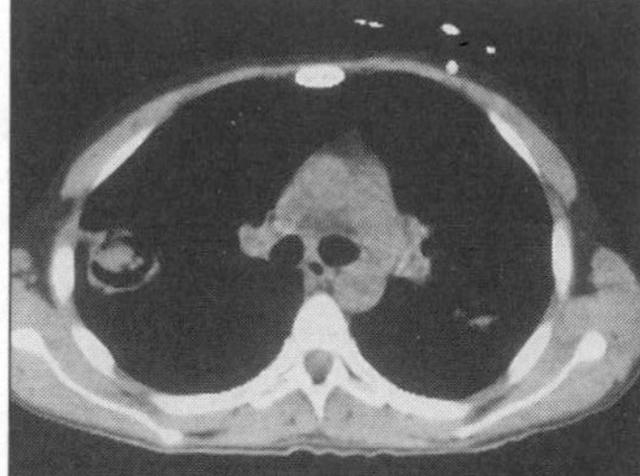

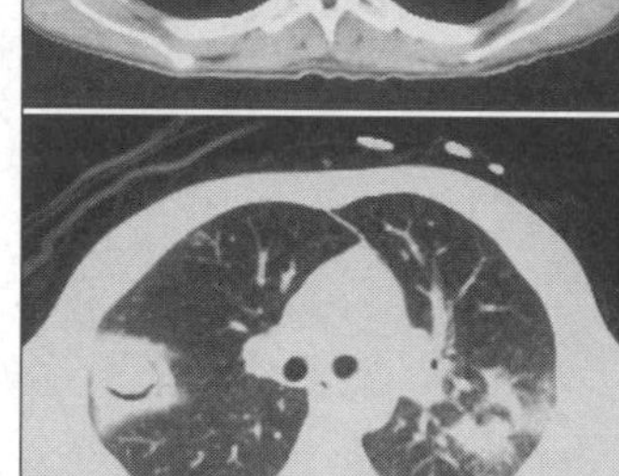

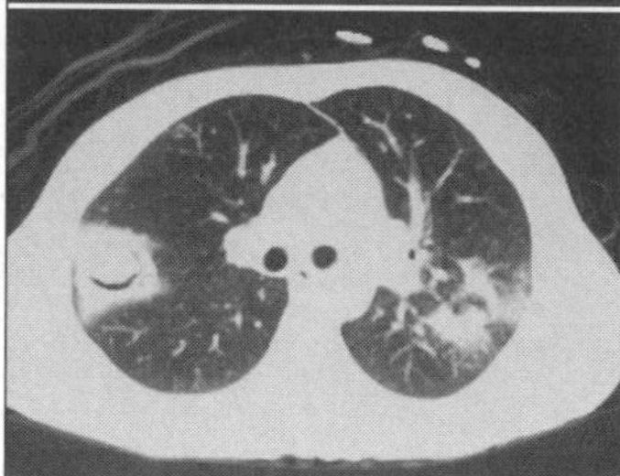

CT of lung with invasive aspergillosis. The mycotic lung sequestrum is usually pleural based and wedged shaped and often shows cavitation.

Complications

• Initially, complications may include those of septicemia, *e.g.*, acute tubular necrosis.

Increased risk of adult respiratory distress syndrome: in patients with *Streptococcus mitis* bacteremia.

Ecthyma gangrenosum in patients with local or disseminated *P. aeruginosa* infection.

Disseminated candidiasis: CT of liver or spleen can be helpful.

Pulmonary infarction or hemorrhage: especially in patients with invasive aspergillosis.

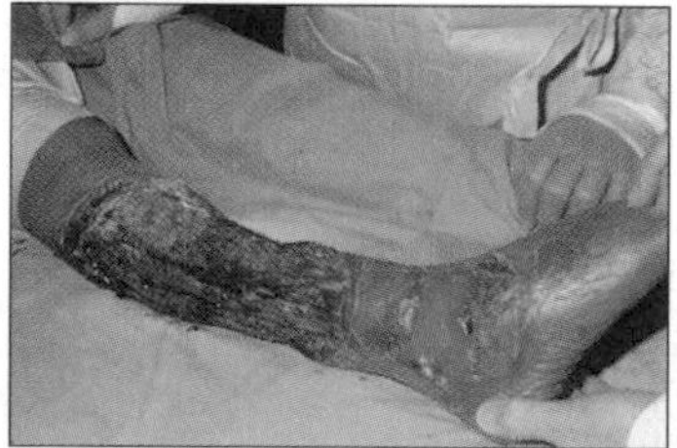

Extensive resection of necrotic tissue of the leg in a child with *Pseudomonas* septicemia and ecthyma gangrenosum.

Differential diagnosis

Reaction to transfusion of blood products.

Drug fever.

Graft-versus-host disease.

Fever associated with underlying disease.

Etiology

Causes of fever

Bacteremia in 20%–30% of patients.

Clinical or nonbacteremic microbiologically documented infection in 30%–40%.

Unexplained in 30%–40%.

Documented focus of infection

Lower respiratory tract (50%).

Upper respiratory tract (20%).

Skin and soft tissue, including perianal (20%–30%).

Urinary tract (<5%).

Predisposing factors for specific infections

Neutropenia: bacterial and fungal.

Lymphopenia: intracellular organisms, *e.g., Toxoplasma gondii, Pneumocystis carinii,* mycobacteria, herpesviruses.

Defects in humoral immunity and splenic hypofunction: encapsulated organisms.

Loss of physical barriers (mucosa, skin): bacteremia, fungemia.

Reservoir of infection (*e.g.*, bronchiectasis): *Pseudomonas* spp.

Geographical considerations: mycobacteria, malaria, strongyloides.

Sources of major pathogens

Staphylococci: skin commensal, cross-infection.

Streptococcus mitis: oral commensal.

Enterobacteriaceae: gut.

Pseudomonas aeruginosa: environment, cross-infection.

Streptococcus pneumoniae: nasopharynx, cross-infection.

Mycobacterium tuberculosis: reactivation.

Pneumocystis carinii: reactivation, possibly cross-infection.

Toxoplasma gondii: reactivation, donor bone marrow.

Candida spp.: oropharynx or gut, cross-infection, parenteral feeding.

Aspergillus spp.: airborne (previous colonization).

Herpes simplex or varicella–zoster virus: reactivation (cross-infection).

Cytomegalovirus: reactivation, blood products.

Epidemiology

• ~1 febrile incident occurs per neutropenic episode (less with quinolone prophylaxis).

Treatment

Diet and lifestyle

• Neutropenic patients must eat a low-pathogen diet but maintain nutrition, *e.g.*, by parenteral route if needed.
• Patients should be given a dental review.
• Hygiene is important for patients and attendants, *e.g.*, hand-washing, cleaning of room and bedding, and i.v. catheter care.
• Water must be treated appropriately to prevent legionella infection.
• Patients must especially avoid exposure to measles and chickenpox; vaccination should be reviewed, but live vaccines must be avoided until immune recovery.

Pharmacological treatment [1,2]

Empirical treatment for pyrexia of unknown origin in neutropenia

• Patients with a fever of 38.5°C or 38°C for 2 h should receive prompt empirical antibiotic treatment: *e.g.*, ceftazidime, or ceftazidime and aminoglycoside, or antipseudomonal penicillin and aminoglycoside. If aminoglycoside was not part of the original regimen and fever persists beyond 24–72 h or clinical deterioration is apparent, add aminoglycoside after reculturing of all potential infection sites. Regardless of initial antibiotic regimen, if fever persists reculture and include vancomycin. Amphotericin B should be added if fever persists beyond 96 h.

Standard dosage	Amphotericin B 1 mg/kg or AmBisome 3–5 mg/kg daily. Ceftazidine 2 g i.v. 8-hourly (adults). Gentamicin 1 mg/kg i.v. 3 times daily. Piperacillin 3–4 g i.v. every 4–6 h. Vancomycin 500 mg i.v. every 6 h or 1 g i.v. every 12 h.
Contraindications	Hypersensitivity; caution in renal impairment; epilepsy, or known intracerebral lesion (imipenem).
Special points	Vancomycin and aminoglycoside dosages may need adjustment.
Main drug interactions	Ototoxicity when combined (uncommon with teicoplanin).
Main side effects	Nephrotoxicity (vancomycin, aminoglycosides, amphotericin). Ototoxicity (vancomycin, aminoglycosides).

Treatment of other specific infections

For most invasive fungal infection: amphotericin B, 0.5–1.5 mg/kg i.v. daily, possibly with 5-flucytosine, or liposomal amphotericin B 1–4 mg/kg daily.
For herpes simplex infection: acyclovir, 5 mg/kg 8-hourly for 7 days.
For varicella-zoster infection: acyclovir, 10 mg/kg 8-hourly for 7 days.
For cytomegalovirus infection: ganciclovir, 5 mg/kg i.v. 12-hourly for 2 weeks, maintained at 5 mg/kg daily for a further 2–3 weeks with immunoglobulin.
For *Pneumocystis carinii* pneumonitis: co-trimoxazole, 120 mg/kg daily in divided doses, with steroids.

Prophylaxis [2]

For gram-negative bacteria: a 4-quinolone, *e.g.*, ciprofloxacin, 250–500 mg orally twice daily, with colistin, 1.5 MU orally.
For gram-positive bacteria: penicillin or macrolide antibiotic.
For mycobacteria (in cases of previous disease, family contact, endemic area): isoniazid 5 mg/kg daily or a 4-quinolone, *e.g.*, ciprofloxacin, 500 mg twice daily.
For legionella: a 4-quinolone, *e.g.*, ciprofloxacin, 500 mg twice daily.
For *Candida albicans* or *Cryptococcus neoformans*: fluconazole, 100–200 mg orally daily.
For *C. glabrata*: amphotericin B suspension, 500 mg orally 6-hourly.
For aspergillosis: air filtration, itraconazole, or amphotericin B, 0.5–1 mg/kg i.v. daily.
For herpes simplex or varicella-zoster virus: acyclovir, 5 mg/kg 8-hourly.
For cytomegalovirus: possibly acyclovir, 10 mg/kg i.v. 8-hourly, ganciclovir (myelosuppression), or foscarnet.
For *Pneumocystis carinii*: co-trimoxazole, 960 mg orally twice daily for 3 days weekly, or aerosolized pentamidine, 150 mg every 2 weeks.
For strongyloidiasis: thiabendazole, 25 mg/kg orally twice daily for 3 days.
For toxoplasmosis: pyrimethamine, 75 mg orally daily (loading dose, 100 mg), with folinic acid, 15 mg 3 times daily, and possibly sulfadiazine, 2 g i.v. or orally 3 times daily.

Treatment aims

To instigate antimicrobial therapy rapidly, using broad-spectrum cidal agents active against the most probable organisms.

Prognosis

• In patients with fever alone, mortality is <5%.
• In patients with fever and pulmonary infiltrates, mortality is 30%–60%.

Follow-up and management

• Subsequent management should take into account the following:
Initial empirical treatment: patients may need addition of a glycopeptide.
Underlying disease and treatment: *Pneumocystis carinii* pneumonia and viral infection (especially cytomegalovirus) with lymphoid disease and bone-marrow transplantation.
Duration of neutropenia: invasive fungal infection increases with time.
Number of previous febrile episodes: increased risk of fungal infection with increased number.
Past history or evidence of latent infection: *e.g.*, invasive aspergillosis, tuberculosis.
Foreign travel, ethnic origin: *e.g.*, risk of malaria, tuberculosis, strongyloidiasis.

Key references

1. Rubin M, Walsh TJ, Pizzo P: Clinical approach to infections in the compromised host. In *Hematology Basic Principles and Practice*. Edited by Hoffman R, Benz E, Shattil S, Furie B, Cohen H. New York: Churchill Livingstone; 1991:1063–1114.
2. Prentice HG, Kibbler CC, MacWhinney PH: Antimicrobial prophylaxis and treatment after chemotherapy or marrow transplantation. In *Recent Advances in Hematology*, vol 6. Edited by Hoffbrand AV, Brenner M. London: Churchill Livingstone; 1991.

Infectious diarrhea

Diagnosis

Symptoms

Liquid stools: >3 movements and over 200 mL per day.

Blood (dysentery): implies active mucosal inflammation.

Abdominal pain: often predefecatory.

Tenesmus: suggests proctitis.

Fever.

Weight loss, malnutrition, dehydration.

Signs

Pyrexia: suggests active mucosal inflammation.

Splenomegaly, rose spots: due to *Salmonella typhi* or *paratyphi* infection.

Borborygmi.

Clinical evidence of dehydration or malnutrition.

Pallor.

Anal rash or excoriation: due to infection by *Enterobius vermicularis* or *Strongyloides stercoralis*.

Investigations

Hematology: peripheral blood eosinophilia suggests invasive helminthic infection.

Fecal microscopy, parasitology, culture: fresh warm specimens yield highest positivity rate for *Entamoeba histolytica*, *Giardia lamblia* (three samples required); stool should also be tested for *Clostridium difficile* toxin and culture.

HIV serology: in patients with risk factors or otherwise negative evaluation [1].

Upper gastrointestinal endoscopy, including duodenal biopsy: for morphology and parasitology in severe cases or when symptoms persist >2 weeks and stool studies are negative.

Small-intestinal radiography: to check for ileocecal tuberculosis (TB) in patients at risk for TB or in those without diagnosis despite extensive evaluation.

Hydrogen breath test: to evaluate for bacterial overgrowth.

Complications

Dehydration, electrolyte disturbance.

Renal failure: due to hypovolemia or sepsis-related acute tubular necrosis.

Anemia: due to hemorrhage.

Gram-negative septicemia: rare.

"Hyperinfection syndrome": due to *Strongyloides stercoralis* infection.

Ileal perforation, hemorrhage: due to salmonellosis.

Mesenteric adenitis or ileitis, nonsuppurative arthritis, ankylosing spondylitis, erythema nodosum, Reiter's syndrome: due to *Yersinia enterocolitica* infection.

Perforation, hemorrhage, Reiter's syndrome, hemolytic uremic syndrome: due to shigellosis.

Acute necrotizing colitis, appendicitis, ameboma, hemorrhage, stricture: due to amebic colitis.

Colonic necrosis: due to pseudomembranous colitis.

Differential diagnosis

Inflammatory bowel disease (usually ulcerative colitis).

Drug-induced diarrhea: laxatives, magnesium compounds, quinidine, prostaglandins.

Lactose intolerance.

Diabetic autonomic neuropathy.

Endocrine-associated diarrhea (*e.g.*, diabetes, hyperthyroidism).

Pheochromocytoma.

Other noninfective causes of bulky, fatty stools (malabsorption): Mediterranean lymphoma (alpha-chain disease), severe malnutrition, intestinal resection, chronic pancreatitis, chronic hepatocellular dysfunction.

Idiopathic diarrhea.

Celiac sprue [2].

Etiology

- Causes include the following:

Travelers' diarrhea: clinical syndrome with many causes including viruses, bacteria, and protozoa.

Food poisoning.

Postinfective malabsorption.

Immunosuppression.

Bacteria: *Aeromonas* spp., *Campylobacter* spp., *Clostridium difficile, Escherichia coli* (including 0157:H7), *Mycobacterium tuberculosis, Plesiomonas shigelloides, Salmonella* spp., *Shigella* spp., *Vibrio* spp., *Yersinia enterocolitica.*

Viruses: adenovirus, astrovirus, Norwalk virus, rotavirus, HIV.

Protozoa: *Entamoeba histolytica, Giardia lamblia, Isospora belli, Cryptosporidium* spp., *Mycobacterium avium-intracellulare.*

Helminths: *Capillaria philippinensis, Enterobius vermicularis, Fasciolopsis buski, Schistosoma mansoni, S. japonicum, Strongyloides stercoralis, Taenia* spp., *Trichuris trichiuria, Ascaris* spp. [3,4].

Epidemiology

- Intestinal infection occurs worldwide.
- Travelers' diarrhea occurs more often in people who have travelled to an area where socioeconomic standards and hygiene are imperfect (including most tropical and subtropical countries), although great geographical variations are found in prevalence rates.

Treatment

Diet and lifestyle

• Food hygiene must be strictly observed: most intestinal infections result from a contaminated environment, commonly food or drink (especially drinking water).

• Avoidance of milk and dairy products frequently diminishes symptoms due to secondary hypolactasia complicating an intestinal infection of any cause.

Pharmacological treatment

• Most infectious diarrheas are self-limiting and require no pharmacological management.

Indications

Travelers' diarrhea: prophylaxis with bismuth subsalicylate; hydration only for loose stools; ciprofloxacin for toxic patients (fever, dehydration) or dysentery, which may require treatment with metronidazole if entamoeba a consideration [5].

Clostridium difficile infection: vancomycin, 125 mg every 6 h for 10 days, or metronidazole, 500 mg 3 times daily for 10 days.

Entamoeba histolytica infection: metronidazole, 500 mg 3 times daily for 10 days.

Giardia lamblia infection: metronidazole, 250–500 mg 3 times daily for 7 days.

Isospora belli infection: trimethoprim-sulfamethoxazole, 160 mg/800 mg 3 times daily for 10 days, then twice daily for 3 weeks.

Salmonella typhi or *paratyphi* infection: ciprofloxacin, chloramphenicol, trimethoprim-sulfamethoxazole, or amoxicillin.

Schistosoma mansoni, japonicum, mekongi, intercalatum, or *matthei* infection: praziquantel.

Strongyloides stercoralis infection: albendazole or thiabendazole.

Cholera, watery (enterotoxigenic) diarrheas: oral rehydration (i.v. in extreme cases, *e.g.*, infection by *Vibrio cholerae*).

Selected regimens

Amoxicillin, 500 mg 3 times daily for 14 days (in *S. typhi* infection, reduced after defervescence).

Ampicillin, 1 g 6-hourly for 14 days.

Chloramphenicol, 50 mg/kg daily in 4 divided doses for 14 days.

Ciprofloxacin, 500–750 mg twice daily for 3 days for severe travelers' diarrhea; for 14 days for *Salmonella* spp.

Albendazole, 400 mg twice daily for 1–3 days; with *S. stercoralis* infection, 3-day course repeated after 3 weeks.

Mebendazole, 100 mg initially (for ascariasis second dose may be needed).

Thiabendazole, 25 mg/kg twice daily for 3 days (longer in "hyperinfection syndrome").

Praziquantel, 40–50 mg/kg initially; for *S. japonicum* infection, 60 mg/kg in three divided doses on a single day.

See manufacturer's current prescribing information for further details.

Treatment aims

To relieve diarrhea, abdominal colic, and other intestinal symptoms.

To rehydrate patient as rapidly as possible, preferably orally.

To ensure bacteriological or parasitic cure.

To return patient's nutritional status to normal, especially when clinically overt malabsorption has accompanied infection.

To prevent recurrences, especially of *Salmonella typhi* or *paratyphi* infections.

To relieve symptoms in untreatable immunosuppressed patients.

Prognosis

• In some severe infections (*e.g.*, shigellosis, *Entamoeba histolytica* colitis), specific chemotherapy results in complete recovery in almost all patients.

• If surgery is necessary for complications, the prognosis is less favorable.

Follow-up and management

• Most intestinal infections are acute; follow-up is unnecessary.

• *Salmonella typhi* or *paratyphi* infections should be followed up in order to establish that the carrier state has not ensued.

• Patients with overt malabsorption as a secondary manifestation of an intestinal infection should be followed up for maintenance therapy and ascertainment of ultimate cure.

Key references

1. Smith PD, *et al.*: Gastrointestinal infections in AIDS. *Ann Intern Med* 1992, **116**:63–77.
2. Gracey M (ed): *Diarrhea*. Boca Raton: CRC Press; 1991.
3. Gorbach SL, Bartlett JG, Blacklow NR (eds): *Infectious Diseases*. Philadelphia: WB Saunders; 1992.
4. Cook GC: *Parasitic Disease in Clinical Practice*. London: Springer-Verlag; 1990.
5. DuPont HL, Ericsson CD: Prevention and treatment of travelers' diarrhea. *N Engl J Med* 1993, **328**:1821–1827.

Diagnosis

Symptoms

Dyspnea: on exertion, progressive.

Cough: usually unproductive and irritating.

Signs

Clubbing: in many patients.

Fine late inspiratory crackles: at lung base, later throughout lungs.

Cyanosis: especially on effort.

Late right ventricular heave, right ventricular gallop, loud pulmonary second sound, raised jugular venous pulse, peripheral edema: signs of cor pulmonale.

Investigations [1,2]

Chest radiography: shows small lung fields, irregular nodular or reticulonodular opacities; often maximal in lower zones, honeycombing in severely ill patients, pulmonary artery enlargement, and cardiomegaly with cor pulmonale.

High-resolution CT: sensitive; may detect disease when chest radiograph normal; characteristically shows subpleural area of increased density, with central sparing; distortion of bronchi and cystic air spaces in advanced disease.

Radionuclide scanning: ^{67}Ga taken up by macrophages appears as hot spots; occasionally used in staging.

Pulmonary function tests: restrictive ventilatory defect, with low lung volumes, decreased lung compliance, and reduced carbon monoxide transfer.

Arterial blood gas analysis: may be normal in patients with mild disease; partial oxygen pressure typically falls on exercise. Severe hypoxia in severe disease.

Bronchoalveolar lavage: increased cell counts in bronchoalveolar fluid; raised lymphocyte count may indicate better response to treatment.

Lung biopsy: open lung biopsy gold standard but inappropriate in very ill or elderly patients; transbronchial, percutaneous, needle biopsy may produce smaller specimens, inadequate for useful histological analysis.

Hematology and biochemistry: usually unhelpful; ESR may be raised; globulin or immunoglobulin (one or more classes) concentrations often raised; 30% of patients positive for rheumatoid or antinuclear antibody.

Complications [3]

Death: ~60% of patients die as direct consequence of fibrosing lung disease (some with terminal infection, others from respiratory failure).

Pulmonary hypertension, right heart failure: clinically evident in some patients.

Lung cancer: apparent excess in patients with interstitial fibrosis (smokers and non-smokers).

Differential diagnosis [4]

• Many conditions of known cause have a tendency to develop into interstitial fibrosis.

Fibrogenic dust inhalation: *e.g.*, silica, asbestos.

Granulomas: due to extrinsic allergic alveolitis, berylliosis, sarcoidosis.

Chronic exudates: *e.g.*, chronic left ventricular failure, drugs, chronic renal failure.

Etiology

• The cause of many interstitial lung diseases is unknown.

• Interstitial fibrosis is characterized by an inflammatory exudate of the alveolar wall, with a tendency to form fibrosis.

• Interstitial fibrosis can occur alone or be associated with connective tissue disorders of unknown cause, *e.g.*, systemic sclerosis, SLE, rheumatoid arthritis, polymyositis.

• Certain drugs, *e.g.*, bleomycin, methotrexate, and amiodarone, can produce a picture similar to that of interstitial fibrosis.

• Certain viral agents, *e.g.*, influenza A2 virus, have been reported as inducing interstitial fibrosis.

Epidemiology

• Interstitial fibrosis is manifest mostly in middle age, often between 50–70 years.

• The prevalence is estimated to be 3–5 in 100 000 population.

Treatment

Diet and lifestyle

- Morbidity is increased, with progressive restriction of daily activities.
- Diet has no effect.

Pharmacological treatment [5]

- The minimum duration of treatment is unknown.

Corticosteroids

- 30%–50% of patients have some symptomatic benefit, at least short-term, from steroids; no more than 20% show objective radiographic or physiological improvement.

Standard dosage	Prednisone, 60 mg daily for 2–3 months; reduced slowly to maintenance dose if condition responsive.
Contraindications	Uncontrolled hypertension, diabetes mellitus, infection, severe osteoporosis.
Main drug interactions	None.
Main side effects	Weight gain, edema, bruising, purple striae in skin (especially of abdomen), moon face, osteoporosis, collapse of vertebrae, diabetes mellitus, hypertension, myopathy (especially proximal girdle muscles), hirsutism, menstrual disturbances, psychotic reactions, cataracts, withdrawal phenomena.

Cyclophosphamide

- Many patients fail to respond to high-dose steroids alone; in patients who continue to deteriorate, low-dose prednisone can be combined with cyclophosphamide, an immunosuppressant drug.

Standard dosage	Cyclophosphamide, 2 mg/kg daily with prednisone.
Contraindications	Severe renal impairment, porphyria.
Special points	Clinical improvement not expected within 2 months of starting treatment.
Main drug interactions	Muscle relaxants.
Main side effects	Hemorrhagic cystitis, bone-marrow suppression, alopecia.

Other drugs

- D-Penicillamine, azathioprine, colchicine, and methotrexate have proved disappointing.

Supportive treatment

Supplemental oxygen.

Diuretics for heart failure.

Opiates for suppression of cough and alleviation of breathlessness.

Treatment aims

To improve quality of life by preventing deterioration of lung function.

To relieve symptoms.

To give maximum supportive care, including counseling, when symptomatic relief not possible.

Other treatments

- Lung transplantation is indicated for patients with rapidly progressive disease and young patients who do not respond to conventional treatment.

Prognosis [6]

- Mortality within 5 years of diagnosis is 50%.
- Probable responders usually have a more cellular histological response.
- Improved survival may be achieved if the disease is detected early and more precise predictors of progression are developed to prevent high-risk patients, in whom more aggressive treatment would be justified.
- The 1-year survival rate after single-lung transplantation is 50%.

Follow-up and management

- The response should be assessed by clinical, subjective, and objective changes in chest radiography and pulmonary function tests.

Key references

1. Schwartz DA, *et al.*: Determinants of progression in idiopathic pulmonary fibrosis. *Am J Respir Crit Care Med* 1994, **149**:444–449.
2. Terriff BA, *et al.*: Fibrosing alveolitis: chest radiography and CT as predictors of clinical and functional impairment at follow-up in 26 patients. *Radiology* 1992, **184**:445–449.
3. Panos R, *et al.*: Clinical deterioration in patients with idiopathic pulmonary fibrosis: causes and assessment. *Am J Med* 1990, **88**:396–404.
4. Muller N: Differential diagnosis of chronic diffuse infiltrative lung disease on high-resolution computed tomography. *Semin Roentgenol* 1991, **26**:132–142.
5. Raghu G: Idiopathic pulmonary fibrosis: a rational clinical approach. *Chest* 1987, **92**:148–154.
6. Schwartz DA, *et al.*: Determinants of survival in idiopathic pulmonary fibrosis. *Am J Respir Crit Care Med* 1994, **149**:450–454.

Intracerebral hemorrhage

Diagnosis

Symptoms

Headache, nausea, vomiting, drowsiness: due to raised intracranial pressure.

Seizure: due to lobar hematoma, in 28%–30% of patients.

Diplopia, gaze impairment, hiccoughs, dysarthia, facial hyperesthesia: due to brain stem hematoma.

Signs

Confusion, coma, papilledema: due to raised intracranial pressure.

Hemiplegia, aphasia, homonymous visual-field defects: due to cortical or subcortical hematomas.

Vertical-gaze palsy, skew deviation of eyes, miotic unreactive pupils: due to thalamic hematoma.

III nerve palsy, skew deviation of eyes: due to midbrain hematoma.

Horizontal-gaze palsy, pin-point reactive pupil, hyperpyrexia: due to pontine hematoma.

Ipsilateral V–VII nerve palsy, ataxia or nystagmus: due to cerebellar hematoma.

Investigations [1]

• Laboratory tests are not diagnostic but may identify underlying abnormalities.

Hematology profile: to identify bleeding disorders.

Clotting profile: to identify disorders of coagulation.

ESR and antinuclear antibody measurement: to identify vasculitic disorders.

CT of brain with bone windows: to identify skull fractures, hemorrhage, hydrocephalus, or edema; after 2 weeks, may be indistinguishable from infarct.

MRI of brain: examination of choice for cavernous angiomas; may help in identifying multiple lesions in patients with intracerebral metastasis.

Four-vessel angiography: to identify aneurysms (causing subarachnoid hemorrhage) or arteriovenous malformations; four-vessel because, in 20%–25% of patients, several aneurysms may be present.

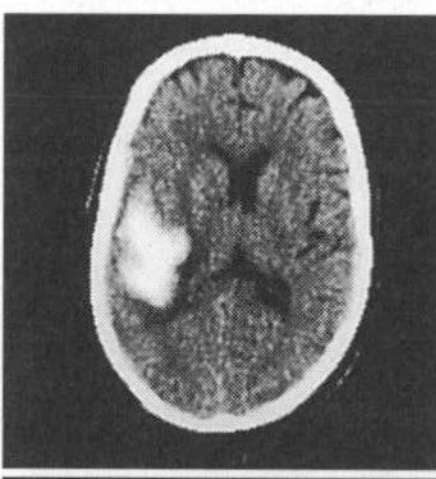

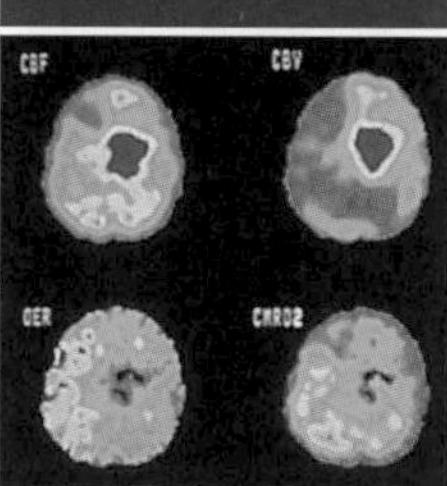

Intracerebral hemorrhage (*top*); fractional images of large arteriovenous malformation (*bottom*).

Complications

Tentorial herniation: with large supratentorial hematoma; herniation from below may occur rarely with large brain stem or cerebellar hematoma.

Foramen magnum herniation: preterminal event with large hematoma.

Hydrocephalus: with ventricular extension of hemorrhage from extrinsic pressure on CSF pathways, especially at aqueduct level and in cerebellar, caudate (75%), and thalamic hemorrhages.

Hyperpyrexia: usually in preterminal pontine hemorrhage.

Seizures: subcortical hematoma, which isolates strip of cortex.

Rebleed and vasospasm: in subarachnoid hemorrhage, risk of bleeding again is 35% within 1 month, with 42% mortality; vasospasm causing cerebral ischemia occurs ~5 days after subarachnoid hemorrhage and may last ≥2 weeks.

Differential diagnosis

Hemorrhagic infarction: usually maximal neurodeficit from onset, raised intracranial pressure improbable, source of emboli present, CT showing mottled attenuation with minimal mass effect.

Subarachnoid hemorrhage: sudden (thunderclap) headache often preceded by warning (sentinel) headache (30%–60%), meningism with possible neck stiffness, photophobia, III (posterior communicating artery aneurysm) or VI nerve palsies, confusion and emotional lability (anterior communicating artery aneurysm).

Hemorrhage into brain tumor: papilledema, multiple-site hemorrhages, mass effect, noncontrasted CT showing high-density hemorrhage surrounding low-density center.

Etiology

• Causes include the following:

Hypertensive intracerebral hemorrhage.

Vascular malformations.

Bleeding into intracranial tumor.

Anticoagulant treatment (8%–11% increased risk) and hemorrhagic disorders.

Sympathomimetic drugs (amphetamine, phenylpropanolamine).

Trauma.

Cerebral amyloid angiopathy (history of dementia in 10%–30%, rare before 55 years).

Granulomatous vasculitis of CNS.

Necrotizing systemic vasculitis.

Epidemiology [2]

• Intracerebral hemorrhage accounts for 10% of all strokes.

• Putaminal hemorrhage is the most usual variety of intracerebral hemorrhage (35%).

• Other common sites include the globus pallidus and pons.

Treatment

Diet and lifestyle

• No special precautions are necessary.

Pharmacological treatment

• Lack of prospective data on intracerebral hemorrhage treatment has led to most patients being treated nonsurgically. A national trial of surgical vs. medical management is currently underway.

For hypertension

• Severe hypertension should be treated to maintain mean arterial pressure between 60 and 70 mm Hg.

• Intravenous beta blockers with additional alpha-blocking action (labetalol) and diuretics are useful.

• Nitroprusside, hydralazine, and calcium antagonists should be avoided in the first week; these are cerebral vasodilators and may worsen intracerebral pressure.

Standard dosage	Labetalol, 2 mg/min i.v. infusion, 50–200 mg total.
Contraindications	Asthma, heart block.
Special points	Upright position must be avoided for 3 h after infusion.
Main drug interactions	Antiarrhythmics.
Main side effects	Postural hypotension.

For seizures

• Routine prophylaxis is not justified.

• Tonic-clonic convulsions need urgent control.

Standard dosage	Diazepam, 10–20 mg i.v., and phenytoin, 1 g i.v. over 30–45 min, with cardiac monitoring.
Contraindications	None of importance.
Special points	May precipitate in 5% glucose solution.
Main drug interactions	None of importance.
Main side effects	Nausea, vomiting, mental confusion.

For coagulopathies

• Patients should be given fresh frozen plasma, vitamin K, or platelet infusion.

For raised intracerebral pressure

• If facilities permit, intracerebral pressure can be monitored, and cerebral perfusion pressure (blood pressure minus intracerebral pressure) can be measured.

• Current techniques for measuring intracerebral pressure are invasive and have a 2%–8% risk of intracranial infection.

• Intracerebral pressure should be maintained <20–25 mm Hg.

Standard dosage	Mannitol, 0.5 g/kg i.v. initially, with furosemide or subsequent albumin infusion.
Contraindications	Congestive cardiac failure, pulmonary edema.
Special points	Mannitol should not be used when serum osmolality is >320 mOsm/L.
Main drug interactions	None of importance.
Main side effects	Chills, fever.

• Hyperventilation is indicated to maintain arterial carbon dioxide concentration at 3.5 kPa; excessive hyperventilation may produce cerebral ischemia.

• Corticosteroids have no role in the management of raised intracerebral pressure caused by hemorrhage.

Treatment aims

To reverse neurodeficit.
To prevent complications.

Other treatments

• Direct evacuation of hematoma, ventricular drainage for hydrocephalus, or surgical obliteration for aneurysm is indicated for the following:
Cerebellar hemorrhage if signs of tegmental compression, hematoma 3 cm in diameter (on CT), hydrocephalus or obliteration of quadrigeminal cisterns.
Lobar hemorrhage (hematoma volume 20–40 mL), with progressive deterioration (100% mortality with medical treatment).
Acute hydrocephalus.
Subarachnoid hemorrhage: direct clipping aneurysms, thrombosis for giant aneurysms.
Hemorrhage from arteriovenous malformation: pre- and intraoperative embolization and staged resection.

Prognosis

• Large hematoma with progressive neurological deficits, coma at presentation, or ventricular extension has poor prognosis (overall mortality, 25%–60%).

• Large pontine hemorrhage is usually fatal within 24–48 h.

• Caudate hemorrhage usually has a benign outcome despite ventricular extension and hydrocephalus.

Follow-up and management

• In patients needing anticoagulation after surgical treatment, aspirin can be started a few days after surgery, warfarin probably after 1 month unless mechanical valve necessitates earlier treatment.

• CT is mandatory if neurological deterioration occurs.

Key references

1. Kase CS: Intracerebral hemorrhage. In *Neurology in Clinical Practice*. Edited by W.G. Bradley, *et al*. Oxford: Butterworth Heinemann; 1991:940–954.
2. Mohr JP, *et al*.: The Harvard cooperative stroke registry: a prospective registry. *Neurology* 1978, **28**:754–762.

Diagnosis

Symptoms

• Criteria for irritable bowel syndrome are continuous or recurrent symptoms for at least 3 months consisting of abdominal pain and disturbed defecation (*i.e.*, at least two of the following: altered stool frequency, form, or passage; passage of mucus).

Abdominal pain: often intermittent, crampy lower abdominal pain; relieved by defecation or passage of flatus; associated with change in frequency or consistency of stool.

Straining, urgency, passage of mucus, feeling of incomplete evacuation.

Loose stools: often in morning or after meals, rarely nocturnal.

Constipation: small, hard stools, difficult to pass.

Abdominal distension: bloating worse after meals and at end of day, relieved by defecation or passage of flatus.

Signs

Variable abdominal tenderness: often over palpable sigmoid colon; frequently present but nonspecific.

• Structural abnormalities such as a mass, ascites, or organomegaly suggest an alternative diagnosis.

Investigations

Screening tests

Full blood count: anemia or leukocytosis suggests an alternative diagnosis.

Liver function tests: abnormal tests suggest an alternative diagnosis.

Thyroid function tests: for myxedema manifest as constipation, or thyrotoxicosis as diarrhea.

Colonic imaging: barium enema or colonoscopy; for new or different symptoms in patients aged >40 years to exclude colonic carcinoma or inflammatory bowel disease. The barium enema or colonoscopy should be normal in patients with irritable bowel syndrome.

Further tests

Small-bowel contrast studies, gastroscopy, abdominal ultrasonography or CT, duodenal or jejunal biopsy or aspiration: in selected cases to exclude Crohn's disease, peptic ulcer, biliary or pancreatic disease.

Colonic biopsy, fecal fat analysis, breath hydrogen test, lactose tolerance test, laxative screening: may be useful in patients with diarrhea predominantly to exclude collagenous colitis, steatorrhea, small-bowel overgrowth, bile-acid malabsorption, or laxative abuse.

Plain abdominal radiography, colonic transit timing, full-thickness colonic biopsy, or defecography: may be useful in patients with constipation predominantly to exclude megacolon, idiopathic slow-transit constipation, neuromuscular gut disorders, obstructed defecation.

Assessment of mental health: a history of previous physical or sexual abuse is relatively common, particularly in women with functional abdominal complaints.

Complications

Increased incidence of colonic diverticulosis: caused by prolonged constipation.

Major physical and psychological morbidity: frequent in intractable cases.

Differential diagnosis

Colonic malignancy.

Inflammatory bowel disease: Crohn's and ulcerative colitis.

Diverticular or celiac disease.

Infections: *e.g.*, by *Giardia* spp.

Pancreatic disorder: *e.g.*, chronic pancreatitis.

Gastric disorders: *e.g.*, peptic ulcer.

Biliary and liver disease: *e.g.*, gallstones.

Congenital or acquired motility disorder, bile-acid malabsorption, bacterial overgrowth, laxative abuse (rarer).

Endometriosis, ovarian malignancy.

Hydronephrosis.

Thyroid disease.

Etiology

• Possible causes include the following:

Abnormal gut motility.

Enhanced visceral sensitivity.

Abnormal central pain perception.

Psychological or psychiatric disorder.

Food allergy or intolerance.

Epidemiology

• Irritable bowel syndrome is common and occurs world wide (10%–20% of population in industrialized countries).

• It occurs more frequently in women.

• Up to 50% of gastroenterological referrals are for irritable bowel syndrome.

Organic or functional bowel disease

• The following features should not be considered part of irritable bowel syndrome without investigation:

Change of bowel habit: new gastrointestinal symptoms in patients aged >40 years.

Weight loss.

Rectal bleeding or nocturnal diarrhea.

Fever.

Abnormal hematology or biochemistry results.

Psychological factors

• 50% of patients have a psychiatric abnormality.

• Anxiety, depression, and personality disorders are common.

• Adverse life events may precede symptoms.

• Psychological factors may determine who consults doctors rather than cause the condition.

Treatment

Diet and lifestyle

- Patients should be encouraged to maintain a high fiber diet.
- A food-intake diary may identify certain foods that often aggravate symptoms.
- Regular exercise improves bowel function.

Pharmacological treatment

- Placebo response rates are high (range, 20%–70%).
- Few drugs have been proved to be of unequivocal benefit; many patients, however, find drugs helpful in controlling symptoms, often preferring "as-required" medication to long-term usage [1,2].
- Treatment should be targeted to predominant complaint.
- Dosage should be as low as possible because patients often report side effects.

Bulking agents

- These are useful mostly for constipation.
- The full effect may not be apparent for several days.

Standard dosage	Bran ispaghula husk, or psyllium titrated to achieve ~1 bowel movement each day. Lactulose, 15 mL twice daily, increased as needed for patients with a major component of constipation; stimulant laxatives are rarely needed for intractable cases.
Contraindications	Intestinal obstruction.
Special points	Patients must take adequate fluid.
Main drug interactions	None.
Main side effects	Distension, flatulence, abdominal pain.

Antispasmodics

- Antispasmodics, either with anticholinergic properties or direct muscle relaxants, are given for pain relief.

Standard dosage	*Anticholinergics:* dicyclomine, 10–20 mg up to 3 times daily, or scopolamine, 20 mg up to 4 times daily. *Direct relaxants:* peppermint oil, 1 capsule up to 3 times daily.
Contraindications	Paralytic ileus, ulcerative colitis. *Anticholinergics:* glaucoma.
Special points	Dosage times should be varied to suit the individual.
Main drug interactions	*Anticholinergics:* disopyramide, cisapride, antidepressants.
Main side effects	*Anticholinergics:* dry mouth, blurring of vision, palpitations, constipation. *Direct relaxants:* heartburn.

Antidiarrheal drugs

- The diarrhea must be confirmed (not pseudodiarrhea or fecal retention with overflow).

Standard dosage	Loperamide, 2–16 mg daily in divided doses or diphenoxylate and atropine, 2 tablets 3–4 times daily; dose adjusted to control symptoms.
Contraindications	Intestinal obstruction, inflammatory bowel disease.
Special points	Night-time dosage might prevent morning diarrhea.
Main drug interactions	*Diphenoxylate/atropine:* anxiolytics and hypnotics.
Main side effects	*Diphenoxylate/atropine:* constipation, dependence.

Other options

Motility stimulants: prostaglandins may be useful in constipation.

Antidepressants: tricyclic antidepressants (*e.g.*, amitriptyline, 25 mg at night) can be helpful, but side effects and excess sedation limit use.

5-HT uptake inhibitors: *e.g.*, fluoxetine, 20 mg daily, effective and less sedating.

Treatment aims

To control or cure the most intrusive complaint.

To treat associated psychological disorders [3].

Other treatments

- Behavioral therapy (hypnotherapy, psychotherapy, relaxation techniques) is effective for some intractable cases.
- Benefit is seen especially in younger patients or those with identifiable psychological disease or stress and recent symptom onset.
- Behavioral therapy is ineffective for older patients or constant or chronic pain sufferers [4].

Prognosis

- This is a chronic relapsing condition.
- >75% of patients respond to treatment over 1 year.
- ~50% have a few symptoms after 5 years.
- Response is better in men, constipation-predominant sufferers, and those with a short history or symptoms after acute diarrhea.

Follow-up and management

- Follow-up is not needed for mild or moderate cases.
- Patients must be monitored for change in symptoms; new or different complaints should be investigated; persistent symptoms do not need further tests.
- Regular, brief review of intractable cases may reduce inappropriate investigation and further referral.

Key references

1. Lynn RB, Friedman LS: Irritable bowel syndrome. *N Engl J Med* 1993, **329**:1940–1945.
2. Thompson WG: Irritable bowel syndrome: pathogenesis and management. *Lancet* 1993, **341**:1569–1572.
3. Camilleri M, Prather CM: The irritable bowel syndrome: mechanisms and a practical approach to management. *Ann Intern Med* 1992, **116**:1001–1008.
4. Heaton KW, *et al.*: Symptoms of irritable bowel syndrome in a British urban community: consulters and non-consulters. *Gastroenterology* 1992, **102**:1962–1967.

Kaposi's sarcoma in AIDS

Diagnosis

Symptoms

Mucocutaneous
Pain, restricted movement: due to flexion contractures and bulk of tumor; late-stage.

Lymphatic
Painful lymphadenopathy and edema.

Pulmonary
• Patients may be asymptomatic; the disease is found *post mortem.*

Dyspnea, hemoptysis, chest pain (pleuritic or dull ache).

Gastrointestinal
• Up to 50% of patients are asymptomatic; the disease is found *post mortem.*

Anorexia, abdominal pain, hematemesis, melena.

Signs

Mucocutaneous
Pink, violacious, purple, brown, or black macule, plaque, or nodule.
Surrounding purple/yellow halo.

Lymphatic
Firm or indurated lymphadenopathy.
Edema of dependent limbs.
Compression of adjacent structures.

Pulmonary
Chest clear or with effusion or scattered rales.
Respiratory failure.

Oral Kaposi's sarcoma in HIV disease

Gastrointestinal
Signs of intermittent or acute bowel obstruction.
Palpable mass.

Other signs
Organomegaly.

Investigations

General
Lymphocyte subset analysis: Kaposi's sarcoma can occur at any stage; tends to be more aggressive in immunosuppressed patients (CD4 count $<200 \times 10^6$/L).
Full blood count: to assess anemia; neutrophil and platelet count needed before chemotherapy.
Skin biopsy: for confirmation.

Pulmonary
Chest radiography: may be normal or reveal infiltrates, nodules, or pleural effusion.
Fiberoptic bronchoscopy: for visualization and biopsy.

Gastrointestinal
Fiberoptic endoscopy or sigmoidoscopy: for visualization and biopsy.
Ultrasonography or CT: with guided biopsy, if disease is not seen by endoscopy.

Complications

Ulceration, infection, immobilization edema.

Gastrointestinal obstruction, hemorrhage.

Respiratory failure.

Differential diagnosis
Purpura, hematoma, angioma, nevus.

Bacillary angiomatosis, dermatofibroma, melanoma.

Etiology
• The cause is unknown, but the following may have a role:

Genetic predisposition (elderly men from eastern Europe and Africa).

Immunosuppression.

HIV infection.

Growth factors and cytokines promoting growth of Kaposi's sarcoma.

Possibly, a transmitted cofactor (perhaps sexually transmitted).

Possibly, a new human herpesvirus.

Epidemiology
• Kaposi's sarcoma occurs in up to 48% of homosexual men with AIDS.

• It is increasing in heterosexual Africans with AIDS, in women who have acquired HIV from bisexual men, and in other risk groups.

• It is rare in children with AIDS.

• It is rarely seen in hemophiliac patients with AIDS.

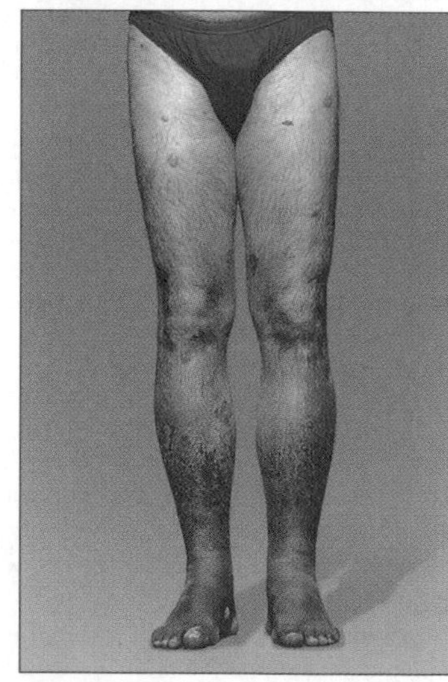

Generalized cutaneous Kaposi's sarcoma.

Treatment

Diet and lifestyle

• No special precautions are necessary.

Pharmacological treatment

• All treatment must be given under specialist supervision.

Intralesional chemotherapy

• Intralesional chemotherapy is indicated for limited mucocutaneous disease.

Standard dosage	Vinblastine into lesion until blanching occurs.
Contraindications	Infection at site.
Main drug interactions	None of importance.
Main side effects	Local pain and ulceration.

Interferon

• Interferons are indicated for good-prognosis Kaposi's sarcoma.

Standard dosage	Interferon-α, i.m. or s.c. daily, possibly with zidovudine.
Contraindications	Bone-marrow suppression, renal or hepatic impairment.
Special points	Lesions may recur after treatment stops.
Main drug interactions	None of importance.
Main side effects	Influenza-like symptoms, neutropenia, anemia.

Bleomycin and vincristine

• These are the first-line chemotherapy in the US for patients with visceral disease or rapidly progressive cutaneous disease.

Standard dosage	Vincristine (or vinblastine if neuropathy develops) and bleomycin every 2 weeks, with hydrocortisone.
Contraindications	Pregnancy and lactation (all), severe lung impairment (bleomycin); caution if patient has a neuropathy.
Main drug interactions	Increased phenytoin concentrations.
Main side effects	*Bleomycin*: rashes, increased skin pigmentation, Raynaud's phenomenon, hypersensitivity reaction, dose-related progressive pulmonary fibrosis. *Vincristine*: alopecia, peripheral and autonomic neuropathy. *Vinblastine*: myelotoxic, neurotoxic (less than vincristine).

Liposomal daunorubicin and doxorubicin

• Liposomal daunorubicin and doxorubicin are currently available within clinical trials or for compassionate use only; they are fairly widely used in the US.

Treatment aims

To achieve cosmetic improvement (limited disease).

To control new lesion development and to treat existing lesions (advancing disease).

To reduce tumor bulk and to treat pain, immobility, and infection (advanced disease).

Other treatments

• Radiotherapy under specialist supervision is the treatment of choice unless control of new lesion is required; it is often combined with chemotherapy.

• Side effects include erythema, increased pigmentation.

Prognosis

• Prognosis is extremely variable; survival may be for months or years.

• Death is often due to other AIDS-defining illnesses.

• Factors indicating poor prognosis include the following:

CD4 count <200 × 10^6/L.

Previous opportunistic infections.

"B" symptoms.

Tumor-associated edema.

Nonnodal visceral Kaposi's sarcoma.

Follow-up and management

• Full blood count must be monitored.

• Patients with limited disease must be followed up every 3 months.

• Patients with extensive disease must be followed up every 1–2 weeks.

General references

Cohen J: Is a new virus the cause of KS? *Science* 1994, **266**:1803–1804.

Lilenbaum RC, Ratner L: Systemic treatment of Kaposi's sarcoma: current status and future directions. *AIDS* 1994, **8**:141–151.

Milliken S, Boyle M: Update on HIV and neoplastic disease. *AIDS* 1993, **7 (suppl 1)**: 203–209.

Diagnosis

Symptoms and signs

• Any organ or tissue can be infected, so the clinical picture can vary enormously.

• The disease follows a biphasic course: the incubation period lasting 7–12 days (range, 2–20 days) is followed by the septicemic phase lasting 4–7 days, which precedes the immune phase lasting 4–30 days.

Anicteric leptospirosis

• This occurs in 90% of patients.

• Onset is abrupt.

Fever, headache, myalgia, malaise, prostration.

Abdominal pain, nausea, vomiting, occasionally diarrhea.

Excruciating headache: usually heralds meningitis in immune stage.

Joint pains, myalgia, conjunctival suffusion, rashes, lymphadenopathy: common findings.

Lymphocytic meningitis: usually lasting a few days, never fatal.

Icteric leptospirosis (Weil's syndrome)

• This form occurs in 10% of patients.

Impaired renal and hepatic function: with anuria and deepening jaundice.

Hepatosplenomegaly, severe hemorrhages into skin, pleura, peritoneum, or gastrointestinal tract.

Vascular collapse and alterations in consciousness.

Myocarditis, hemorrhage, adult respiratory distress syndrome, multiorgan failure: causing death in 10%–20% of icteric patients.

Investigations

• Diagnosis is confirmed by isolation of the organism or detection of a rise in antibody titers.

Isolation: special media needed; organisms isolated from blood or CSF during septicemic phase and from urine during third week in untreated patients.

Serology: slide agglutination tests unreliable; antibodies appear in 6–12 days, reach maximum in 4 weeks, can be suppressed by antibiotic treatment; enzyme-linked immunosorbent assay IgM test detects antibodies from day 5 of illness; microagglutination test is specific and identifies infecting serotype.

Full blood count and coagulation screen: to identify bleeding disorder and thrombocytopenia.

Liver function tests: usually normal except for raised bilirubin.

Serum creatinine measurement: to identify degree of renal impairment.

CSF analysis: to confirm lymphocytic meningitis.

Complications

Uveitis 6–12 weeks after original illness and chronic persistent leptospiruria: extremely rare.

Transplacental transmission, with fetal death and abortion: has occurred.

Differential diagnosis

Influenza-like illness, viral infections, aseptic meningitis, encephalitis.

Enteric-fever-like illness.

Infective hepatitis, other causes of jaundice.

Atypical pneumonia, rickettsioses.

Septicemia, nephritis.

Leukemia, thrombocytopenic purpura, meningococcal disease.

Etiology

• In the US, prevalent serotypes of pathogenic leptospires, *Leptospira interrogans*, are *icterohaemorrhagiae*, *australis*, *autumnalis*, and *canicola*.

• Wild and domestic animals, especially rats (*icterohaemorrhagiae*) and cattle.

• Contact of mucous membranes or abraded skin with infected animal tissue or urine or contaminated water or soil can lead to transmission.

Epidemiology

• People at risk include farmers, dairyworkers, abattoir workers, veterinarians, and those working or engaged in recreational pursuits on or in natural inland waters.

Treatment

Diet and lifestyle

• Rodents must be controlled in and around human habitations.

• Contamination of living, working, and recreational areas by infected urine should be prevented.

• Cuts should be covered by waterproof dressings and protective clothing worn.

• Immersion in natural inland waters should be avoided.

• Participants should shower after swimming, canoeing, windsurfing, or waterskiing.

• Safety cards should be issued to people at risk to show medical staff if illness occurs.

• Patients should be educated on modes of transmission and preventive measures.

• Domestic animals, especially cattle and dogs, should be immunized.

Pharmacological treatment

Antibiotics

• Antibiotics can influence the course of the disease only if given in the first week.

• Intensive treatment is needed for severe infections.

Standard dosage Penicillin G, 900 mg; ampicillin, 1 g; or erythromycin, 500 mg, all parenterally 4 times daily for 1 week.
Amoxicillin, 500 mg orally 3 times daily, or doxycycline, 100 mg twice daily for 1 week.

Contraindications Hypersensitivity; oral agents should be avoided in pregnancy, infancy, and childhood.

Special points *Penicillin:* can induce a short-lived exacerbation with pyrexia and hypotension: this Jarisch-Herxheimer reaction is regarded as a sign of leptospiral lysis.

Main drug interactions *Penicillins:* inactivate aminoglycoside in syringe.
Erythromycin: potentiates digoxin, warfarin, and carbamazepine.
Doxycycline: affects anticoagulant treatment.

Main side effects *Parenteral agents:* anaphylactic reaction, gastrointestinal reactions (rare).
Amoxicillin: erythematous rash in patients with glandular fever.
Doxycycline: photosensitivity (rare), permanent teeth discoloration.

For symptoms

Prompt correction of electrolyte imbalance.

Fresh blood, platelets, or clotting factors for hemorrhage.

Meperidine or morphine for severe pain.

Diazepam and phenytoin for seizures.

Steroids for thrombocytopenia.

Hemodialysis for renal failure.

Treatment aims

To alleviate symptoms.

Prognosis

• Most cases are mild and often undiagnosed; patients recover spontaneously.

• In Weil's syndrome with hepatorenal involvement, mortality is 10%–20%.

• No ill effects are seen after renal or hepatic involvement in surviving patients.

• Death without jaundice is extremely rare.

• Reinfection by a different serotype is possible.

Follow-up and management

• Supportive treatment includes analgesics, sedation, and antiemetics.

• Renal and cardiac function must be monitored daily.

General references

Ferguson IR: Leptospirosis surveillance: 1990–1992. *Commun Dis Rep* 1993, 3:R47–R48.

Ferguson IR: Leptospirosis update. *BMJ* 1991, **302**:128–129.

Diagnosis

Symptoms

• Usually, acute lymphoblastic leukemia has a short history of 2–3 months.

Tiredness and dyspnea: due to anemia.

Recurrent infections: due to leukopenia.

Bruising and bleeding: due to thrombocytopenia.

Symptoms of hyperviscosity: if leukocyte count is very high (*e.g.*, >200×10^9/L).

Joint and bone pain: less common than in children.

Signs

• Often no physical signs are manifest.

Pallor.

Evidence of infection.

Purpura or bruising.

Lymphadenopathy or hepatosplenomegaly.

Investigations

General

Full blood count (with Romanowsky's or Wright-Giemsa stained film): diagnosis may be evident from careful morphological examination; leukemic blasts not always seen in peripheral blood; platelet count and hemoglobin may be low or normal.

Bone-marrow aspiration: blasts should be >30% to make the diagnosis.

Blood urea nitrogen, creatinine, electrolytes, calcium, phosphate, urate measurement: important initial investigations before starting treatment, particularly if leukocyte count is high.

Chest radiography: to look for mediastinal mass, seen in 70% of patients with T-cell acute lymphoblastic leukemia (ALL; high risk of tumor lysis syndrome if this is present).

Lumbar puncture with CSF cytology: important initial investigation to detect CNS involvement (unusual at presentation).

Special

• These tests help to confirm the diagnosis;: confirming that blasts are lymphoid in origin is occasionally difficult on light microscopy.

• They also help to categorize the disease more fully, giving additional prognostic information.

Cytochemistry: helps to differentiate ALL from acute myeloblastic leukemia (*e.g.*, negative reaction with Sudan black).

Immunophenotyping: identifies origin of blast cell using panel of cell-surface "markers"; useful markers include TdT (all subtypes positive except B ALL), CD10 (identifies common ALL antigen), CD19 (positive in B-lineage ALL), CD2 (positive in T-lineage ALL).

Cytogenetics: direct examination of chromosomes at metaphase can identify translocations in ~70% of patients with ALL; this can identify poor-risk patients, *e.g.*, those with t(9,22) or Philadelphia-positive ALL, which has bad prognosis; may provide a marker that can be used to detect early relapse.

Complications

• Most complications are related to bone-marrow failure (cytopenia) due to the disease or, more often, to the intensive treatment needed.

Differential diagnosis

Acute myeloid leukemia:

Aplastic anemia: diagnosis of acute lymphoblastic leukemia might not be obvious initially if presenting leukocyte count is low and bone-marrow aspirate "dry."

Lymphoblastic lymphoma: predominantly lymphomatous presentation, with <25% blasts in bone marrow; distinction may be arbitrary in adults because treatment is often the same.

Etiology

• The cause of acute lymphoblastic leukemia is unknown; it is presumed to be due to genetic mutations, the risk of which is increased by DNA damage, *e.g.*, due to radiation or DNA repair defects.

• Victims of exposure to ionizing radiation have a higher incidence of leukemia, but this is more often myeloid than lymphoid in origin.

Epidemiology

• Acute lymphoblastic leukemia is uncommon in adults, particularly in those aged >30 years.

• Patients aged >15 years are defined as adults because they constitute a separate group with much poorer remission and survival rates.

Classification [1]

Morphological

• Based on appearance on light microscopy, the French–American–British (FAB) classification divides acute lymphoblastic leukemia (ALL) into L1, L2, and L3.

• This has little correlation with prognosis or immunophenotype, except L3 morphology with B-cell ALL.

Immunological

• On the basis of expression of surface antigens by the blast cells, ALL is divided into T lineage (early T precursor and T cell ALL) and B lineage (early B precursor, common ALL, pre-B ALL, and B cell ALL).

Treatment

Diet and lifestyle

• Nutrition must be maintained.

• Psychological support should be provided to patients and their relatives, especially if a young family is involved; financial support should be considered if earnings are disrupted.

• Patients must take precautions against infection during neutropenia.

Pharmacological treatment

Principles

• Treatment should be given under specialist supervision, within the context of a clinical trial if possible to allow adequate evaluation and the development of new treatments.

• Initial treatment involves several blocks of inpatient treatment.

Induction: remission (*i.e.*, <5% blasts in bone marrow) can be achieved in ~80% of adults usually within 1 month of starting treatment; agents include steroids, vincristine, and anthracyclines.

Consolidation: usually follows quickly after induction, and new chemotherapeutic agents should be introduced; optimum duration and intensity of treatment have not yet been established.

CNS-directed treatment: often described as "CNS prophylaxis"; CNS leukemia occurs in ~50% of patients in hematological remission if no specific treatment directed at the CNS is given; possible treatments include cranial irradiation, intrathecal methotrexate, or high-dose i.v. methotrexate (which crosses the blood–brain barrier).

Maintenance therapy: continuous treatment for ~2 years improves outcome; usual treatment involves weekly methotrexate and 6-mercaptopurine, with monthly courses of vincristine and steroids.

Supportive treatment: particularly important in the early stages of treatment; includes allopurinol, adequate hydration, blood-product support, and timely use of antimicrobial treatment.

General complications of treatment

Myelosuppression (inevitable).

Hair loss.

Compromise or loss of fertility.

Infection, particularly during neutropenia: empirical treatment is often needed for bacterial, viral, or fungal infection.

Nausea and vomiting: may be easy to control.

Complications of specific drugs

Vincristine: extravasation injury, alopecia, muscle and jaw pain, urinary retention, dysphagia, peripheral neuropathy.

Prednisone: Cushing's syndrome and other steroidal side effects (including psychiatric).

L-Asparaginase: thrombotic episodes, pancreatitis, anaphylaxis.

Daunorubicin: extravasation injury, cardiomyopathy, bone-marrow suppression, vomiting, gut toxicity.

Cytarabine: gut and bone-marrow toxicity, erythema, cerebellar toxicity in high doses.

Thioguanine: hepatic and bone-marrow toxicity, rashes.

VP16 epipodophyllotoxin: gut and bone-marrow toxicity.

Methotrexate: renal, hepatic, and gut dysfunction; bone-marrow suppression; mucositis (depending on dose and mode of treatment); affects intellect.

Mercaptopurine: bone-marrow suppression, rashes, hepatic dysfunction.

Treatment aims

To maximize chance of cure, with minimal toxicity.

Other treatments [2]

Allogeneic bone-marrow transplantation

• Adults should receive allograft in first complete remission if they have a matched sibling donor and are aged 20–50 years; this is particularly indicated in Philadelphia-positive disease (incurable by drugs alone).

Autologous bone-marrow transplantation

• The role is less well established; by definition, it is available to more patients but will probably be less effective because of lack of "graft-versus-leukemia effect."

Prognosis

• Despite best available treatment, overall survival in adult disease is poorer than in childhood disease; studies indicate a 5-year leukemia-free survival of 20%–35% in unselected patients.

• Poor prognostic factors include increasing age, high leukocyte count at presentation (>30 × 10^9/L), t(9,22), and failure to reach complete remission after 1 month of treatment.

Follow-up and management

• After discharge the patient must be seen regularly for full blood count; if on maintenance therapy, the dose may need adjustment.

• Prophylactic co-trimoxazole is usually given during this time.

Relapsed disease

• ~70% of patients relapse; the risk varies from 40% for young adults to >80% for patients aged >50 years.

• Treatment depends on age, duration of initial remission, and previous treatment.

• Relapsed disease is not curable by conventional chemotherapy.

Key references

1. Bain BJ: *Leukaemia Diagnosis: A Guide to the FAB Classification.* London: Gower Medical Publishing; 1990.
2. Ramsay NKC, Kersey JH: Indications for bone marrow transplantation in acute lymphoblastic leukaemia. *Blood* 1990, **75**:815–818.

Leukemia, acute lymphoblastic in children ALL

Diagnosis

Symptoms

• A constellation of symptoms is seen, many nonspecific and related to bone-marrow failure.

**Easy bruising, bone pain, fevers, pallor, lethargy, anorexia, malaise:** due to bone-marrow failure.

Abdominal distention: due to hepatosplenomegaly.

Shortness of breath, facial swelling: due to mediastinal mass; unusual.

Headache, vomiting: due to CNS disease; unusual.

Overt bleeding: due to bone-marrow failure; unusual.

Signs

Pyrexia, mucosal bleeding, skin purpura, pallor, congestive heart failure (rare): due to bone-marrow failure.

Hepatosplenomegaly, lymphadenopathy, upper trunk and facial edema with distended superficial veins, skin infiltrates, testicular enlargement: due to leukemic "mass."

Cranial nerve palsies (III, V, VI, VII), papilledema, fundal hemorrhages, leukemic infiltrates: due to CNS disease (rare).

Investigations

Full blood count: shows pancytopenia, normal counts, or isolated raised leukocyte count.

Blood film: shows possible presence of leukemic blasts.

Bone-marrow morphology: confirms diagnosis in conjunction with cytochemistry and immunophenotyping (mature B cell varieties treated on lymphoma-type protocols).

Chest radiography: for mediastinal mass.

Lumbar puncture: for CNS disease.

Blood urea nitrogen, creatine, electrolytes, and urate analysis.

Liver function tests: for liver failure (rare).

Complications

Early

• Early complications are usually related to drug side effects or further bone-marrow suppression.

Tumor lysis syndrome, associated with hyperkalemia, hyperuricemia, hyperphosphatemia, renal dysfunction.

Infection of all types.

Bleeding.

Anemia.

Vomiting, hair loss, peripheral neuropathy and myopathy, mucositis.

Late

Learning difficulties: *e.g.*, problems with short-term memory or concentration; due to cranial radiation.

Cardiotoxicity: due to anthracycline treatment.

Cataracts, sterility, growth and hormone problems: due to cyclophosphamide treatment and total body irradiation for bone-marrow transplantation.

Secondary malignancies: due to epipodophyllotoxins.

Differential diagnosis

Lymphadenopathy

Infections: *e.g.*, infectious mononucleosis.

Lymphomas or other tumors.

Hepatosplenomegaly

Leishmaniasis.

Macrophage, metabolic, storage, or autoimmune disorders.

Lymphomas.

Bone-marrow failure

Aplastic anemia.

Myelodysplasia.

Macrophage disorders.

Autoimmune disorders.

Bone-marrow tumor: *e.g.*, neuroblastoma.

Infections: *e.g.*, tuberculosis, visceral leishmaniasis.

Etiology [1]

• The cause is unknown but is presumed to be a genetic mutation.

• Increased risk is associated with the following:

Down's syndrome.

Fanconi's anemia.

Bloom's syndrome.

Ataxia telangiectasia and various immunodeficiency disorders.

• The effects of irradiation or electromagnetic fields are unconfirmed.

Epidemiology [1]

• Acute lymphoblastic leukemia is the most common malignant disease of childhood.

• A peak incidence at 2–5 years accounts for 20% of all leukemia.

• Slightly more boys than girls are affected.

• 85% of childhood leukemia is acute lymphoblastic.

Treatment

Diet and lifestyle

• Specialist support is needed for children and their families, including siblings, both in hospital during treatment and after discharge.

• Maintenance of nutrition is important.

Pharmacological treatment

• Treatment should be given under specialist supervision, in the context of a clinical trial if possible to allow adequate evaluation and the development of new treatments.

Treatment choice [2–5]

For high-risk patients (slow remitters, near haploid, Philadelphia-chromosome positive, older boys with high leukocyte counts, usually $>100 \times 10^9$/L): transplantation in first remission.

For patients at high risk of CNS disease relapse (leukocyte count $>50 \times 10^9$/L): cranial irradiation or high-dose i.v. methotrexate.

For lower-risk patients (leukocyte count $<50 \times 10^9$/L): continuing intrathecal or high-dose methotrexate.

For patients with CNS disease at diagnosis: craniospinal or cranial irradiation and continuing intrathecal methotrexate.

For infants <6 months: intensive multiagent treatment.

Principles

Induction: usually vincristine, asparaginase, steroids; remission in 97% of patients.

Consolidation: intensive treatment with some different drugs from induction course to eradicate "resistant clones."

CNS-directed treatment: to eradicate disease in CNS sanctuary site.

Consolidation: as for second step; two or three consolidations may be needed.

Continuation of treatment up to 2 years: to eradicate minimal residue disease.

Complications of specific drugs

Vincristine: extravasation injury, alopecia, muscle and jaw pain, urinary retention, dysphagia, peripheral neuropathy

Prednisone: Cushing's syndrome and other steroidal side effects (including psychiatric).

L-Asparaginase: thrombotic episodes, pancreatitis, anaphylaxis.

Daunorubicin: extravasation injury, cardiomyopathy, bone-marrow suppression, vomiting, gut toxicity.

Cytarabine: gut and bone-marrow toxicity, erythema, cerebellar toxicity in high doses.

Thioguanine: hepatic and bone-marrow toxicity, rashes.

VP16 epipodophyllotoxin: gut and bone-marrow toxicity.

Methotrexate: renal, hepatic, and gut dysfunction, bone-marrow suppression, mucositis (depending on dose and mode of treatment); affects intellect.

Mercaptopurine: bone-marrow suppression, rashes, hepatic dysfunction.

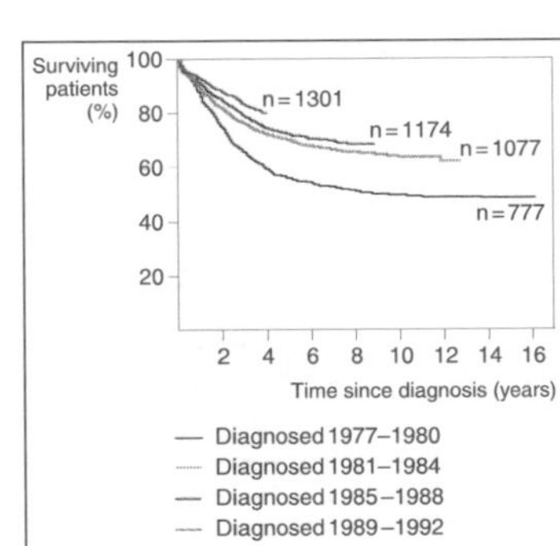

Survival rates of patients with acute lymphoblastic leukemia 1977–1992.

Treatment aims

To cure patient at least cost (toxicity of specific drugs and complications).

Other treatments

Transplantation.

Cranial irradiation.

See Pharmacological treatment *for indications.*

Prognosis

• Adverse prognostic features include failure to remit after 1 month of treatment, Philadelphia-chromosome positive, near haploid, older age, male sex, high leukocyte count, infants <6 months.

Follow-up and management

• Patients on continuation treatment should be followed up every 1–2 weeks, depending on blood count.

• After completion of treatment, all patients should be followed indefinitely; for the first 6 years, they must be checked carefully for signs of relapse (organomegaly, testicular swelling, low blood count, blasts on film) and endocrine, growth, intellectual, and cardiac late effects.

• Prophylactic co-trimoxazole should be given for pneumocystis.

• Advice should be given on returning to school and when normal childhood immunization can be given.

Key references

1. Greaves MF: Speculations on the cause of childhood acute lymphoblastic leukemia. *Leukemia* 1988, **2**:120–125.
2. Chessell JM: Treatment of childhood acute lymphoblastic leukemia: present issues and future prospects. *Blood Rev* 1992, **6**:193–203.
3. Eden OB, *et al.*: Report to the MRC: results of MRC UKALL VIII. *Br J Haematol* 1990, **78**:187–196.
4. Hann IM: CNS directed therapy in childhood. *Br J Haematol* 1992, **82**:2–5.
5. Hann IM, *et al.*: UKCCSG MACHO chemotherapy for B stages IV NHL & B-ALL. *Br J Haematol* 1990, **76**:359–364.

Diagnosis

Symptoms

• Some patients are symptom-free.

Lethargy, irritability, fatigue, reduced exercise tolerance: symptoms of anemia.

Infection: due to leukopenia.

Spontaneous bleeding or bruising: symptom of thrombocytopenia.

Signs

Pallor, infections, bruises, petechiae.

Lymphadenopathy or hepatosplenomegaly: occasionally.

Gum hypertrophy, skin infiltration: features of monocytic leukemia.

Hemorrhagic manifestations: feature of promyelocytic leukemia.

Investigations

Full blood count: often shows reduced hemoglobin; thrombocytopenia frequent; leukocyte count $>100 \times 10^9$/L unusual, associated with poor response to treatment; presentation with count $<3.0 \times 10^9$/L common; differential leukocyte count usually abnormal, with neutropenia and presence of "blast cells" (large cells, ~1.5–2 times diameter of erythrocytes; usually have large nuclear:cytoplasmic ratio [less common with acute myeloid leukemia]; nucleus may contain at least one nucleolus [usually large single nucleus in monoblast]; blasts may show features of maturation, *e.g.*, cytoplasmic granulation, Auer dies, or monocytic features); numerical thrombocytopenia confirmed morphologically.

Bone-marrow analysis: increased proportion of blast cells; conventionally, >30% of bone-marrow cellularity to distinguish from the blastic forms of myelodysplasia.

Cytochemistry: useful to confirm myeloid or monocytic origin of blast cells; Sudan black, chloroacetate esterase, or myeloperoxidase stains.

Immunophenotyping: most reliable method of determining hematopoietic lineage of origin; expression of CD33 or CD15 indicates some myeloid maturation; CD34 and HLA DR earlier nonlymphoid markers, providing important objective methods for distinguishing myeloid from lymphoid leukemia; antigens are expressed on normal cells, but "leukemia-specific" or aberrant phenotypes have been identified that will probably be useful for monitoring remission status when normal antigens are inappropriately expressed on leukemic cells.

Cytogenetics: many structural chromosome abnormalities have been described; relationship between prognosis and cytogenic abnormality, *e.g.*, better prognosis with FAB M3 (usually has 15:17 translocation), some M2s (8:21 translocation), and inverted 16; worse prognosis with abnormalities or deletions of chromosomes 5 and 7.

Molecular genetics: molecular probes for the 15:17 and 8:21 translocations now available; polymerase chain reaction detection of minor cell populations therefore possible; such technology will be important in assessing quality of remission.

Complications

Overwhelming infection.

Bleeding: especially intracranial in promyelocytic leukemia.

Differential diagnosis

Any cause of pancytopenia.

Etiology

• The risk is increased in the following:

Radiation exposure.

Chemotherapy for cancer, *e.g.*, Hodgkin's disease.

Chronic myeloproliferative disorders or myelodysplasia.

Epidemiology

• Acute myeloid leukemia is the most common form in adults.

• The median age of presentation is ~60 years.

• The male:female ratio is equal.

• The prevalence increases with age (*e.g.*, 1 in 10^5 in children, up to 3 in 10^5 in patients >70 years).

Classification

• Based on morphological appearance, acute myeloid leukemia is divided into FAB (French–American–British) types M0–7 .

• The M3 type (promyelocytic) has a high chance of remission and a lower risk of relapse.

• Although valuable in standardizing terminology, this classification has limited prognostic power.

Treatment

Diet and lifestyle

• Nutrition must be maintained.

• Psychological support should be provided to patients and their relatives, especially if a young family is involved; financial support should be considered if earnings are disrupted.

• Patients must take precautions against infection during neutropenia.

Pharmacological treatment

Supportive

• Infection can be prevented by expert nursing care; isolation in a single room with air filtration; mouth care; vigilance of temperature, mucous membranes, perineum, and central-line site.

• Infection can be treated, after appropriate bacteriological, fungal, and viral samples have been taken, by rapid introduction of i.v. antibiotics (usually aminoglycoside and ceftazidime or penicillin with anti-pseudomonal activity).

• If a response occurs within 48 h, treatment should be continued for 3–5 days; in cases of no or incomplete response and no bacteriological guidance, vancomycin should be added; if further failure, i.v. amphotericin should be added. (*See* Infections in hematological malignancy *for details.*)

For coagulopathy

• Coagulation factor deficiency should be corrected by appropriate blood products or vitamin K supplements.

• Severe coagulopathy, including disseminated intravascular coagulation, can be a dominant feature in promyelocytic leukemia (FAB M3), needing specific attention.

• All-*trans*-retinoic acid (ATRA) can be effective in correcting the defect (usually within 2–3 days).

• Blood-product support is essential, but fibrinolytic inhibition (tranexamic acid) and heparin have become less widely used.

Chemotherapy [1,2]

• Treatment should be given under specialist supervision.

• If induction of remission and consolidation phases are sufficiently intense, maintenance should be of no benefit.

• Drugs include anthracyclines, cytosine arabinoside, thioguanine, and etoposide; side effects include cardiotoxicity.

• Intensive supportive care is needed during remission induction, but most patients achieve complete remission with one course.

• An extra course may be needed for less intensive approaches, and more supportive care may be needed overall in all patient groups.

Treatment aims

To restore normal bone-marrow function.

To establish prolonged remission or cure.

Other treatments

Allogeneic bone-marrow transplantation

• The risk of relapse is reduced from 60% to 15%.

• Treatment-related mortality of 30% is due to toxicity, infection, pneumonitis, and graft-versus-host disease.

• Treatment may result in infertility and late cataracts (in 10%–15% of patients).

• Allogeneic transplantation is available only to 10%–15% of patients.

Autologous bone-marrow transplantation

• Autologous transplantation is indicated for patients <55 years without a sibling donor.

Advantages: less toxicity, no graft-versus-host disease, available to more patients, low procedure-related mortality (6%–8%).

Disadvantages: potential for the harvested marrow to be contaminated, lack of graft-versus-leukemia effect.

Prognosis [1,2]

• Current schedules achieve remission in 80% of patients <55 years (range, 90% in children to 70% in those in fifth decade); in older patients, remission rates of 60% should be achieved.

• 30%–40% of patients <55 years treated by chemotherapy alone and 20% of older patients remain in remission at 5 years.

• Allogeneic bone-marrow transplantation cures 50%–60% of recipients; autologous transplantation cures 45%–55% of recipients.

• Treatment failure >5 years is rare after bone-marrow transplantation but occurs in chemotherapy patients, although at a much lower rate than in the first 2–3 years.

Follow-up and management

• 2–3 weeks after recovery from hypoplasia induced by chemotherapy, the bone marrow should be checked for remission status.

General references

Burnett AK, Lowenberg B: Treatment options for remission in acute myeloid leukemia. In *Hematological Oncology,* vol 1. Cambridge: Cambridge University Press; 1991.

Foon KA, Gale RP: Therapy for acute myelogenous leukemia. *Blood Rev* 1992, **6**:15–25.

Diagnosis

Symptoms

• 70% of patients are asymptomatic, the diagnosis being made on incidental blood count.

Enlarged lymph nodes or discomfort in left upper quadrant of abdomen: in 20%.

Symptoms of anemia: uncommon.

Bruising or bleeding: rare.

Weight loss, fever unassociated with infection, night sweats: "B" symptoms; very unusual and often signal transformation to high-grade lymphoma.

Signs

Lymphadenopathy in cervical, axillary, or inguinal regions: in 30% of patients.

Mild to moderate splenomegaly: in 10%.

Hepatomegaly: rare.

Anemia: unusual.

Purpura: rare.

Investigations [1]

Full blood count: shows lymphocytosis $>5 \times 10^9$/L, mature monomorphic small lymphocytes with smear cells.

Lymphocyte marker analysis: shows sparse surface immunoglobulin of a single light chain (κ or λ); $CD5^+$, $CD19^+$, $CD20^+$, $CD23^+$, $CD37^+$, $CD3^-$, $CD10^-$, $CD22^-$.

Serum immunoglobulin measurement: reduced concentration in all classes; IgM paraprotein in 5% of patients.

Direct antiglobulin test: positive in 10%.

Bone-marrow trephine analysis: interstitial, nodular, or diffuse infiltration by small lymphocytes.

Karyotyping: trisomy 12 in 30%, deletion 13q14 in 25%.

Leukapheresis specimen from chronic lymphocytic leukemia with Romanowsky's stain, showing small monomorphic lymphocytes with occasional prolymphocytes and smear cells.

Complications

Autoimmune hemolytic anemia: in 10% of patients, more in stage C.

Autoimmune thrombocytopenia, neutropenia, pure erythrocyte aplasia: in <2%.

Infection: due to hypogammaglobulinemia in a few patients.

Shingles: in 25%.

Transformation to prolymphocytic leukemia or high-grade lymphoma: in 10% and 2% (Richter's syndrome), respectively.

Pneumococcal pneumonia.

Differential diagnosis

Prolymphocytic leukemia.

Hairy cell leukemia.

Splenic lymphoma with villous lymphocytes.

Large granular lymphocytic leukemia.

Sézary syndrome and adult T-cell lymphoma/leukemia.

Follicle center cell lymphoma and mantle cell lymphoma.

Etiology

• The cause is unknown.

• No association has been found with radiation or retroviruses.

Epidemiology

• Chronic lymphocytic leukemia is the most common leukemia in western Europe and North America.

• It is increasingly common with age, the median age at presentation being 69 years.

• The male : female ratio is 2:1, but, because women live longer, in the elderly population, ~50% of patients are female.

• A slight familial tendency has been found.

Staging

Rai (US)

Stage 0: lymphocytosis alone.

Stage I: with lymphadenopathy

Stage II: with spleno- or hepatomegaly.

Stage III: with anemia; hemoglobin 110 g/L.

Stage IV: with thrombocytopenia; platelets 100×10^9/L.

Binet (Europe) [2]

Stage A: no anemia or thrombocytopenia; <3 lymphoid areas* enlarged.

Stage B: no anemia or thrombocytopenia; 3 or more lymphoid areas* enlarged.

Stage C: hemoglobin 100 g/L or platelets 100×10^9/dL.

*Cervical, axillary, or inguinal lymph nodes; spleen; and liver.

Treatment

Diet and lifestyle

- Patients should be encouraged to lead a normal life.

Pharmacological treatment

- All treatment should be given under specialist supervision.
- Stage A patients should not receive chemotherapy.

Alkylating agents

- Chlorambucil is the mainstay of treatment.
- The response rate is 50%.

Standard dosage Chlorambucil, continuous oral dose or intermittently every 4 weeks.
Cyclophosphamide, orally or i.v. every 2–3 weeks.

Contraindications None.

Main drug interactions None established.

Main side effects Nausea and bone-marrow suppression, drug rash (in 5% of patients on chlorambucil), alopecia (cyclophosphamide).

Nucleoside analogues

- Fludarabine is a purine analogue that produces responses in up to 50% of patients resistant to chlorambucil.
- 2-Chlorodeoxyadenosine is a similar agent.

Standard dosage Fludarabine, i.v. daily for 5 days every 28 days.

Contraindications None.

Special points Less bone-marrow suppression than chlorambucil, but profound T lymphocytopenia, which predisposes to infection by viruses, fungi, or protozoa.

Main drug interactions None established.

Main side effects Bone-marrow suppression, immunosuppression.

Other options

Prednisone: for patients with autoimmune complications; effects a redistribution of lymphocytes from tissue to blood and may be useful in thrombocytopenic patients beginning treatment with alkylating agents.

CHOP chemotherapy (cyclophosphamide, doxorubicin, vincristine, prednisone): may be more effective than chlorambucil in Stage C cases.

Immunoglobulin replacement therapy: for patients with recurrent infections whose serum immunoglobulin concentration is <4 g/L.

Treatment aims

To relieve symptoms.

To prolong life in stage B or C patients.

Other treatments

- Leukapheresis may be used to prevent or treat hyperleukocytosis in patients with very high leukocyte counts (>500 × 10^9/L) or to control the leukocyte count in drug-resistant patients.

Prognosis

- Stage A patients have the same prognosis as age- and sex-matched controls.
- Median survivals achieved with chlorambucil are 12 years for stage A, 5 years for stage B, and 2 years for stage C patients.

Follow-up and management

- Patients should be observed to determine whether the disease is progressive; patients whose disease is static and who are asymptomatic may safely be observed.
- Progressive disease should be treated by chlorambucil.
- All patients need long-term follow-up, the frequency being determined by the pace of the disease.

Key references

1. Litz CE, Brunning RD: Chronic lymphoproliferative disorders: classification and diagnosis. *Clin Haematol* 1993, 6:767–783.
2. Binet JL: Treatment of chronic lymphocytic leukaemia. *Clin Haematol* 1993, 6:867–878.

Diagnosis

Symptoms

• 25% of patients are asymptomatic.

Fatigue, weight loss, weakness: in 25%.

Bruising or infections: in 25%.

Abdominal fullness or discomfort: in 25%.

Signs

Moderate to massive splenomegaly: in 75% of patients.

Lymphadenopathy: rarely.

Hepatomegaly: occasionally.

Signs of infection, bleeding, or bruising.

Investigations

Full blood count: shows normochromic, normocytic anemia, neutropenia, monocytopenia, thrombocytopenia, "hairy" leukocytosis. Hairy cells are large lymphocytes with open nucleus, with loose, lacy chromatin and one or two distinct nucleoli; the cytoplasm is pale blue-grey, with fine, hair-like projections; usually few are found in blood, but they number $>10 \times 10^9$/L in 10% of patients.

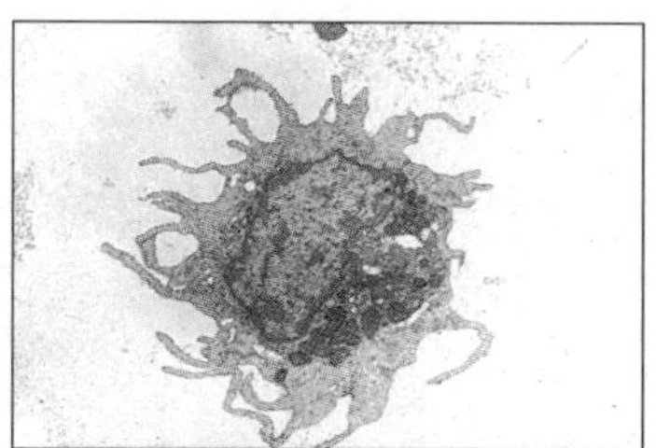

Hairy cell on transmission electron microscopy.

Bone-marrow trephine: shows diffuse or patchy infiltration of leukemic cells, characteristic pale halos of cytoplasm surrounding monotonous, bland nuclei.

Cell marker analysis: moderately positive for surface immunoglobulin of a single light chain class; CD11c$^+$, CD19$^+$, CD20$^+$, CD25$^+$, CD37$^+$, CD3$^-$, CD15$^-$, CD10$^-$; tartrate-resistant acid phosphatase positive.

Complications

Infections: neutropenia and monocytopenia render patients susceptible to infection, so both bacterial and more atypical infections are seen; fungal, protozoan, and mycobacterial organisms are implicated.

Vasculitis: microscopic polyarteritis in 5% of patients.

Differential diagnosis

Tumors with similar "hairy" cytoplasmic projections: *e.g.*, splenic lymphoma with villous lymphocytes, hairy cell variant, and monocytoid B-cell lymphoma (may be distinguished by careful morphological examination and cell markers).

Other causes of isolated splenomegaly with hypersplenism.

Etiology

• The cause is unknown, although, in one case of the rare T-cell hairy cell leukemia, the human T-cell lymphotrophic virus II retrovirus was isolated.

Epidemiology

• This is a rare leukemia, with an incidence of 1 in 500 000 population.

• The male : female ratio is 4 : 1.

• The median age at presentation is 55 years (range, 20–90 years).

Treatment

Diet and lifestyle

• Patients should be encouraged to live as normal a life as possible.

Pharmacological treatment [1]

• Treatment should be given under specialist supervision.

2-Chlorodeoxyadenosine

Standard dosage 0.1 mg/kg/day by continuous infusion for 7 days.

Main side effects Fever and infection during the first month following therapy, decline in the neutrophil and platelet counts, which generally reverse by the end of the fourth week.

• This is currently the drug of choice in the US.

• It may be capable of producing long-term complete remissions.

• Side effects include myelotoxicity (intense hematological support needed early in treatment to prevent death from hemorrhage or infection), and the risk of fungal, viral, or protozoan infection due to $CD4^+$ T-cell suppression (similar to 2′deoxycoformycin).

Additional agents

α-Interferon

Standard dosage α-Interferon, 3 MU 3 times weekly usually for 2 years, is effective in 80% of patients.

Contraindications Hypersensitivity, severe renal failure, hepatic or myeloid dysfunction.

Special points Early in treatment, cytopenias may be exacerbated, with risk of hemorrhage or infection.
Antibodies to interferon-α occur in 50% of patients but only occasionally cause treatment failure.

Main drug interactions No information available.

Main side effects Mild influenza-like symptoms (improve with time).

2′Deoxycoformycin

• This inhibitor of adenosine deaminase produces a higher rate of complete remissions than interferon (up to 80%); early studies suggest that most remissions are prolonged beyond 4 years.

Standard dosage 2′Deoxycoformycin, 4 mg/m^2 weekly for 3 weeks, then on alternate weeks for 6 weeks.

Contraindications Low glomerular filtration rate; caution in renal dysfunction.

Main drug interactions No information available.

Main side effects Risk of fungal, viral, or protozoan infections due to $CD4^+$ T-cell suppression.

Treatment aims

To allow patient to lead symptom-free life.

To attempt, particularly in younger patients, long-term remission, albeit at some early risk from increased pancytopenia.

Other treatments

• Splenectomy was the mainstay of treatment before effective drugs were available; it is still used in patients with the following:
Important splenomegaly and cytopenias.
Relatively little bone-marrow involvement.
Intolerance of pharmaceutical intervention.
Laparotomy for other reasons.

Prognosis

• With modern treatment, most patients have a normal lifespan.

• Only a few patients achieve complete remission after interferon treatment, but most achieve sufficient hematological improvement to make their disease of no consequence to them.

• Relapse occurs progressively 1–2 years off treatment.

Follow-up and management

• All patients should be followed up indefinitely.

• Treatment should be reintroduced if symptoms or blood count warrants it.

Key reference

1. Lill MCC, Golde DW: Treatment of hairy cell leukaemia. *Blood Rev* 1990, **4**:238–244.

Liver failure, fulminant

Diagnosis

Symptoms

Lethargy, nausea, vomiting: prodromal symptoms of viral hepatitis.

Abdominal pain, hematemesis: common after acetaminophen overdose.

Drowsiness or confusion: in grades 1 and 2 encephalopathy.

Restlessness, agitation: possibly aggressive; in grade 3.

Unresponsiveness: in grade 4.

Signs

Jaundice: common but not always manifest at presentation.

Encephalopathy of varying severity: asterixis, fetor hepaticus late features.

Liver size: typically normal, although hepatomegaly may be seen in severe hepatitis, Budd–Chiari syndrome.

Ascites: late finding.

Systemic hypertension, decerebrate posturing, hyperventilation: indicating cerebral edema.

Acute fatty liver of pregnancy: a consideration in pregnant patients.

Investigations

History: of toxin (amanita mushrooms, carbon tetrachloride) or drug exposure (*e.g.*, acetaminophen, isoniazid, NSAIDs).

Prothrombin time or INR measurement: prolongation (in the absence of disseminated intravascular coagulation or vitamin K deficiency) indicates severe hepatic dysfunction.

Hemoglobin measurement: hemolytic anemia suggests Wilson's disease.

Serum bilirubin measurement: prognostic significance in non–acetaminophen-induced cases.

Serum creatinine measurement: urea underestimates renal impairment; prognostic significance in acetaminophen-induced cases.

Glucose measurement: hypoglycemia indicates poor prognosis.

Acetaminophen measurement.

Hepatitis A serology: to detect IgM anti-hepatitis A virus.

Hepatitis B and D serology: to detect IgM anti-core, hepatitis B surface antigen, anti-hepatitis D virus.

Hepatitis C antibody: often negative in fulminant non-A, non-B viral hepatitis.

Ceruloplasmin and 24-hour urinary copper excretion: low and high, respectively, in Wilson's disease.

CMV, Epstein-Barr serology.

Ultrasonography: to assess liver size and texture.

Complications

• All of the following are late complications, mainly occurring in patients with advanced encephalopathy.

Hypoglycemia.

Renal failure.

Cerebral edema [1].

Bleeding, infection.

Respiratory failure.

Hypotension.

Differential diagnosis

Acute decompensation of chronic liver disease.

Reye's syndrome.

Other metabolic encephalopathy.

Etiology

• Causes include the following:

Acetaminophen ingestion.

Hepatitis A, B, B/D, or E virus infection, seronegative hepatitis (non-A, non-B, non-C), halothane hepatitis, idiosyncratic drug reactions.

Pregnancy-related, Budd–Chiari syndrome, autoimmune liver disease, malignancy, mushroom poisoning [2,3].

Epidemiology

• Fulminant liver failure complicates 0.1%–4.7% of hospitalized patients with viral hepatitis, depending on the cause.

Classification

Fulminant liver failure

Acute liver failure with encephalopathy in a patient presumed to have a normal liver within 8 weeks of the onset of illness.

Hyperacute liver failure

Encephalopathy within 7 days of onset of jaundice, characterized by high incidence of cerebral edema; despite this, many patients survive with medical management.

Subacute liver failure

Encephalopathy 8–12 weeks after onset of jaundice, low incidence of cerebral edema and less severe prolongation of prothrombin times, but poor prognosis [4,5].

Treatment

Diet and lifestyle

• Referral to a liver transplant center is required.

• Parenteral or enteral nutritional support is usually needed.

• Survivors return to a normal diet and lifestyle, unless they are recipients of liver grafts, in which case they need lifelong follow-up and immunosuppressive treatment.

Pharmacological treatment

N-acetylcysteine

• Administration should begin as soon as possible and optimally within 12 h of ingestion of acetaminophen [6].

Standard dosage	N-acetylcysteine, 140 mg/kg loading dose, followed by maintenance dose of 70 mg/kg orally every 4 h.
Contraindications	Hypersensitivity.
Main drug interactions	None.
Main side effects	Occasional hypersensitivity reactions; vomiting and aspiration should be watched for.

Gastric protection

• H_2 antagonists or sucralfate to reduce the incidence of gastrointestinal bleeding.

Standard dosage	Ranitidine, 50 mg i.v. 8-hourly. Sucralfate, 1 g orally 6-hourly.
Contraindications	Hypersensitivity.
Main drug interactions	None relevant.
Main side effects	*Ranitidine:* thrombocytopenia.

Lactulose

• This is often ineffective and recommended only in patients with grade 1 or 2 encephalopathy.

Standard dosage	Lactulose, 30 mL 8-hourly; doses titrated to three bowel movements daily.
Contraindications	Gastrointestinal obstruction.
Main drug interactions	None relevant.
Main side effects	Nausea, flatulence, abdominal discomfort.

Treatment aims

To anticipate and treat complications.

Other treatments

• Liver transplantation must be considered early in patients with progressive fulminant hepatitis.

Prognosis

• Most patients who do not progress beyond grade 2 encephalopathy survive.

• Survivors make complete recoveries; progression to chronic liver disease is unusual.

Follow-up and management

• Long-term medical follow-up is rarely needed, except in liver-graft recipients.

• Psychiatric and social support is important in overdose cases.

Key references

1. Blei AT, *et al.*: Complications of intracranial pressure monitoring in fulminant hepatic failure. *Lancet* 1993, **341**:157–158.
2. Lee WM: Acute liver failure. *N Engl J Med* 1993, **329**:1862–1872.
3. Fingerote RJ: Fulminant hepatic failure. *Am J Gastroenterol* 1993, **88**:1000–1010.
4. O'Grady JG, Schalm SW, Williams R: Acute liver failure: redefining the syndromes. *Lancet* 1993, **342**:273–275.
5. O'Grady JG, Portmann BC, Williams R: Fulminant hepatic failure. In *Fulminant Hepatic Failure.* Edited by Schiff E, Schiff L. Philadelphia, JB LIppincott; 1993:1077–1090.
6. Harrison PM, *et al.*: Improvement by N-acetylcysteine of hemodynamics and oxygen transport in fulminant hepatic failure. *N Engl J Med* 1991, **324**:1853–1857.

Diagnosis

Symptoms

Cough, hemoptysis, breathlessness, hoarseness.

Chest pain, lymphadenopathy.

Weight loss, general malaise.

Intellectual impairment, headache, focal neuropathy, tremor.

Signs

- Signs are not always manifest.

Lung nodule or mass.

Lobar or lung collapse, consolidation, pleural effusion, monophonic wheeze.

Cervical lymphadenopathy, hepatomegaly, local chest-wall tenderness, Horner's syndrome, neurological deficit.

Finger clubbing, cerebellar degeneration, peripheral neuropathy.

Investigations [1]

For diagnosis

Chest radiography: shows mass, collapse, distal infection, abscess, adenopathy, metastases.

Sputum cytology: shows malignant cells.

Bronchoscopy: tumor often directly visible; operability can be assessed, and samples obtained for cytology and histology.

Pleural aspiration and biopsy: primary test if effusion present; malignant cells indicate inoperable tumor.

For staging

Bronchoscopy: to assess presence of central disease.

CT of thorax: to assess presence of hilar or mediastinal adenopathy.

Mediastinoscopy: to evaluate lymphadenopathy.

Biochemistry: may indicate bone or liver involvement; sodium and calcium disturbance may occur without metastasis.

Liver ultrasonography: disease often spreads to liver.

CT of brain: disease often spreads to brain.

Pulmonary function tests: to assess ability to tolerate lung resection.

Complications

Lobar collapse, obstruction of superior vena cava.

Pneumonia, abscess.

Pain, pleural effusion.

Pericardial effusion, direct invasion.

Metastases: especially bone, brain, liver, adrenal glands.

Local neurological invasion, neuropathies.

Cushing's syndrome, inappropriate antidiuretic hormone secretion, hypercalcemia.

Recurrent venous thrombosis.

Clubbing, hypertrophic osteoarthropathy.

Differential diagnosis

Simple pneumonia.

Benign tumor or cysts.

Tuberculosis.

Pulmonary metastases.

Other causes of lung abscess.

Other causes of pleural effusion.

Etiology [2]

- Causes include the following:

Cigarette smoking: lung cancer was rare in the 19th century, and its increase is closely linked to the increasing popularity of cigarettes in the 20th century.

Atmospheric pollution: increased rates in urban areas.

Radioactivity: radon, uranium.

Manufacturing: chromate, asbestos, nickel, arsenic, haematite.

Epidemiology

- Lung cancer is the most common fatal cancer in men and women in the U.S.
- The rate of lung cancer mortality is increasing.

Treatment

Diet and lifestyle

• Anorexia is a common feature; no specific diet is needed.

• Patients should be encouraged to be active.

• Most patients stop smoking after diagnosis, but this does not alter prognosis significantly.

Pharmacological treatment [3,4]

• Chemotherapy is the treatment of choice for small-cell cancer; various regimens are available.

• No satisfactory regimen has yet been found for large-cell tumors (*i.e.*, adenocarcinoma, squamous-cell or anaplastic tumors).

• The local oncology service should be consulted.

Nonpharmacological treatment [3,4]

Surgical resection

• Surgical resection is possible in only a few patients.

• It is limited by the frequent involvement of mediastinal nodes and central structures.

• Adequate lung function is needed (forced expiratory volume in 1 s >1.2 L for lobectomy, >1.5 L for pneumonectomy).

• Surgical resection is rarely appropriate for small-cell lung cancer (usually has extensive central disease, even if endoscopically resectable).

Radiotherapy [5]

• Palliative radiotherapy is useful in the management of hemoptysis and bony deposits.

• Radiation therapy can achieve local control of primary tumor and may improve survival.

• "Local" (endobronchial) radiotherapy, a novel experimental treatment, has yet to show any superiority to palliative external beam radiotherapy.

Endobronchial laser resection [6]

• This is a palliative procedure for tracheal or main bronchus disease.

• It is available in only a few specialist centers.

Treatment aims

To identify patients who can be treated surgically.

To identify patients with small-cell cancer and treat them by chemotherapy.

To provide palliative treatment, guided by symptoms, to the remaining patients.

Prognosis

• Prognosis is generally poor unless the tumor is resectable.

• When disease is technically resectable, the 5-year survival rate is ~28%.

Follow-up and management

• Surgical cure is possible in 5%–10% of patients.

• In patients who are inoperable, the main goal is palliation.

• Local symptoms are usually best treated by radiotherapy.

Key references

1. Lillington G: Management of solitary pulmonary nodules. *Dis Mon* 1991, **37**:279–318.
2. Capewell S, *et al.*: Lung cancer in young men. *Resp Med* 1992, **86**:499–502.
3. Murren J, Buzaid A: Chemotherapy and radiation for the treatment of non–small-cell lung cancer. *Clin Chest Med* 1993, **14**:161–200.
4. Matthay R, ed: Lung Cancer. *Clin Chest Med* 1993, **14**:1–203.
5. Hazuka MB, Bunn PA: Controversies in the nonsurgical treatment of stage III non-small cell lung cancer. *Am Rev Resp Dis* 1992, **145**:967–977.
6. Pierce RJ: Lasers, brachytherapy and stents – keeping airways open. *Resp Med* 1991, **85**:263–265.

Diagnosis

Symptoms

• Patients may be asymptomatic.

Acute disease

• Symptoms occur 3–32 days after tick bite.

Influenza-like illness: malaise, pyrexia, myalgia, arthralgia, sore throat.

Rash.

Stiff neck.

Photophobia.

Chronic disease

• Symptoms occur weeks or months later.

Headache, stiff neck, photophobia, confusion, concentration and memory impairment.

Chest pain.

Joint pain and swelling.

Abdominal pain, tenderness, diarrhea.

Rashes.

Signs

Acute disease

Pyrexia, tender muscles or joints, inflamed throat.

Erythema chronicum migrans: characteristic rash (~5 cm), red macule or papule at site of tick bite, enlarges peripherally with central clearing over several weeks; metastatic lesions may develop; can last months.

Lymphadenopathy.

Meningism.

Erythema chronicum migrans.

Chronic disease

Meningitis, encephalitis, cranial neuritis (especially Bell's palsy), radiculoneuritis, peripheral neuropathies.

Atrioventricular block, myopericarditis.

Arthritis.

Hepatomegaly, splenomegaly.

Acrodermatitis chronica atrophicans: vivid red lesions becoming sclerotic or atrophic.

Acrodermatitis chronicum atrophicans.

Investigations

Microscopy, histopathology, and culture: lack sensitivity and not widely available but may be diagnostic.

Serological tests: widely available but not diagnostic (support clinical diagnosis); IgM tests positive 3–6 weeks after infection, may persist for many months, but may not be reproducible; IgG tests positive 6–8 weeks after infection, may remain positive for years, but more reproducible so are mainstay of diagnosis; immunofluorescence tests and enzyme linked immunosorbent assays most widely available.

• False-negative antibody results may occur early in illness, with antibiotic treatment, or due to immune complexes; a negative antibody test does not exclude the diagnosis. False-positive results are due to other spirochete infections, other infections, or the test; Western blotting may distinguish true- from false-positive results.

Complications

CNS abnormalities.

Cardiac conduction disturbances.

Oligoarthritis.

Differential diagnosis

Erythema chronicum migrans

Erythema marginatum.

Erythema multiforme rheumaticum.

Granuloma annulare.

Lymphadenopathy

Infectious mononucleosis.

Cytomegalovirus.

Toxoplasmosis.

Neurological symptoms

Infectious diseases.

Toxoplasmosis.

Guillain–Barré syndrome.

Multiple sclerosis.

Cardiac symptoms

Infectious diseases.

Chronic heart disease.

Digitalis use.

Arthritis

Rheumatoid arthritis.

Reactive arthritis.

Other dermatological symptoms

Erythema nodosum.

Circulatory insufficiencies.

Lymphoma.

Etiology

• Infection is transmitted by tick bites, usually *Ixodes scapularis* in the US.

• The causative organism is *Borrelia burgdorferi*, a spirochete.

Epidemiology

• Lyme disease is found in the USA, Europe, Russia, China, Japan, and Australia.

• Occurrence parallels distribution and infection in ticks (0%–25%).

• In forested areas, 5%–10% of the population have antibodies.

• Infection peaks in June and July.

• It is found in patients of all ages but especially in the most active and those exposed to ticks.

Treatment

Diet and lifestyle

• No special precautions are necessary.

Pharmacological treatment

Criteria for treatment

• The risk depends on infected tick attachment: <24 h, little risk; 48 h, 50% risk; 72 h, almost certain infection.

• Infection occurs in ~10% of people bitten by infected ticks, so empirical treatment is not justified in areas where infected ticks are rare.

• Erythema chronicum migrans must be treated; acute disease with positive serology and chronic disease when other causes are excluded warrant treatment.

• Treatment should be considered in anxious patients with possible infection but without high expectation of success.

• Asymptomatic individuals with positive serology probably should not be treated.

For acute disease

Standard dosage	Doxycycline, 200 mg orally daily for 14 days. Amoxicillin, 500 mg 3 times daily for 14 days.
Contraindications	*Doxycycline:* pregnancy, lactation, children <12 years, SLE, porphyria. *Amoxicillin:* penicillin hypersensitivity.
Main drug interactions	*Doxycycline:* anticoagulants, antiepileptics, oral contraceptives. *Amoxicillin:* anticoagulants, oral contraceptives.
Main side effects	*Doxycycline:* nausea, vomiting, diarrhea, headache. *Amoxicillin:* nausea, diarrhea, rashes.

• Erythromycin and clarithromycin are less effective but can be used in penicillin-sensitive children.

For chronic disease

• Chronic disease may be cardiac, neurologic, or rheumatologic.

Standard dosage	Ceftriaxone, 2 g i.v. or i.m. daily for 14–21 days. Penicillin G, 3 g i.v. 4 times daily for 14–21 days.
Contraindications	*Ceftriaxone:* hypersensitivity to cephalosporin. *Penicillin:* hypersensitivity.
Main drug interactions	*Ceftriaxone:* anticoagulants, probenecid. *Penicillin:* anticoagulants, oral contraceptives.
Main side effects	*Ceftriaxone:* gastrointestinal complaints, allergic reactions, rashes, hematological disturbance, liver dysfunction. *Penicillin:* sensitivity reactions, especially urticaria, angioedema, anaphylaxis.

Treatment aims

To kill organism.

To prevent disease progression.

To alleviate symptoms.

Prognosis

• Despite antibiotic treatment, symptoms recur in 50% of patients, although severity and duration are greatly reduced; occasionally, recurrent symptoms may last several years.

• Acute Lyme disease and carditis have good prognosis.

• Cranial nerve palsies and meningitis have good prognosis; radiculoneuritis, peripheral neuropathy, encephalitis, and encephalomyelitis usually have a favorable outcome, but a tendency toward chronic or recurrent disease is seen.

• Arthritis often resolves, but response may be slow, often needing further treatment.

• In chronic disease, recurrence is not usual.

Follow-up and management

• Patients may need careful monitoring for months or years, depending on the severity of the symptoms.

General references

Guy EC: The laboratory diagnosis of Lyme borreliosis. *Review of Medical Microbiology* 1993, **4**:89–96.

Magid D, *et al.*: Prevention of Lyme disease after tick bites. *N Engl J Med* 1992, **327**:534–541.

Rahn DW, Malawista SE: Recommendations for diagnosis and treatment. *Ann Intern Med* 1991, **114**:472–481.

Weber K, Pfister H: Clinical management of Lyme borreliosis. *Lancet* 1994, **343**:1017–1020.

Malaria

Diagnosis

Symptoms

• The diagnosis may be overlooked, especially if a travel history is not obtained. A brief stopover in an endemic area is sufficient to allow inoculation with the parasite.

• Illness usually occurs 1–4 weeks after mosquito bite but may be delayed for weeks or even years.

Uncomplicated malaria

Fever: usually rapid onset; rigors, malaise, headache, and myalgia followed by profuse sweating; fever paroxysms every 2–3 days develop in some patients.

Nausea, vomiting, anorexia, diarrhea, cough: possible early symptoms.

Complicated falciparum malaria

Altered consciousness, convulsions, oliguria, jaundice, respiratory distress, hemorrhage.

Signs

• Fever is usual; it may, however, be intermittent, so some patients are afebrile when first seen. Occasionally, patients remain afebrile throughout the illness.

Uncomplicated malaria

Fever: either continuous or episodic.

Rigors.

Moderately enlarged liver or spleen.

Complicated falciparum malaria

Confusion.

Delirium.

Coma.

Acidosis.

Pallor.

Jaundice.

Shock syndrome.

Investigations

Urgent

Blood films: thick and thin, stained with Giemsa for malaria parasites, to identify species of malaria and density of parasitemia; a single blood film may be negative in malaria; repeat films may reveal parasites.

Blood glucose profile: repeated at intervals.

Hemoglobin and full blood count: regularly, because hemoglobin may fall rapidly.

In severe falciparum malaria

Urine output, plasma urea, creatinine, electrolytes, and arterial blood gas analysis: to identify renal failure and respiratory distress syndrome.

Platelet count: if $<50 \times 10^9$/L, bleeding time, serum fibrinogen, and fibrin degradation products should be checked to identify disseminated intravascular coagulation.

Chest radiography: peripheral shadows indicate pulmonary edema or adult respiratory distress syndrome.

Blood culture: for bacterial pathogens in patients with shock.

Complications

• Complications occur only with *Plasmodium falciparum* malaria; they are more likely if treatment is delayed.

Cerebral malaria: altered consciousness with or without convulsions.

Extreme prostration.

Shock.

Hypoglycemia.

Lactic acidosis.

Intravascular hemolysis.

Jaundice.

Severe anemia.

Disseminated intravascular coagulation.

Respiratory distress syndrome.

Acute renal failure.

Differential diagnosis

Uncomplicated malaria

Influenza or any viral upper respiratory tract infection.

Hepatitis, gastroenteritis.

Complicated falciparum malaria

Fulminant hepatitis.

Meningitis, encephalitis.

Leptospirosis, heat stroke, ketoacidosis.

Septicemia or septic shock.

Pneumonia or pulmonary edema.

Acute tubular necrosis.

Etiology

• Malaria is a protozoal infection transmitted by mosquitoes.

• Four parasite species infect humans: *Plasmodium falciparum, P. vivax, P. malariae,* and *P. ovale.*

• Only *P. falciparum* malaria progresses to complicated disease, which may be fatal.

Epidemiology

• 1–3 million children die of malaria annually throughout the world.

Treatment

Diet and lifestyle

• Travelers to endemic areas should remember the following points:
• Mosquito bites can be prevented by using permethrin-impregnated bed-net or sleeping in well screened buildings, wearing long sleeves and trousers in evenings or after dark, and applying insect repellent containing diethyl toluamide (DEET) for journeys into swamp or jungle (Mosigard is an alternative).
• Antimalarial prophylactic drugs appropriate to the area to be visited should be taken.
• Immediate diagnosis and treatment should be sought for any fever developing during or after travel.
• A supply of antimalarial drugs suitable for immediate treatment of possible malaria should be taken on any journey far from medical services.

Pharmacological treatment

For malaria due to *Plasmodium vivax, P. malariae*, or *P. ovale*

• Oral treatment should be given when possible. Doses are for chloroquine base.

Standard dosage Chloroquine phosphate or sulfate, 600 mg (child, 10 mg/kg) on days 1 and 2; 300 mg (child, 5 mg/kg) on day 3.

Contraindications Rare hypersensitivity.

Special points *P. vivax* acquired in southeast Asia may be resistant to chloroquine: alternative treatment is Fansidar, 3 tablets once daily (adults).

Main drug interactions None of importance.

Main side effects Rare hypotension, pruritus in blacks.

For malaria due to *P. vivax or P. ovale*

Chloroquine as above and primaquine, 15 mg (child, 0.25 mg/kg) daily for 15 days to eliminate dormant hepatic parasites: contraindicated in glucose-6-phosphate dehydrogenase deficiency; status must be checked before primaquines prescribed.

For uncomplicated malaria due to *P. falciparum*

• Treatment is needed urgently because complications may develop quickly; in non-endemic countries (*e.g.*, US), hospital admission is advised, at least for initiation of treatment. Oral treatment is recommended when possible.

Standard dosage Quinine sulfate salt, 600 mg (child, 10 mg/kg) 3 times daily for 7 days, with doxycycline, 100 mg twice daily for 7 days.
Alternatively, mefloquine, 500 mg orally, repeated after 6 h.

Contraindications *Quinine*: caution in cardiac disease.
Doxycycline: pregnancy.
Mefloquine: pregnancy, beta blocker treatment, history of epilepsy or chronic neurological disease.

Main drug interactions *Quinine:* may potentiate cardiotoxic effect of other cardiac drugs.

Main side effects *Quinine:* hypoglycemia (especially in pregnancy), hypotension, tinnitus (always).

For *P. falciparum* malaria with complications

• This is a medical emergency: immediate hospital admission is vital, preferably with intensive care facilities.

Standard dosage Quinine dihydrochloride salt, 20 mg/kg (up to 1400 mg) i.v. infusion in saline solution over 4 h, then 10 mg/kg over 4 h for each dose every 12 h; changed to oral treatment as soon as possible.
Alternatively, quinidine gluconate.

Contraindications Caution in elderly patients or those with cardiac disease.

Special points First dose 10 mg/kg if quinine, mefloquine, or halofantrine taken in preceding 24 h.
When condition satisfactory, Fansidar can be added.

Main drug interactions None of importance.

Main side effects None of importance.

Treatment aims

To support patients with complicated disease while drugs eliminate parasites.

To clear blood of parasites.

To eliminate liver-stage dormant parasites (*Plasmodium vivax, P. ovale*).

Prognosis

• Full recovery is expected for patients with nonfalciparum infection.
• Prompt correct treatment of *Plasmodium falciparum* malaria should result in cure.
• After complications have developed, the mortality in falciparum malaria is 10%–40%, determined by the extent and severity of the complications and the quality of intensive care offered.
• Recovery from renal failure or coma is usually complete; a few patients have neurological sequelae after cerebral malaria.

Follow-up and management

• Patients must be told to report promptly with any fever because recrudescence or relapse may occur.
• Organ complications must be followed up in their own right.
• Hemoglobin concentrations must be adequately restored and maintained; this must be monitored.

General references

Bradley D, *et al.*: Prophylaxis against malaria for travellers from the United Kingdom. *BMJ* 1993, **306**:1247–1252.

Molyneux ME, Fox R: Diagnosis and treatment of malaria in Britain. *BMJ* 1993, **306**:1175–1180.

World Health Organization: Severe and complicated malaria. *Trans R Soc Trop Med Hyg* 1990, **84 (suppl 2)**:1–65.

Diagnosis

Symptoms

Fever: for 3–4 days.
Rash.
Systemic upset; "misery."
Unproductive cough.
Catarrh.
Conjunctivitis.

Signs

Prodromal period before rash

Fever.

Enanthema, Koplik's spots: pathognomic small greyish-white spots on reddened mucous membranes, notably the buccal mucosa.

Rash: maculopapular, blotchy, not itchy; starts on face and behind ears; spreads downwards over a few days; lasts ~5 days; almost invariably stains (persisting discoloration that does not blanch on pressure) from erythrocyte leakage during active rash.

Associated with development of rash

Reddened throat.
Bronchitic cough.
Conjunctivitis.
Lymph-node enlargement.

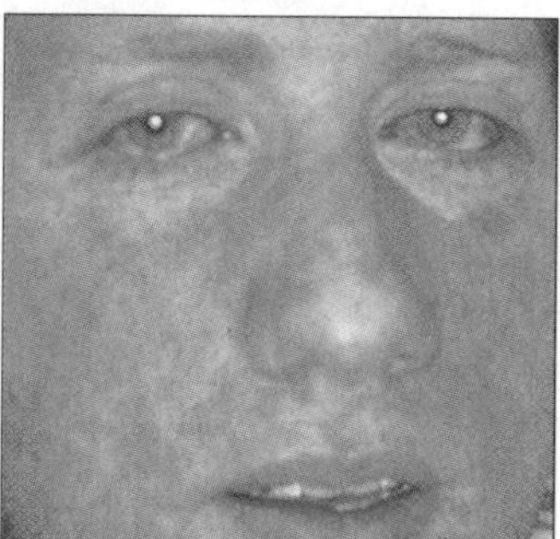

Blotchy rash of measles and conjunctivitis.

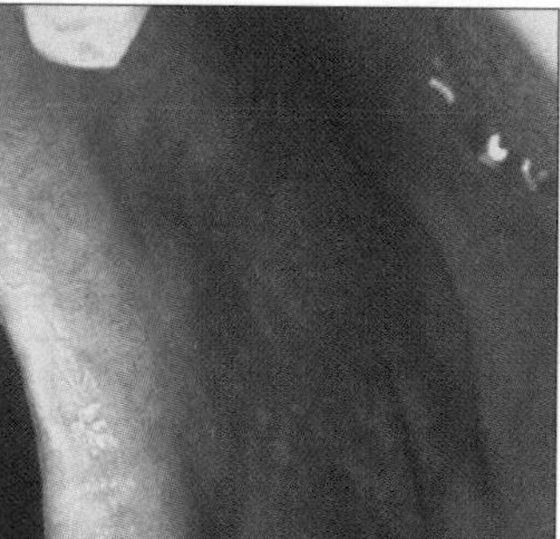

Koplik's spots in measles.

Investigations

• The clinical picture is usually diagnostic.

Throat swab or nasopharyngeal aspirate: measles virus may be grown (technically difficult).
Immunofluorescent staining of throat secretions: may identify measles virus.
Serology: measles-specific IgM may be present in blood early in illness.
Paired sera examination: may show diagnostic rises in antibody (about fourfold).

Complications

• Complications are more severe in old or very young patients.

Measles bronchiolitis: when rash heaviest on trunk.
Secondary bacterial pneumonia and otitis media: in ~15%, especially children.
Febrile convulsions: in children, especially during prodrome.
Post–acute measles encephalitis: immune-mediated, at about day 6 of illness.
Subacute sclerosing panencephalitis: caused by persisting measles virus infection in nervous system, usually fatal; develops several years after acute infection.
Gastroenteritis: in malnourished children can lead to kwashiorkor and acute vitamin A deficiency.
Thrombocytopenia.
Giant-cell pneumonia or measles encephalitis: progressive in immunocompromised patient.

Differential diagnosis

Drug rashes: do not usually evolve from above downwards, may be itchy, only occasionally stain, often not associated with fever.

Rubella: patients not usually ill, rash not usually blotchy.

Adenovirus or enterovirus infection.

• Koplik's spots are not a feature in any of the above.

Etiology

• Measles is caused by measles virus, an RNA virus.

• Transmission is by respiratory droplets.

Epidemiology

• Measles occurs worldwide.

Infectivity

• Measles is highly infectious: patients are infectious for about 4 days before the rash and until the rash has stained.

• Active infection without illness and a rash is extremely rare.

• Immunity after an attack is for life.

• Maternally derived antibodies protect babies for about the first 6 months of life.

• There is no infective carrier state.

Mean incubation period

To febrile illness: 10 days.

To rash: 14 days.

Treatment

Diet and lifestyle

• Patients should be isolated during the period of infectivity, which usually lasts from the onset of symptoms until the rash has stained.

Pharmacological treatment

Symptomatic

Analgesics, *e.g.*, acetaminophen.

Antibacterial drugs for bacterial complications.

• Ribavirin may be of benefit for giant-cell pneumonia.

Prophylactic

Vaccination by live virus preparation in second year of life as MMR: may cause mild measles-like illness.

Pooled human immunoglobulin: protective if given shortly after exposure.

• Vaccination and pooled human immunoglobulin can be given together if vaccination of vulnerable patients (*e.g.*, those with cystic fibrosis) is desired.

• Vitamin A deficiency (clinical or subclinical) increases the severity, complications, and risk of death from measles.

• In countries where the measles fatality rate is 1% or more, vitamin A should be given in all cases; elsewhere, it should be given in severe cases.

Treatment aims

To relieve symptoms.

To treat complications promptly.

Prognosis

• Most patients make a full recovery and are immune thereafter.

Follow-up and management

• No follow-up is necessary.

General references

Anonymous: Measles surveillance. *Commun Dis Rep CDR Wkly* 1993, **3**:21.

Dales LG, *et al.*: Measles epidemic from failure to immunize. *West J Med* 1993, **159**:455–464.

Makhene MK, Diaz PS: Clinical presentations and complications of suspected measles in hospitalized children. *Pediatr Infect Dis J* 1993, **12**:836–840.

Tohani VK, Kennedy FD: Vaccine efficacy in a measles immunisation programme. *Commun Dis Rep CDR Rev* 1992, **2**:R59–R60.

Diagnosis

Symptoms

Headache.
Neck and back pain and stiffness.
Vomiting.
Photophobia.
Fever.
Altered level of consciousness.
Seizures.

• Atypical clinical manifestations may occur in very young, elderly, or immunocompromised patients (highest-risk groups).

Signs

Nuchal rigidity: on flexion only, not on lateral rotation.

"Meningeal cry": high-pitched, in infants.

Kernig's sign: pain and hamstring spasm on passive knee extension with hip flexed.

Brudzinski's sign: spontaneous knee and hip flexion on attempted neck flexion.

Cranial nerve palsies and other focal signs.

Deteriorating level of consciousness: in up to 25% of patients.

Papilledema, bulging fontanelle in infants: indicating raised intracranial pressure.

Fever, tachycardia, shock, evidence of primary source of infection: *e.g.*, pneumonia, endocarditis, sinusitis, otitis media.

Rash: in ~50% of patients with meningococcal infections, sometimes briefly erythematous before becoming petechial or purpuric.

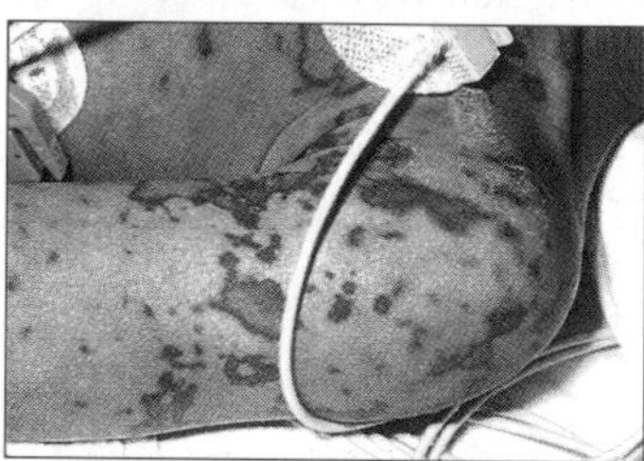

Purpuric rash of meningococcal meningitis.

Investigations

Lumbar puncture: in untreated acute bacterial meningitis, reveals turbid CSF under raised pressure, neutrophilic pleocytosis (hundreds or thousands of cells/μL), protein concentration usually >1 g/L, glucose concentration low. Specific tests for causative organisms include Gram stain, culture, sensitivity testing, fungal and tubercular microscopy and culture, and bacterial antigen immunoassay. Contraindications include papilledema, deteriorating level of consciousness, and focal neurological signs; prepuncture cranial CT is needed in such patients to exclude mass lesion.

Full blood count: to detect neutrophil leukocytosis.

Coagulation screen and fibrin degradation product analysis: for disseminated intravascular coagulation.

Electrolyte analysis: to detect hyponatremia.

Blood culture: may be positive when CSF sterile.

Chest and skull (sinus) radiography: to identify primary source of infection.

Complications

Seizures, focal CNS signs, raised intracranial pressure, subdural effusion, cerebral or subdural abscess formation, hydrocephalus (obstructive or communicating).

Septic shock, disseminated intravascular coagulation with adrenal hemorrhage: Waterhouse–Friderichsen's syndrome, complication of meningococcal meningitis.

Inappropriate antidiuretic hormone secretion: in <10% of patients.

Arthritis: septic or immune complex, in <10% of meningococcal infections.

Behavioral disturbances, mental retardation, hearing loss, epilepsy, cranial nerve palsies, visual and motor deficits: long-term complications (more usual in *S. pneumoniae* infections; <30% of patients).

Differential diagnosis

• Few patients, even with severe headache and fever, have meningitis.

Viral meningitis, especially enteroviruses, mumps.

Intercurrent infections, especially influenza A and B with meningism.

Cranial infections: cerebral abscess, sinusitis, throat infections.

Noninfective meningitis: subarachnoid hemorrhage, leukemic infiltration, Mollaret's meningitis (recurrent fever, meningeal signs, and CSF pleocytosis).

Autoimmune diseases, vasculitis.

Chemical meningitis, *e.g.*, intrathecal drugs.

Etiology

• 70%–90% of cases of bacterial meningitis are due to one of three organisms:

Neisseria meningitidis.

Haemophilus influenzae (type b).

Streptococcus pneumoniae.

• Other organisms found in specific at-risk groups include the following:

Enterobacteriaceae, group B streptococci in neonates.

Listeria monocytogenes in neonates and immunocompromised patients.

Mycobacterium tuberculosis in patients from developing countries and immunocompromised patients.

Staphylococci in patients with head trauma or neurosurgical shunts.

Epidemiology

• The incidence of bacterial meningitis is ~5–10 in 100 000 annually in developed countries.

• The three common organisms have characteristic patterns of occurrence: *Neisseria meningitidis* in epidemics, *Haemophilus influenzae* in children <5 years, *Streptococcus pneumoniae* in patients aged >40 years (especially alcoholic, splenectomized, and sickle-cell anemic patients).

Treatment

Diet and lifestyle

• No special precautions are necessary.

Pharmacological treatment

General management

• Bacterial meningitis may prove fatal within hours; successful treatment depends on early diagnosis and i.v. administration of appropriate antibiotics in antimeningitic doses (intrathecal antibiotics not recommended); until the causative organism and its antibiotic sensitivities have been identified, broad-spectrum agents should be used (*e.g.*, ampicillin and ceftriaxone).

• If lumbar puncture is delayed by the need for prepuncture CT, antibiotic treatment should be started before the scan, after blood cultures.

• Treatment should ideally be bactericidal with a high therapeutic ratio, the drug penetrating the CSF in adequate concentrations; very high i.v. doses may be needed despite damage to the blood–brain barrier in meningitis.

• Adjunctive corticosteroids are indicated when bacterial organisms are present on Gram stain or in the setting of increased intracranial pressure.

Against *Neisseria meningitidis, Streptococcus pneumoniae*, and *Haemophilus influenzae*

Standard dosage — *Adults:* ceftriaxone, 2 g every 12 h for 10 days.

Contraindications — Cephalosporin hypersensitivity; caution in renal impairment, history of allergy.

Special points — Other options include cefotaxime, ceftriaxone, and chloramphenicol.

Main drug interactions — None.

Main side effects — Sensitivity reactions.

Against penicillin-susceptible pneumococcus or established meningococcus

Standard dosage — *Adults:* Penicillin G, 14.4 g (24 MU) i.v. daily in divided doses (usually 4 MU initially, then 2 MU 2-hourly; can be relaxed to 4- or 6-hourly regimen with evidence of clinical improvement, usually within 48–72 h); treatment should continue for 7 days after the patient has become afebrile (14 days for *S. pneumoniae* infection).
Children and infants: Penicillin G, 100–300 mg/kg daily depending on age, according to manufacturer's current prescribing information.

Contraindications — Penicillin hypersensitivity; caution in renal impairment, history of allergy.

Special points — Other options include cefotaxime, ceftriaxone, and chloramphenicol.

Main drug interactions — None.

Main side effects — Sensitivity reactions.

Prevention

• Chemoprophylaxis (using rifampicin or ciprofloxacin) is indicated for household contacts and index patients before hospital discharge.

• Immunization against *Haemophilus influenzae* infection (using *H. influenzae* type b vaccine) is recommended routinely for children at the ages of 2, 3, and 4 months.

Treatment aims

To secure survival and prevent persistent neurological complications.

To reduce the of recurrence by treating any predisposing cause.

To prevent spread to close contacts.

Prognosis

• Mortality is ~10% overall, 5%–10% from *Haemophilus influenzae* infection, 5%–10% from *Neisseria meningitidis* infection, and 10%–30% from *Streptococcus pneumoniae* infection.

• Long-term sequelae are 9%–22%, 4%–6%, and 14%–40%, respectively.

Follow-up and management

• Repeat lumbar puncture to monitor treatment is not necessary if the patient is improving.

• Bacteriological relapse needs immediate reinstitution of treatment.

• Adults should be reviewed at 3 months, children at 6–12 months, and neonates for longer to detect any long-term sequelae.

Causes of treatment failure

Wrong diagnosis: *e.g.*, tuberculosis, abscess.

Wrong drug: poor CSF penetration, antimicrobial resistance.

Wrong route: intraventricular instillation needed for ventriculitis with "resistant" infections.

Poor-risk patient: extremes of age, immunocompromise.

Unrecognized complication: treatable raised intracranial pressure, abscess or ventriculitis, subdural effusion or abscess (treatable); vasculitis, cerebritis (less treatable).

Shock.

General references

Finch RG, Mandragos C: Corticosteroids in bacterial meningitis. *BMJ* 1991, **302**:607–608.

Quagliarello V, Scheld WM: Bacterial meningitis: Pathogenesis, pathophysiology and progress. *N Engl J Med* 1992, **327**:864–872.

Tunkel AR, Wispelweg B, Scheld M: Bacterial meningitis: recent advances in pathophysiology and treatment. *Ann Intern Med* 1990, **112**:610–623.

Diagnosis

Symptoms

• Symptoms are usually chronic, usually <3 weeks, but can be acute.

Immunosuppression: with CD4 counts $<100 \times 10^9$/L.

Headache: in 81% of patients.

Fever: in 77%.

Nausea or vomiting: in 44%.

Photophobia: in 27%.

Seizures: in 5%; can be the presenting feature.

Signs

• No signs are reported in >50% of patients.

Abnormal mental status: in 28%.

Focal neurological signs and papilledema: rare; may be present if the patient has cryptococcus.

Extraneural involvement: in 20%, with pulmonary infiltrates, skin lesions, and prustatic involvement.

Investigations

• Cryptococcal antigen in blood is positive in 90% of patients.

CT or MRI: should be performed before lumbar puncture to exclude a mass lesion if focal neurological signs are present; usually shows no abnormality or cerebral atrophy; communicating hydrocephalus infrequent; low-density lesions, scattered and symmetrical, sometimes seen, attributed to cryptococci.

CSF culture: to establish diagnosis; usually shows mononuclear pleocytosis (<70% leukocytes) and raised protein; glucose may be low, sometimes the only abnormality; india-ink preparation can show cryptococci; cryptococcal antigen positive in 95% of patients; cryptococcus can be cultured from other sites (sputum, blood, bone marrow).

Other investigations: abnormal liver function, low albumin concentration, or hyponatremia in 20%; lymphopenia common in peripheral blood.

Complications

Death: during the acute illness despite treatment (up to 30% of patients); sometimes due to other overwhelming systemic infections or progression of the meningitis with seizures, cranial nerve palsies, stupor, and coma.

Cerebral cryptococcomas: *i.e.*, cryptococcal abscesses; rare.

Differential diagnosis

Viral and tuberculous meningitis.

Cerebral toxoplasmosis.

Cerebral lymphoma.

Benign headaches (migraine, tension, depression).

Meningitis due to hysteria.

Etiology

• Cryptococcus is a yeast present in high quantities in the environment.

• Infection is acquired by inhalation.

• The spread to the CNS is hematogenous.

Epidemiology

• Most cases of cryptococcal meningitis are AIDS-related.

• Cryptococcal meningitis is found in 2%–12% of AIDS patients in different clinical series.

• It is the most frequent cause of meningitis.

Treatment

Diet and lifestyle

• No special precautions are necessary.

Pharmacological treatment

Initial treatment

• The established initial treatment is by amphotericin B and flucytosine.

• Treatment of the first episode fails in 20%–40% of patients.

Standard dosage	Amphotericin B, 0.75 mg/kg i.v. daily, and flucytosine, 50 mg/kg daily. Usual course is 15 mg/kg total.
Contraindications	Renal failure, pregnancy, breast-feeding, old age.
Special points	Hepatic and renal function, blood count, electrolytes, and drug concentrations must be monitored.
Main drug interactions	*Amphotericin B:* increased risk of nephrotoxicity with cyclosporin, aminoglycosides; antagonizes miconazole.
Main side effects	*Amphotericin B:* nausea, vomiting, fever, nephrotoxicity. *Flucytosine:* diarrhea, bone-marrow suppression.

Adjunctive 5-Fluorocytosine

• This agent may improve the outcome when added to amphotericin.

Standard dosage	5F-C, 150 mg/kg daily.
Contraindications	Hepatitis, vomiting.
Main drug interactions	None.
Main side effects	Vomiting, hepatitis, bone marrow suppression.

Maintenance treatment

• ~50% of HIV-seropositive patients with cryptococcal meningitis relapse without maintenance treatment.

• The relapse rate can be markedly reduced with fluconazole.

Standard dosage	Fluconazole, 200 mg orally daily for life.
Contraindications	Possibly breast-feeding, pregnancy, children.
Special points	Can be used for initial treatment i.v. or orally at 400 mg daily in mildly ill patients who are not obtunded. Itraconazole is a useful alternative.
Main drug interactions	Enhances warfarin, phenytoin, theophylline, cyclosporin, sulfonylureas; reduces rifampin.
Main side effects	Diarrhea, bone-marrow suppression.

Treatment aims

To eradicate cryptococcal infection.

Prognosis

• 30%–50% of patients do not respond to treatment.

Follow-up and management

• Patients should be closely followed, particularly for the first year when relapses are more common.

General references

Bozzette SA, *et al.*: A placebo controlled trial of maintenance therapy with fluconazole after treatment of cryptococcal meningitis in the acquired immmunodeficiency syndrome. California Collaborative Treatment Group. *N Engl J Med* 1991, **324**:580–584.

Chuck SL, Sande MA: Infections with *Cryptococcus neoformans* in the acquired immunodeficiency syndrome. *N Engl J Med* 1989, **321**:794–799.

Saag MS, *et al.*: Comparison of amphotericin B with fluconazole in the treatment of acute AIDS-associated cryptococcal meningitis. *N Engl J Med* 1992, **326**:83–89.

Weinke T, *et al.*: Cryptococcosis in AIDS patients: observations concerning CNS involvement. *J Neurol* 1989, **236**:38–42.

Diagnosis

Definition

Migraine with aura (classic migraine): characterized by aura followed by episodic unilateral throbbing headache, with nausea, photophobia, and phonophobia; auras usually last 10–20 min but can persist for up to 1 h; laterality of neurological disturbance not related to side of ensuing headache.

Migraine without aura (common migraine): characterized by episodic unilateral or bilateral headache, gastrointestinal upset, photo- or phonophobia, but no aura.

• Migraine headaches are paroxysmal, lasting from a few hours up to 3 days, but with periods of complete relief between attacks.

Cluster headache: 90% of sufferers men; paroxysmal very severe unilateral periorbital pain lasting 0.5–2 h, once or twice daily (often at night) for weeks, with months or years of relief between bouts; usually associated with Horner's syndrome, lacrimation and nasal stuffiness ipsilateral to pain.

Ophthalmoplegic migraine: recurrent attacks of III or VI cranial-nerve palsies associated with headache; resolution of deficit may be delayed by several days.

Retinal migraine: monocular visual loss involving scotoma or altitudinal defect followed by headache.

Hemiplegic migraine: recurrent attacks of hemiparesis of rapid onset followed by headache; weakness may last hours.

• Migraine variants are diagnoses of exclusion; other more serious causes of the clinical picture (*e.g.*, stroke, aneurysmal leak, transient ischemic attack) must be excluded, especially if the pain is severe, before the diagnosis is accepted.

Symptoms

• The aura of classic migraine may be visual (in 50% of patients) or sensory (in 30%) or occasionally may involve dysphasia or motor deficit.

Visual auras: teichopsia, fortification spectra, fragmentation, scotoma, homonymous hemianopia.

Transient tingling or numbness: sensory symptoms; upper limbs more frequently involved than lower limbs.

Signs

• Common migraine may have no signs.

• The scotomas, hemianopia, and sensorimotor phenomena of classic migraine may be detected if the aura is still present at the time of examination.

• Prolonged deficit requires exclusion of other causes.

Investigations [1]

• Investigation is not needed if the diagnosis of migraine is well founded; it is needed when the diagnosis is in doubt and in patients with residual neurological deficit after migraine.

• Investigation including the following is aimed at excluding alternative diagnoses:

ESR measurement: for temporal arteritis.

Radiography, MRI: for cervical spondylosis.

CT or MRI: for tumor, vascular malformation, hydrocephalus.

CSF analysis: for subarachnoid bleed, arteritis.

Angiography: for aneurysmal bleeding.

Complications

Complicated migraine: rarely, residua from migraine auras continue as permanent deficits or stroke.

Dehydration.

Migrainous infarction: rare, usually posterior parietal or occipital.

Differential diagnosis

Tension headache: continuous dull, pressure-like pain over vertex or around head; lasts weeks to years; nausea occasional, vomiting rare; may coexist with migraine to produce pattern of constant headache with episodic exacerbations.

Temporal arteritis: in patients usually aged >65 years with unilateral temporal pain and tenderness; visual disturbances may occur before blindness; high ESR.

Local disease: *e.g.*, glaucoma, sinusitis, naso-pharyngeal lesions, vascular abnormalities.

Tumor: cerebral tumors usually manifest with epilepsy, focal neurological deficits, clouded consciousness, and rarely headache, although this may develop later.

Hemorrhage: abrupt onset of severe head-ache, usually occipital and associated with neck stiffness and photophobia; aneurysms may produce pressure effects; no history of recurrent similar headaches.

Arteriopathies: SLE may manifest with migraine; polyarteritis nodosa may produce headache and transient neurological deficits.

Etiology

• Migraine is probably due to a combination of genetic predisposition and environmental triggers (*e.g.*, stress, certain foods) causing changes in neurotransmitter release (5-HT), with alteration in cerebral blood flow and pain in the distribution of the trigeminal nerve.

Epidemiology [2]

• The prevalence is ~5% in men and 12%–15% in women, although some investigators have quoted prevalence rates as high as 60%–70%.

• The incidence increases from puberty to young adulthood; onset >50 years is unusual.

Treatment

Diet and lifestyle

• Dietary precipitants, *e.g.*, chocolate, cheese, coffee, red wine, should be avoided in sensitive patients.

• Stress is a common precipitant of migraine: appropriate measures may reduce the frequency of attacks.

• Oral contraceptives are best avoided; they are contraindicated in migraine with focal neurological deficits.

Pharmacological treatment

• Many patients treat attacks satisfactorily with rest, darkness, and simple analgesics, including naproxen, Midrin.

For migraine with and without aura: acute

• Patients with gastrointestinal disturbance and more severe headache may benefit from a combination of analgesic and antiemetic; the antiemetic not only reduces vomiting but increases gastric emptying thereby improving absorption of the analgesic.

• More severe attacks unresponsive to this treatment may be treated by sumatriptan or ergotamine.

Standard dosage Sumatriptan, 25–100 mg orally at onset or 6 mg s.c. by auto-injector.
Ergotamine in varying doses according to route.

Contraindications *Sumatriptan:* patients >65 years or with history of coronary disease; to be avoided in children or hemiplegic migraine.
Ergotamine: vascular disease, active infection, hemiplegic migraine.

Special points *Sumatriptan:* effective in 60% at 2 h and 80% at 4 h.
Ergotamine: maximum dose of preparation must not be exceeded because of risk of vasospasm.

Main drug interactions *Sumatriptan:* ergotamine, monoamine oxidase inhibitors, lithium.
Ergotamine: beta blockers, methysergide, and sumatriptan all increase risk of vasospasm.

Main side effects *Sumatriptan:* chest pain or tightness, light-headedness, transient pain at site of injection.
Ergotamine: nausea, vomiting, headache (possibly due to overuse), tingling, chest tightness.

For common and classic migraine: prophylactic

• Beta blockers or 5-HT antagonists should be considered for ≥2 attacks a month; 6–12 months' effective treatment may allow withdrawal at original frequency.

Standard dosage Propranolol, 60–160 mg long-acting daily may be sufficient; larger doses occasionally needed.
May also use nadolol or metaprolol.
Tricyclic antidepressants: amitriptyline, nortriptyline.

Contraindications *Beta blockers:* asthma, cardiac failure, heart block.

Main drug interactions *See manufacturer's current prescribing information.*

Main side effects *Beta blockers:* bradycardia, heart failure, bronchospasm, fatigue, depression.
Tricyclic antidepressants: dry mouth, orthostasis, fatigue, weight gain.

For cluster headache: acute

Sumatriptan or ergotamine.
Oxygen (>40%), if not contraindicated.
Prednisolone, 60 mg (occasionally helpful).

For migrainous neuralgia: prophylactic

Short-term sumatriptan or ergotamine before predicted onset of attack.
Lithium and methysergide in refractory patients: regular monitoring of lithium concentrations and checking of thyroid function needed; methysergide used intermittently (4–5 months every 6 months) to reduce risk of retroperitoneal fibrosis.

Treatment aims

To provide adequate relief from symptoms.

To adjust treatment appropriately to severity and frequency of attacks.

To minimize effect of migraine on work and leisure activities.

Prognosis

• Most patients respond well to acute or prophylactic treatment, or both.

• The frequency of migraine often declines with age but only occasionally does migraine disappear.

Follow-up and management

• Regular follow-up in hospital is not required for uncomplicated migraine.

• GPs should assess the response to treatment until appropriate and successful treatment is established.

• Prophylactics should be continued for 6–12 months before withdrawal.

Key references

1. Dalessio DJ: Diagnosing the severe headache. *Neurology* 1994, **44 (suppl 3)**:S6–S12.
2. Baumel B: Migraine. *Neurology* 1994, **44 (suppl 3)**:S13–S17.

Mitral regurgitation

Diagnosis

Symptoms [1]

• Symptoms are often mild or absent.

Dyspnea: due to pulmonary congestion.

Fatigue: due to low cardiac output.

Palpitation: due to atrial fibrillation.

Fluid retention: in late-stage disease.

Signs

Irregular pulse: if patient is in atrial fibrillation.

Low-amplitude pulse pressure.

Raised venous pressure.

Parasternal heave: right ventricular hypertrophy and systolic left atrial expansion.

Laterally displaced and hyperdynamic apical impulse.

Pansystolic murmur.

Third heart sound.

Loud pulmonary second sound: if patient has pulmonary hypertension.

Investigations

ECG: shows broad bifid P wave (P mitrale), atrial fibrillation.

Chest radiography: shows pulmonary congestion, left atrial enlargement, cardiac enlargement, pulmonary artery enlargement (if severe and long-standing).

Echocardiography and Doppler ultrasonography: large left atrium, large left ventricle, increased fractional shortening, regurgitant jet (Doppler), leaflet prolapse (floppy valve or flail leaflet).

Transesophogeal echocardiography: may give better visualization of valve apparatus.

Cardiac catheterization: large "V" wave in wedge trace, angiographic evidence of mitral regurgitation.

Complications

Systemic embolism.

Pulmonary hypertension, right heart failure.

Endocarditis.

Differential diagnosis

Floppy mitral valve: late systolic murmur and midsystolic click [2].

Hypertrophic cardiomyopathy: ECG and echocardiographic evidence of left ventricular hypertrophy.

Etiology

• Causes include the following:

Rheumatic disease.

Floppy mitral valve.

Chordal rupture.

Papillary muscle dysfunction or rupture.

"Functional" disorder, *i.e.*, secondary to dilated, poorly contracting left ventricle.

• Floppy valve and chordal rupture are associated with connective tissue abnormalities, papillary muscle dysfunction and rupture with coronary artery disease.

Epidemiology

• The increasing availability of echocardiography may result in more patients with mitral regurgitation being found.

Treatment

Diet and lifestyle

• Patients should avoid being overweight, stop smoking, and maintain normal activities, if possible.

Pharmacological treatment

Digoxin

• If the patient is in atrial fibrillation, digoxin is indicated for control of ventricular rate (less easy than with mitral stenosis).

Standard dosage Digoxin, 0.5 mg loading dose, repeated after 8 h; maintenance dose usually 0.25 mg daily.

Contraindications Caution in patients who are elderly, relatively small, or renally impaired (reduced dosage).

Main drug interactions Diuretic-induced hypokalemia enhances effect of digoxin.

Main side effects Nausea, vomiting, diarrhea, yellow discoloration to vision (xanthopsia), bradycardia.

Diuretics

• Diuretics are indicated to relieve pulmonary congestion.

Standard dosage Furosemide, 20–80 mg daily with potassium supplements or potassium-sparing agent (particularly if patient is also taking digoxin).

Contraindications None.

Special points May precipitate attacks of gout in susceptible patients and may interfere with diabetic control.

Main drug interactions Digoxin.

Main side effects Hypokalemia, dehydration.

Vasodilators

• Vasodilatation is used to reduce regurgitant factor by reducing afterload unless systemic blood pressure is low.

Standard dosage Angiotensin-converting enzyme (ACE) inhibitors, *e.g.*, enalapril, 5–20 mg twice daily, or captopril, 12.5–50 mg 3 times daily.
Calcium antagonists, *e.g.*, nifedipine, 5–20 mg 3 times daily.
Hydralazine, 12.5–50 mg 3 times daily.
Initially given at night to avoid immediate hypotensive effects.

Contraindications Hypotension.

Special points *ACE inhibitors*: treatment best started in hospital if patient taking large dose of diuretic or other vasodilator at same time.

Main drug interactions *ACE inhibitors:* potassium-sparing diuretics or supplements.

Main side effects *ACE inhibitors*: hypotension, renal dysfunction, dysgeusia (taste dysfunction), rashes, dry unproductive cough.
Calcium antagonists: flushing, headache, fluid retention.
Hydralazine: hypotension, headache, lupus-like syndrome (rare).

Anticoagulants

• Anticoagulants are indicated to reduce the risk of systemic embolism in patients with moderate to severe mitral regurgitation, atrial fibrillation, and dilated left atrium.

Standard dosage Warfarin, 10 mg daily for 3 days; maintenance dose depends on regular checks of INR.

Contraindications Bleeding tendency.

Main drug interactions Any drug that displaces warfarin from protein-binding sites or increases liver enzyme activity may cause alteration in the INR and thus necessitate dose adjustment.

Main side effects Increased bleeding tendency.

Treatment aims

To achieve normal functional capacity.

To perform surgical repair prior to development of left ventricular dysfunction owing to chronic volume overload.

Other treatments

Surgical mitral valve repair or replacement [3,4].

Prognosis

• Prognosis is good unless pulmonary artery pressures have been chronically high or left ventricle is severely impaired.

Follow-up and management

• Drug treatment needs regular review to ensure that it has not become inadequate.

Key references

1. Braunwald E: Mitral regurgitation: physiological, clinical, and surgical considerations. *N Engl J Med* 1969, **281**:425–432.
2. Devereux RB, *et al.*: Mitral valve prolapse: causes, clinical manifestations, and management. *Ann Intern Med* 1989, **111**:305–317.
3. Cohn LH: Surgery for mitral valve regurgitation. *JAMA* 1988, **260**:2883–2887.
4. Galloway AC, *et al.*: Long-term results of mitral valve reconstruction with Carpentier techniques. *Circulation* 1988, **78**(suppl I):I-97–105.

Diagnosis

Symptoms

Fatigue: insidious onset; due to low cardiac output [1].

Dyspnea, orthopnea: due to pulmonary congestion.

Palpitation: due to atrial fibrillation.

Signs

Irregular pulse: in atrial fibrillation.

Loud (palpable) first heart sound.

Opening snap: if valve is mobile.

Mitral diastolic murmur: long if severe.

Raised venous pressure.

Parasternal heave: right ventricular hypertrophy.

Loud pulmonary second sound.

Investigations

ECG: shows broad bifid P wave
(P mitrale), usually atrial fibrillation if disease advanced.

Chest radiography: shows left atrial enlargement, pulmonary congestion, prominent pulmonary arteries (in pulmonary hypertensive patients).

Echocardiography and Doppler ultrasonography: show thickened mitral valve with reduced movement, large left atrium, reduced left ventricular filling rate, reduced mitral valve area.

Cardiac catheterization: shows raised right heart pressures and an end-diastolic gradient from pulmonary artery wedge pressure (or left atrium if transseptal puncture done) to left ventricle.

Complications

Systemic embolism: from left atrium.

Pulmonary hypertension, right heart failure.

Endocarditis: unusual.

Differential diagnosis

Left atrial myxoma: physical signs may be identical (echocardiography confirms diagnosis).

Etiology

• Causes include the following:

Rheumatic disease.

Congenital abnormality (rare).

Epidemiology

• The occurrence of mitral stenosis is decreasing in developed countries as a result of the declining incidence of rheumatic fever.

Treatment

Diet and lifestyle

• Patients should avoid being overweight, give up smoking, and maintain normal activities, if possible.

Pharmacological treatment

Digoxin

• If the patient is in atrial fibrillation, digoxin is indicated for control of ventricular rate.

Standard dosage	Digoxin, 0.5 mg loading dose, repeated after 8 h; maintenance dose usually 0.25 mg daily, adjusted according to serum digoxin concentration.
Contraindications	Caution in patients who are elderly, relatively small, or renally impaired (reduced dosage).
Main drug interactions	Diuretic-induced hypokalemia enhances effect of digoxin.
Main side effects	Nausea, vomiting, diarrhea, yellow discoloration to vision (xanthopsia), bradycardia.

Diuretics

• Diuretics are indicated for dyspnea or fluid retention.

Standard dosage	Furosemide, 20–80 mg daily with potassium supplements or potassium-sparing agent (particularly if patient is also taking digoxin).
Contraindications	None.
Special points	May precipitate attacks of gout in susceptible patients and may interfere with diabetic control.
Main drug interactions	Digoxin.
Main side effects	Hypokalemia, dehydration.

Anticoagulants

• Anticoagulants are mandatory if the degree of stenosis is high, even if the patient is still in sinus rhythm.

Standard dosage	Warfarin, 10 mg daily for 3 days; maintenance dose depends on regular checks of INR.
Contraindications	Bleeding tendency.
Main drug interactions	Any drug that displaces warfarin from protein-binding sites or increases liver enzyme activity may cause alteration in INR and thus necessitate dose adjustment.
Main side effects	Increased bleeding tendency.

Treatment aims

To achieve normal exercise capability and normal functional capacity.

Other treatments

Balloon valvuloplasty if valve is mobile and not heavily calcified [2].

Surgical valvotomy or replacement.

Prognosis

• The prognosis is good unless pulmonary hypertension is chronic.

Follow-up and management

• Restenosis may occur after valvotomy or valvuloplasty.

• Drug treatment may become inadequate and indicate intervention eventually.

• Patients should have prophylactic treatment against endocarditis (*see* Endocarditis *for details*).

Key references

1. Wood P: An appreciation of mitral stenosis. *BMJ* 1954, **1**:1051–1055.
2. Abascal VM, *et al.*: Echocardiographic evaluation of mitral valve structure and function after percutaneous mitral valvuloplasty. *J Am Coll Cardiol* 1988, **12**:606–615.

Diagnosis

Definition

• Motor neuron disease is one of many motor neuron disorders. The term covers amyotrophic lateral sclerosis (the most common form), progressive muscular atrophy, and progressive bulbar palsy (thought to be variants of the same disorder).
• The disorder is progressive and is characterized by degeneration of cortical, brain stem, and spinal-cord motor neurons.

Symptoms [1]

Cramps or fasciculations: may precede other symptoms by months.
Asymmetrical weakness or wasting of proximal or distal upper limb muscles: presenting symptom in 40%–60% of patients with upper limb involvement and 20% with lower limb involvement (unilateral foot drop common).
Dysarthria: presenting complaint in 25%–30%, usually followed by limb involvement; 70%–80% presenting with limb involvement develop dysarthria, culminating in anarthria.
Dysphagia: accompanying dysarthria.
Shortness of breath: usually due to diaphragmatic weakness.
Minor sensory symptoms: occasionally.
Changes in character and behavior: in 5%–10%.
Frontal-lobe dementia: rarely.

Signs

Typical disease

Fasciculations, wasting, depressed reflexes: lower motor neuron signs.
Spasticity, slowing of alternating movements, brisk tendon reflexes, Babinski responses: upper motor neuron signs.

• Typical motor neuron disease has lower and upper motor neuron signs in several regions (cranial nerves, arms, legs), with evidence of disease progression.
• Signs are usually asymmetrical in the early stages, with no evidence of sensory signs or bladder or bowel involvement.

Bulbar involvement

Emotional lability, with uncontrolled laughter and crying, brisk jaw jerk, spasticity of facial muscles, spastic dysarthria, dysphagia, spasticity of tongue: indicating upper motor neuron involvement (pseudobulbar palsy).
Wasting of facial and jaw muscles, fasciculation and wasting of tongue, nasal speech, dysphagia, bovine cough: indicating lower motor neuron involvement (bulbar palsy).

Investigations

• Laboratory results are usually normal (creatine kinase activity may be 2–3 times normal).

Electromyography: shows widespread anterior horn cell damage; nerve conduction studies usually normal; electrophysiology supports clinical diagnosis and excludes root and plexus lesions or motor neuropathy; characteristic abnormalities include fibrillation potentials and positive sharp waves, fasciculations, abnormal motor units of increased amplitude and duration.
MRI or myelography: may be needed to exclude spinal cord or root compression; MRI may show altered signal in posterior limb of internal capsule in region of degenerating corticospinal tract fibers.
Muscle biopsy: sometimes needed to exclude other diagnoses in atypical cases; confirms denervation, with small angular fibers and prominent fiber type grouping.

Complications

Depression: social and emotional isolation, especially in patients with severe dysarthria.
Dysphagia: leading to weight loss, malnutrition, dehydration, and aspiration.
Bronchopulmonary infections: related to aspiration and ventilatory muscle weakness.
Venous thrombosis and pulmonary embolism.
Constipation: due to pelvic and abdominal wall weakness and poor fluid intake.
Ventilatory failure: usual cause of death.

Differential diagnosis

Myasthenia gravis with bulbar onset.
Post poliomyelitis muscular atrophy syndrome.
Cervical myelopathy.
Intramedullary spinal cord lesions.
Motor neuronopathy.
Late-onset spinal muscular atrophy.
Kennedy's syndrome.
Late-onset hexosaminidase A deficiency.

Etiology [2,3]

• 5%–10% of patients have a family history suggesting autosomal-dominant inheritance.
• Point mutations of the gene encoding Cu/Zn superoxide dismutase on chromosome 21q are present in 10%–20% of families.
• X-linked bulbospinal neuronopathy (Kennedy's syndrome) is caused by a mutation of the gene encoding the androgen receptor.
• The cause of sporadic motor neuron disease is unknown; free radical damage and excitotoxicity have been implicated.

Epidemiology

• The incidence of motor neuron disease in Europe and North America is 2 in 100 000.
• The prevalence is 3–6 in 100 000.
• The male : female ratio is 1.5:1.
• The peak onset in sporadic disease is at 60 years, about a decade earlier in familial disease.
• The incidence may be increasing, especially in older age groups.

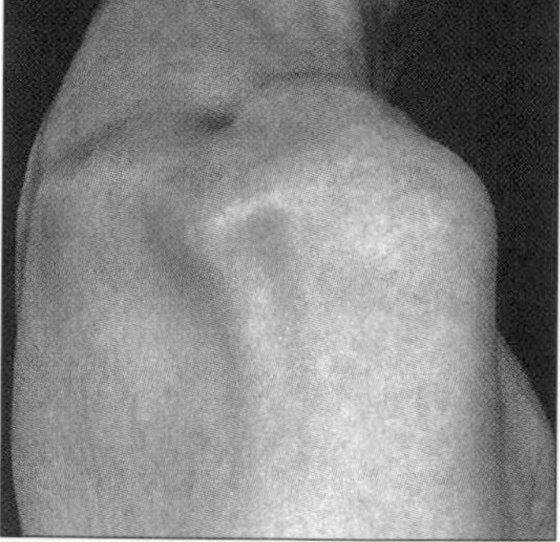

Marked muscle wasting around the shoulder girdle in a patient with motor neuron disease.

Treatment

Diet and lifestyle

• Dietary advice is needed for patients with dysphagia and those who are being treated by percutaneous endoscopic gastrostomy.

Pharmacological treatment

Symptomatic medications

Benzhexol, hyoscine (orally or transdermal patches), atropine for drooling.

Quinine for cramps.

Baclofen, dantrolene sodium, diazepam for spasticity.

Amitriptyline, dothiepin, fluoxetine for depression.

Lactulose, danthron for constipation (with increased fluid intake).

Opiates, diazepam for symptomatic relief of dyspnea.

• The antiglutamate agent riluzole may slow disease progression; a definitive trial is in progress.

Potential therapy

Riluzole may be useful in slowing the course of bulbar disease, but it is not yet widely available [4].

Nonpharmacological treatment

Physical therapy.

Counseling for depression.

Percutaneous endoscopic gastrostomy for dysphagia (best considered early).

Radiotherapy to the parotid glands for excess saliva.

Assisted ventilation for respiratory failure: techniques available include nasal intermittent positive airway pressure ventilation, a rocking bed, a cuirasse, or, in exceptional circumstances, a tracheostomy and intermittent positive pressure ventilation.

Treatment aims

To maintain patient's independence and quality of life.

To alleviate symptoms.

Prognosis

• 80%–90% of patients develop upper and lower motor neuron signs at some stage.

• 10% show only lower motor neuron signs (progressive muscular atrophy).

• The median survival is 4 years (2 years for bulbar onset).

• 5%–10% of patients survive for 5 years or more; a few live for 15 years or more.

• Patients with only lower motor neurone signs tend to have a better prognosis than those with typical motor neuron disease.

Follow-up and management

• A multidisciplinary neuro-care team approach is recommended; the team comprises neurologist, physical therapist, occupational therapist, speech therapist, dietitian, social worker, and other relevant health-care workers. Each patient may be allocated a "key worker" to integrate the activities of the team.

• Communication and other aids should be provided, and the home adapted.

• Patients might require referral to a hospice.

Patient support

Amyotrophic Lateral Sclerosis Association,
21021 Ventura Blvd. Suite 321
Woodland Hills, CA 91364;
phone (818) 340-7500 or (800) 782-4747.

Key references

1. Leigh PN, Ray-Chaudhuri K: Motor neurone disease. *J Neurol Neurosurg Psychiatry* 1994, **57**:886–896.
2. Rosen DR, *et al.*: Mutations in the Cu/Zn superoxide gene are associated with familial amyotrophic lateral sclerosis. *Nature* 1993, **362**:59–62.
3. Zeman S, *et al.*: Excitatory amino acids, free radicals and the pathogenesis of motor neurone disease. *Neuropath Appl Neurobiol* 1994, **20**:219–231.
4. Bensimon G, Lacomblez V, Meininger V, the ALS/Riluzole Study group: A controlled trial of riluzole in amyotrophic lateral sclerosis. *N Eng J Med* 1994, **330**:585–591.

Diagnosis

Symptoms

• Up to 10% of patients are asymptomatic.

Anorexia, weight loss.
Bone pain, back pain, pathological fracture.
Anemia, purpura, infection: symptoms of bone-marrow failure.
Polyuria, nocturia, pruritus: symptoms of renal failure.
Abdominal pain, anorexia, polyuria, polydipsia, constipation: symptoms of hypercalcemia.
Infection: due to hypogammaglobulinemia.
Visual symptoms, confusion, dyspnea, bleeding manifestations, polyneuropathy: symptoms of hyperviscosity.
Cardiac failure and edema: due to increased plasma oncotic pressure or viscosity.

Signs

Anemia, purpura.
Bony tenderness: over sites of lytic deposits.
Infections: especially skin, respiratory tract, and urinary tract.
Skin and soft tissue deposits: particularly in IgD myeloma.
Proteinuria.
Peripheral neuropathy: due to paraprotein deposition.
Hepatosplenomegaly and lymphadenopathy: rare; suggest an IgM paraprotein or amyloidosis.

• Diagnosis requires the presence of >10% abnormal plasma cells in bone marrow and one of the following: bone lesions, serum paraprotein, and urine paraprotein.

Investigations [1]

Full blood count: to check for anemia or bone-marrow failure.
ESR measurement: characteristically raised, often exceeds 100 mm/h.
Complete biochemical screening: including creatinine, creatinine clearance, serum calcium (alkaline phosphatase usually normal), albumin.
Skeletal survey: preferred to isotope bone scan, to show osteolytic lesions, vertebral collapse or osteoporosis.
Serum protein electrophoresis, immunoelectrophoresis, serum and urine analysis: to measure immunoglobulin concentrations, paraprotein quantification, and urinary Bence Jones protein.
β_2-Microglobulin and CRP measurement: to assess prognosis.
Bone-marrow aspiration and trephine biopsy: to show infiltration by malignant plasma cells and to assess normal bone-marrow reserve.
Microbiological cultures: if signs of infection.
Plasma cell labeling index, immunophenotype analysis, cytogenetic and DNA studies: if available, for further characterization of disease and prognosis.
MRI: a sensitive indicator of skeletal disease, especially good for detecting deposits around spine.

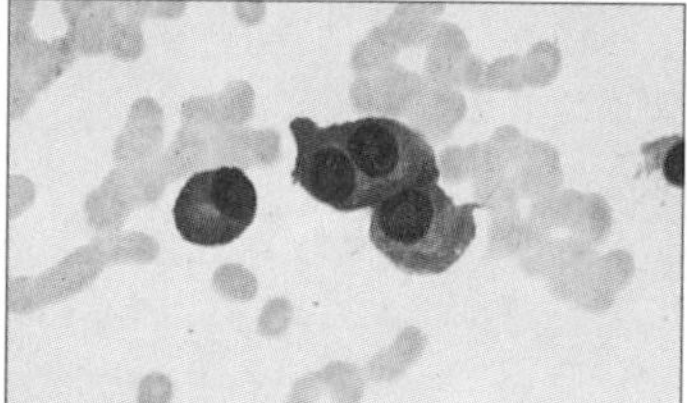

Plasma cells infiltrating bone marrow.

Complications

Renal failure, hypercalcemia, hyperviscosity syndrome.

Infection: most common cause of death.

Pathological fracture and spinal-cord compression.

Polyneuropathy, cardiac and renal failure, macroglossia, skin infiltration: in 5%–10% of patients, caused by amyloidosis.

Differential diagnosis

Metastatic carcinoma: hypercalcemia, lytic lesions, but normal alkaline phosphatase differentiates.

Polymyalgia rheumatica, temporal arteritis: anemia, high ESR, but no paraprotein.

Other causes of renal failure.

Benign monoclonal gammopathy: but paraprotein is <30 g/L, with normal concentrations of other immunoglobulins, anemia, renal failure, lytic lesions all absent, little or no Bence Jones proteinuria and no progression on follow-up.

Solitary plasmacytoma, primary amyloidosis, other lymphoproliferative disorders (*e.g.*, Waldenström's macroglobulinemia, non-Hodgkin's lymphoma).

Etiology [1]

• The cause is largely unknown, but risk factors include the following:

Ionizing radiation, organic chemical exposure, chronic antigenic stimulation, chronic inflammatory disease.

Genetic predisposition: acquired genetic mutations to oncogenes may promote tumor growth, and certain cytokines (*e.g.*, interleukin-6) may function as growth factors.

Epidemiology [1]

• Multiple myeloma forms ~1% of all malignancies, 10%–15% of all hematological malignancies.

• The median age at diagnosis is 71 years.

• The incidence is rising gradually.

• The disease occurs more often in blacks.

• The male:female ratio is ~5:3.

Staging [1]

Stage I: hemoglobin >10 g/dL, normal calcium, normal skeletal survey or solitary plasmacytoma, low paraprotein (IgG <50 g/L, IgA <30 g/L, urinary Bence Jones protein <4 g/24 h).

Stage II: neither stage I nor stage III.

Stage III: hemoglobin <8.5 g/dL, hypercalcemia, advanced skeletal disease, high paraprotein (IgG >70 g/L, IgA >50 g/L, urinary Bence Jones protein >12 g/24 h).

Subclassification: A, normal creatinine; B, raised creatinine.

Treatment

Diet and lifestyle

- Patients may need a diet appropriate for the degree of renal failure.
- Cooked food is needed for severely neutropenic patients.
- Patients should avoid bone damage, *e.g.*, heavy lifting.

Pharmacological treatment

Supportive treatment

- Careful supportive care is important, *e.g.*, the following:

Hydration and promotion of diuresis in renal failure and before chemotherapy.

Appropriate antibiotics or antifungal agents.

Adequate analgesia.

Blood component support.

Treatment of hypercalcemia (*e.g.*, biphosphonates): pamidronate may also reduce progression of bone disease and relieve pain.

Chemotherapy [2]

- Oral chemotherapy is the simplest protocol and involves melphalan and prednisone for 4–7 days every 4–6 weeks.
- Intravenous combination chemotherapy generally leads to a more rapid response, with higher complete remission rates, but the survival advantage over melphalan and prednisone is marginal and probably occurs only in patients aged <70 years. Current regimens include the following:

ABCM (doxorubicin, BCNU, cyclophosphamide, melphalan).
VBMCP (vincristine, BCNU, melphalan, cyclophosphamide, prednisone).
VAD (vincristine, doxorubicin by continuous i.v. infusion over 4 days with oral dexamethasone; standard for relapsed patients, also has a place in induction).

- α-Interferon, s.c. 3 times weekly, may improve combination therapy response rates and may prolong remission ("plateau" phase) and overall survival.
- Relapsed patients can be given cyclophosphamide orally or i.v. weekly, high-dose steroids (dexamethasone or methylprednisolone), and melphalan, single i.v. dose (high or intermediate).
- VAD gives responses in up to 40% of patients, and cyclosporin (to block multiple drug resistance) combined with VAD may be even more effective. High-dose cyclophosphamide with etoposide and granulocyte–macrophage colony-stimulating factor is valuable in VAD-resistant myeloma.

Complications of treatment

- Chemotherapy is immunosuppressive and myelotoxic.
- Growth factor support (granulocyte- and granulocyte–macrophage colony-stimulating factor) elevates the leukocyte count to reduce infective complications due to leukopenia, but also causes bone pain.
- Recombinant erythropoietin reduces erythrocyte transfusion requirement, particularly in renal failure.
- VAD and cyclophosphamide are preferred in renal failure because they are metabolized primarily by the liver.
- Antibacterial and antifungal prophylaxis with blood component support (principally platelets) is needed for myeloablative and intensive chemotherapy regimens.
- Hair loss, nausea, vomiting, mucositis (i.v. melphalan); bone demineralization (prednisone); and fatigue, fever, and anorexia (α-interferon) also occur.
- NSAIDs may accelerate renal failure if used for pain relief.

Treatment aims

To achieve normal immunoglobulin and blood counts and to relieve bone pain.

Other treatments

- The following are indicated for primary nonresponders, relapsed patients, or those with local complications.

Radiotherapy: relieves pain from lytic lesions; systemic activity against tumor but often leads to prolonged pancytopenia.

Internal fixation of pathological fractures.

Allogeneic bone-marrow transplantation: after conditioning by high-dose cyclophosphamide and total-body radiotherapy; for patients <50 with histocompatible sibling.

Autologous bone-marrow transplantation or peripheral blood stem cell infusion: intensive treatment for patients <60 years, after high-dose chemotherapy.

Plasma exchange: for hyperviscosity syndrome.

Dialysis.

Prognosis

- In untreated patients, the median survival is <1 year; with treatment, it rises to 3–4 years.
- β_2-Microglobulin concentrations correlate well with prognosis (<6 mg/L good, 6–12 mg/L intermediate, >12 mg/L poor prognosis).
- Raised CRP, poor response to treatment, age >75, skin or soft tissue involvement, and advanced stage indicate poor prognosis.
- Disappearance of paraprotein and restoration of normal immunoglobulin (complete remission) or normal blood counts with stable paraprotein ("plateau" phase) are achieved after 4–6 cycles of chemotherapy in >85% of patients.

Follow-up and management

- Full blood count, renal function, β_2-microglobulin and serum and urine paraprotein concentrations should be assessed regularly (every 1–2 months) to monitor the disease and the effects of treatment.
- Patients should be checked for opportunistic infection and new skeletal abnormalities.

Key references

1. Barlogie B, ed: Multiple Myeloma. *Hematol Oncol Clin North Am* 1992, **6**:211–484.
2. Alexanian R, Dimopoulos M: The treatment of multiple myeloma. *N Engl J Med* 1994, **330**:484–489.

Diagnosis

Symptoms

Relapsing and remitting

• 90% of patients initially have relapses and remissions of neurological disturbance attributable to CNS white matter lesions, including the following:

Visual loss.	**Weakness.**	**Urinary urgency.**
Diplopia.	**Incoordination.**	**Pain.**
Vertigo.	**Paresthesia.**	**Impotence.**

Progressive

• Progressive disease takes two forms.

Primary, in 10%: progressive from onset without remission.

Secondary, in 50%: progressive after an initially relapsing and remitting course.

Signs

• Signs are variable but include the following:

Optic atrophy.

Ophthalmoplegia.

Nystagmus.

Weakness: hemiparesis or paraparesis.

Sensory loss.

Investigations

• The diagnosis is primarily clinical and depends on the demonstration of two or more necessarily separate CNS lesions in a patient with a history of two characteristic episodes.

• Investigations provide invaluable support, but none of the abnormalities is specific to multiple sclerosis.

Evoked potentials: especially visual and somatosensory, to detect subclinical involvement and provide evidence for demyelination.

MRI: to detect subclinical involvement and the characteristic pattern of lesions.

CSF analysis: for electrophoresis to show oligoclonal IgG, present in 90% of patients.

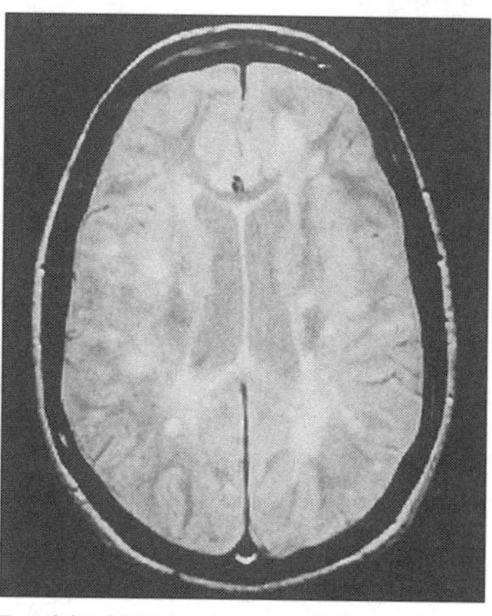

T_2 weighted MRI showing areas of abnormal signal in the cerebral hemispheres in a patient with multiple sclerosis.

Complications

Visual loss, paresis, tremor, incontinence: due to persistent neurological deficit.

Significant cognitive impairment: may occur late.

Differential diagnosis

Relapsing and remitting

Collagen vascular disease.

Neurosarcoidosis.

Lyme disease.

Progressive

Compression: *e.g.*, tumor, craniocervical anomaly.

Spinocerebellar degeneration.

Motor neuron disease.

Etiology

• Causes include the following:

Genetic predisposition: HLA association,but probably additional factors.

Extrinsic factor: probably infective, possibly viral.

Epidemiology [1]

• 60 in 100 000 population in the US are affected by multiple sclerosis.

• 20% of patients have an affected relative.

• Multiple sclerosis is diagnosed in patients under the age of 10 or over the age of 40 in only 13% of cases.

Treatment

Diet and lifestyle

• Patients should be assessed for functional limitations to determine appropriate modifications in lifestyle (neurorehabilitation, physical therapy, occupational therapy).

• Exposure to heat or fever worsens the motor symptoms temporarily.

Pharmacological treatment [2]

For symptoms

Standard dosage *For spasticity:* baclofen initially, 5 mg 3 times daily; maximum 100 mg daily.
For urinary frequency, urgency, and incontinence: oxybutynin, 5 mg 2–3 times daily.

Contraindications *Baclofen:* peptic ulceration.
Oxybutynin: bladder outflow obstruction, glaucoma.

Main drug interactions *Baclofen:* muscle relaxants.
Oxybutynin: antimuscarinics.

Main side effects *Baclofen:* weakness, sedation enhanced by alcohol.
Oxybutynin: antimuscarinic effects.

• For impotence, patients should be referred to a specialist for intracorporal pharmacotherapy.

For relapse

• Steroids are indicated when functional impairment is significant.

Standard dosage Methylprednisolone, 1 g in 250 mL normal saline solution i.v. over 30 min daily for 3 days.
Alternatively, oral steroids, although value uncertain: 3-week course, starting at 60 mg daily.

Contraindications Hypertension, diabetes, peptic ulceration, systemic infection, history of tuberculosis, osteoporosis, history of psychiatric disorder.

Special points Frequent use should be avoided.

Main drug interactions Other drugs causing hypokalemia, drugs inducing liver enzymes.

Main side effects Fluid retention, hypokalemia, depression, psychosis, hypertension, glucose intolerance, peptic ulceration, osteoporosis.

For prophylaxis

Standard dosage Beta interferon, 8 million IU s.c. every other day, to reduce relapses in some patients with relapsing-remitting disease.

Contraindications Hypersensitivity.

Main side effects Fatigue, malaise, flu-like symptoms, injection site reactions, sometimes depression.

To modify the course

• Much interest is being taken at present in the use of beta interferon. The published evidence, however, shows only a modest reduction in relapse rate but a more marked effect on MRI activity. Beta interferon has not, however, been shown to affect the rate of progression of neurological impairment. Until more information is available, the widespread use of beta interferon cannot be recommended.

Treatment aims

To alleviate symptoms.

To control relapse.

To modify course.

Prognosis

• Prognosis is very variable, ranging from death in a few months to survival without disability for 50 years.

• At least one-third of patients have little disability after 15 years.

Follow-up and management

• Follow-up depends on the condition of the patient.

• In complete remission, regular follow-up is not needed.

• When significant disability is present, assessment in a comprehensive neurological rehabilitation clinic is useful as the condition changes.

Patient support

National Multiple Sclerosis Society,
733 3rd Ave., New York, NY 10017-3240;
phone (212) 986-3240 or (800) FIGHT-MS

Key references

1. Matthews WB, *et al.* (eds): *McAlpine's Multiple Sclerosis.* Edinburgh: Churchill Livingstone; 1991.
2. McDonald WI: New treatments for multiple sclerosis. *BMJ* 1995, **310**:345–346.

Diagnosis

Symptoms

Painless muscle weakness increasing with exercise ("fatigue").

Drooping eyelids (one or both) and double vision.

- Weakness may characteristically also affect smiling, swallowing, chewing, speaking, neck muscles, arm elevation, elbow extension, hand movements, walking, and breathing.
- Symptoms are worst at the end of the day.

Signs

Fatiguable ptosis.

Variable limitation of eye movement.

Impaired eye closure.

Snarling smile.

Nasal speech.

Fatiguable weakness of affected muscles.

Wasting: rare.

Brisk tendon reflexes.

Investigations

Serum acetylcholine receptor antibody analysis: raised titer specific for myasthenia gravis.

Edrophonium (Tensilon) test: if patient is seronegative.

Clinical electrophysiology: increased decrement; increased jitter on single fiber study.

CT of thymus: for thymoma.

Striated muscle antibody analysis: positive in 90% of patients with thymoma, 50% of patients with generalized myasthenia gravis.

Complications

Myasthenic crisis: acute respiratory or bulbar symptoms.

Cholinergic crisis: due to excess anticholinesterase treatment; causing hypersalivation, lacrimation, increased sweating, vomiting, and miosis; can also cause weakness and respiratory failure.

Local or pleural spread of thymoma.

Differential diagnosis

Lambert–Eaton myasthenic syndrome.

Congenital myasthenia gravis.

Chronic fatigue syndrome.

Etiology

- Antibodies to muscle acetylcholine receptors (AChRs) cause receptor loss.
- Immune response genes influence susceptibility.
- Penicillamine may induce AChR antibodies and typical myasthenia gravis.
- Placental transfer of AChR antibodies causes neonatal myasthenia gravis in the offspring of 12% of mothers with the disease [1].
- "Seronegative" myasthenia gravis is antibody-mediated: the antigenic target is not known.

Epidemiology

- The prevalence is 8–9 in 100 000 people.
- The annual incidence is 0.4 in 100 000.
- All races are susceptible; restricted ocular myasthenia gravis is more frequent in Asian patients.
- The disease is manifest from infancy to extreme old age.

Clinical classification [2,3]

- The clinical subgroup influences treatment selection; typical features are shown below.

Early onset (50%)

Symptom distribution: generalized.
Age at onset: <40 years.
Thymus pathology: hyperplasia.
Acetylcholine receptor (AChR) antibody titer: high.

Late onset (25%)

Symptom distribution: generalized or ocular.
Age at onset: >40 years.
Thymus pathology: atrophy/normal.
AChR antibody titer: low.

Seronegative (15%)

Symptom distribution: ocular or generalized.
Age of onset: any.
Thymus pathology: atrophy/normal.
AChR antibody titer: absent.

Thymoma (10%)

Symptom distribution: generalized.
Age at onset: any.
Thymus pathology: thymoma.
AChR antibody titer: intermediate.
Increased frequency of striated muscle antibody.

Treatment

Diet and lifestyle

• No special precautions are necessary.

Pharmacological treatment [4]

Management strategy

• The following treatments are helpful, usually in this order:

Anticholinesterase for immediate symptom control.
Plasma exchange in severe cases (*see* Other treatments).
Thymectomy in some patients (*see* Other treatments).
Prednisone.
Azathioprine.
Plasma exchange.
Other immunosuppressive treatment (cyclosporin, cyclophosphamide).

Anticholinesterase

• This provides symptomatic relief in all patients.

Standard dosage Pyridostigmine, 30–120 mg 5 times daily.
Propantheline, 15 mg 3-4 times daily, if necessary, to control adverse gastrointestinal effects.

Contraindications Intestinal or urinary obstruction.

Main drug interactions Antiarrhythmics (quinidine), antibacterials (aminoglycosides, clindamycin, lincomycin and polymyxins), antimalarials (chloroquine), beta blockers (propranolol), lithium, muscle relaxants.

Main side effects Diarrhea, abdominal cramps, increased salivation, nausea and vomiting.

Prednisone

For generalized disease of moderate severity unresponsive to other treatments (inpatients).

Standard dosage *Outpatients:* prednisone, 5 mg single dose on alternate days, increased by 5 mg at weekly intervals to controlling dose or 0.75–1 mg/kg/day, whichever is lower.
Inpatients: prednisone, 10 mg single dose on alternate days, increased by 10 mg increments to controlling dose or 1–1.5 mg/kg/day.
In both groups, dose should be tapered by 5 mg/month when remission is established and adjusted to define effective minimal dose.

Contraindications Osteoporosis, diabetes.

Main drug interactions Antibacterials, *e.g.*, rifampicin, antiepileptics.

Main side effects Initial exacerbation of myasthenic symptoms, adrenal suppression, diabetes, osteoporosis, avascular necrosis of femoral head, mental disturbance, weight gain, cushingoid features, cataracts.

Azathioprine

• Azathioprine is indicated in combination with prednisone for generalized moderate or severe disease (inpatients).

Standard dosage Azathioprine, 2.5 mg/kg/day orally.

Contraindications Myelosuppression.

Special points Full blood count and liver function tests weekly for 8 weeks, every 1–3 months thereafter.

Main drug interactions Allopurinol enhances toxic effect.

Main side effects Myelosuppression, hepatotoxicity, gastrointestinal symptoms, rashes, B-cell lymphoma (very rare).

Treatment aims

To allow patient to recover strength.

Other treatments

Plasma exchange

• Plasma exchange is indicated for the following:

Symptomatic control in severe cases.
Myasthenic crisis.
Preparation for thymectomy.
After thymectomy while awaiting response.
Recurrently, in severe myasthenia gravis, while awaiting response to immunosuppressive drug therapy.

Thymectomy (by median sternotomy)

• Thymectomy is indicated for the following:

Thymoma (because of risk of local spread).
Early-onset generalized myasthenia gravis (outcome in subsequent 1–2 years 25% remission, 50% improvement, 25% neutral).

Prognosis

• Most patients achieve substantial improvement or full recovery.

Follow-up and management

• In patients treated by immunosuppressive drugs, continuing low-dose treatment and regular follow-up is usually needed to maintain disease control.

Key references

1. Shillito P, Vincent A, Newsom-Davis J: Congenital myasthenic syndromes. *J Neuromusc Dis* 1993, **3**:183–190.
2. Newsom-Davis J: Myasthenia gravis. *Med Int* 1992, **100**:4168–4171.
3. Penn AS, *et al.* (eds): Myasthenia gravis and related disorders. *Ann N Y Acad Sci* 1993, **681**:1–611.
4. Verma P, Oger J: Treatment of acquired autoimmune myasthenia gravis. *Can J Neurol Sci* 1992, **19**:360–375.

Diagnosis

Symptoms

• Symptoms of disseminated *Mycobacterium avium* or *M. intracellulare* infection may be difficult to distinguish from those of other opportunistic infections associated with HIV infection.

• Disseminated infection may be asymptomatic.

Systemic

Fever: with or without sweats.

Anorexia and malaise.

Weight loss: often associated with anemia and neutropenia.

Gastrointestinal

Chronic diarrhea and abdominal pain: resulting from *M. avium-intracellulare* invasion of the colon or small bowel or bulky retroperitoneal lymph nodes infected by *M. avium-intracellulare.*

Signs

Weight loss, oral candidiasis, cutaneous Kaposi's sarcoma: evidence of underlying HIV infection and other HIV-associated complications.

Weight loss, anemia, hepato(spleno)megaly: indicating disseminated disease.

Localized or cutaneous abscesses, endophthalmitis, arthritis.

Investigations

Blood culture: using lysis/centrifugation or radiometric technique, yield increased (from 60% to almost 100%); 5–50 days needed for blood cultures to become positive.

Biopsy: diagnosis of disseminated *M. avium-intracellulare* infection made by isolation or culture from any normally sterile site (blood, bone-marrow, lymph-node, and liver biopsy best); negative blood cultures unusual with positive histology from lymph-node, liver, or bone-marrow biopsy; stains may show acid-fast bacilli before blood cultures become positive, thus suggesting diagnosis.

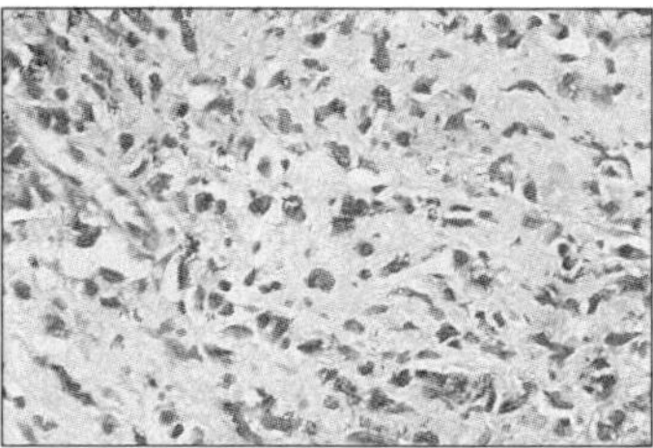

Lymph-node biopsy. Numerous clumps of acid-fast bacilli are seen within the tissue. There is no granulamatous response. Magnification × 400.

• Isolation of *M. avium-intracellulare* from sputum and bronchoalveolar lavage may occur but is not diagnostic of disseminated infection.

Complications

None.

Differential diagnosis

Progression of HIV or other systemic opportunistic infection.

Etiology

• Two closely related species, *Mycobacterium avium* and *M. intracellulare*, known as *M. avium* complex, cause widely disseminated infection in AIDS patients: up to 30% have disseminated infection diagnosed before death, and about 50% are found to have it at postmortem examination.

• Disseminated infection occurs exclusively in patients with advanced HIV disease and CD4 counts $<100 \times 10^6$/L.

• The host defect in AIDS patients allowing dissemination is probably macrophage dysfunction.

• The source of invasion in AIDS patients may be gastrointestinal; large numbers of mycobacteria within macrophages of the small bowel lamina propria suggest that the bowel is the portal of entry.

Epidemiology

• *M. avium-intracellulare* is ubiquitous in the environment, being found in water, soil, animals, and dairy products.

Pathogenesis and pathology

• Almost all AIDS patients with disseminated *M. avium-intracellulare* have positive blood cultures (in contrast to those with stool, urine, or respiratory secretion colonization).

• Mycobacteremia usually ranges from 10^1 to 10^4 colony-forming units/mL blood.

• In patients with disseminated infection, the liver, spleen, and lymph nodes are found at postmortem examination to contain up to 10^{10} colony-forming units/g tissue.

• Histology of involved organs reveals absent or poorly formed granulomata and mycobacteria within macrophages. Little tissue destruction is seen, despite heavy mycobacterial load.

Treatment

Diet and lifestyle

• No special precautions are necessary.

Pharmacological treatment

• *Mycobacterium avium-intracellulare* is resistant to many antituberculous drugs at concentrations achievable in plasma, yet >50% of strains can be inhibited by achievable concentrations of amikacin, azithromycin, ciprofloxacin, clarithromycin, clofazimine, cycloserine, ethambutol, ethionamide, or rifabutin.

• Single-agent treatment (*e.g.*, by clarithromycin) is of temporary benefit only: fever, anorexia, and mycobacteremia return rapidly; combination therapy is more effective.

• A two-drug regimen with clarithromycin and ethambutol is recommended with or without a third drug (clofazimine).

• Additional agents may be used if the standard two- or three-drug regimens have failed or have resulted in toxicities.

Standard dosage
Ethambutol, 15 mg/kg orally once daily, with clarithromycin, 500–1000 mg orally twice daily.
Ciprofloxacin, 500 mg orally twice daily, and clofazimine, 100 mg orally once daily can be added. Ciprofloxacin and rifabutin are used in case of toxicities or failure.
Amikacin, 7.5 mg/kg i.v. once daily, may be added for patients with refractory fever or anorexia. Treatment is given for 2–4 weeks.

Contraindications
Previous drug hypersensitivity.
Rifabutin: jaundice, porphyria.
Ethambutol: renal impairment, optic neuritis.
Clarithromycin: porphyria, hepatic or renal failure.

Special points
Drug levels must be monitored.
Palliative glucocorticoids (oral prednisolone, 1–2 mg/kg daily) may be given to patients with very advanced HIV disease who have profound anorexia and weight loss, without adversely affecting prognosis.

Main drug interactions
Rifabutin: induces hepatic microsome enzyme activity and so increases metabolism of azole drugs; interacts with fluconazole or clarithromycin to produce uveitis in 30% of patients if >300 mg of rifabutin are given daily.
If steroids are given with an antibacterial regimen containing rifampin or rifabutin, the dose should be doubled to take into account the hepatic microsome-inducing effects of the drugs.

Main side effects
Rifabutin: nausea and vomiting, diarrhea, anorexia; body fluids become orange-red.
Ethambutol: optic neuritis, red–green color blindness, peripheral neuritis.
Ciprofloxacin: nausea and vomiting, abdominal pain, diarrhea, headache, photosensitivity, arthralgia, myalgia.
Clarithromycin: nausea and vomiting, abdominal pain, diarrhea.
Clofazimine: nausea, giddiness, headache, diarrhea; skin and urine colored terracotta red.

• Rifabutin, 300 mg orally once daily given as primary prophylaxis reduces the risk of developing *M. avium-intracellulare* bacteremia by half but does not improve survival. It is indicated for persons with CD4 cell counts <100/mm^3.

Treatment aims

To reduce mycobacteremia or fever and transfusion requirements.

• Cure is not achievable.

Prognosis

• Survival in AIDS patients with disseminated *Mycobacterium avium-intracellulare* infection is shorter (median, 4.1 months) than in comparable patients (with similar CD4 counts) without disseminated infection (median, 11 months).

•The presence of *M. avium-intracellulare* in gastrointestinal secretions strongly predicts the subsequent development of disseminated infection.

Follow-up and management

• Treatment is for life.

General references

Jacobson MA: Mycobacterial disease. In *The Medical Management of AIDS*, edn 3. Edited by Sande MA, Volberding PA. Philadelphia: WB Saunders; 1992:284–296.

Masur H: Recommendations on prophylaxis and therapy for disseminated *Mycrobacterium avium* complex disease in patients infected with the human immuno-deficiency virus. *N Engl J Med* 1993, **329**:898-904.

Scoular A, French P, Miller RF: *Mycobacterium avium intracellulare* infection in the acquired immunodeficiency syndrome. *Br J Hosp Med* 1991, **46**:295–300.

Diagnosis

Symptoms

• Chronic myeloid leukemia is usually manifest in chronic phase; it transforms spontaneously to an accelerated phase and then to an acute blastic phase normally within 3–6 years of diagnosis (range 0–10 years).

• Polycythemia vera, essential thrombocythemia, and primary myelofibrosis are manifest more insidiously and evolve more slowly.

• Symptoms are an incidental finding in many patients.

Abdominal pain and distention: also due to renal occlusive disease in polycythemia vera.

Spontaneous bleeding: including hematuria, bruising, visual disturbances.

Sweats, weight loss.

Priapism: in chronic myeloid leukemia.

Pruritus: in chronic myeloid leukemia.

Symptoms of hyperviscosity syndrome: in polycythemia vera.

Gout.

Peptic ulceration and hypertension: in polycythemia vera.

Signs

Splenomegaly.

Ecchymoses, retinal hemorrhages.

Weight loss.

Hepatomegaly: occasionally.

Investigations

Full blood count: raised leukocyte count (20 to >500 × 10^9/L); increased numbers of blasts, promyelocytes, neutrophils, eosinophils, basophils; low neutrophil alkaline phosphatase content in chronic myeloid leukemia; variable anemia; thrombocytosis especially in essential thrombocythemia; raised hemoglobin, packed-cell volume, and erythrocyte mass in polycythemia vera.

Bone-marrow analysis: hypercellular, loss of fat spaces; increased megakaryocyte count, especially in essential thrombocythemia; variable amounts of fibrosis in chronic myeloid leukemia; increased reticulin and collagen in myelofibrosis; in chronic myeloid leukemia, all dividing cells have a Philadelphia chromosomal translocation, designated t (9;22) (q34;q11), bringing into apposition parts of the *bcr* gene normally on chromosome 22q with the bulk of the *abl* proto-oncogene normally present on chromosome 9q.

Biochemistry: uric acid raised, especially in myelofibrosis; increased vitamin B_{12} and vitamin B_{12}-binding protein.

Complications

"Blast" transformation: in chronic myeloid leukemia; blast cells may be myeloid or lymphoid.

Changes between groups: *e.g.*, polycythemia vera to myelofibrosis.

Vascular or thrombotic complications: in polycythemia vera.

Gout: especially in myelofibrosis.

Renal tubular obstruction.

Splenic infarction: in chronic myeloid leukemia.

Retinal hemorrhages: in chronic myeloid leukemia.

Gonadal failure: due to busulfan.

Differential diagnosis

Leukocytosis

Infections.

Allergic conditions.

Bone-marrow invasion by cancer.

Splenomegaly

Malaria, visceral leishmaniasis.

Acute leukemia, lymphoma.

Gaucher's disease.

Thalassemia syndromes.

Portal hypertension.

Etiology

• Causes include the following:

Acquired abnormality in hematopoietic stem cells: such stem cells and their progeny carry a Philadelphia chromosome (22q-) with the *bcr/abl* chimeric gene in chronic myeloid leukemia.

Idiopathic disease.

Association with previous radiation exposure occasionally in chronic myeloid leukemia.

Epidemiology

• Chronic myeloid leukemia occurs in ~1 in 100 000 annually worldwide.

Treatment

Diet and lifestyle

• Patients may live normal lives during the chronic phase of chronic myeloid leukemia.

Pharmacological treatment [1]

• Drug treatment is indicated for polycythemia vera (hydroxyurea, radioactive phosphorus [^{32}P]), myelofibrosis (hydroxyurea, busulfan), and essential (primary) thrombocythemia (hydroxyurea, busulfan, Anagrelide [imidazole-2,1-b, quinazolin-2-1 is currently undergoing phase II and III FDA investigations, but is available for compassionate purposes], ^{32}P, supportive measures, *e.g.*, dipyridamole, aspirin).

• α-Interferon (given daily or on alternate days by injection) controls hematological features in 70%–80% of patients and induces some degree of Philadelphia chromosome negativity in the bone-marrow in 10%–20%; it is the drug of first choice [2].

• Hydroxyurea is easier to tolerate.

• Busulfan should not be used in patients aged <50 years but can be used for older patients or those who cannot take hydroxyurea.

Nonpharmacological treatment

Bone-marrow transplantation [3]

• Transplantation is indicated for chronic myeloid leukemia; if applicable, it should be done within 1 year of diagnosis.

• Allogeneic bone-marrow transplantation is indicated for patients aged <55 years with HLA-identical siblings (~15% of all patients).

Treatment of other disorders

Polycythemia vera: venesection.

Myelofibrosis: splenic irradiation, splenectomy (in selected patients).

Treatment aims

To cure the patient.

To prolong life without cure.

To prevent or alleviate symptoms.

To maintain leukocyte count in normal range.

To re-establish Philadelphia chromosome-negativity with interferon treatment.

Prognosis

• The median duration of chronic phase diseases is 4 years and of survival with conventional treatment is 4.3 years.

• A few patients survive >10 years in chronic phase.

• The 5-year disease-free survival after bone-marrow transplantation is about 65%; most of these patients are cured; the procedure-related mortality is 15%–20%, and the relapse rate 10%–15%.

Follow-up and management [1]

• Regular follow-up is needed if the patient is on chemotherapy or interferon.

• Bone marrow must be checked annually for progressive fibrosis or cytogenetic evolution.

• Patients should have the usual follow-up for bone-marrow transplantation.

Key references

1. Goldman JM: Management of chronic myeloid leukemia. *Blood Rev* 1994, **8**:21–29.
2. Kantarjian HM, *et al.*: Chronic myelogenous leukemia: a concise update. *Blood* 1993, **82**:691–703.
3. Soutar RL, King DJ: Bone-marrow transplantation. *BMJ* 1995, **310**:31–36.

Myocardial infarction

Diagnosis

Symptoms

Chest pain: typically precordial, often with radiation to left or right arm, throat, lower jaw, epigastrium, or back; usually severe; crushing or vice-like; pain often described as indigestion-like, may be relieved by belching.

Breathlessness: common, often without cardiac failure.

Malaise, nausea, vomiting, syncope, apprehension, sweating.

Signs

• Few cardiovascular signs may be apparent on acute presentation.

Malaise, pallor, sweating, restlessness.

Pyrexia: usually developing the day after infarction.

Unexpectedly slow or rapid pulse.

Raised jugular venous pressure: only with significant right ventricular failure.

Third or fourth heart sounds, dyskinetic apical impulse: indicating significant myocardial dysfunction.

Chest crackles: may indicate left ventricular failure.

New murmurs or pericardial rub: may be heard in patients with complications.

• Many patients present with sudden cardiac death.

Investigations

12-lead ECG: often sufficient to establish diagnosis; adjunctive tests may be necessary for confirmation if infarction is minor or if ECG shows pre-existing abnormalities, *e.g.*, previous infarction, conduction abnormalities (especially left bundle branch block).

Chest radiography: to check for pulmonary congestion.

Cardiac enzymes evaluation: creatine kinase, aspartate transaminase, and lactate dehydrogenase rise characteristically after myocardial infarction; creatine kinase MB cardiospecific isoenzyme may be helpful with skeletal muscle damage.

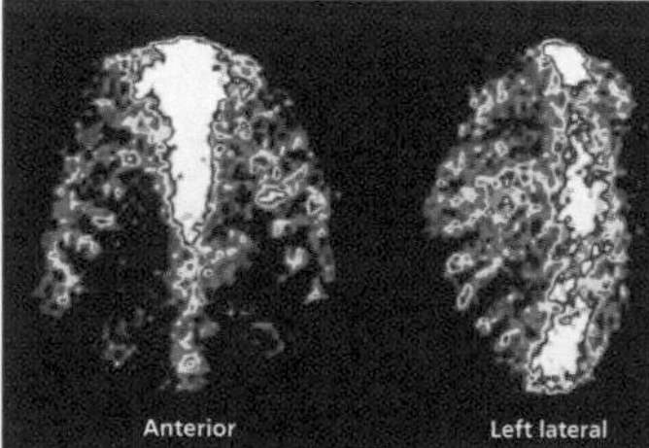

Abnormal uptake of pyrophosphate in the heart indicating recent myocardial infarction.

Echocardiography: to assess wall motion abnormalities, ventricular septal defect, regurgitation, and mural thrombus.

Scintigraphy: ^{99m}Tc pyrophosphate scan may detect myocardial infarction 4 h to 7 d after onset.

Complications

Left ventricular failure.

Cardiogenic shock.

Bradyarrhythmias.

Tachyarrhythmias.

Cardiac rupture.

Pericarditis.

Acute ventricular septal defect.

Acute mitral regurgitation.

Systemic emboli.

Aneurysm formation.

Differential diagnosis

Angina without infarction.

Pericarditis.

Esophageal or gastrointestinal pain.

Aortic dissection.

Pulmonary embolus.

Musculoskeletal or nonspecific chest pain.

Etiology

Causes

Thrombotic occlusion of a coronary artery, related to rupture of an atherosclerotic plaque and subsequent intraluminal hemorrhage.

Risk factors

Increasing age.

Family history.

Hypertension.

Diabetes mellitus.

Lack of exercise.

Male gender.

Smoking.

Hyperlipidemia.

Thrombotic tendency (fibrinogen).

Obesity.

Surgical menopause at young age.

Epidemiology

• 10–17 in 1000 men aged 40–69 years sustain myocardial infarction.

• In the US >500 000 myocardial infarctions occur per year.

Treatment

Diet and lifestyle

• Patients must give up smoking, reduce weight, take up regular exercise, and achieve low fat, low cholesterol diet.

Pharmacological treatment

Immediate treatment

Analgesia: i.v. morphine sulfate.
Oxygen.
Aspirin: 325 mg orally initially, then maintenance dose 75–325 mg daily.
Nitrates: particularly in patients with continuing ischemia.
Beta blockade: atenolol or metoprolol i.v. and then orally, except in patients with left ventricular failure, pulse rate <70/min, or blood pressure <100 mm Hg.

Thrombolytic treatment

• Treatment should be given as soon as possible, unless contraindicated.

• It is indicated for all suitable patients within 12 h of onset of symptoms.

• Maximum benefit is with large myocardial infarction and early administration (especially <4 h).

• The value is proven for patients with acute myocardial infarction and ST elevation or bundle branch block; no benefit has been shown in patients with ST depression or normal ECG.

• rt-PA is more effective than streptokinase but is much more expensive; it should be used in patients for whom streptokinase is unsuitable and particularly for patients presenting within 4–6 h of symptom onset and large infarction such as those with anterior infarction, hypotension, and/or persistent sinus tachycardia.

Standard dosage	Streptokinase, 1.5 MU over 1 h. rt-PA, 15 mg bolus, then 50 mg in 30 min, then 40 mg in 60 min, followed by i.v. heparin [1].
Contraindications	Possible aortic dissection, active peptic ulceration, recent surgery, hemorrhagic diathesis, possible pregnancy, subarachnoid hemorrhage, cardiovascular accident with residual defect, recent transient ischemic attack, unconscious patient, severe hypertension, systemic thrombus (*e.g.,* aortic aneurysm, left atrial clot), prolonged or traumatic resuscitation, recent central venous or arterial puncture. Few contraindications are absolute.
Special points	Streptokinase should be avoided in patients with known allergy or those who have been treated between 5 days and 1 year previously.
Main side effects	Hemorrhage (treated by tranexamic acid, 1 g slow i.v. injection, and fresh frozen plasma to restore clotting factor).

Nonpharmacological treatment

Primary coronary angioplasty (PCA) [2]

• May be more effective than thrombolytic therapy in establishing antegrade coronary flow and relieving fixed coronary obstruction.

• Should be performed only when:
Experienced interventional team can be readily mobilized.
Cardiac surgical back-up is available.
Perceived time delay from presentation to open artery will not exceed 60–90 min.
It can be done at cardiac center of excellence with high volume interventional program.

• Primary PCA is a reasonable option only in a small minority of U.S. hospitals because few have a catheterization laboratory, cardiac surgery is performed only at a few, and most lack a sufficient volume of experience.

Follow-up treatment

• Secondary prevention is needed for all patients.

Beta blockers: *e.g.*, atenolol, 25–50 mg twice daily, or metoprolol, 50–100 mg daily.

Angiotensin-converting enzyme (ACE) inhibitors: *e.g.*, captopril titrated to maximum tolerated dose, if possible 50 mg 3 times daily (12.5 mg 3 times daily by hospital discharge); indicated for all patients with left ventricular ejection fractions <40% [3].

Treatment aims

To relieve pain and other symptoms.
To salvage threatened myocardium by opening occluded cornary artery.
To prevent and treat complications.

Other treatments

Early coronary angiography for patients with:
• Electrical or hemodynamic instability.
• Stuttering course.

Prognosis

• In-hospital mortality after acute myocardial infarction is ~10%; subsequent mortality is higher than for age-matched control populations [4].
• Mortality is falling because of therapeutic advances and changes in the natural history.
• Poor prognosis is indicated by advanced age, severe left ventricular dysfunction, and multivessel coronary disease.
• Coronary artery bypass grafting may improve prognosis in some high-risk groups.
• Coronary angioplasty is treatment of choice in cardiogenic shock.

Follow-up and management

• Risk factors, *e.g.*, hyperlipidemia, hypertension, or diabetes, should be controlled.
• Exercise testing is needed to check for residual ischemia, followed by coronary angiography if the test is positive.

Key references

1. GUSTO Investigators: An international randomized trial comparing four thrombolytic strategies for acute myocardial infarction. *N Engl J Med* 1993, **329**:673–682.
2. Grines CL: A comparison of immediate angioplasty with thrombolytic therapy for acute MI. *N Engl J Med* 1993, **328**:673–679.
3. Pfeffer MA *et al.*: Effect of captopril on mortality and morbidity in patients with left ventricular dysfunction after myocardial infarction. *N Engl J Med* 1992, **327**:669–677.
4. DAVIT-II: Effect of verapamil on mortality and major events after acute myocardial infarction. *Am J Cardiol* 1990, **66**:779–785.

Diagnosis

Symptoms

Weakness: principally affecting proximal muscles in arms and legs; 15%–30% of these patients have associated arthralgias, Raynaud's phenomenon, or myalgia; painless weakness is common [1].

Unusual, severe manifestations: interstitial lung disease, pulmonary hypertension, ventilatory failure, heart block or arrhythmias, dysphagia [2].

Skin rashes.

• Patients with dermatomyositis, especially men aged >45 years, may have an accompanying tumor, causing various symptoms, *e.g.*, weight loss [3].

Signs

Muscle wasting: principally of proximal muscles.

Loss of muscle reflexes: in late-stage disease.

Heliotrope rash: lilac discoloration around eyelids.

Gottron's papules: small raised reddish plaques over knuckles.

Erythematous rash: over face, upper chest, and arms, usually on extensor surfaces.

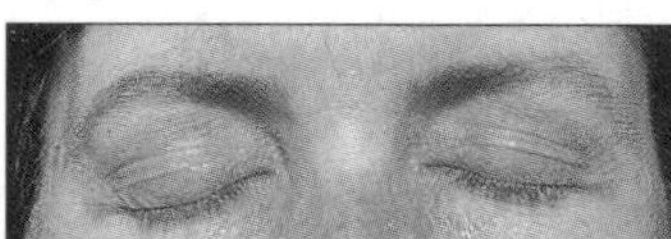

Classic heliotrope rash on the eyelids of a patient with dermatomyositis.

Investigations

Key investigations

Creatine kinase, aldolase measurement: concentration 5–30 times upper limit of normal but not disease-specific; concentrations higher in many patients with muscular dystrophy [4].

Electromyography: to check for insertional irritability and small polyphasic potentials.

Muscle biopsy: needle or open surgical technique; classic changes are inflammation, with mononuclear cell infiltrate composed mainly of lymphocytes (some macrophages and plasma cells), with muscle-fiber necrosis, and, in chronic cases, replacement of muscle fibers by fat and fibrous tissue; changes often patchy, and up to 20% of patients may have relatively normal appearance.

Other investigations

Measurement of other enzymes: *e.g.*, transaminase concentrations may be raised [4].

24-h urine creatine excretion measurement: may be high; more sensitive but less specific than raised creatine kinase.

Myoglobin measurement: appears to reflect disease activity.

Autoantibody analysis: weak positive antinuclear antibody reaction in 60%–80% of patients with myositis; antibodies to transfer RNA synthetase enzymes have been found to be virtually disease-specific, notably the anti-Jo-1 antibody.

Complications

Interstitial lung fibrosis, arthritis, Raynaud's phenomenon: in patients with Jo-1 antibody.

Cardiac or respiratory failure: rare; caused by rapidly progressive myositis.

Underlying neoplasm: muscle disease often intractable until tumor identified and treated.

Recurrent falls and danger of major internal trauma: caused by an unusual, steroid-resistant form of myositis, associated with inclusion bodies.

Differential diagnosis

Muscular dystrophy.
Osteomalacia.
Rhabdomyolysis.
Drug-induced inflammatory disease (including D-penicillamine).
Metabolic myopathies (*e.g.*, McArdle's disease).
Inclusion body myositis [1].

Etiology

• Inflammatory muscle diseases are part of the family of autoimmune rheumatic diseases.

• Causes include the following:
Hormonal component.
Immunogenetic predisposition: HLA B8 and DR3 associated with myositis, principally in whites; DR3 linked to Jo-1 antibody.
Environmental factors: increased risk of developing myositis at different times of year found in one study.
Viruses, *e.g.*, picornaviruses and retroviruses: may be triggering factors; link between myositis and HIV has been suggested.

Epidemiology

• The annual incidence of myositis is 5 in one million population.

• The prevalence is 5–8 in 100 000.

• The female:male ratio is 2–3:1 overall and 9:1 in patients with an associated autoimmune rheumatic disease.

Factors suggesting malignancy [1,3]

Dermatomyositis in male patients.
Age >45 years.
Weight loss.
Poorer than expected response to treatment.
Absence of autoantibodies.
Unexplained historical, physical, or laboratory abnormalities.

Dermatomyositis or polymyositis? [1]

Dermatomyositis
Onset: childhood to old age.
Skin rash, microvascular injury.
Perifascicular atrophy common.
Endomysial infiltration less common.
Surrounded and invaded fibers less than in polymyositis.
Anti-Jo-1 in 5%, other antisynthetases at least as much as in polymyositis.

Polymyositis
Onset: adulthood.
No skin rash or microvascular injury.
Perifascicular atrophy uncommon.
Endomysial infiltration common.
Surrounded and invaded fibers frequent.
Anti Jo-1 in 30%.

Treatment

Diet and lifestyle

• Exercise and activity are limited during the inflammation.

• No special diet is necessary.

Pharmacological treatment

Corticosteroids

• After the diagnosis has been established, treatment should be initiated quickly [1,2,5,6].

Standard dosage Prednisone, 1 mg/kg daily initially (usually 60–80 mg); continued until creatine kinase returned to near normal (usually 1–3 months); then reduced to 5–10 mg daily over following 3 months.

Contraindications Severe osteoporosis.

Main drug interactions None.

Main side effects Osteoporosis, increased risk of infection, diabetes, hypertension.

Other immunosuppressants

• These are indicated in patients who have not shown a response to high-dose steroids after 1 month or who cannot tolerate them [5,6].

Standard dosage Azathioprine, 2–3 mg/kg.
Methotrexate, up to 15 mg weekly.

Contraindications *Methotrexate:* abnormal liver function, major renal disease, porphyria.

Main drug interactions *Methotrexate:* many analgesics and antibacterials.

Main side effects Bone-marrow suppression, liver damage.

Other options

• Oral or occasionally i.v. cyclophosphamide has been used in severely affected patients, occasionally combined with steroids and methotrexate or azathioprine.

• Reports of the use of cyclosporin in myositis are conflicting, and it is not widely used in this disease.

• Intravenous gammaglobulin may be used.

Nonpharmacological treatment

Plasmapheresis.

Total lymph-node irradiation and thoracic duct drainage in severe cases.

Physical therapy and hydrotherapy.

Treatment aims

To control disease as soon as possible.

To maintain reasonable degree of mobility.

To reduce treatment to smallest dose needed after 3–4 months of aggressive therapy to avoid side effects (*e.g.*, intercurrent infection or osteoporosis).

Prognosis

• ~20% of patients recover fully.

• 10%–20% die as a direct result of the disease or as a consequence of its treatment.

• Most patients are left with some muscle weakness.

• Patients who respond most slowly to initial treatment have the poorest prognosis.

Follow-up and management

• Patients must be followed for several years.

• Regular clinical examination, creatine kinase measurement, and formal muscle strength testing are needed.

• Physical therapy and hydrotherapy help to keep the range of joint movement normal and to maintain muscle power.

Key references

1. Dalakas MC: Polymyositis, dermatomyositis, and inclusion-body myositis. *N Engl J Med* 1992, **325**:1487–1498.
2. Targoff IN: Polymyositis and dermatomyositis: adult onset. In *Textbook of Rheumatology.* Edited by Maddison P, *et al.* Oxford: Oxford University Press; 1993:794–821.
3. Sigurgeirsson B, *et al.*: Risk of cancer in patients with dermatomyositis or polymyositis. *N Engl J Med* 1992, **326**:363–367.
4. Bohlneyer, *et al.*: Evaluation of laboratory tests as a guide to diagnosis and therapy of myositis. *Rheum Dis Clin North Am* 1994, **20**:845–856.
5. Plotz PH, *et al.*: Current concepts in the idiopathic inflammatory myopathies polymyositis, dermatomyositis and related disorders. *Ann Intern Med* 1989, **111**:143–157.
6. Joffe MM, *et al.*: Drug therapy of the idiopathic inflammatory myopathies. predictors of response to prednisone, azathioprine and methotrexate in a comparison of their efficacy. *Am J Med* 1993, **94**:379–387.

Diagnosis

Symptoms and signs

Acute interstitial nephritis

• This is usually manifest as acute (potentially reversible) nonoliguric renal failure, less often as acute on chronic renal failure.

• The clinical picture may be dominated by the disease process for which an offending drug was administered or by features of extrarenal infection.

Fever, skin rash, and eosinophilia: in 30% of cases associated with drug allergy; NSAID-associated cases may be complicated by nephrotic syndrome.

Arthralgias and lymphadenopathy.

Anterior uveitis and granulomatous infiltration of other organs: in a small group of patients with idiopathic disease.

Chronic interstitial nephritis

• This usually manifests insidiously as chronic (irreversible) renal failure.

• The clinical picture may be dominated by features of an underlying disease process or by the condition for which analgesics were taken.

• No specific features allow differentiation from other causes of chronic renal failure.

Investigations

Full blood count: with differential for eosinophilia in acute interstitial nephritis.

Blood urea nitrogen, creatinine clearance, 24-h urinary protein excretion measurement: to quantify renal function.

Blood cultures and other specific serological tests: if systemic infection, connective tissue disease, or vasculitis suspected (casts, eosinophiluria).

Microscopy and culture of midstream urine.

Urinary Bence Jones protein and serum protein electrophoresis: to screen for myeloma.

Ultrasonography of urinary tract and plain abdominal radiography: in all patients.

Intravenous urography: in patients with adequate renal function (serum creatinine <250 μmol/L) in whom papillary necrosis or reflux nephropathy is suspected, except in diabetic patients with significant renal impairment (serum creatinine >150 μmol/L) and myeloma.

Renal biopsy: in all patients with renal impairment and normal sized, non-hydronephrotic kidneys on ultrasonography, except those in whom diagnosis is apparent from clinical features (*e.g.*, prerenal cause of acute tubular necrosis) or previous investigations (*e.g.*, intravenous urographic diagnosis of reflux nephropathy or papillary necrosis); renal biopsy is dangerous in patients with small kidneys - a careful history provides more reliable diagnostic clues in these.

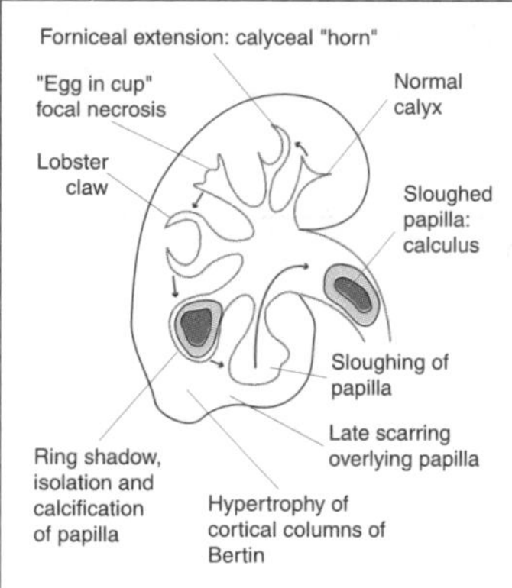

Radiographic features and progression of analgesic nephropathy.

Complications

Acute interstitial nephritis

• The major complications are those of acute renal failure.

Chronic interstitial nephritis

• The major complications are those of chronic renal failure.

Salt wasting, renal tubular acidosis, occasionally Fanconi's syndrome.

Symptomatic anemia inappropriate to level of renal function: in patients with analgesic nephropathy.

Differential diagnosis

Acute interstitial nephritis

Other causes of acute renal impairment, especially rapidly progressive glomerulonephritis (either idiopathic or associated with systemic vasculitis).

Chronic interstitial nephritis

All other causes of chronic renal failure.

Etiology

Causes of acute interstitial nephritis

Drug hypersensitivity: beta lactam antibiotics (*e.g.*, methicillin, ampicillin), other antibiotics (*e.g.*, sulfonamides, rifampicin), NSAIDs (*e.g.*, fenoprofen, indomethacin), diuretics (*e.g.*, thiazides, furosemide), and other miscellaneous drugs (*e.g.*, phenindione, phenytoin, allopurinol).

Infections: complicating urinary tract infection (especially in diabetic patients) or complicating extrarenal infection (*e.g.*, with streptococci, legionella, brucella, leptospira, mycoplasma, *Toxoplasma* spp., infectious mononucleosis, hantavirus).

Immunological disorders: interstitial lesions sometimes overshadow glomerular.

Idiopathic.

Causes of chronic interstitial nephritis

Toxic and metabolic: analgesics, lithium, cisplatinum, lead, cadmium, hypercalcemia.

Granulomatous: sarcoidosis, tuberculosis, drugs.

Immunological: associated with primary glomerular disease, Sjögren's syndrome, transplant rejection.

Miscellaneous: reflux nephropathy, post-obstructive, myeloma, sickle cell disease, radiation nephritis, Balkan nephropathy, hereditary.

Causes of papillary necrosis

Analgesic nephropathy, sickle cell disease, diabetes mellitus, obstruction with infection, tuberculosis, cryoglobulinemia.

Epidemiology

• The true incidence of acute interstitial nephritis is unknown.

• Renal biopsy studies suggest that it accounts for up to 8% of cases of acute renal failure; this is almost certainly an underestimate.

• 20%–40% of patients being treated for end-stage renal failure have primary tubulointerstitial disease.

Treatment

Diet and lifestyle

• Patients who habitually abuse analgesics may benefit from psychological support and counseling.

• Occupational health measures have helped to limit industrial exposure to heavy metals.

• Patients with chronic renal failure have accelerated atherogenesis; smoking should be discouraged, and a diet low in saturated fat recommended.

• Patients with drug-related interstitial nephritis should be advised never to take the same or a related drug in the future.

Pharmacological treatment

• Patients may present with features of severe uremia and need stabilization by urgent dialysis before definitive investigation and treatment can safely be carried out.

For acute interstitial nephritis

Drug-associated: withdrawal of offending drug; prednisolone, 40 mg daily, with rapid tapering according to response, may hasten resolution.

Infection-associated: antibiotic treatment tailored to causative organism; steroids not indicated at least until infection is controlled.

Idiopathic disease associated with uveitis: steroids as for drug-associated disease dramatically improve renal and ocular lesions.

For chronic interstitial nephritis

Toxin-induced: withdrawal of causative agents.

Reflux nephropathy: childhood urinary tract infection must be eradicated by appropriate antibiotics; this should be followed by long-term low-dose chemoprophylaxis until reflux is resolved or renal growth complete.

Sarcoidosis: long-term steroid treatment, using minimum dose to maintain stable renal function. *See* Sarcoidosis *for details.*

Tuberculosis: antituberculous chemotherapy; concurrent use of low-dose steroids may limit renal scarring. *See* Tuberculosis, extrapulmonary *for details.*

Myeloma: referral to hematologist or oncologist recommended for institution of appropriate treatment regimen; hypovolemia must be avoided; allopurinol to prevent acute urate nephropathy. *See* Multiple myeloma *for details.*

For analgesic nephropathy

Withdrawal of offending drugs.

Provision of psychological support.

Monitoring and treatment of the following:
Hypertension: antihypertensive agents (diuretics often inappropriate).
Salt wasting: oral slow sodium may improve glomerular filtration rate.
Renal tubular acidosis: oral sodium bicarbonate.
Inappropriate anemia (gastrointestinal blood loss): misoprostol, iron supplements.
Early renal osteodystrophy: alpha calcidol and calcium carbonate.
Frequent urinary tract infection: prolonged treatment for upper tract infections.
Obstruction due to sloughed papillae: nephrostomy or double-J stents.
Increased incidence of urothelial tumors: regular urine cytology.
Increased atheromatous renovascular disease.

Treatment aims

Acute interstitial nephritis

To provide dialysis support if needed, pending restoration of normal renal function.

Chronic interstitial nephritis

To stabilize renal function.

To reduce rate of progression and complications of chronic renal failure.

To institute renal replacement therapy when necessary.

Prognosis

Acute interstitial nephritis

• Normal renal function is recovered in many patients by prompt treatment.

Chronic interstitial nephritis

• Withdrawal of offending toxins or specific treatment (when possible) may stabilize or improve renal function (occasionally).

• When renal damage has been severe (serum creatinine, >300 µmol/L), progression to end-stage renal disease is probable; even in chronic glomerular disease, the degree of interstitial damage is the major correlate of progression.

Follow-up and management

Acute interstitial nephritis

• When recovery of renal function is incomplete, long-term follow-up is needed.

Chronic interstitial nephritis

• Long-term follow-up is needed.

• Control of hypertension slows progression.

• Salt wasters (5%–10%) need supplements of sodium chloride or bicarbonate.

• Phosphate binders (*e.g.*, calcium carbonate) help prevent secondary hyperparathyroidism; hypercalcemia must be avoided.

• Preparations for renal replacement therapy should be made in good time.

General references

Cameron JS: Allergic interstitial nephritis: clinical features and pathogenesis. *Q J Med* 1988, **66**:97–115.

Nath KA: Tubulointerstitial changes as a major determinant in the progression of renal damage. *Am J Kidney Dis* 1992, **20**:1–17.

Stewart JH, ed: Analgesic and NSAID-induced kidney disease. In *Oxford Monographs on Clinical Nephrology,* vol 2. Oxford: Oxford Medical Publications; 1993.

Diagnosis

Symptoms

• Acute herpetic neuralgia merges into postherpetic neuralgia (persistent neuralgia at 3 months after acute eruption).

• The patient's emotional state, environmental temperature, and fatigue may all affect the severity of postherpetic neuralgia.

Continuous pain: often burning, raw, severe aching, or tearing.

Superimposed spontaneous paroxysmal pains: stabbing, shooting, or shock-like in many patients.

Pain in dermatome: often throughout affected dermatome but usually particularly severe within part of dermatome.

Pain accompanied by unpleasant skin sensitivity: hyperalgesia, and allodynia, sometimes with hyperpathia; these evoked pains are the most troublesome symptoms of postherpetic neuralgia for many patients.

Associated depression: common.

Weakness: caused by shingles affecting a limb dermatome at the same segmental level as the rash; on the trunk, anterior horn cell involvement may be present but difficult to detect and is clinically minor.

Signs

Scarring: usually; variable degree in affected dermatome; depigmented.

Hypoesthesia in the scars, variable hyperalgesia, allodynia, and hyperpathia: in remainder of dermatome.

Investigations

• No investigation is needed in most patients.

• In younger patients, shingles, either isolated or with generalized zoster, may be a symptom of immunosuppression, particularly associated with lymphoma: appropriate investigation of such patients is needed.

Complications

Depression: common, sometimes severe.

Weakness in a limb: when an appropriate dermatome is affected.

Differential diagnosis

Other causes of sensory ganglion and root disease, including diabetes, Sjögren's disease.

Etiology

• Reactivation of herpes varicella zoster virus causes acute shingles.

• Corticosteroid treatment for an unrelated condition sometimes precipitates shingles.

• The mechanism of postherpetic neuralgia includes peripheral and CNS factors (abnormal impulse generation, partial deafferentation and loss of normal inhibition).

• Histopathology in postherpetic neuralgia shows damage to peripheral nerve, dorsal root ganglion, sensory root, and dorsal horn atrophy [1].

Epidemiology

• The female : male ratio is 3 : 2.

• The overall incidence of postherpetic neuralgia at 1 year is ~3% of all patients with acute shingles.

• The most common sites are the mid-thoracic dermatomes and the ophthalmic division of the trigeminal nerve: it may occur in any dermatome.

• Postherpetic neuralgia is rare after shingles in patients aged <50 years and becomes more common with increasing age >50 years.

Treatment

Diet and lifestyle

• No special precautions are necessary.

Pharmacological treatment

• No treatment for patients with acute shingles has yet been proved to prevent the development of postherpetic neuralgia. Treatment remains unsatisfactory.

Local

• Possibilities for local treatment must always be exhausted because simple measures may give partial relief and avoid the side effects so often seen with systemic drug treatment in this mainly elderly patient population.

• Treatments include the following:

Local anesthetic ointment (5% lidocaine) 3 times daily: sometimes effective.

Capsaicin, 0.075% ointment 3 times daily: causes initial burning but helps some patients significantly.

• Local anesthetic, peripheral nerve or root blocks, and sympathetic blocks (occasionally) may temporarily relieve postherpetic neuralgia but has no long-term benefit.

Systemic

Standard dosage	Amitriptyline, 10–25 mg at night, gradually increased to 75–150 mg at night, as tolerated.
Contraindications	Recent myocardial infarction, heart block, mania, porphyria.
Special points	Up to maximum tolerated doses have been consistently shown in controlled trials to provide partial relief of postherpetic neuralgia.
Main drug interactions	Sedation enhanced by other sedatives.
Main side effects	Drowsiness, constipation, urinary hesitancy, dry mouth, blurred vision, postural hypotension, tachycardia, sweating, tremor.

• Opioids may be useful in refractory cases [2].

Treatment aims

To relieve pain.

Other treatments

Local measures

• Cold packs applied for 15–20 min several times daily may produce partial analgesia, sometimes lasting a few hours after a single application.

• Transcutaneous electrical nerve stimulation, acupuncture, vibration, ultrasound may each be helpful in some patients.

Psychological measures

• Counseling by a clinical psychologist about coping strategies may help some patients.

Prognosis

• Most patients with troublesome postherpetic neuralgia at 1 year have the condition lifelong, although some patients slowly improve over long periods.

• After acute shingles, persistent, troublesome neuralgia gradually decreases over several months at least.

Follow-up and management

• ~50% of patients with postherpetic neuralgia benefit from regular long-term follow-up; the role of a sympathetic doctor who is prepared to listen should not be underestimated, even when all treatment options have apparently been exhausted.

• Many patients can be discharged from follow-up when treatment leads to partial relief of pain.

Key references

1. Bennett GJ: Hypotheses on the pathogenesis of herpes zoster associated pain. *Ann Neurol* 1994, **35** (suppl):S38–S41.
2. Paggagallo M, Campsall JN: Chronic opioid therapy as alternative treatment for postherpetic neuralgia. *Ann Neurol* 1994, **35** (suppl):S54–S56.

Diagnosis

Symptoms

Pain: unilateral shooting, shock-like, usually from upper lip to eye or from corner of mouth to ear; rare in ophthalmic division; paroxysmal, lasting <1 min but may occur frequently; occurs spontaneously but often triggered by innocuous facial or oral stimulation, *e.g.*, touching face, washing or shaving, brushing teeth, eating, talking, and drinking; bouts last weeks to months, with remissions of months to years; may become chronic in some patients; rarely develops on contralateral side; in chronic trigeminal neuralgia, some patients complain of background aching pain.

Signs

• Idiopathic trigeminal neuralgia has no signs.

Trigeminal sensory impairment: caused by a compressive lesion of the trigeminal root; such lesions may rarely lead to trigeminal neuralgia.

Investigations

• Investigation is not usually needed.

CT or MRI: in patients being considered for surgical treatment or in whom sensory impairment is present (symptomatic trigeminal neuralgia; rare).

Complications

Depression.

Differential diagnosis

• No other facial pain has the same stereotyped paroxysmal nature.

• Migrainous neuralgia, atypical facial pain, or ophthalmic postherpetic neuralgia should not cause confusion.

Etiology

• The mechanisms of this unique paroxysmal neuropathic pain are poorly understood but involve peripheral and central factors.

• The following may play a role:

Mild compression of the trigeminal root by a blood vessel, usually an ectatic superior cerebellar artery, in chronic sufferers.

Minor degenerative changes in nerve ganglion or root.

Epidemiology

• The female:male ratio is 3:1.

• Onset usually occurs after the age of 50 years.

• The disease is associated with multiple sclerosis, but most young patients (<50 years) with trigeminal neuralgia do not develop multiple sclerosis.

Treatment

Diet and lifestyle

• No special precautions are necessary.

Pharmacological treatment

Carbamazepine

• Carbamazepine is the drug of choice.

Standard dosage	Carbamazepine, 100 mg twice daily initially, increased to a dose that controls pain or to maximum tolerated dose.
Contraindications	Hypersensitivity.
Special points	Blood level monitoring often helpful.
Main drug interactions	Sedation enhanced by other sedatives.
Main side effects	Drowsiness, nausea, ataxia, hypersensitivity rash, neutropenia.

Other drugs

• Phenytoin, tricyclic antidepressants, and baclofen are also often helpful.

Treatment aims

To alleviate pain until onset of remission.

Other treatments

Surgery

• Surgery is indicated for patients who have unremitting pain or who are unresponsive to or intolerant of medical treatment.

Controlled thermocoagulation gangliolysis

• This is a minimally invasive procedure, suitable for elderly, frail patients.

• It is effective, usually giving pain relief of at least 1–2 years, with low risk.

• It can be repeated if necessary.

• Morbidity includes facial sensory impairment; in rare instances, this is severe enough to lead to anesthesia dolorosa and neuroparalytic keratitis.

Microvascular decompression

• This is effective, often permanently, and thus is more suitable for younger patients.

• Morbidity is the same as for thermocoagulation but also includes deafness and brain stem damage (rare).

Prognosis

• Some patients have bouts lasting weeks, with remissions of years.

• Some develop chronic trigeminal neuralgia.

Follow-up and management

• Frequent follow-up is needed until the pain is controlled.

• Withdrawal of treatment must be supervised to assess whether remission has occurred.

General references

1. Loeser JD: Tic douloureux and atypical face pain. In *Textbook of Pain,* edn 3. Edited by Wall PD, Melzack R. Edinburgh: Churchill Livingstone; 1994:699–710.

Neuropathy, peripheral

Diagnosis

Symptoms

General

Distal numbness.

Paresthesia, burning, lancinating pain.

Progressive distal weakness and wasting.

Foot and hand deformities, neuropathic ulcer, neuropathic arthropathy.

Of autonomic neuropathy

Impotence, orthostatic hypotension, dry eyes or mouth, urinary or fecal incontinence, nausea and vomiting, constipation or diarrhea.

Signs

General

Distal hyporeflexia, weakness, stocking-glove sensory loss.

Muscle weakness and wasting.

Reduced or absent tendon reflexes.

Sensory ataxia, neuropathic tremor.

Nerve thickening.

Of autonomic neuropathy

Anhidrosis, unreactive or asymmetric pupils, postural hypotension (fall of 30 mm Hg in systolic and 15 mm Hg in diastolic pressure).

Investigations

Full blood count.

ESR measurement.

Glucose tolerance test: if random and fasting samples give equivocal results.

U&E analysis.

Liver function test.

Measurement of thyroid-stimulating hormone, vitamin B_{12}, serum protein electrophoresis, autoantibodies.

DNA analysis: for hereditary demyelinating neuropathies; chromosome 17 duplication in a subgroup of patients with HMSN type 1 (HMSN 1A); chromosome 17 deletion associated with hereditary liability to pressure palsies (tomaculous neuropathy).

Urinalysis: for glucose, Bence Jones protein, porphyrins.

CSF analysis: raised protein concentration in inflammatory neuropathies.

Nerve conduction studies: diagnosis confirmed by slowing of motor or sensory conduction velocities (moderate in axonal type, marked in demyelinating type) and reduction in sensory action potential amplitude (small in axonal neuropathy).

Electromyography: characteristic pattern in denervated muscle.

Sensory threshold recording: thermal (useful in patients with small-fiber neuropathy) and vibration.

Imaging: screening for malignancy in patients with suspected paraneoplastic neuropathy; skeletal survey for suspected myeloma; chest radiography for suspected sarcoidosis.

Nerve biopsy: done in operating room under strict aseptic conditions using local anesthetic; fascicular biopsy limits degree of sensory loss; full thickness biopsy indicated for suspected vasculitis; used to discover cause of progressive neuropathy not revealed by detailed investigation or to confirm presence of vasculitis, leprous neuropathy, or inflammatory infiltrates; sensory nerves (sural, superficial peroneal, superficial radial) usually biopsied.

Bone-marrow biopsy: for vitamin B_{12} deficiency or myeloma.

Formal autonomic function tests, endoscopy, colonoscopy, barium studies, urodynamic studies: for autonomic neuropathy.

Complications

Burns, cuts, bruising, neuropathic ulcers: unnoticed when sensory loss is severe.

Distal weakness.

Differential diagnosis

- The differential diagnosis depends on the cause.

Combined systems degeneration (B_{12}, folate).

Polyradiculopathy.

Etiology

Causes of sensory polyneuropathy

Diabetes, uremia, hypothyroidism.

Amyloidosis.

Paraneoplastic, paraproteinemic.

Thallium, isoniazid, vincristine, cisplatin, metronidazole.

Sjögren's syndrome.

Leprosy.

HIV, Lyme borreliosis infection.

Hereditary sensory and autonomic neuropathies.

Fabry's disease.

Vitamin B_{12} deficiency.

Causes of sensorimotor polyneuropathy

Hereditary motor and sensory neuropathies.

Alcohol.

Acute or chronic inflammatory demyelinating polyradiculoneuropathy.

Vasculitis.

Paraproteinemic, paraneoplastic.

Diabetes, uremia, hypothyroidism, acromegaly.

Sarcoidosis.

Causes of motor neuropathies

Acute or chronic inflammatory demyelinating polyradiculoneuropathy.

Porphyria, diphtheria, lead.

Hereditary motor neuropathies [1].

Causes of focal and multifocal neuropathies

Entrapment and compression syndromes [2].

Polyarteritis nodosa, connective tissue disorders.

Wegener's granulomatosis.

Lymphomatous and carcinomatous infiltration, neurofibromatosis.

Tuberculoid leprosy, herpes zoster, HIV, Lyme borreliosis.

Sarcoidosis: especially facial nerve.

Hereditary liability to pressure palsies.

Multifocal motor neuropathy with conduction block.

Epidemiology

- The epidemiology depends on the cause.

Treatment

Diet and lifestyle

- Patients with alcoholic neuropathy should abstain from drinking alcohol.
- Postural hypotension can be relieved by raising the foot of the bed.

Pharmacological treatment

For focal and multifocal neuropathies

For vasculitis: prednisone, 60 mg daily orally; azathioprine can be introduced to enable dose of steroids to be reduced; degree of immunosuppression and duration of treatment depend on clinical response.

For protection against peptic ulceration: H_2 antagonists.

For alcoholic neuropathy: vitamin B supplements.

For herpes zoster infection: acyclovir, 800 mg orally 5 times daily for 1 week.

- Leprosy should be treated under specialist supervision.

For autonomic neuropathy

For postural hypotension: fludrocortisone, 100–400 mg, or ephedrine, 15–60 mg daily.

For gastroparesis: erythromycin, 125 mg daily; cisapride, 10 mg 3 times daily; domperidone, 10–20 mg 3 times daily; or metoclopramide, up to 10 mg 3 times daily.

For diarrhea: diphenoxylate (Lomotil), loperamide (Imodium), codeine phosphate.

For impotence: penile intracavernous papaverine injection

For painful neuropathy

- Treatment is extremely difficult and often unsatisfactory.

Regular simple analgesic, *e.g.*, acetaminophen, 1 g 4 times daily.

For burning diffuse pain and paresthesia: amitriptyline, 25-75 mg at night or desipramine, 25-75 mg daily.

For shooting pain: carbamazepine, 100 mg at night, increasing slowly to 600 mg daily in divided doses; mexiletine, 100-400 mg daily may be worth trying.

For postherpetic neuralgia or diabetes: topical capsaicin, 0.075% after lesions have healed.

For chronic inflammatory demyelinating polyradiculoneuropathy

For acute disorder: *see* Guillain–Barré syndrome.

For mild to moderate disease: prednisone, 60 mg/day, tapering as possible; azathioprine may be added for steroid-sparing effect.

For progressive disease or relapses: i.v. immunoglobulin, 0.4 g/kg/day for 5 days and possible replacement of azathioprine with either cyclosporin titrated to leukocytes or cyclophosphamide [3].

Treatment aims

- Treatment aims depend on the type of neuropathy.

Treat dysesthesias or pain, orthostasis.

Other treatments

For focal and multifocal neuropathies

Conservative: wrist and foot support, elbow pad.

Surgical decompression:

Median and ulnar nerve entrapment with evidence of wasting or weakness of denervated muscles.

For persistent sensory symptoms when conservative measures have failed.

For chronic inflammatory demyelinating polyradiculoneuropathy

Plasma exchange for progressive neuropathy unresponsive to immunoglobulin.

Prognosis

- Prognosis depends on the underlying cause of the neuropathy.

Follow-up and management

- Regular follow-up is needed to assess progression.
- Patients requiring immunosuppression need frequent follow-up.

Key references

1. Lupski JR, *et al.*: DNA duplication associated with Charcot–Marie–Tooth disease type 1A. *Cell* 1991, **66**:219–232.
2. Chance PF, *et al.*: DNA deletion associated with hereditary neuropathy with liability to pressure palsies. *Cell* 1993, **72**:143–151.
3. van Doorn PA, *et al.*: High dose intravenous immunoglobulin treatment in chronic inflammatory demyelinating neuropathy: a double blind, placebo controlled, crossover study. *Neurology* 1990, **40**:212–214.

General reference

Dyck PJ, Thomas PK: *Peripheral Neuropathy*, edn 3. Philadelphia: WB Saunders; 1993.

Non-Hodgkin's lymphoma

Diagnosis

Symptoms

Lymph node in neck, axilla, or groin, noticed by patient as unexplained "lump": the most common presenting symptom.

• The disease may be seen in multiple sites at presentation.

• Systemic symptoms (*e.g.*, the "B" symptoms of Hodgkin's disease) are less common than in Hodgkin's disease.

• Symptoms may relate to the anatomical site of disease, *e.g.*, superior vena cava obstruction due to mediastinal nodes or to primary lymphomas at extranodal sites (*e.g.*, CNS, gastrointestinal tract).

• Primary extranodal non-Hodgkin's lymphoma occurs much more often than extranodal Hodgkin's disease.

Signs

Palpable lymphadenopathy: careful examination of all nodal areas essential.

Hepatomegaly and splenomegaly: possibly.

Signs of other organ involvement: *e.g.*, pleural effusion as a result of pulmonary parenchymal involvement, skin involvement (rarely).

Investigations

• Initially, investigations must be directed at confirming the diagnosis.

• A good sample of tissue that has not been placed in formalin is needed.

• The diagnosis may be apparent on routine staining with hematoxylin and eosin or Giemsa.

• Immunohistochemistry, especially markers for T and B lymphocytes and leukocyte common antigen, is vital in subclassification and may help to distinguish undifferentiated lymphomas from carcinoma.

• Subsequent investigations must be systematic and thorough to enable accurate localization of disease and if possible to estimate disease volume.

Full blood count: usually normal.

U&E analysis: as a baseline.

Liver function tests: may be abnormal if liver is involved.

Lactate dehydrogenase measurement: useful marker of disease bulk and activity.

Chest radiography: to rule out hilar or mediastinal nodes or intrapulmonary disease.

CT of chest and abdomen: to rule out node or organ involvement.

Bone-marrow examination: trephine is particularly important.

Examination of postnasal space and tonsillar fossa.

Lumbar puncture with cytology: in high-grade disease only.

Complications

Recurrent or atypical infections.

Autoimmune hemolysis and thrombocytopenia.

Bone marrow failure.

Gastrointestinal bleeding or perforation: obstructive jaundice.

Differential diagnosis

Other causes of lymphadenopathy: *e.g.*, Hodgkin's disease.

Infective causes: *e.g.*, toxoplasmosis, glandular fever, Epstein–Barr virus.

Etiology

• The cause is unknown, but the following may have a role:

Epstein–Barr virus: associated with endemic Burkitt's lymphoma in Africa.

Adult T-cell leukemia–lymphoma: associated in all cases with human T-cell lymphotropic virus.

HIV infection: particularly primary CNS non-Hodgkin's lymphoma (rare in other settings).

Epidemiology

• The median age of onset is 50 years.

• Intermediate- or high-grade disease is more common in younger patients.

Classification [1]

• Non-Hodgkin's lymphomas constitute a diverse group of disorders arising from different cell types, usually T and B lymphocytes; the wide spectrum of disease biology is reflected by the varying clinical presentations, responses to treatment, and overall outcomes.

• Various schemes for classification have been proposed and developed; the most useful are those that can be used to predict clinical behavior and prognosis.

• Classifications include the following:

Rappaport.

Lukes-Collins.

Lennert: the Kiel classification.

The Working Formulation (used here): an international attempt to provide a translation from one classification to another, now widely used in its own right; non-Hodgkin's lymphoma is divided into low, intermediate, and high grades, each having different treatment and prognosis.

Staging

• Patients may be staged I–IV according to the Ann Arbor system originally developed for Hodgkin's disease (*see* Hodgkin's disease).

• Staging is less useful than for Hodgkin's disease because, with the exception of stage 1 disease, all patients with non-Hodgkin's lymphoma should receive chemotherapy.

Treatment

Diet and lifestyle

• Many patients maintain a fairly normal lifestyle during treatment, but some are unwell and need multiple hospital admissions.

Pharmacological treatment

• Treatment should take place in the context of a clinical study whenever possible.

• It should be given by a specialist hematologist or oncologist.

For intermediate-grade non-Hodgkin's lymphoma

• Treatment should begin as soon as investigation is completed.

• These lymphomas are usually sensitive to many chemotherapy drugs, and many effective combination regimens may be curative.

• Stage 1 disease may be treated successfully by radiotherapy alone, but localized disease is very unusual in non-Hodgkin's lymphoma.

• The standard treatment is by CHOP (cyclophosphamide, doxorubicin, vincristine, prednisone), usually given on a monthly cycle for 6 months; other regimens including additional drugs, *e.g.*, PACEBOM (prednisone, doxorubicin, cyclophosphamide, etoposide, bleomycin, vincristine, methotrexate), are given more intensively, reducing total time taken for treatment, but none has been shown to be superior to CHOP [2].

• Allopurinol, 300 mg daily, should be given for at least the first month.

• Main side effects include hair loss, nausea (often preventable), and myelosuppression (for which dose reductions may be needed during subsequent cycles).

For low-grade non-Hodgkin's lymphoma

• These lymphomas are also sensitive to chemotherapy, but, although they usually do not behave aggressively clinically, they are usually considered incurable by standard treatment.

• A conservative approach is often advocated, particularly in elderly asymptomatic patients, because early treatment has no survival advantage.

• 50% of patients may avoid treatment for up to 3 years.

• In truly localized low-grade disease, radiotherapy may give long-term remission.

• Patients may respond well to treatment and often may have considerable periods when no treatment is needed.

• Initial treatment is usually by oral chlorambucil, best used cyclically rather than continually.

• Combination chemotherapy, *e.g.*, chlorambucil with prednisone, vincristine, and possibly anthracycline, is sometimes used but has no proven advantage.

• Interferon-α has just been licensed for low-grade disease, but its indications and benefits are not yet clear.

• The new agents fludarabine and 2-chlorodeoxyadenosine may be of value in relapsed disease.

• Main side effects of chlorambucil include myelosuppression and mild nausea.

For high-grade non-Hodgkin's lymphoma

• Lymphoblastic and Burkitt's lymphomas are very aggressive clinically and often manifest with widespread disease, including bone-marrow and CNS involvement; they need intensive leukemia-style treatment, usually involving very myelosuppressive inpatient regimens and CNS-directed prophylaxis.

Treatment aims

To cure patient, with minimum toxicity.

To palliate if cure is not possible.

Other treatments

• High-dose treatment and autologous bone-marrow transplantation are indicated for the following:

Intermediate grade: age <60 years, relapsed disease still sensitive to chemotherapy.

Low grade: criteria difficult to define because long-term follow-up is needed to assess benefit because of the indolent nature of the disease.

• Allogeneic transplantation may have a role for young patients with high-grade disease.

Prognosis

Low grade

• At 5 years, ~70% of patients are still alive, but few are in complete remission; most patients eventually die of their disease.

• In many patients, the disease ultimately transforms to high grade and becomes refractory to chemotherapy.

Intermediate and high grades

• The complete remission rate is ~85% in patients with limited disease, ~55% with extensive disease.

• Overall disease-free survival is ~40% and depends on several factors; poor prognostic factors include stage III or IV disease, high lactate dehydrogenase concentration, failure to attain complete remission on first-line treatment, and older age.

Follow-up and management

• During treatment, regular follow-up is needed, including examination and full blood count before each course of chemotherapy; toxicity must be monitored, and complications treated.

• After treatment is completed, full restaging should take place: if the patient is in complete remission, regular follow-up should be continued to detect early relapse.

Key references

1. Falzon M, Isaacson PG: Histological classification of the non-Hodgkin's lymphoma. *Blood Rev* 1990, **4**:111–115.
2. Armitage JO: The place of third generation regimens in the treatment of adult aggressive non-Hodgkin's lymphoma. *Ann Oncol* 1991, **2 (suppl 1)**:37–41.

Diagnosis

Symptoms

Social embarrassment.

Shortness of breath on mild exercise.

Pain in back, hips, or knees: especially in middle-aged women.

Infertility, menstrual irregularity.

Pain associated with angina, gallstones, varicose veins.

Heat-intolerance.

Signs

Weight:height ratio >30 kg/m²: definitive diagnosis.

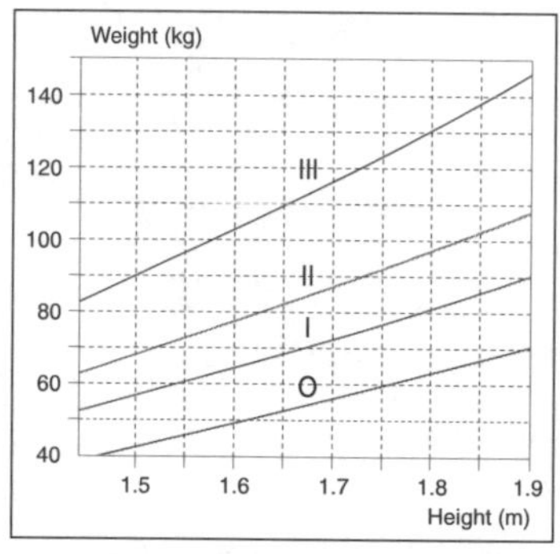

Relation of weight and height for desirable range (O) and mild (I), moderate (II), and severe (III) obesity.

Investigations

• Often no investigation is needed; elaborate endocrine tests are counterproductive because they wrongly imply a probable metabolic basis for obesity.

24-h urine cortisol measurement: for Cushing's syndrome.

Measurement of thyroid-stimulating hormone or free thyroxine: for hypothyroidism if clinically indicated.

Complications

Hypertension, impaired glucose tolerance or non–insulin-dependent diabetes mellitus: common in grade II (moderate) and III (severe) obesity; risk of hypertension or diabetes greater with positive family history or central fat distribution (waist : hip circumference ratio >0.93 in men, >0.83 in women).

Myocardial infarction [1].

Gallstones.

Hiatal hernia.

Osteoarthritis.

Varicose veins.

Infertility.

Increased liability to cancer: colon, rectum, prostate in men; breast, endometrium, ovary in women.

Differential diagnosis

Genetic disorders in children of short stature.

Hyperphagia caused by hypothalamic damage (in adults) or depressive illness.

Cushing's syndrome: alters fat distribution.

Hypothyroidism.

Etiology

• Obesity is caused by greater energy intake than output.

• Familial clustering is seen, partly due to genetic factors and partly to lifestyle.

Epidemiology

• In the US population aged 16–64 years, the prevalence is 28% in men, 30% in women; it is inversely related to social class.

• The prevalence is lower in Canada and Europe.

• The worldwide prevalence is increasing.

Treatment

Diet and lifestyle [2]

• The mainstay of treatment is a reduction in dietary energy, especially from fat, sugar, and alcohol.

• The loss of 1 kg/week of adipose tissue requires an energy deficit of 4.2 MJ/day (1000 kcal/day).

• Physical exercise promotes fitness but is ineffective alone in causing weight loss.

• The help of a dietitian should be sought, and regular (monthly) supportive counseling is essential.

Pharmacological treatment [2]

• Long-term results of drug treatment are disappointing; a short course of anorectic drugs does not assist subsequent weight loss.

• Drugs designed to inhibit the absorption of energy from the gut or stimulate the metabolic rate have not yet been shown to be clinically useful.

Treatment aims

To maintain an average rate of weight loss of 0.5–1 kg/week until "desirable" ratio of weight : height is achieved.

To maintain reduced weight indefinitely.

To restore patient's self-esteem.

Other treatments

Gut bypass surgery: intended to cause malabsorption; not generally used because metabolic complications can be severe and prolonged [3].

Gastric stapling or jaw wiring: to restrict intake; can cause massive weight loss.

"Apronectomy": useful to remove excess skin after weight loss but not an effective primary treatment [3].

Psychotherapy: role unclear; obese people have no specific psychopathology but often have exogenous depression and eating disorders caused by ill advised "crash" diets.

Prognosis

• Substantial weight loss can be achieved by well supervised dieting in 1–2 years and brings great health benefits, especially in young patients.

• Maintenance of weight loss requires constant vigilance: a nylon waist cord provides a warning of unwanted weight regain.

Follow-up and management

• A reasonable target weight (*i.e.*, in grade I) and rate of weight loss (*i.e.*, 0.5–1.0 kg/week) should be set.

• The following errors must be avoided: unrealistic expectations about targets; dietetic incompetence by doctor or patient; misinformation about "wonder cures"; mutual recrimination between doctor and patient from failure to appreciate that dieting is tedious and difficult.

Key references

1. Manson JE, *et al.*: A prospective study of obesity and risk of coronary heart disease in women. *N Engl J Med* 1990, **322**:822–829.
2. Garrow JS: Treatment of obesity. *Lancet* 1992, **340**:409–413.
3. Anonymous: Gastrointestinal surgery for severe obesity. NIH Consensus Development Conference; March 25–27, 1991. Washington: National Institutes of Health; 1991.

Obsessive-compulsive disorder

Diagnosis

Symptoms

Obsessions: involuntary unwanted intrusive thoughts, images, or impulses; accompanying feelings of anxiety.

Compulsions: repetitive behaviors, *e.g.*, checking, cleaning, or mental actions, *e.g.*, praying, counting, performed in order to reduce distress.

Ruminations: obsessional thoughts without overt compulsions; compulsions are covert.

Signs

• Patient at some point recognizes obsessional thoughts as intrusive and inappropriate; compulsive behavior as excessive or unreasonable.

• Patients recognize obsessive thoughts as products of their own mind.

Investigations

• The aim is to allow formulation of problems and to assess suitability for treatment by assessing depression, drug and alcohol abuse, psychosis, and organic causes.

Behavioral analysis: problems reviewed in detail, *e.g.*, using Lazarus mnemonic (*see box*); in addition, maintaining factors, avoidance behaviors, full psychiatric and medical history, and mental state must be elicited; self-monitoring by patient over time, *e.g.*, with diary, used at initial assessment stage and then to monitor subsequent changes, useful for measuring duration and frequency of problem behaviors.

Questionnaires: specific questionnaires used to measure problem and monitor progress during treatment.

Behavioral tests: help therapist to observe problem behavior directly, *e.g.*, test for patient with "fear of contamination by germs" would be to ask him or her to touch a contaminated area, *e.g.*, carpet, and to note the rituals performed, such as checking, washing.

Complications

Episodes of depression: frequent, although suicide rate lower than that of other depressive patients.

Differential diagnosis

Phobia.
Eating disorders.
Obsessive-compulsive personality disorder.
Psychotic disorder.
Tic or movement disorder.
Organic or substance-induced disorder.
Hypochondriasis.

Etiology

• Causes may include the following:

Biological theories

Reduction in neurotransmitters, particularly 5-HT in the limbic system.
Gross brain disease: abnormal activity in the limbic system, abnormality in frontal lobe and basal ganglia system, or feedback system between limbic area and central connections.
Increased genetic concordance more probable in monozygotic than dizygotic twins.

Psychoanalytic theories

Regression to anal eroticism.
Defense mechanisms: isolation, undoing, and reaction formation.
Protection against underlying psychosis.

Sociological theories

Environment: modelling.
Life events: bereavement, head injury.
Strict religious training.

Behavioral and cognitive theories

Learned response to specific situations.
Theory of prepotency.

Epidemiology

• The male :female ratio is equal.

• Obsessive-compulsive disorders usually affect people in early adult life.

• They are seen in different cultures.

• Large-scale epidemiological surveys in the US have shown a 6-month incidence of 1.3%–2.0% and a lifetime incidence of 1.9%–3.3%.

Lazarus mnemonic

For rapid behavioral assessment
B = behavior.
A = affect.
S = sensations.
I = imagery.
C = cognitions.
I = interpersonal relationships.
D = drugs.

Treatment

Diet and lifestyle

• No special precautions are necessary.

Pharmacological treatment [1,2]

• Drugs can be useful in many cases, especially when patient is depressed or obsessions are prominent.

Standard dosage
Clomipramine, 150–250 mg daily.
Fluvoxamine, 100 mg daily, increased to 300 mg daily.
Fluoxetine, 20 mg daily, increased to 60 or 80 mg daily.
Sertraline, 50–200 mg daily.
Paroxetine, 20–50 mg daily.

Contraindications
Clomipramine: myocardial infarction, heart block, severe liver disease, pregnancy.
Fluvoxamine, fluoxetine: pregnancy, lactation, epilepsy, severe renal failure.

Special points
Many patients relapse on stopping the drug; treatment may need to be continued for years.

Main drug interactions
Clomipramine: monoamine oxidase inhibitors, barbiturates, alcohol, anticholinergics, local anesthetics, cimetidine, antihypertensives, estrogen.
Fluvoxamine: propranolol, theophylline, phenytoin, warfarin, monoamine oxidase inhibitors, alcohol, lithium, tryptophan.
Fluoxetine: monoamine oxidase inhibitors, tryptophan, lithium.

Main side effects
Clomipramine: significant anticholinergic effects, *e.g.*, dry mouth, blurred vision, constipation, urine retention.
Sexual disturbances, *e.g.*, impotence, common.
Specific 5-HT reuptake inhibitors: lower overall incidence of adverse effects than clomipramine.
Nausea, headaches, and sexual disturbance.
Initial agitation.

Nonpharmacological treatment [3,4]

Behavioral and cognitive therapy

• This is often the treatment of choice, especially when compulsions are prominent; combined treatment with medications can enhance outcome [5,6].

Exposure and response prevention: should be prolonged, *in vivo*, graduated (as far as the patient can tolerate), and self-imposed.

Other techniques: modelling, shaping, prompting and pacing, and thought-stopping.

Habituation training: deliberate thought evocation, writing the thought down repeatedly, and listening to a loop tape.

Cognitive therapy: overvalued ideation may be amenable.

Psychosurgery

Stereotactic limbic leukotomy or capsulotomy; for patients with severe obsessive-compulsive disorder who have not responded to other forms of treatment (rarely used).

Psychodynamic psychotherapy

• This is only useful for patients with obsessional traits, not for obsessive-compulsive disorders.

Treatment aims

To reduce or abolish obsessional thoughts and actions.

To decrease restrictions in lifestyle.

To reduce depression and anxiety.

Prognosis

• Success rates have ranged from 75% to 85% of patients.

• The outcome for obsessional ruminations is less favorable.

• Gains are maintained for at least 4 years.

Follow-up and management

• Follow-up appointments are generally 1, 3, and 5 months after discharge.

• Patients are educated to become their own therapists, to draw up their own program, and to use the principles when they encounter difficulties.

Causes of treatment failure

Depression.

Overvalued ideation.

Exposure sessions too short.

Neutralizing by seeking reassurance, etc.

Noncompliance.

Key references

1. Rasmussen SA, *et al.*: Current issues in the pharmacologic management of obsessive compulsive disorders. *J Clin Psychiatry* 1993, **54**(suppl 6):4–9.
2. Greist JH, *et al.*: Efficacy and tolerability of serotonin transport inhibitors in obsessive-compulsive disorder. A meta-analysis. *Arch Gen Psychiatry* 1995, **52**:53–60.
3. Baer L: Behavior therapy for obsessive compulsive disorder in the office-based practice. *J Clin Psychiatry* 1993, **54**(suppl 6):10–15.
4. Foa EB: *Stop Obsessing*. New York: Bantam; 1991.
5. Greist JH: An integrated approach to treatment of obsessive compulsive disorder. *J Clin Psychiatry* 1992, **53**(suppl 4):38–41.
6. Cottraux J, *et al.*: A controlled study of fluvoxamine and exposure in obsessive-compulsive disorder. *Int Clin Psychopharmacol* 1990, **5**:17–30.

Diagnosis

Symptoms

• Many patients are asymptomatic.

• Women have more symptoms than men.

• Symptoms occur more frequently in large, weight-bearing joints.

• They are often phasic and are not always progressive; muscle weakness and psychological status are often better predictors of symptoms or functional impairment than structural damage [1].

Pain: typically on use.

Stiffness after inactivity: "gelling" common.

Functional impairment: particularly of gait; a major problem.

Signs

• Signs are often discordant with symptoms.

Bony swelling, deformity, crepitus, restriction of movement: bony swelling may be marked in interphalangeal joints (Heberden's and Bouchard's nodes).

Joint-line tenderness.

Local heat, effusion: occasional inflammatory features, particularly in crystal-related osteoarthritis or developing finger nodes.

Investigations

• Osteoarthritis is principally a clinical diagnosis. Often occuring in middle-aged or elderly patients, the question is not usually whether it is present but whether it is the cause of current symptoms; only clinical examination can answer this.

General

Radiography: may show structural change, *e.g.*, loss of joint space (cartilage), osteophytosis, sclerosis, cysts, osteochondral bodies.

Premature osteoarthritis

• Onset occurs before the age of 55 years [1].

Ferritin measurement: for hemochromatosis.

Calcium, phosphate, alkaline phosphatase measurement: for hyperparathyroidism.

Urine homogentisic acid measurement: if ochronosis suspected.

Lateral spine radiography: for spondyloepiphyseal dysphasia.

Pituitary studies: if acromegaly suspected.

Acute flare

Synovial fluid examination: for sepsis and crystals.

"Locking"

Arthroscopy or MRI: for loose bodies (osteochondral), meniscal lesions.

Complications

Acute crystal synovitis: mainly calcium pyrophosphate crystals.

Septic arthritis.

Loose-body formation.

Avascular necrosis.

Differential diagnosis

• Periarticular lesions may coexist and may be the prime source of symptoms.

Polyarticular osteoarthritis
Inflammatory arthropathies.
Gout.

Poor bone response and destruction
Charcot's arthropathy.
Sepsis.

Acute crystal-related oligoarthritic osteoarthritis
Sepsis.
Gout.
Inflammatory arthropathy.

Etiology

• Osteoarthritis probably has many causes; recognized factors include the following:
Obesity.
Age.
Occupational trauma.
Genetics: nodal osteoarthritis, (spondylo-) epiphyseal dysplasia, type II collagen abnormalities.
Metabolic or endocrine disorders: hemochromatosis, hyperparathyroidism, ochronosis, acromegaly [1].
Previous joint disease or damage.

Epidemiology

• Osteoarthritis is strongly age-related.

• It is the most common cause of locomotor disability.

• Nodal osteoarthritis may manifest with florid polyarticular disease and Heberden's nodes in menopausal women.

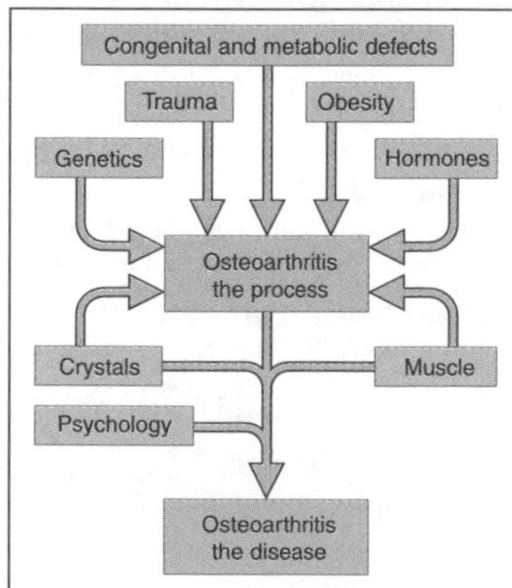

Factors leading to progression of osteoarthritis.

Treatment

Diet and lifestyle

• Patients should be encouraged to take control of the condition.

• Physical activity should be encouraged, *e.g.*, aerobic fitness and muscle strengthening.

• Biomechanical factors, *e.g.*, obesity, varus knee deformity, should be tried (wedge insoles, shock-absorbing footwear, use of cane).

Pharmacological treatment

Analgesics

• These are often sufficient [2].

• Compound preparations with opiates may only increase adverse effects, without improving symptom control.

Standard dosage	Acetaminophen, 1 or 2 650-mg tablets orally every 6–8 h, as required [2].
Contraindications	Liver disease.
Main drug interactions	None.
Main side effects	Rare, except in overdosage when hepatic failure may ensue.

NSAIDs

• NSAIDs may be tried [1,3].

• Use should be regularly reviewed.

Standard dosage	Depends on agent; lowest dose needed for benefit.
Contraindications	Active peptic ulceration, hypersensitivity, renal impairment (relative).
Special points	Patients show marked variation in response to different drugs.
Main drug interactions	Warfarin.
Main side effects	Gastrointestinal ulceration, anemia, renal dysfunction, skin rashes.

Intra-articular steroids

• Local corticosteroids are indicated for short-term relief of inflammatory episodes or coexistent periarticular lesions.

Standard dosage	Depends on agent and joint; in large joints, generally no more than 3-monthly; in small joints, yearly.
Contraindications	Septic arthritis, hypersensitivity (rare).
Special points	Longer-acting steroids provide more benefit.
Main drug interactions	None.
Main side effects	Occasional facial flushing, deterioration of diabetic control.

Topical antirheumatics

• These include NSAIDs and capsaicin ointment.

• Their role is controversial, but they are probably effective.

• Contraindications include sensitive or broken skin.

Nonpharmacological treatment

• Arthroplasty is particularly helpful for patients with disease of hips, knees. Indications include exercise/activity limitation, sleep disturbance, poor quality of life secondary to joint pain.

Treatment aims

To relieve pain.

To maintain functional ability.

Other treatments

Arthroplasty: for patients with persistent pain or marked functional impairment.

Prognosis

• Many patients show phasic symptoms, and some improve with time.

• Symptoms may remain static for years.

Follow-up and management

• Follow-up is usually in a primary care setting.

• The aims are to determine the need for further intervention as a result of deterioration in symptoms or function and to monitor treatment, particularly by NSAIDs to assess the need for continued use and the development of adverse effects.

Key references

1. Brandt K: The pathogenesis of osteoarthritis. *Rheumatol Rev* 1991, **1**:3–11.
2. Bradley JD, *et al.*: Comparison of an anti-inflammatory dose of ibuprofen, an analgesic dose of ibuprofen, and acetaminophen in the treatment of osteoarthritis of the knee. *N Engl J Med* 1991, **325**:87–91.
3. Brandt KD: NSAID's in the treatment of osteoarthritis. Friends or foes? *Bull Rheum Dis* 1993, **42**:1–4.

Diagnosis

Symptoms [1]

Primary or secondary amenorrhea: erratic menstruation or oligomenorrhea in earliest phases.

Delayed puberty.

Infertility.

Hot flushes, vaginal dryness and dyspareunia, thin skin, and scalp hair loss: symptoms of estrogen deficiency.

Signs [1]

• Few signs are manifest, particularly shortly after onset of amenorrhea.

Incomplete pubertal maturation: indicating primary amenorrhea.

Atrophic vaginal mucosa.

Features of Turner's syndrome: short stature, webbed neck.

Investigations

For the disorder

Serum follicle-stimulating hormone (FSH) measurement: persistently raised concentration (>25 IU/L); in women with possible incipient ovarian failure (erratic cycles and moderately raised serum FSH [10–25 IU/L]), care must be taken to ensure sampling was not done during a preovulatory gonadotropin surge (risk of false-positive results) [2].

Progestogen challenge test: negative, indicating estrogen deficiency; determination of estrogen state (of the endometrium) helps to screen for other causes of raised FSH concentration; no value for measuring estradiol.

For the underlying cause

Autoimmune profile: including antiovarian antibodies.

Chromosome analysis: to check for aneuploidy (45XO, 47XXX, 46XY).

Laparoscopy: if streak ovaries seen, possibility of conception is ruled out; if ovaries "normal," biopsy unhelpful; conception has been recorded in women with no follicles at histology.

For assessment of bone state

Radiography for bone age: if delayed in girls with primary amenorrhea, ultralow-dose estrogen should be used to achieve maximum height (ethinyl estradiol, 2 μg daily).

Bone densiometry: no clinical value.

Complications

Infertility: almost all women affected are sterile.

Unwanted pregnancy: fertility returns unexpectedly in a small proportion of women.

Osteoporosis or atraumatic fractures: resulting from estrogen deficiency [3].

Cardiovascular disease: effect of estrogen deficiency on lipid state.

Gonadal neoplasia: in women with gonadal dysgenesis and 46XY karyotype.

Differential diagnosis

• Gonadotropin-secreting pituitary adenomas are rare; the distinguishing feature is estrogenization.

Spurious elevation of follicle-stimulating hormone.

Polycystic ovarian syndrome.

Etiology

• Causes include the following:

Gonadal dysgenesis: *e.g.*, Turner's syndrome, pure gonadal dysgenesis.

Autoimmune: antiovarian antibodies.

Infection: mumps.

Irradiation or chemotherapy.

Extensive ovarian surgery: for endometriosis or recurrent cysts.

Idiopathic premature menopause.

Polycystic ovarian syndrome.

Treated galactosemia.

17α -hydroxylase deficiency (non–salt wasting congenital adrenal hyperplasia).

Epidemiology

• The lifetime risk (before 40 years) is 0.6%.

• ~5% of cases of anovulation, 10% of amenorrhea, and 2% of oligomenorrhea are due to ovarian failure.

Treatment

Diet and lifestyle

• Advice about increasing dietary calcium and the risk of atraumatic fractures should be given to women with long-standing untreated amenorrhea.

• Women not wishing to conceive should be warned of the small risk of conception.

Pharmacological treatment

• Sex-steroid therapy alleviates symptoms of estrogen deficiency and prevents osteoporosis and cardiovascular disease.

• Estrogen is the active agent; progestogens are used to prevent endometrial neoplasia.

• Standard hormone replacement preparations are not contraceptive; women who wish to avoid the small risk of conception should use low-dose combined oral contraceptive (ethinyl estradiol, 20 μg; desogestrel, 150 μg).

Standard dosage Depends on patient's needs.

Contraindications Undiagnosed abnormal menstruation.

Special points *Transdermal estradiol patches:* poor absorption in young women because of thick skin.
Progestogens: third-generation agent should be used to avoid deleterious effect on lipids.

Main drug interactions Anticonvulsants, warfarin.

Main side effects *Estrogen:* nausea (avoided by slow introduction).
Progestogen: premenstrual symptoms.

Treatment aims

To avoid general health risks.
To achieve conception.

Other treatments

Laparoscopic gonadectomy

• If gonads are found on laparoscopy of the internal genitalia, they should be removed laparascopically.

• If streak gonads only are found, no further action is needed.

• If gonads are not evident, the inguinal canal should be explored.

For infertility [4]

• Ovarian failure represents end-organ failure for which the chances of resumption of ovulation (spontaneous or induced) are small and difficult to predict.

• Several methods of inducing ovulation have been described, but, for most women, in-vitro fertilization with donated oocytes offers the only realistic chance of a pregnancy.

• Fostering, adoption, and surrogacy can also be considered.

Prognosis [4]

• The results from one trial of estrogen and human menopausal gonadotropin treatment in 91 women with hypergonadotropic amenorrhea are as follows:
34 patients ovulated.
19 conceptions.
10 miscarriages (53% of conceptions).
1 stillbirth.
8 viable births.

Follow-up and management

• Yearly review is necessary to ensure compliance with hormone replacement therapy.

Key references

1. Rebar RW, *et al.*: Clinical features of young women with hypergonadotrophic amenorrhea. *Fertil Steril* 1990, **53**:804–810.
2. Cahill DJ, *et al.*: Spurious elevation of follicle-stimulating hormone. *Acta Obstet Gynecol Scand* 1992, **71**:388–389.
3. Davies MC, *et al.*: Bone mineral loss in young women with amenorrhea. *BMJ* 1990, **301**:790–793.
4. Check JH, *et al.*: Ovulation induction and pregnancies in 100 consecutive women with hypergonadotrophic amenorrhea. *Fertil Steril* 1990, **53**:811–817.

Diagnosis

Symptoms

Weight loss: in 90% of patients.

Pain: in 80%.

Anorexia: in 60%.

Lethargy: in 40%.

Pruritus: in 40%.

Diabetes mellitus: in 15%.

Acute pancreatitis: in 5%.

Acute cholangitis: in 2%.

Deep-vein thrombosis: in 1%.

Signs

Jaundice: in 85% of patients.

Cachexia: in 70%.

Hepatomegaly: in 60%.

Palpable gallbladder: Courvoisier's sign in 40%.

Epigastric mass: in 15%.

Ascites: in 10%.

Abdominal tenderness: in 5%.

Trousseau's syndrome: migratory thrombophlebitis in <1%.

Virchow's node: firm fixed node in left supraclavicular fossa in <1%.

Splenic-vein thrombosis: gastric fundus varices in <1%.

Investigations

Full blood count: to detect anemia or leukemoid reaction.

Clotting studies: prothrombin time may be prolonged but should correct after vitamin K, 10 mg i.m.

Liver function tests: to confirm "obstructive" jaundice; alkaline phosphatase often elevated and albumin low.

Ultrasonography: to confirm dilated bile ducts and to localize disease (75% accuracy); increased detection of small tumors with endoluminal ultrasonography (90%–100% accuracy).

Endoscopic retrograde cholangiopancreatography: 90%–95% accuracy; brush or pancreatic juice cytology positive in 60%–70% of cases.

Contrast-enhanced CT: 80%–90% accuracy [1].

Laparoscopy: to detect small metastatic lesions otherwise missed [2].

Percutaneous biopsy: 80%–93% accuracy; should not be used in patients with potentially resectable tumors.

Serum marker analysis: *e.g.*, CA-19-9, CA-125; many influenced by jaundice and have poor sensitivity for "early" pancreatic cancer.

Complications

• The symptoms and signs are complications in themselves.

Massive gastrointestinal hemorrhage: caused by erosion into duodenum.

Gastric outlet obstructions/gastroparesis.

Differential diagnosis

Obstructive jaundice
Bile-duct stones, ampullary tumor, tumors of the biliary tract, benign bile duct strictures, metastatic disease, duodenal cancer.

Hepatic jaundice
Chronic hepatitis, sclerosing cholangitis, congestive heart failure.

Cachexia
Gastric, colorectal, or ovarian cancer.

Other pancreatic disease
Chronic pancreatitis (may coexist), non-functioning endocrine tumors, metastases to pancreas.

Etiology

• The cause is largely unknown, but the following may have a role:

Smoking: relative risk, ~2.0 (compared with relative risk of lung cancer, ~20).

Diets high in total or animal fat.

Genetic predisposition (rare): familial colonic and pancreatic cancer, hereditary chronic pancreatitis, familial adenomatous polyposis, Peutz–Jeghers disease, von Hippel–Lindau disease, Lynch II, ataxic telangiectasia.

Long-standing chronic pancreatitis [3].

Epidemiology

• The incidence varies widely according to country and ethnicity, the highest incidences being in central and northern Europe, North America, and Australasia.

• The incidence standardized by age is 8–11 in 100 000 women and 10–12.5 in 100 000 men.

• Pancreatic cancer occurs less in premenopausal women, but the difference between men and women decreases with age.

• The mean age of presentation is 67 years for women and 63 years for men.

Pathology

• 70%–80% of pancreatic cancers arise in the head of the gland, the rest in the body or tail or diffusely located; <6% are multicentric.

Duct cell origin: 95%.

Acinar cell origin: 2%.

Uncertain histogenesis: 2%.

Nonepithelial tumors: 1%.

Treatment

Diet and lifestyle

• No special precautions are necessary.

Pharmacological treatment

Before surgery or endoscopy

• The following are needed initially before resection or relief of jaundice (surgical or nonsurgical):

Correction of anemia, optimization of nutritional status.

Vitamin K, 10 mg i.m. daily for 3 days.

Crystalloid solution, 1–2 L i.v. for at least 24 h before any procedure.

Antibiotic cover for any procedue requiring instrumentation of the biliary tract.

For pain

• In up to 30% of patients, the disease is so advanced that conservative management is most appropriate (*i.e.*, pain relief and palliative care).

• NSAIDs may precipitate acute renal failure.

• Patients can be given morphine slow-release orally, i.v., or by epidural infusion using a portable pump; this may cause constipation, nausea, and drowsiness.

Nonpharmacological treatment

• The choice of treatment to relieve jaundice depends on age, tumor burden, and local expertise.

• In-hospital mortality figures are comparable for the different techniques, although endoscopic methods are probably superior.

• Patients who are potential surgical candidates must be appropriately staged (ultrasonography, CT, laparoscopy), with the help of a radiologist and surgeon.

Surgical resection

• Resection is possible in 10%–15% of patients, with a hospital mortality of 3%–10% [4,5].

Endoscopic stents

• Stents are most useful in patients with symptoms caused by biliary tract obstruction (*i.e.*, pruritis).

• Expandable metal stents need fewer changes and are recommended for patients with an expected better survival rate.

Percutaneous internal stenting

• The complication rate is higher than for endoscopic stents.

Surgical bypass

• Bypass is a consideration for young patients with low tumor burden.

• Duodenal bypass may also be used to avoid obstruction from growth into duodenum (10%–15%).

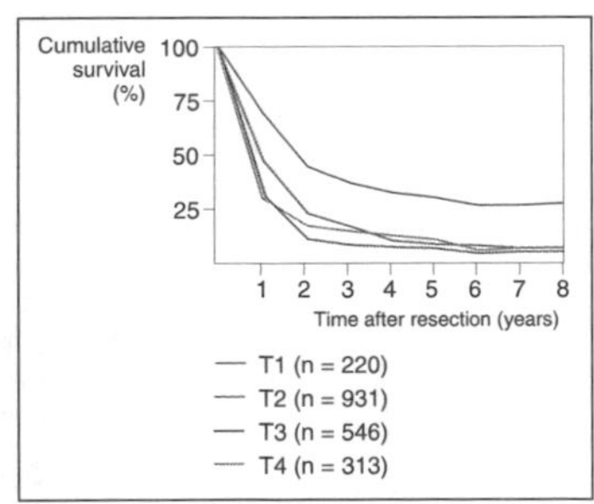

Survival rates after resection for pancreatic cancer stages T1–T4, based on data from the Japanese Pancreatic Cancer Registry.

Treatment aims

To relieve jaundice, duodenal obstruction, weight loss, and pain [6].

Prognosis

• Cure is rarely possible, but a drainage procedure often results in the best palliation.

• After palliative treatment, mean survival is 3–6 months.

• After resection, mean survival is 12–18 months, and the 5-year survival rate is 5%–15%; the survival rate may be increased by adjuvant radiochemotherapy.

Follow-up and management

• Patients who have had resection may be suitable for postoperative adjuvant external beam radiotherapy followed by chemotherapy for 6–24 months.

• After palliative treatment, stents may need to be changed, gastric bypass may be needed for duodenal obstruction, and patients may need pain control.

• Localized recurrence may be worth re-resecting in some patients.

Key references

1. Klöppel G, Maillet B: Classification and staging of pancreatic non-endocrine tumors. *Radiol Clin North Am* 1989, **27**:105–115.
2. Warshaw AL: Implications of peritoneal cytology for staging of early pancreatic cancer. *Am J Surg* 1991, **161**:26–30.
3. Lowenfels AB, *et al.*: Pancreatitis and the risk of pancreatic cancer. *N Engl J Med* 1993, **328**:1433–1437.
4. Russell RCG: Surgical resection for cancer of the pancreas. *Clin Gastroenterol* 1990, **4**:889–916.
5. Warshaw AL, *et al.*: Pancreatic carcinoma. *N Engl J Med* 1992, **326**:455–465.
6. Cotton PB: Management of malignant bile duct obstruction. *J Gastroenterol Hepatol* 1990, **Suppl 1**:63–67.

Pancreatitis, acute

Diagnosis

Symptoms

Epigastric pain: sudden onset; radiation into back; may become increasingly severe.

Anorexia, nausea, vomiting.

Fever: less common.

Signs

Tachycardia, diaphoresis, peritonitis: mild; usually in upper abdomen.

Generalized peritonitis, shock, respiratory failure, "septic" picture.

Turner's sign, Cullen's sign: ecchymosis on flanks and periumbilically, respectively; signs of intra-abdominal hemorrhage.

Peripheral fat necrosis: uncommon (more frequent in alcohol-induced pancreatitis).

Jaundice: especially in gallstone-induced pancreatitis.

Tetany (hypocalcemia).

Investigations

Amylase measurement: serum concentration >100 IU/dL; elevated lipase more specific and sensitive (both may be falsely elevated in renal failure).

Chest radiography (erect): to exclude gastrointestinal perforation.

Ultrasonography: to determine as soon as possible whether gallstones are causative (~80% sensitive); useful in following course of acute fluid collections (*i.e.*, pseudocysts and abscesses).

Serum transaminase, alkaline phosphatase, and bilirubin measurement: elevations raise the possibility of biliary pancreatitis.

Arterial blood gases: hypoxia indicates poor prognosis.

Contrast-enhanced CT: extent of necrosis accurately determined in 85%–90% of cases; only for clinically severe or suspected "silent" pancreatitis.

Fine-needle aspiration: for biopsy of necrotic tissue and Gram stain and culture to ascertain presence of infected necrosis.

Endoscopic retrograde cholangiopancreatography: to ascertain presence of gallstones or choledocholithiasis requiring endoscopic extraction and other causes in biliary tree or pancreas; in severe pancreatitis, disruption of main pancreatic duct suggests significant central necrosis; also indicated in cases of pancreatic trauma.

Complications

• At least one systemic complication occurs in 25%–30% of patients [1].

Cardiovascular, respiratory, and renal failure.

Uremia, hyperglycemia, hypocalcemia.

Acute cholangitis: may coexist with gallstone pancreatitis in 5%–10%.

Disseminated intravascular coagulation, major hematological abnormalities: in 1%–5%.

Acute fluid collections: occur early, in 30%–50% with severe disease and often in patients with mild disease.

Pancreatic necrosis: clinically significant in 3%–5%; up to 70% are infected necroses; lesser degrees (<30% of the gland) often occur in clinically mild pancreatitis.

Pseudocysts: in 15%–20%, although only 33%–50% of these become clinically significant; develop 4 weeks after attack.

Abscess: in 1%.

Death: in 8%–20%.

Differential diagnosis

Abdominal catastrophe: any perforation of gastrointestinal tract, ruptured aneurysm, ectopic pregnancy, mesenteric infarction, ovarian cyst torsion.

Myocardial infarction.

Acute cholecystitis.

Hyperamylasemia.

• Serum amylase concentrations may be raised in most of the above.

• Other conditions include intestinal obstruction, salpingitis, Crohn's disease, afferent loop obstruction after gastrectomy, appendicitis, pregnancy, protein-bound hyperamylasemia (macroamylasemia, lymphoma, AIDS), various tumors, salivary gland disease, renal failure, diabetic ketoacidosis.

Etiology

• Causes include the following:

Alcohol in 50%.

Biliary disorders in 30%–60% of patients: gallstones, cholesterolosis, "sludge," ascariasis, sclerosing cholangitis, choledochocele, tumors.

Complication of endoscopic retrograde cholangiopancreatography.

Penetrating duodenal ulcer.

Hyperlipidemia in 1%–5%: types I (30%), IV (15%), and V (30%–40%).

Unusual causes in 1%–5%: obstructive (pancreas divisum, strictures, tumors), trauma, ischemia, infections (viruses, bacteria, parasites), drugs (azathioprine, L-asparaginase, warfarin), vasculitides, transplantation, hypercalcemia, scorpion bites [2].

Epidemiology

• Gallstone-induced pancreatitis occurs more often in elderly people and women.

• Typically, 30–60 in 10^5 population are affected annually.

• The incidence is increasing.

Treatment

Diet and lifestyle

• During acute illness, patients should not be allowed to take liquids or solids orally.

• Once pancreatitis has resolved, patients must eat regular meals; prolonged starvation followed by large meals must be avoided.

Pharmacological treatment

• Supportive care involves the following:

Intravenous fluid: crystalloid and colloid (up to 12 L may be sequestered in the first 24–48 h).

Nasogastric suction for symptomatic relief of nausea and vomiting.

Pain relief (morphine should be avoided if possible).

Calcium supplementation as needed.

Monitoring and treatment of diabetes mellitus as needed.

Pressor support: if systolic blood pressure <100 mm Hg or renal perfusion inadequate despite fluid replacement.

Antibiotics: for patients with gallstone pancreatitis.

• Glucagon, antiproteases (*e.g.*, aprotinin), somatostatin, and peritoneal lavage are of no value.

Nonpharmacological treatment

Oxygen administration: if oxygen saturation in arterial blood <90%; large pleural effusions should be tapped.

Hemodialysis: for renal failure refractory to fluid replacement and inotropic support.

Endoscopic retrograde cholangiopancreatography and endoscopic sphincterotomy: for patients with severe pancreatitis in patients in whom biliary tract disease is suspected.

Infected necrosis is a strong indication for surgery.

Drainage: for large pseudocysts (>6 cm), persisting in size, expanding, or causing symptoms; repeated percutaneous tapping increases risk of infection and abscess; percutaneous or endoscopic drainage can be used for pseudocysts, although surgical internal drainage is preferred in many patients; abscess may be treated by external drainage; abscess must not be confused with infected pancreatic necrosis with expansive retroperitoneal spread of necrosis and infection [3,4].

Treatment aims

To provide supportive care.

To prevent further attacks.

To reduce complications and underlying disorders (*e.g.*, hyperlipidemia).

Prognosis

• The mortality is 8%–20% overall, <2% for endoscopic sphincterotomy for gallstones, <20% for necrosectomy, <5% for pseudocysts, <5% for abscess.

• Most patients recover after management in hospital with fluid replacement.

• Recurrent attacks are highly probable if alcohol abuse continues or if hyperlipidemia is not treated.

• Unless cholecystectomy or endoscopic sphincterotomy is performed in patients with gallstones, 10%–40% suffer recurrent attacks [2].

Follow-up and management

• Further attacks can be prevented by laparoscopic cholecystectomy (for gallstones) or endoscopic sphincterotomy, stopping alcohol intake, treating hyperlipidemia and other underlying disorders.

• Follow-up is needed only in patients in whom the cause has not been identified or treated or in those who have had extensive surgery for necrosis.

Key references

1. Bradley EL III: A clinically based classification system for acute pancreatitis. *Arch Surg* 1993, **128**:586–590.
2. Steinberg W: Acute pancreatitis. *N Engl J Med* 1994, **330**:1198–1210.
3. Poston GJ, Williamson RCN: Surgical management of acute pancreatitis. *Br J Surg* 1990, **77**:5–12.
4. Fernandez del Castillo C, Rattner DW, Warshaw AL: Acute pancreatitis. *Lancet* 1993, **342**:475–479.

Diagnosis

Symptoms

• Chronic pancreatitis usually evolves over 5–20 years; symptoms, signs, and complications vary during this period [1].

Abdominal pain: in 90% of patients.

Weight loss: in 80%.

Diarrhea or steatorrhea: in 40%.

Diabetes mellitus: in 40%.

Acute pancreatitis: in 40%.

Signs

Marked weight loss: in 40% of patients.

Greasy stool: in 10% on rectal examination.

Epigastric mass: in 10%.

Anemia: in 5%.

Jaundice: in 5%.

Investigations

Chest radiography: for effusion, mediastinal pseudocyst.

Abdominal radiography: for pancreatic calcification.

Ultrasonography: for parenchymal changes, duct dilatation, calcification, pseudocysts, ascites.

Contrast-enhanced CT: highly sensitive for calcification; also useful to evaluate for inflammatory mass, ductal dilation, pseudocysts, ascites.

Endoscopic retrograde cholangiopancreatography: for changes in main duct and side branches ("minimal change pancreatitis"), stones (calcified and noncalcified) and protein plugs in duct, pseudocysts, fistulas.

Blood glucose measurement and glucose tolerance test.

72-h fecal fat determination or pancreatic function tests: pancreatic secretion collection and measurement of enzymes and bicarbonate after stimulation by creatine kinase-secretin to assess exocrine function.

Serum amylase, lipase measurement: concentrations raised in acute exacerbations of pancreatitis.

Endoscopic ultrasonography: classic changes of chronic pancreatitis may be observed.

Complications

Pancreatic exocrine insufficiency.

Pancreatic endocrine insufficiency.

Acute pancreatitis and sequelae.

Duodenal ulcer.

Common bile duct obstruction: secondary biliary cirrhosis (rare).

Duodenal obstruction.

Pseudocysts: pancreatic, intra-abdominal, mediastinal.

Pancreatic ascites.

Pleural effusion.

Pancreatic abscess.

Pancreatic pseudoaneurysm.

Splenic vein thrombosis: gastric fundus varices.

Complications of alcohol and drug abuse.

Bleeding into the pancreatic duct.

Exocrine pancreatic cancer.

Differential diagnosis

Recurrent acute pancreatitis without chronic pancreatitis.

Idiopathic hypertrophy of head of pancreas.

Secondary pancreatic inflammation (duodenal ulceration).

Pancreatic cancer.

Etiology

• Causes include the following:

Alcohol in 60%–80% of patients.

Obstruction in 10%: ampullary stenosis, pancreas divisum, annular pancreas, stricture (trauma, tumor), irradiation, pancreatitis.

Idiopathic in 10%.

Hereditary (chronic familial pancreatitis).

Malnutrition (tropical pancreatitis).

Cystic fibrosis.

Hypercalcemia.

• Many of these causes are associated with decreased pancreatic stone protein (reducing calcium-protein precipitation).

Epidemiology

• In industrialized countries, the incidence largely depends on alcohol consumption (other factors have a modifying effect): 1–10 in 100 000 population are affected annually.

• Chronic pancreatitis occurs more often in men than in women; the ratios vary from 10:1 to 2:1.

• The incidence is increasing in all countries.

Treatment

Diet and lifestyle

- Patients should eat regular meals and abstain from alcohol.
- Use of medium-chain triglycerides is occasionally helpful.

Pharmacological treatment

For the underlying cause

See Peptic ulceration *and* Diabetes mellitus *for details.*

- For exocrine insufficiency, pancreatic enzyme therapy consisting of 28,000 IU of lipase administered over a 4-h postprandial period and titrated to symptoms (steatorrhea, weight); concomitant H_2-receptor antagonists may improve the activity of enzyme supplements [2].

For pain

- Self-titration of pancreatic supplements containing proteases may reduce mild or moderate pain (despite the absence of overt steatorrhea) [3].
- Simple analgesics or NSAIDs can be used.
- Celiac plexus block with steroids can be considered, repeated if necessary.

Nonpharmacological treatment

Main pancreatic duct drainage

- Endoscopic sphincterotomy and stone extraction are suitable in only a few patients; stenting of strictures may be helpful in select cases [4].
- Pancreaticojejunostomy or transduodenal sphincteroplasty are alternatives to endoscopic treatment; draining alone is usually insufficient in the presence of extensive parenchymal calcification, inflammation, and pain [5–8].

Surgery for pain

- Surgery is a consideration in patients with intractable pain.
- For nondiabetic patients or those having an operation for the first time, treatment should be conservative and only "dominant" disease resected.
- For patients with diabetes or previous surgery, extensive surgery may be required.
- Preservation of the stomach, pylorus, duodenum, and spleen is almost always possible.

Treatment aims

To eliminate cause.
To relieve pain.
To delay disease progression (duct drainage).
To treat malabsorption.

Prognosis

- The disease is not always progressive.
- Pain and calcification occur after 5–10 years, and both may subsequently regress, but this is unpredictable.
- The long-term survival may be poor: up to 50% of patients die within 7 years.
- Causes of late death include chronic pancreatitis itself (40%), malignancy (20%), sudden death (suicide, cardiovascular disease; 20%).

Follow-up and management

- All patients must be followed up to control endocrine and exocrine function and pain and to ascertain the need for operation or reoperation.

Key references

1. Steer ML, *et al.*: Chronic pancreatitis. *N Engl J Med* 1995, **332**:1482–1490.
2. Gold EB, Cameron JL: Chronic pancreatitis and pancreatic cancer. *N Engl J Med* 1993, **328**:1485–1486.
3. Ihse I, Permerth J: Enzyme therapy and pancreatic pain. *Acta Chir Scand* 1990, **156**:281–283.
4. Greenen JE, Rolny P: Endoscopic management of pancreatic disease. *Baillières Clin Gastroenterol* 1991, **5**:155–182.
5. Malfertheiner P, Dominquez-Munoz JE, Büchler M: Diagnosis and staging of chronic pancreatitis. In *Standards in Pancreatic Surgery.* Edited by Beger HG, *et al.* Berlin: Springer-Verlag; 1993:297–313.
6. Nealon WH, Thompson JC: Progressive loss of pancreatic function in chronic pancreatitis is delayed by main pancreatic duct decompression. *Ann Surg* 1993, **217**:458–466.
7. Watanapa P, Williams RC: Pancreatic sphincterotomy and sphincteroplasty. *Gut* 1992, **33**:865–867.
8. Beger HG, Büchler M, Bittner R: The duodenum preserving resection of the head of the pancreas (DPRHP) in patients with chronic pancreatitis and an inflammatory mass in the head. *Acta Chir Scand* 1990, **156**:309–315.

Diagnosis

Symptoms

Panic

Recurrent attacks of severe unprovoked anxiety: starting suddenly, reaching a peak within a few minutes, and lasting at least 20 min, with at least four of the following:

Palpitations.
Stomach churning.
Hot or cold flushes.
Shaking or trembling.
Choking or difficulty breathing.
Fear of dying.
Feelings of unreality.
Fear of losing control.
Sweating.
Chest pain or discomfort.
Feeling dizzy, unsteady, lightheaded, or faint.
Paresthesias (numbness or tingling sensations).

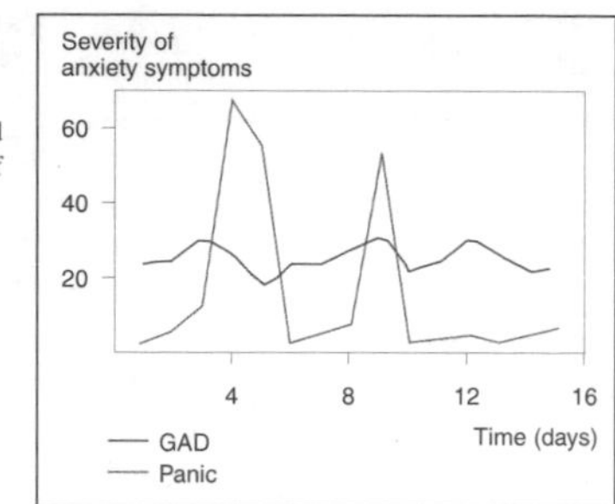

Course of pure panic disorder and pure generalized anxiety disorder (GAD).

Generalized anxiety disorder

Relatively persistent anxiety: at least 6 months, associated with worrying and apprehension about events and other matters that do not justify excessive worry; the anxiety and worry are associated with at least three of the following symptoms:

Restlessness: feeling keyed up or on edge.
Being easily fatigued.
Difficulty concentrating or mind going blank.
Irritability.
Muscle tension.
Sleep disturbance: difficulty falling or staying asleep or restless, unsatisfying sleep.

Signs

Panic

• Physicians seldom see a panic attack *in vivo* because patients usually feel more secure in a medical setting. Features present on examination include the following:

Fear of having a panic attack.
Reassurance that a heart attack or other physical catastrophe is not imminent.
Wish to be physically examined.
Physiological evidence of anxiety: usually no different from generalized anxiety disorder.

Generalized anxiety disorder

Furrowed brow, hunted look, lack of confidence: evidence of long-standing anxiety.
Tachycardia: pulse 80–100 beats/min.
Sweating.
Dilated pupils.
Observed tremor.

Investigations

• Investigations should not be entered into lightly in patients with anxiety disorders because they may cause hypochondriacal concern and increased anxiety. If, however, anxiety appears for the first time in middle age or later, it may have an organic cause.

Thyroid function tests, full blood screening, neurological assessment: may sometimes be indicated if anxiety is episodic, diurnally varied, or linked to specific somatic symptoms persistently; epilepsy and pheochromocytoma are rare but remediable causes of anxiety.

Complications

Alcohol dependence: with persistent anxiety (alcohol provides temporary relief).
Hypochondriasis: due to anxiety about bodily complaints.
Agoraphobia: due to persistent severe anxiety, particularly after panics in public places.
Social phobia: due to self-consciousness of anxiety attacks.

Differential diagnosis

Adjustment disorder, pheochromocytoma, thyrotoxicosis: anxiety related to physical disease.

Post-traumatic stress: anxiety due to major unusual event (*e.g.*, rape, major disaster).

Hypochondriasis, somatoform disease: anxiety due entirely to fear of disease or preoccupation with bodily symptoms.

Organic psychoses, schizophrenia, affective psychoses: anxiety due to psychotic symptoms, e.g. delusions or hallucinations.

Agoraphobia, social or simple phobias: anxiety due to specific stimuli, accompanied by avoidance of the stimuli.

Mixed anxiety and depressive disorder, depressive episode: anxiety due to depressive symptoms.

Substance abuse disorders: anxiety due to alcohol or drug abuse.

Etiology

• The immediate cause of anxiety in panic and generalized anxiety disorder is unknown.

• The episodes of anxiety are unfocused or "free-floating" (generalized anxiety disorder) or spontaneous (panic).

• Both disorders are associated with life changes and events and may sometimes be a delayed reaction to the events.

• A genetic component is possible.

Epidemiology

• Panic attacks are most frequent in the 15–24-year age range and have an annual prevalence of ~2% in this group, with ~1% in the total population.

• Generalized anxiety disorder is much more common, with an annual prevalence of ~6%.

Treatment

Diet and lifestyle

• A good square meal is sometimes said to be the best tranquillizer in the world; unsurprisingly therefore, some anxious people resolve their anxiety by overeating and getting fat. This may relieve their anxiety (good studies show that fat people are less anxious generally than thin people) but does not improve their health overall.

• Because anxious people fear trouble around every corner, they often restrict their lifestyles; this is seen to its extreme in the housebound agoraphobic.

Pharmacological treatment [1]

• The patient's view must be taken into account: some refuse drug treatment, others are equally negative about psychological treatment.

• Less effective treatments, *e.g.*, beta blockade and relaxation training, should be avoided in patients with panic disorder.

• Combined drug and psychological treatments are acceptable and may even be more effective than individual treatments alone.

• Patients must be warned against self-medication with alcohol for anxiety and pain: it provokes worse symptoms in the longer term.

• The duration of treatment should be set in advance, whenever possible.

Standard dosage Benzodiazepines, *e.g.*, diazepam, 2–10 mg daily; alprazolam, 0.25–6.0 mg daily.
Buspirone, 10–60 mg daily.
Beta blockers, *e.g.*, propranolol, 40–120 mg daily.
Tricyclic antidepressants, *e.g.*, imipramine, 100–150 mg daily [2].
Specific 5-HT reuptake inhibitors, *e.g.*, fluoxetine, 20 mg daily.

Contraindications *Benzodiazepines:* caution with previous or present evidence of dependent personality or behavior.

Special points *Benzodiazepines:* rapid and more effective in short term than other treatments, but tolerance and dependence makes them generally unsuitable for regular treatment; may interfere with success of behavior therapy.
Beta blockers: useful if somatic symptoms of anxiety are prominent but not severe (more useful in generalized anxiety disorder).
Tricyclic antidepressants: more effective than benzodiazepines when given for more than 4 weeks, but slow onset of antianxiety effects [2].

Main drug interactions Additive effects with alcohol.

Main side effects Sedation (not beta blockers).

Nonpharmacological treatment

Psychological treatments [3]

Relaxation training: of some value (but less than other more intensive therapies) and can be very cheap.

Cognitive therapy: effective in both disorders, may be superior to other psychological treatments; aimed at altering unproductive dysfunctional thinking that helps to generate and maintain anxiety; patients with panic disorders learn to decatastrophize thinking, so that attacks are avoided.

Behavior therapy: effective in treating maladaptive behaviors associated with anxiety, mainly by gradual exposure to more adaptive situations.

Combination therapies: cognitive behavior therapy, anxiety management training.

Hypnosis and alternative therapies (yoga, meditation): sometimes useful but not as effective as cognitive and behavior therapies.

Treatment aims

To alleviate symptoms.

To teach patient to recognize anxiety early.

To teach patient stress management and relaxation techniques.

Prognosis

• Prognosis is generally good except when symptoms begin early in adult life and are associated with personality disturbance.

Follow-up and management

• Drug treatment is best regarded as a temporary measure, except in patients who are persistently anxious; long-term treatment should be psychological because relapse is less likely and self-esteem is improved.

Key references

1. Brown CS, *et al.*: A practical update on anxiety disorders and their pharmacologic treatment. *Arch Intern Med* 1991, **151**:873–884.
2. Tyrer P, Hallstrom C: Antidepressants in the treatment of anxiety disorder. *Psychiatr Bull* 1993, **17**:75–76.
3. Durham RC, Allan T: Psychological treatment of generalized anxiety disorder: a review of the clinical significance in outcome studies since 1980. *Br J Psychiatry* 1993, **163**:19–26.

Diagnosis

Symptoms

Tremor: in ~70% of patients; unilateral and usually noted in hand first; may be seen in jaw or leg. Most often unilateral at onset.

Poverty of movement, difficulty initiating movements and with repetitive movements: *e.g.*, shuffling gait, drooling, difficulty turning in bed, micrographia, softness of voice, constipation.

Rigidity: *e.g.*, poor balance, falls, muscle stiffness, pain.

Signs

Tremor: asymmetric, resting, "pill-rolling" at 3–5 Hz; usually disappears on intention; increased by anxiety; possibly postural tremor at 6–8 Hz.

Rigidity and bradykinesia: stooped, flexed posture; shuffling gait with poor swing of affected arm; cogwheel rigidity, may be enhanced by synkinesis; immobile facies, reduced blink and swallowing rates; rigidity usually noted first in axial muscles, *e.g.*, neck and shoulder.

Investigations

• No tests are available for Parkinson's disease; the diagnosis is based on clinical features alone.

• Investigation is indicated only if the diagnosis is in doubt or presentation is atypical.

Testing of autonomic function: patients with multiple system atrophy may show abnormalities.

MRI: can show abnormal hypointensity in the putamen of patients with multiple system atrophy.

Copper and ceruloplasmin measurement: in all patients with young-onset or atypical Parkinson's disease.

Complications

Depression, anxiety.

Postural imbalance: with falls and trauma.

Cognitive and psychiatric problems: frontal lobe dysfunction, bradyphrenia, fluctuating confusional state (dementia in 25% of patients); possible overlap with other syndromes, *e.g.*, diffuse Lewy body disease, senile dementia of Lewy body type.

Complications of L-dopa: dyskinesias, motor fluctuation.

Differential diagnosis

Drug-induced parkinsonism: *e.g.*, phenothiazines, butyrophenones; usually symmetrical and reversible.

Essential tremor: bilateral; absent at rest, exacerbated by intention, or maintaining posture; improved by alcohol; possible family history; should be treated with beta blockers or primidone when necessary.

Multiple system atrophy or progressive supranuclear palsy: symptoms and signs usually symmetrical; tremor less usual; falls frequent; additional features, *e.g.*, pyramidal or cerebellar deficits, gaze palsies, or autonomic involvement including postural hypotension, and bladder dysfunction.

Wilson's disease: 40% present with neurological features, mainly parkinsonism and hypokinetic dysarthria; liver cirrhosis or psychiatric disease also occur; Kayser–Fleischer rings visible by slit lamp in most; low serum ceruloplasmin, high urinary copper; liver biopsy shows high copper and evidence of liver cell damage; should be treated with penicillamine.

Toxin-induced parkinsonism (*e.g.*, carbon monoxide).

Mitochondrial disorders; abnormal movements, usually dystonia or chorea.

Etiology [1]

• >80% dopamine depletion occurs in the striatum at presentation; neurons are lost in the substantia nigra (dopaminergic), locus caeruleus (noradrenergic), and substantia innominata (cholinergic). Intracytoplasmic inclusions, Lewy bodies, are found in surviving neurons.

• The cause of Parkinson's disease is not known, but environmental toxins and genetic susceptibility may play a role alone or in combination.

Epidemiology

• The incidence is ~20 in 100 000, with an overall prevalence of 150 in 100 000 (500 in 100 000 for those aged >50 years).

• The male : female ratio is equal.

• Parkinson's disease occurs world wide but is possibly less frequent in China and Africa than in the United States and Europe.

Treatment

Diet and lifestyle

• Maintaining activity is important: a multidisciplinary approach, with physical therapy, occupational therapy, speech therapy, and social work contact is helpful; patients and caregivers may need support.

• Dietary protein should be reduced during the day; a main meal at night allows more predictable absorption of L-dopa.

Pharmacological treatment [2]

At diagnosis

• Most neurologists advocate selegiline, although early use is debated.

Standard dosage Selegiline (Eldepryl), 5 mg twice daily.

Contraindications Possible interaction with tricyclic antidepressants or 5-HT reuptake inhibitors.

Special points May delay requirement for L-dopa, although mechanism of action uncertain; some symptomatic benefit.

Main drug interactions Concurrent L-dopa dose may need to be decreased 20%–50%; should not be administered with tricyclic antidepressants.

Main side effects Gastrointestinal upset, hypotension, confusion.

At review

• Treatment is essentially symptomatic.

• L-Dopa has medium to long-term side effects, so treatment is prescribed when clinical features interfere with life.

• Tremor and bradykinesia respond well, postural instability less well.

• The use of controlled-release L-dopa offers some improvement in patients with medium to advanced disease, especially in decreasing "off time"; transition to these drugs should be gradual because the bioavailability is different from that of the standard preparations; some neurologists use controlled-release preparations early to provide a more "physiological" prolonged drug exposure to dopaminergic neurons.

• Dopaminergic agonists may be used alone (early) or in combination with L-dopa.

Standard dosage L-Dopa with a dopa decarboxylase inhibitor, initially at low dose and frequency, *e.g.*, 100 mg twice or three times daily; increased as necessary.
Dopaminergic agonists, *e.g.*, bromocriptine or pergolide in low doses initially and built up gradually.

Contraindications *L-Dopa:* closed angle glaucoma.
Dopaminergic agents: hypotension, cardiac arrhythmias.

Special points *L-Dopa:* generally, frequent small doses (up to every 2–3 h) are better than infrequent large doses.
Dopaminergic agents: may be used alone, but tolerance to these drugs develops quickly.

Main drug interactions *Dopaminergic agents:* combination with L-dopa may improve control and potentially delay onset of side effects associated with L-dopa.

Main side effects *L-Dopa:* gastrointestinal upset, postural hypotension, confusion, hallucination, dyskinesias and dystonia (excess L-dopa), fluctuations, including dyskinesias, freezing, and unpredictable "on-offing" in 50%–60% of patients 3–5 years after starting treatment; neuropsychiatric side effects best treated by dose modification, but clozapine may be used (possible development of agranulocytosis).
Dopaminergic agents: hypotension, hallucinations, confusion, gastrointestinal symptoms.

• Amantidine or anticholinergics may be useful adjunctive medications for tumor.

Treatment aims

To improve functional disability.

To avoid or minimize drug-related side effects.

To treat fluctuations when present.

Other treatments

• Fetal implant therapy continues to be developed, but substantial and sustained benefit has not yet been shown.

• Adrenal implants are rarely performed and are of questionable efficacy.

• The benefit of antioxidant treatment has not yet been shown.

• Posteroventral pallidotomy may be useful in selected patients to improve tremor, rigidity, and motor fluctuations.

Prognosis

• Parkinson's disease progresses at variable rates.

• Patients with dementia have a significantly worse prognosis.

Follow-up and management

• The need for symptomatic treatment should be assessed.

• Correct use and titration of drugs should be monitored.

• Medical and support needs should be assessed.

Key references

1. Calne DB: Treatment of Parkinson's disease. *N Engl J Med* 1993, **329**:1021–1027.

2. Marsden CD: Parkinson's disease. *J Neurol Neurosurg Psychiatry* 1994, **57**:672–681.

Diagnosis

Symptoms

• Often no symptoms are manifest.

Mild feverish illness: in children.

Mild feverish illness with arthralgia or arthritis: in adults.

Symptoms of an aplastic crisis: in patients with hemolytic anemias or occasionally normal people; onset usually acute but self-limiting.

Symptoms of persistent severe anemia: in immunosuppressed patients.

Signs

• The illness, when accompanied by a rash, is known as erythema infectiosum, fifth disease, or slapped cheek syndrome.

Rash: usually seen in children; appears on cheeks, giving slapped-cheek appearance; lasts 1 week; recurs for several months on exposure to sun or wind; variable but often reticular maculopapular rash may also develop on arms and legs but rarely affects palms or soles.

Lymph-node enlargement: in adults.

Arthralgia or arthritis: often involving wrists and knees in adults; can occur without rash; usually last 2–4 weeks, occasionally longer.

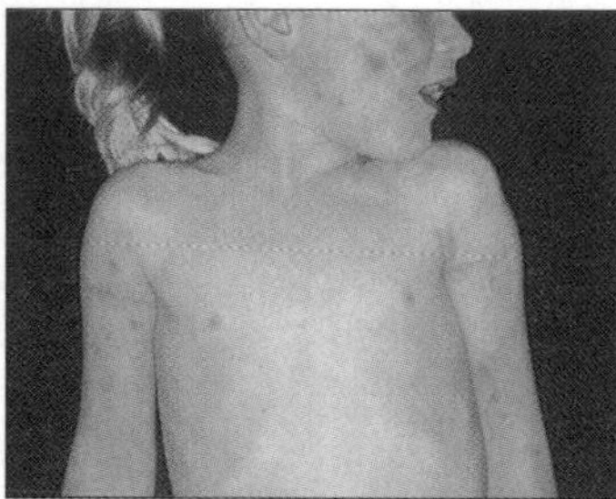

Slapped-cheek appearance of parvovirus B19 infection and reticular rash on arms.

Investigations

Serology: IgM specific to parvovirus B19 manifest in early illness; parvovirus B19 IgG antibody develops early in illness and falls within 1–2 months.

Complications

Aplastic crisis.

Fetal anemia, hydrops fetalis, and death: especially during second trimester, although effect on pregnancy uncertain; about one-third of pregnant women with primary infection transmit it to fetus.

Differential diagnosis

Scarlet fever: parvovirus has no oral stigmata.

Measles: no Koplik's spots or marked syndrome in parvovirus infection.

Rubella, enteroviral infections, cytomegalovirus, Epstein–Barr virus, toxoplasmosis.

Etiology

• Infection is by parvovirus B19.

• Transmission is by respiratory droplets.

Epidemiology

• Infection occurs worldwide.

• Most infections are in spring or early summer.

Infectivity

• Parvovirus B19 is moderately infective.

• Immunity is apparently for life after an acute episode.

Mean incubation period

To the mild febrile illness: 6–8 days.

To the rash: 17–18 days.

Treatment

Diet and lifestyle

• People known to be infected should avoid contact with pregnant women.

Pharmacological treatment

Analgesics, *e.g.*, acetaminophen.

NSAIDs for reactive arthralgia.

Treatment aims

To relieve symptoms (if any).

Prognosis

• Prognosis is good in acquired illness.

• Mortality is 9%in recognized fetal infections.

Follow-up and management

• Follow-up is not needed.

General references

Gay NJ, *et al.*: Age specific antibody prevalence to parvovirus B19: how many women are infected in pregnancy? *Comm Dis Rep* 1994, **4**:R104–R107.

Pattison JR: Human parvovirus B19. *BMJ* 1994, **308**:149–150.

Diagnosis

Symptoms

Pericarditis

Mild to severe precordial pain: on inspiration or worse on inspiration; may radiate to neck and shoulders; worse on coughing, swallowing, or sneezing; improved by leaning forward.

Dyspnea, nausea.

Tamponade

Precordial discomfort: occasionally, due to large effusions.

Cough, hoarseness, tachypnea, dysphagia: due to pressure.

Malaise, cyanosis, dyspnea, sweating, anxiety, hypotension: rapidly developing.

Signs

Pericarditis

Fever.

Pericardial, often pleuropericardial, coarse rub: best heard at left sternal edge with patient leaning forward; may come and go over minutes to hours, may decrease with development of effusion.

Initially normal venous pressure.

Tamponade

Tachycardia: nearly always present.

Low blood and pulse pressures.

Pulsus paradoxus: pulse may disappear on inspiration; may occur in asthma.

Raised venous pressure: with prominent "y" descent and no "x" descent; may increase on inspiration [1].

Investigations

• For any pericardial disease, the underlying cause must always be sought.

Pericarditis

Full blood count, ESR and U&E measurement.

Antistreptolysin O titer, antineutrophil factor, rheumatoid factor analysis.

Cardiac enzyme tests: enzymes may be normal or increase, but creatinine phosphokinase MB probably not significantly increased unless accompanying myocarditis.

Paired viral antibody screening: increase in neutralizing antibodies (up to 4 times) within 3–4 weeks of onset.

Mantoux test.

ECG: changes throughout all leads; raised ST segment, inverted T waves only in some patients, pericardial effusion (low-voltage QRS and T wave in large effusions), electrical alternans (caused by heart swinging about).

Chest radiography: normal unless pericardial fluid >250 mL; cardiac contour may be globular, with no congestion in lungs.

Tamponade

Echocardiography: essential in any patient in whom pericardial fluid is suspected (*e.g.*, cardiomegaly on chest radiography with hypotension); right ventricular collapse characteristic of tamponade.

Complications

Relapsing or constrictive pericarditis, pericardial effusion and tamponade: complications of pericarditis.

Hypotension, renal failure: complications of tamponade.

Differential diagnosis

Pericarditis

Extension of infarct after infarction.

Myocardial infarction, unstable angina, ulcer dyspepsia, acute aortic dissection, spontaneous pneumothorax, pleurisy, pulmonary embolus.

Tamponade

Cardiomyopathy or constrictive pericarditis.

Etiology

Causes of pericarditis

Viral: may be associated with pleurisy.

Immune or collagen diseases: SLE, scleroderma.

Rheumatic fever, rheumatoid athritis.

Myocardial infarction or cardiac surgery.

Metabolic: uremia, myxedema.

AIDS, opportunistic infections (*e.g.*, tuberculosis).

Association with neoplasia, particularly lymphomas, leukemia, carcinoma of bronchus or breast.

Causes of tamponade

Any of the above, but particularly the following:

Carcinoma of bronchus or breast.

Uremia.

Cardiac surgery.

Viral infection (in young patients).

Epidemiology

• The incidence at post-mortem examination is 2–6%.

• The clinical incidence is <1 in 100 hospital admissions.

• More men than women are affected.

• The disorder may recur after treatment but is usually a one-off event, depending on the cause.

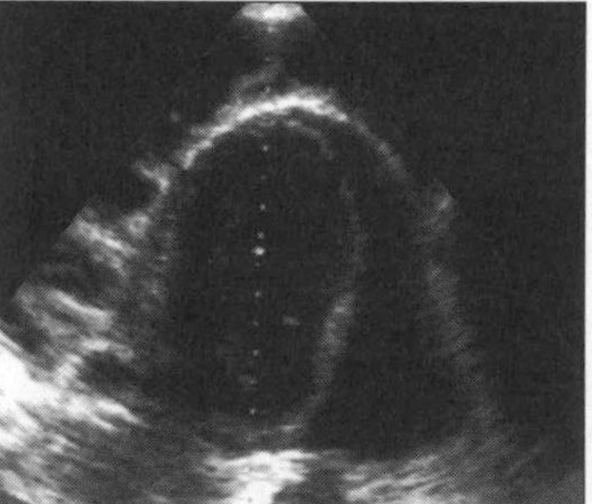

Pericardial space containing fluid (*top center*); bright pericardium (*mid center*); left ventricle (*lower center*); fibrinous strands in pericardial fluid (*lower left*).

Treatment

Diet and lifestyle

- No special dietary precautions are necessary.
- Overactivity is contraindicated until the symptoms have resolved.

Pharmacological treatment

- Drugs are indicated for pericarditis.
- Aspirin usually settles both pain and fever; indomethacin is particularly useful in preventing recurrence; a short course of steroids may be needed.
- Specific treatment is needed for any related condition.

Standard dosage
Aspirin, 300–600 mg every 3–4 h.
Indomethacin, 50–200 mg in divided doses (adults).
Prednisolone, 30 mg for 2–3 weeks, then reduced depending on symptoms.

Contraindications
Aspirin: peptic ulceration, hypersensitivity.
Indomethacin: peptic ulceration.
Prednisolone: osteoporosis, history of gastrointestinal symptoms, tuberculosis, pregnancy.
Caution in renal or hepatic impairment.

Main drug interactions
All: warfarin.
Indomethacin: aspirin, steroids.
Prednisolone: aspirin.

Main side effects
Aspirin: dyspepsia.
Indomethacin: gastrointestinal problems, including bleeding.
Prednisolone: hypertension, peripheral edema, potassium loss, hyperglycemia.

Nonpharmacological treatment

- For tamponade, pericardial aspiration may be life-saving with large effusions.
- As much fluid as possible should be drained; blood-stained effusions usually signify malignancy, but all samples should be sent for cytology and bacteriology.
- Recurrent effusions may need balloon pericardotomy or surgical drainage.
- Chemotherapy can be started if malignant disease has been confirmed.

Treatment aims

To prevent adverse hemodynamic changes of tamponade.
To diagnose and treat underlying condition.

Prognosis

- Prognosis depends on the underlying condition: it is good for viral pericarditis but poor for malignant pericardial effusion [2,3].
- Patients with viral pericarditis usually recover completely in 1–2 weeks.

Follow-up and management

- Regular echocardiographic follow-up is necessary for pericardial effusions.

Key references

1. Fowler NO: Cardiac tamponade. A clinical or an echocardiographic diagnosis. *Circulation* 1993, **87**:1738–1741.
2. Friman G, Fohlman J: The epidemiology of viral heart disease. *Scand J Infect Dis* 1993, **88**:7–10.
3. Spodick DH: Pericarditis in systemic diseases. *Cardiol Clin* 1990, **8**:709–716.

Diagnosis

Definition [1]

• Personality disorders are dysfunctional patterns of thinking and behavior that reflect persistent ways of relating to self and others, which deviate markedly from the norm and are invariably accompanied by impairment of social role or major subjective distress.

•The specific personality disorders that appear in adolescents can be broadly categorized into three main areas:

Flamboyant: histrionic, emotionally unstable (borderline or impulsive), dissocial.

Eccentric: paranoid/schizoid.

Fearful: anancastic, anxious/avoidant, dependent.

• Others are acquired later in life and arise as a result of organic insult, psychiatric illness, or catastrophic stress.

Symptoms and signs

Suspicion, oversensitivity, querulousness, unforgiving: paranoid.

Emotional coldness, solitude, social insensitivity: schizoid.

Impulsiveness, emotional instability, poor self-control: emotionally unstable (impulsive or borderline).

Obsessions, perfectionism, rigidity, self-doubt: anancastic.

Social sensitivity, apprehension, feelings of social inferiority: anxious, avoidant.

Reliance on others, subordination of own needs, fear of abandonment: dependent.

Callousness, irresponsibility, blaming others, aggressiveness: dissocial.

Dramatics, suggestibility, seeking center stage, shallowness: histrionic.

Investigations

History: should be corroborated with other sources if possible (with patient's permission): personality characteristics of parents, early development, adverse life events and upbringing; school/social services (history of neglect, impoverishment, or abuse); legal sources (e.g. probation office); spouse, cohabitee (partners may also have personality disorders); employer.

Standardized questionnaires: usually time-consuming but highly reliable; patients are asked tightly worded questions covering specific areas of personal and social function in order to avoid biased judgement on the part of the therapist; this is particularly important in the case of disorders with antisocial characteristics.

Munich Checklist for ICD-10: a good alternative [2].

EEG: finding may be abnormal in patients with dissocial disorder.

Complications

High suicide rate.

Self-harming behavior: may lead to frequent presentations in a wide variety of health-care settings, *e.g.*, emergency departments, medical wards.

Alcohol addiction and drug abuse.

Harm to others: *e.g.*, violent assault or sexual abuse of children.

Differential diagnosis

Comorbidity with mental illness (AXIS I): cross-sectional studies show that ~40% of patients also manifest AXIS I disorders when they present in clinical settings.

Schizotypal disorder: frequently overlaps with borderline and schizoid disorders.

Prodromal or residual phase of schizophrenia.

Affective disorders: hypomania may mimic dissocial disorder; depression is frequent in patients suffering from borderline disorder.

Etiology

• Causes include the following:

Genetic inheritance.

Abnormal developmental biology.

Failure to negotiate critical stages of emotional development.

Childhood trauma: sexual abuse is a more frequent feature in borderline disorders.

Social theories: abnormal parenting or lack of an appropriate role model.

Epidemiology

• Schizoid personality disorder appears to be rare because sufferers avoid society.

• The prevalence in the general population is 2%–6%; in primary care settings, 15%–34%; in psychiatric outpatients, 20%–40%; in psychiatric inpatients, 40%–60%; in forensic settings, 50%–90%.

Treatment

Diet and lifestyle

• No special precautions are necessary.

Pharmacological treatment [3]

• All drugs must be used with caution because of the dangers of overdose and abuse.

• Neuroleptics, *e.g.*, thioridazine or haloperidol in low doses, can alleviate symptoms, *e.g.*, hostility, anger, suspiciousness, and depressed mood, in borderline or dissocial conditions.

• Monoamine oxidase inhibitors may be useful in borderline conditions.

• Long-term use of benzodiazepines must be avoided because of the probability of addiction; they may cause paradoxical disinhibition.

• Mood stabilizers (lithium and carbamazepine) are most useful if there is evidence of mood swings or family history of affective disorder.

Nonpharmacological treatment

Psychotherapy

• Interpretative psychotherapies for flamboyant disorders are effective in mild to moderate conditions.

Behavior or cognitive therapy

• This is being developed but is not widely available; it is similar to therapies used in the treatment of depression and anxiety.

Supportive therapy

• This includes social support and is most useful for patients with severe disruptive personality disorders.

• Patients are encouraged to find practical solutions to present problems, *e.g.*, relationship difficulties, accommodation, other personal needs.

Group therapy

• Group therapy may help patients with some forms of personality disorders.

• It includes the use of therapeutic communities.

Treatment aims

To alleviate subjective distress and reduce impact of dysfunctional behavior.

Prognosis [4]

• Prognosis is usually poor in severely affected patients, but most improve with age (4th or 5th decade); improvement is more noticeable for the flamboyant group.

• The outcome is invariably worse when comorbid mental illness is present.

• Good prognostic features include intelligence and the presence of positive adaptive traits, *e.g.*, candor and introspectiveness.

Follow-up and management

• No treatment has universally proven effectiveness; the most useful approach is based on long-term supportive contact and crisis intervention when needed.

• Patients tend to arouse strong feelings in therapists; staff working in crisis situations particularly need regular support.

Danger

• Most patients with personality disorders are no more dangerous than unaffected people.

• A few people with severe disorders, especially those with paranoid or dissocial traits, can exhibit considerable aggression towards others; safety and surveillance is paramount in such circumstances.

• In community settings, the police should be involved to make the situation safe.

• Admission to secure units or forensic facilities may be needed.

Key references

1. Anonymous: *ICD-10 Classification of Mental and Behavioural Disorders. Clinical Descriptions and Diagnostic Guidelines*. Geneva: World Health Organization; 1992.
2. Bronisch T, *et al.*: The Munich diagnostic checklist for the assessment of DSM–III-R personality disorders for use in routine clinical care and research. *Eur Arch Psychiatry Clin Neurosci* 1992, **242**:77–81.
3. Stein G: Drug treatment of personality disorders. *Br J Psychiatry* 1992, **166**:67–84.
4. Stone M: Long term outcome in personality disorders. *Br J Psychiatry* 1993, **162**:299–313.

Diagnosis

Symptoms

Sore throat: with difficulty swallowing.
Concurrent coryza, laryngitis, productive cough: suggesting viral cause.
Malaise, fever, headache: common.

Signs

General

Injected mucous membranes of pharynx, tonsils, conjunctivae, and tympanic membranes.
Enlarged tonsils: sometimes with exudates.
Enlarged cervical lymph nodes.

Streptococcal infection

Grey exudates in tonsillar follicles.
Enlarged injected tonsillar and peri-tonsillar area.
Coated tongue with fetor.
Enlarged, tender cervical nodes.
Occasional meningismus.
Diffuse punctate erythema, flushed cheeks, circumoral pallor, reddened mucous membrane, white then red strawberry tongue: signs of scarlet fever.

Infectious mononucleosis

Prolonged fever: often for 10–14 days.
Nasal voice/"fish mouth" breathing.
Enlarged lymph nodes and splenomegaly.
Palatal petechiae and clean tongue.
Enlarged tonsils: sometimes almost meeting in middle, with confluent white exudates.
Faint maculopapular rash.

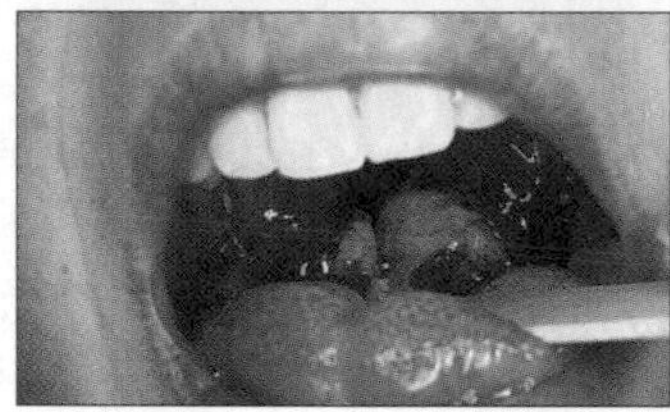

Streptococcal follicular tonsillar exudates (top) and confluent exudates (bottom) in infectious mononucleosis.

Coxsackie A virus

5–10 small aphthoid ulcers: scattered over oral cavity.
Firm vesicular lesions: along sides of fingers and on feet (usually few).
Papular lesions: especially on feet and lower legs, occasionally up to buttocks.

Diphtheria

Toxic, listless, tachycardia due to myocarditis: fever usually low-grade or nonexistent.
Adherent whitish membrane: spreading from tonsils to oropharynx or oral cavity.
Enlarged anterior cervical lymph nodes: with surrounding edema.

Investigations

Throat swab: to check for streptococcal infection and diphtheria; usually not needed for viral infections.
Differential leukocyte count: elevated neutrophil leukocytosis indicates streptococcal infection; elevated, many atypical mononuclear cells indicate infectious mononucleosis.
Serology: for Epstein–Barr virus, mycoplasma.

Complications

Peritonsillar abscess, reactive phenomena (rheumatic fever, glomerulonephritis, erythema nosodum, Henoch–Schönlein purpura): with streptococcal infection.
Respiratory obstruction, hepatitis, splenic rupture: with infectious mononucleosis.
Nerve palsies, myocarditis: with diphtheria.
Erythema multiforme: with *Mycoplasma pneumoniae* infection.

Differential diagnosis

• Differential diagnosis depends on the underlying cause.

Etiology [1]

• Causes include the following:

Pharyngitis with nonspecific features
Viral infection, especially adenoviruses, enteroviruses, influenza or parainfluenza virus, Epstein–Barr virus.
Beta-haemolytic *streptococcus pyogenes* group A, C, or G.
Mycoplasma pneumoniae, Corynebacterium diphtheriae, Neisseria gonorrhoeae.

Pharyngitis with clinically recognizable features
Streptococcus pyogenes infection: cause of follicular tonsillitis, scarlet fever.
Epstein–Barr virus infection: cause of infectious mononucleosis.
Coxsackievirus infection: cause of hand, foot, and mouth disease (A16), herpangina (A).
Corynebacterium diphtheriae infection: cause of diphtheria.

Epidemiology

• Very common disease of adults and children.
• Adenoviral infection is the most common viral type identified in children with respiratory illnesses, which are more prevalent in crowded conditions.
• Enteroviral infection usually occurs in late summer or early autumn, with one or two types dominating (out of >70).
• Some influenza virus activity is usual each winter, with some larger outbreaks.
• Epstein–Barr virus circulates throughout childhood but is usually only manifest symptomatically in teenagers and young adults.
• Streptococcal infection occurs in late winter and early spring, especially in school children.
• Very few cases of diphtheria occur in the US each year.

Treatment

Diet and lifestyle

• Infants should be breast-fed and subsequently provided with adequate nutrition throughout childhood.

• Respiratory secretions must be disposed of hygienically.

Pharmacological treatment [2]

• Immunization should be given as nationally recommended: *e.g.*, against diphtheria, influenza A.

• Symptomatic treatment is indicated for presumed viral infections: *e.g.*, throat lozenges, acetaminophen.

Antibiotics

• Penicillins are effective against streptococcal and diphtherial infections [3,4].

Standard dosage	Penicillin G, 1.2 MU i.m. Phenoxymethylpenicillin, 500 mg orally 6 hourly.
Contraindications	Hypersensitivity.
Special points	Erythromycin, 250 mg 6 hourly, or new macrolides are other options.
Main drug interactions	None.
Main side effects	Sensitivity reactions, diarrhea.

Antitoxin

• Antitoxin should be given immediately on clinical suspicion of diphtheria.

Standard dosage	Antitoxin 20 000–100 000 units i.v. (depending on disease severity).
Contraindications	Hypersensitivity (epinephrine should be available).
Special points	Test dose is needed before full dose because of equine origin of antitoxin.
Main drug interactions	None.
Main side effects	Sensitivity reactions, including serum sickness.

Treatment aims

To provide symptomatic relief.
To reduce infectivity.
To prevent rheumatic fever (in streptococcal infections).
To neutralize circulating toxins of diphtheria promptly.

Other treatments

Drainage of peritonsillar abscess, indicated by marked inferior and posterior displacement of tonsil.
Tracheostomy for respiratory obstruction.
Tonsillectomy in children with recurrent tonsillitis that disrupts schooling.

Prognosis

• Full rapid recovery is usual.
• Occasionally, patients suffer from post-viral fatigue, especially after influenza, Epstein–Barr, or enteroviral infections.
• Mortality from diphtheria is 5%–10%; survivors usually recover completely.

Follow-up and management

• Patients who have apparently recovered from streptococcal tonsillitis may continue to have enlarged and tender cervical nodes that subsequently spread infection as cellulitis or septicemia.
• Patients with diphtheria should be followed up after 2–6 weeks for late nerve palsies and myocarditis.

Notification

• Diphtheria and scarlet fever are legally notifiable diseases in the US.

Key references

1. Vukmir RB: Adult and pediatric pharyngitis: a review. *J Emerg Med* 1992, **10**:607–616.
2. Goldstein MN: Office evaluation and management of the sore throat. *Otolaryngol Clin North Am* 1992, **25**:837–842.
3. Kline JA, Runge JW: Streptococcal pharyngitis: a review of pathophysiology, diagnosis, and management. *J Emerg Med* 1994, **12**:665–680.
4. Blumer JL, Goldfarb J: Meta-analysis in the evaluation of treatment for streptococcal pharyngitis: a review. *Clin Ther* 1994, **16**:604–620.

Diagnosis

Symptoms

• Symptoms are usually paroxysmal, resulting from tumor release of catecholamines with stimulation of adrenergic receptors.

• If asked, patients often report a feeling of "impending doom"; up to 20%, however, are asymptomatic; flushing is not typical.

Headache: in 80% of patients.

Sweating: in 70%.

Palpitations: in 70%.

Pallor: in 40%.

Nausea: in 40%.

Tremor: in 30%.

Weakness: in 30%.

Anxiety: in 20%.

Epigastric pain: in 20%.

Chest pain: in 20%.

Dyspnea: in 20%.

Constipation: in 10%

Signs

Hypertension: in >90% of patients (sustained in 60% or paroxysmal in 30%); malignant hypertension possible, retinopathy common, paradoxically postural hypotension (secondary to reduction in plasma volume) frequent.

Supraventricular tachycardia, myocardial ischemia and infarction, cardiomyopathy, and heart failure.

Fever, weight loss.

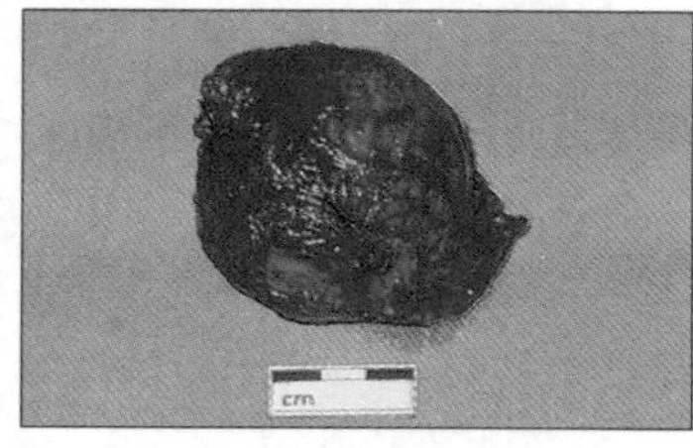

Operative specimen of a pheochromocytoma.

Investigations [1–3]

To establish the diagnosis

• Plasma catecholamines and provocative tests are of limited value.

Urinalysis: to measure metanephrines, free catecholamines (epinephrine, norepinephrine), vanillylmandelic acid; 24-h collection using an acid-containing bottle mandatory (30 ml 6N HCl); possible false-positive results due to interfering medications (propranolol, labetalol, methyldopa, clonidine withdrawal).

To localize the disorder

• These investigations should be done only after biochemical diagnosis has been made.

CT or MRI of abdomen: >95% specificity, >55% sensitivity.

^{131}I-meta-iodobenzylguanidine scintigraphy, imaging of other regions (thorax, head and neck): to detect extra-abdominal tumors; can be considered if imaging of abdomen negative; successful localization after scintigraphy with ^{131}I-somatostatin has been reported.

Complications

Diabetes mellitus.

Hypercalcemia: suggesting a malignant pheochromocytoma or multiple endocrine neoplasia.

Malignant pheochromocytoma: in 10% of patients.

Myocardial infarction.

Pulmonary edema.

Cerebrovascular accident.

Paralytic ileus.

Differential diagnosis

Thyrotoxicosis, hypoglycemia, migraine.

Labile "essential" hypertension, tachyarrhythmia, angina.

Anxiety neurosis.

Cerebellar tumors (rare).

Etiology [1,2]

• Pheochromocytomas are tumors of chromaffin tissue, secreting predominantly norepinephrine (85%).

• The cause of sporadic cases is unknown.

• Familial causes include the following:

Multiple endocrine neoplasia type II: hyperparathyroidism, medullary thyroid cancer.

Neurofibromatosis.

Von Hippel–Lindau disease: cerebellar or retinal hemangioblastoma, renal carcinoma.

Epidemiology

• Pheochromocytoma is found in 0.1% of hypertensive patients.

Treatment

Diet and lifestyle

- No special precautions are necessary.

Pharmacological treatment [2–4]

Alpha blockade

- Alpha blockers should always precede beta blockers.

Standard dosage Phenoxybenzamine, 20 mg orally twice daily, increasing by 20 mg every second day to 200 mg daily maximum.

Contraindications None.

Special points Control of hypertension and paroxysms with abolition of postural hypotension monitored to assess response.
Hypertensive crises can be treated by phentolamine, 2–5 mg i.v.

Main drug interactions None.

Main side effects Postural hypotension, tachycardia, inhibition of ejaculation, nasal congestion, gastrointestinal irritation, fatigue.

Beta blockade

- Tachycardia can be treated by propranolol. Unopposed beta blockade, however, should be avoided, as should combined alpha and beta blockade preparations.

Standard dosage Propranolol, 40 mg 3 times daily, increased as needed to 240 mg daily maximum.

Contraindications Severe asthma, heart failure (possibility of catecholamine-induced cardiomyopathy).

Special points None.

Main drug interactions Verapamil reduces myocardial contractility; phenytoin or rifampicin increases clearance; cimetidine reduces clearance.

Main side effects Bradycardia, atrioventricular block, claudication, tiredness, vivid dreams, bronchospasm, gastrointestinal disturbances.

For malignant disease

- Patients can be given therapeutic doses of ^{131}I metaiodobenzylguanidine, chemotherapy, or alpha or beta blockade.

Treatment aims

To normalize blood pressure.

To eradicate tumor.

Other treatments

Resection of metastatic deposits, when possible, for patients with malignant disease.

Adrenalectomy for patients with an adrenal tumor.

- Inadequate surgical preparation can result in precipitous hypertension during induction for surgery and severe hypotension after removal of the tumor; this is minimized by alpha and beta blockade for at least 2 weeks before surgery and the use of plasma volume expanders if needed.
- During surgery, patients can be given i.v. phentolamine or nitroprusside for hypertensive episodes.

Prognosis

- Blood pressure is restored in 70% of patients postoperatively.
- Failure to lower blood pressure may reflect a second tumor, operative damage to renal vasculature, or secondary hemodynamic changes in a hypertensive patient.
- The 5-year survival rate for patients with malignant disease is 35%.

Follow-up and management

- Urinary catecholamine excretion should be measured 1 week postoperatively and, if normal, annually for 5 years.

Key references

1. Bravo EL: Evolving concepts in the pathophysiology, diagnosis, and treatment of pheochromocytoma. *Endocr Rev* 1994, **15**:356–368.
2. Gifford RJ, Manger WM, Bravo EL: Pheochromocytoma. *Endocrinol Metab Clin North Am* 1994, **23**:387–404.
3. Werbel SS, Ober KP: Pheochromocytoma. Update on diagnosis, localization, and management. *Med Clin North Am* 1995, **79**:131–153.
4. Raum WJ: Pheochromocytoma. *Curr Ther Endocrinol Metab* 1994, **5**:172–178.

Diagnosis

Symptoms

• Platelet disorders may be manifest by bleeding or discovered incidentally in an otherwise asymptomatic patient.

Bruising.

Bleeding: usually mucosal, *e.g.*, gingival, nasal, gastrointestinal, menorrhagic; occasionally retinal (loss of vision) or intracranial (headache); after surgical procedures.

Deafness: in some familial disorders.

Signs

Petechiae, purpura, bruises.

Retinal hemorrhages.

Thrombosis and skin microinfarcts: in thrombotic thrombocytopenic purpura.

Capillary bleeding.

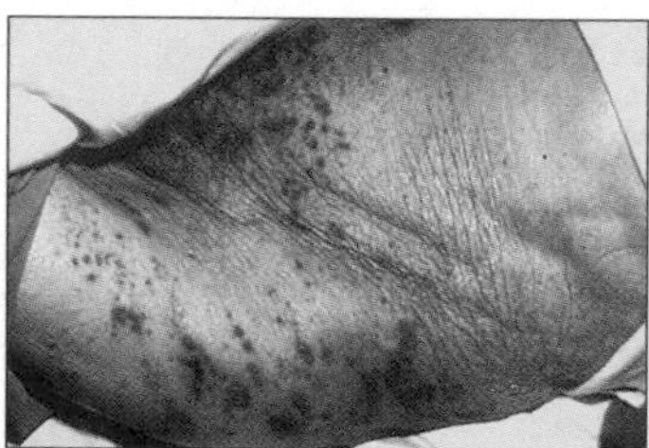

Purpura due to thrombocytopenia.

Investigations

• Initial investigations are used to identify primary platelet disorder and to exclude von Willebrand's disease in patients with a strong family history and lifelong bleeding disorder.

Full blood count: platelet count and mean platelet volume, to exclude other hematological disease and pseudothrombocytopenia due to clumping or EDTA (ethylenediaminetetraacetic acid)-induced aggregation.

Microscopic examination of film: for platelet morphology, to detect erythrocyte or leukocyte abnormality.

Coagulation screening: to exclude primary coagulopathy

Biochemistry profiles: to identify renal or hepatic disease.

Platelet function tests: bleeding time, if prolonged, suggests platelet function disorder or von Willebrand's disease (drugs that affect platelet function, *e.g.*, aspirin, should be avoided for 10 days before testing); spontaneous *in vitro* aggregation and response to ADP (adenosine diphosphate), collagen, and ristocetin should be recorded; if abnormal, response to other agonists (*e.g.*, epinephrine, thrombin, arachidonate) should be assessed; release reaction of radiolabeled 5-HT (5-hydroxytryptamine); measurement of platelet adenine nucleotides; hereditary and some acquired platelet disorders have characteristic aggregation responses.

Bone-marrow aspiration and biopsy: in most patients with thrombocytopenia, to assess number and structure of megakaryocytes and bone-marrow function.

Platelet serology: in posttransfusion purpura and in neonates with alloimmune thrombocytopenia, to identify specific antiplatelet antigen antibodies.

Platelet-associated immunoglobulin measurement: nonspecific, often increases in immune thrombocytopenias.

Flow cytometry: to quantify platelet membrane glycoproteins, using monoclonal antibodies to detect hereditary disorders.

Complications

Iron-deficiency anemia: caused by menorrhagia or recurrent epistaxis or gastrointestinal bleeding.

Neurological impairment or death: caused by intracranial bleeding.

Differential diagnosis

Bleeding disorders

Von Willebrand's disease.

Fibrinogen disorders.

Purpura

Vasculitis: *e.g.*, Schönlein-Henoch syndrome.

Amyloid.

Senile purpura.

Scurvy.

Steroid treatment.

Collagen disorders (*e.g.*, Ehlers–Danlos syndrome).

Hereditary hemorrhagic telangiectasia (does not cause purpura but can lead to low platelet count in extreme forms).

Etiology [1]

• Causes include the following:

Decreased production

Bone-marrow failure: leukemia, metastatic tumor, idiopathic aplasia, infiltration, abnormal production, myelodysplasia, aplastic anemia, drugs (predictable, *e.g.*, cytotoxic drugs, or idiosyncratic reactions).

Increased consumption

Immune: autoimmune (idiopathic, post-viral, HIV, associated with other autoimmune disorders), alloimmune against platelet-specific antigens, *e.g.*, HPA-1.

Drugs: *e.g.*, quinine, heparin, sulfonamides, rifampin.

Coagulopathy: disseminated intravascular coagulation, thrombotic thrombocytopenic purpura.

Hypersplenism and splenomegaly.

Hereditary

Platelet membrane glycoprotein abnormalities, *e.g.*, Bernard-Soulier and Glanzmann's diseases.

Platelet storage pool abnormalities.

Other abnormalities, *e.g.*, May–Hegglin anomaly.

Acquired

Platelet storage pool defects: *e.g.*, aspirin, uremia, ethanol, cirrhosis, myeloproliferative disorders.

Epidemiology

• Acquired disorders of platelet function are common and are associated with disorders such as chronic renal failure or the ingestion of aspirin.

• Chronic idiopathic thrombocytopenic purpura is relatively common (one group suggests that 0.18% of patients admitted to hospital in a 10-year period had the disease).

Treatment

Diet and lifestyle

• Patients should avoid trauma and contact sports.

Pharmacological treatment

For immune thrombocytopenia

• In children, the onset is usually acute and often follows a viral infection; spontaneous recovery is common, and treatment is given to those with severe or life-threatening bleeding to elevate the platelet count. In adults, the onset is more insidious, and it almost never remits spontaneously.

Standard dosage	*Children:* immunoglobulin, 0.4 g/kg i.v.daily (in 4–6 h) for 5 days (sometimes 1.0 g/kg daily for 2 days); or prednisone 1 mg/kg. *Adults:* prednisone, 1 mg/kg daily initially until maximum response, then tailed off.
Contraindications	*Prednisone:* active infection, diabetes mellitus.
Main drug interactions	*See manufacturer's current prescribing information.*
Main side effects	*Immunoglobulin:* headache, hypertension tachycardia. *Prednisone:* hypertension, diabetes mellitus, osteoporosis.

• Adults who do not respond or who relapse when steroids are reduced should be considered for splenectomy.

• Other treatments for adults failing steroids or splenectomy include i.v. immunoglobulin, azathioprine, vinca alkaloids, danazol, high-dose dexamethasone, or vitamin C.

For platelet functional defects [2]

• The bleeding tendency is often mild, and specific treatment (platelet transfusion, arginine vasopressin [DDAVP]) is needed for major hemorrhage or to cover surgical procedures. Antifibrinolytic agents may be helpful to control minor bleeding; antiovulatory treatment may be needed for menorrhagia.

Standard dosage	One single donor platelet pack/10 kg body weight or one platelet pheresis pack should raise the platelet count by 20–40 × 10^9/L. DDAVP, 0.4 µg/kg i.v. in 100 mL 0.9% saline solution in 15–20 min. Tranexamic acid, 0.5–1.0 g 3 times daily orally or i.v. Aminocaproic acid, 2–4 g 4 times daily, orally.
Contraindications	*DDAVP:* coronary artery disease. *Tranexamic acid:* history of thromboembolism.
Special points	*DDAVP:* ineffective in Glanzmann's thrombasthenia.
Main drug interactions	*See manufacturer's current prescribing information.*
Main side effects	*Platelet transfusion:* allergic reactions, HLA or alloimmunization in multitransfused patients; hepatitis B (rare) or C transmission. *DDAVP:* nausea, tremor, vomiting, angina, myocardial infarction. *Tranexamic acid:* nausea, vomiting, diarrhea.

For bone-marrow disorders

• The risk of spontaneous hemorrhage increases when the platelet count is <10 × 10^9/L. Prophylactic platelet transfusions are given to maintain the count above this level during the treatment of acute leukemia or aplastic anemia or during bone-marrow transplantation.

• In chronic thrombocytopenia due to bone-marrow failure, platelet transfusions are given for symptomatic bleeding.

For thrombotic thrombocytopenic purpura [3]

Supportive therapy of medical complications, *e.g.*, hemodialysis. Plasma exchange with fresh frozen plasma replacement (1.5 times plasma volume) for 7 days. Additional treatments include aspirin, dipyridamole, methylprednisone, and vincristine.

For alloimmune thrombocytopenia, neonatal and posttransfusion

Antigen-negative platelet transfusion, i.v. immunoglobulin, prednisone, or plasma exchange.

Treatment aims

To cure or alleviate symptoms, depending on underlying disease.

Other treatments

• Splenectomy is indicated for immune thrombocytopenia (not in children <6 years).

• Vaccination by Pneumovax and against *Haemophilus influenzae* type b and *Neisseria meningitidis* serogroups A and C should be given 1–2 weeks before surgery.

Lifelong antipneumococcal prophylaxis (*e.g.*, penicillin V, 250 mg twice a day) is recommended for splenectomized patients.

Prognosis

• Up to 90% of children with idiopathic thrombocytopenic purpura remit spontaneously, with 50% recovering in 1 month.

• 80% of adults with idiopathic thrombocytopenic purpura remit after treatment by steroids alone or after splenectomy.

• The bleeding tendency in patients with hereditary platelet defects varies.

• In patients with acquired platelet function defects, the prognosis is related to the underlying disease.

• Mortality in patients with untreated thrombotic thrombocytopenic purpura is up to 90%; 60%–80% respond to treatment, reducing mortality to ~30%.

• Alloimmune thrombocytopenias are self-limiting but potentially fatal.

Follow-up and management

• The frequency of follow-up depends on the clinical severity and stability of the underlying disorder.

Key references

1. George JN, Shattil SJ: The clinical importance of acquired abnormalities of platelet function. *N Engl J Med* 1991, **324**:27–38.
2. Bolan CD, Alving BM: Pharmacologic agents in the management of bleeding disorders. *Transfusion* 1990, **30**:541–551.
3. Rock GA, *et al.*: Comparison of plasma exchange with plasma infusion in the treatment of thrombotic thrombocytopenic purpura. *N Engl J Med* 1991, **325**:393–397.

Diagnosis

Symptoms

• Patients are often asymptomatic if the effusion is small.

Breathlessness.

Chest pain: increased on deep inspiration or movement.

Positional discomfort or pain: with large effusions, causing mediastinal shift.

Symptoms of underlying disease.

Fever.

Signs

• Signs are clinically detectable only if the volume is ≥300 mL; loculated effusion may be very difficult to detect.

Decreased movement of chest wall on affected side.

Dull percussion note: "stony dull."

Absent breath sounds in area of dullness.

Occasional bronchial breathing at upper margin of area of dullness.

Displaced trachea: large effusions only.

Investigations [1,2]

Chest radiography: to assess extent of effusion and possible underlying disease.

Ultrasonography: if doubt about nature of shadowing and to define loculated area for aspiration.

Aspiration: for cytology, Gram stain and Ziehl–Neelsen stain for acid-fast bacilli, culture, protein content, lactate dehydrogenase (LDH), cell count and differential, pH, glucose.

• Comparison of pleural protein content and LDH to plasma protein and LDH is essential to distinguish between transudative and exudative effusions [3].

Pleural biopsy: in experienced hands, much more reliable for diagnosis of tuberculosis and malignancy than simple aspiration.

Repeat radiography: after drainage of effusion, to visualize underlying lung.

Thoracoscopy: if doubt remains, to obtain better samples for histology.

CT: for visualizing loculated effusions and pleural and parenchymal disease.

Complications

Constrictive fibrosis of pleura and restricted lung function: caused by empyema and postpneumonic effusions.

Iatrogenic secondary infection.

Iatrogenic pneumothorax.

Unilateral pulmonary edema: after injudiciously rapid drainage.

Hemorrhage: damage to intercostal vessels, especially after pleural biopsy.

Differential diagnosis

Infections: postpneumonic, tuberculosis.

Inflammation: pancreatitis, rheumatoid arthritis, SLE, polyarteritis nodosa.

Primary malignancy: mesothelioma.

Secondary malignancy: bronchogenic carcinoma, metastatic spread (especially breast, stomach, pancreas), lymphoma.

Infarction secondary to pulmonary embolism.

Etiology [4]

• Causes include the following:

Exudates

Unknown in ~20%, despite extensive investigation.

Infections: viral pleurisy, bacterial pneumonia, tuberculosis, empyema.

Secondary malignancy or secondary cancer (*e.g.*, lung, breast, stomach), leukemia or lymphoma.

Vascular: pulmonary infarction.

Collagen disorders: rheumatoid arthritis.

Primary pleural malignancy (mesothelioma).

Transudates

Congestive heart failure, hypoalbuminemia (nephrotic syndrome and hepatic cirrhosis), constrictive pericarditis.

Abdominal disease: subphrenic abscess, pancreatitis.

Epidemiology

• Pleural effusion is frequently found with lung cancer and after pneumonia.

• Tuberculosis is declining in importance but remains one of the most common causes of pleural effusion world wide.

• Mesothelioma is rare but is associated with asbestos exposure.

Treatment

Diet and lifestyle

• No special precautions are necessary.

Pharmacological treatment

Principles

• The principal aim is to treat any underlying cause and to treat the local problem by drainage, possibly with chemical pleurodesis.

• For transudates, the underlying disease must be treated.

• For infective causes (empyema, pneumonia), systemic antibiotics are indicated and intercostal drainage is essential; surgical drainage and decortication of pleura can be done if thick pleural rind develops.

• For tuberculosis, standard oral antituberculosis chemotherapy is indicated. The effusion should be aspirated to dryness. Tube drainage and surgery should be avoided if possible. *See* Tuberculosis, pulmonary *for details.*

• For malignant effusions, pleural effusion indicates inoperability; treatment is guided by symptoms. Intermittent aspiration is usually helpful. Tube drainage is the best method of preventing recurrence and achieving pleurodesis. In mesothelioma, tube drainage is best avoided if possible because of the risk of seeding tube tract [5,6].

• Pulmonary infarcts usually resolve without needing drainage.

• For noninfective nonmalignant causes, the effusion should be drained to dryness and followed with repeated chest radiographs.

• Pulmonary infarcts usually resolve without needing drainage, but formal anticoagulation with warfarin is usually appropriate (*see* Pulmonary embolism *for details*).

Chemical pleurodesis [6]

• Chemical pleurodesis is best done by specialists, who can consider the advantages and disadvantages in each individual case. It is usually reserved for malignant pleural effusions.

Standard dosage Doxycycline, 500 mg or minocycline, 300 mg in 50 mL saline, after pleural fluid has been drained. A second dose may be given after 72 h.
Bleomycin, 60 units is an acceptable alternative for malignant effusions.

Contraindications Transudate, bronchopleural fistulas, infection.

Main drug interactions None.

Main side effects Local pain, transient fever.

Treatment aims

To achieve resolution of pleural effusion without residual fibrosis or functional deficit.

Prognosis

• Prognosis varies widely according to the underlying cause.

• If cleared by drainage, most bacterial effusions resolve, leaving some pleural scarring, which may need surgery if severe.

• Malignant effusions have poor prognosis, and treatment is mainly palliative, guided by symptoms.

Follow-up and management

• Serial chest radiographs should be taken, usually at 4–6 week intervals to assess recurrence.

• Lung function tests are needed to assess residual restrictive deficit if radiographic changes persist.

Key references

1. Collins TR, Sahn SA: Thoracentesis: complications, patient experience and diagnostic value. *Chest* 1987, **91**:817–819.
2. Bone R: The techniques of diagnostic and therapeutic thoracentesis. *J Crit Illness* 1990, **5**:371–379.
3. Light R, *et al.*: Pleural effusions: the diagnostic separation of transudates and exudates. *Ann Intern Med* 1972, **77**:507–513.
4. Sahn S: The pleura. *Am Rev Respir Dis* 1988, **138**:184–234.
5. Keller SM: Current and future therapy for malignant pleural effusion. *Chest* 1993, **103 (suppl)**:635–675.
6. Sahn S: Pleural effusion in lung cancer. *Clin Chest Med* 1993, **14**:189–200.

Pneumocystis carinii pneumonia in AIDS

Diagnosis

Symptoms

Fever, fatigue, weight loss: for weeks or months before respiratory symptoms develop.

Nonproductive cough, shortness of breath: initially on exertion, then at rest with disease progression.

• The absence of respiratory symptoms does not exclude *Pneumocystis carinii* pneumonia, especially in patients who are receiving prophylaxis or who have had previous episodes of infection.

Signs

Wasting, fever, diffuse lymphadenopathy, oral candidiasis, hairy leukoplakia, cutaneous Kaposi's sarcoma: general signs of immunosuppression secondary to HIV infection.

Tachypnea, dry rales: revealed by auscultation, but often no pulmonary abnormalities.

Splenomegaly, fundal abnormalities: rare extrapulmonary signs of infection.

Investigations

• *Pneumocystis carinii* pneumonia occurs in HIV-infected individuals who have a CD4 lymphocyte count $<200 \times 10^6$/L.

Full blood count: to exclude anemia.

Plain chest radiography: may show diffuse interstitial infiltration, sensitive but non-specific indicator of disease; various other appearances, including lobar infiltrate, occur.

Arterial oxygen tension measurement: hypoxia commonly occurs.

Exercise oximetry: a useful noninvasive test.

Sputum analysis: obviates need for routine bronchoscopy if laboratory is experienced; sputum induced by inhaled nebulized hypertonic saline solution; samples stained by Grocott and immunofluorescent stains.

Fiberoptic bronchoscopy: reserved for patients whose induced sputum test results are not diagnostic.

Complications

Pneumothorax.

Restrictive lung disease.

Extrapulmonic *Pneumocystis carinii* infection.

Adult respiratory distress syndrome.

Differential diagnosis

Bacterial pneumonia.

Pulmonary Kaposi's sarcoma.

Pulmonary tuberculosis.

Toxoplasmosis.

Pulmonary lymphoma.

Symptomatic anemia.

Asthma.

Cytomegalovirus pneumonitis.

Lipid interstitial pneumonitis.

Histoplasmosis.

Aspergillosis.

Etiology

• The pneumonia is caused by infection by *Pneumocystis carinii* (possibly a fungus or protozoan).

• Acquisition may be common early in life (and controlled by the immune system) or occur shortly before the disease develops.

Epidemiology

• Most children have serological evidence of previous *Pneumocystis carinii* infection by the age of 4 years; the disease was first recognized because of epidemics in orphanages after World War II.

• The disease is the most common AIDS opportunistic infection in people with HIV-induced immunosuppression, with no difference between genders or among races, although it occurs significantly less often in many developing countries.

Treatment

Diet and lifestyle

Not applicable.

Pharmacological treatment

Treatment of the disease

• Most treatment is based on inhibition of folic acid metabolism.

• The most effective agent is trimethoprim/sulfamethoxazole (TMP/SMX); in less severely ill patients, oral treatment may be used.

• Unfortunately, up to 40% of patients fail to complete a treatment course because of allergic or toxic side effects.

• Alternative treatment includes atovoquone, clindamycin and primaquine, trimethoprim and dapsone or pentamidine either i.v. or inhaled. The choice of therapy depends upon the severity of illness.

• Corticosteroids have been shown to reduce mortality and the risk of respiratory failure in patients presenting with partial arterial oxygen pressure <8 kPa. The subsequent use of antiretrovirals has been shown to improve survival.

Standard dosage	TMP/SMX, 15 mg/kg i.v. every 6 hours.
Contraindications	Hypersensitivity.
Special points	Full blood count, U&E monitoring, and liver function tests must be done.
Main drug interactions	None.
Main side effects	Nausea and vomiting (antiemetic can be given), skin rash, leukopenia, thrombocytopenia, raised liver function tests.

Prophylaxis

• Primary prophylaxis is recommended in patients with clinical evidence of immunosuppression (*e.g.*, buccal candidiasis) or other opportunistic infections or laboratory evidence (CD4 count $<200 \times 10^6$/L).

• Secondary prophylaxis should be offered to patients who have had previous episodes of *Pneumocystis carinii* pneumonia.

Standard dosage	TMP/SMX, 1 tablet daily. Alternatively, dapsone, 100 mg daily, or pentamidine, 300 mg inhaled every month.
Contraindications	Allergy to sulfonamides or trimethoprim.
Special points	Cotrimoxazole may also reduce the incidence of subsequent toxoplasmosis and bacterial infection.
Main drug interactions	None.
Main side effects	Skin rash, nausea and vomiting, leukopenia, thrombocytopenia, raised liver function tests.

Treatment aims

To treat pneumonia.

To return patient's quality of life.

To suppress future infection.

Prognosis

• Mortality for the first episode of *Pneumocystis carinii* pneumonia is <10% but is higher for subsequent attacks.

Follow-up and management

• Full blood count should be done after treatment because anemia is common.

• Patients should be followed up at least monthly.

General references

Masur H: Prevention and treatment of *Pneumocystis* pneumonia. *N Engl J Med* 1992, **327**:1853–1860.

Miller RF, Mitchell DM: AIDS and the lung: update 1992. 1. *Pneumocystis carinii* pneumonia. *Thorax* 1992, **47**:305–314.

Moe AA, Hardy WD: *Pneumocystis carinii* infection in the HIV-seropositive patient. *Infect Dis Clin North Am* 1994, **8**:331–364.

Diagnosis

Symptoms

Common

• Onset may be abrupt or over days.

Cough: with sputum, which may be purulent, in two-thirds of patients.

Fever: possibly with rigors and diaphoresis.

Pleuritic chest pain.

Dyspnea.

Less common

Hemoptysis, vomiting, diarrhea, myalgia.

Mental confusion: especially in patients with severe pneumonia and in elderly patients.

Signs

Pyrexia.

Mental confusion, cyanosis, hypotension: suggesting severe illness.

Raised respiratory rate: suggesting severe illness.

Dullness on percussion.

Increased vocal fremitus.

Crackles.

Bronchial breathing: egobronchophony and whispering pectoriloquy; in one-third of patients.

Investigations [1]

To confirm diagnosis

Chest radiography: shows consolidation or infiltrates.

To assess severity

Arterial blood gas analysis: low partial oxygen pressure, raised partial carbon dioxide pressure, low pH.

Full blood count: leukocyte count <4 or >20 × 10^9/L indicates high risk.

To assess cause

Blood culture: for bacteremia.

Sputum Gram stain and culture.

Pleural-fluid Gram stain and culture: if fluid present.

Serology: acute and convalescent sera for antibodies to viruses, chlamydia, mycoplasma, *Coxiella* spp., and legionella.

Bronchoscopy: for lower respiratory secretions; often needed in immunocompromised patients but rarely in others.

Complications

Empyema, lung abscess, pulmonary embolus, adult respiratory distress syndrome.

Acute renal failure, hemolysis.

Sepsis.

Differential diagnosis

Pulmonary edema.

Exacerbation of chronic bronchitis.

Pulmonary embolus.

Lung cancer.

Etiology [2,3]

• Pneumococcal infection is the cause of 50%–80% of community-acquired pneumonias.

• Gram-negative organisms (*e.g.*, *Escherichia coli* and *Pseudomonas* spp.) are the cause of 50% or more of nosocomial pneumonias.

• Anaerobic bacteria (*e.g.*, bacteroides) are important in aspiration pneumonia.

• Immunocompromised patients may be infected by a huge range of microorganisms, *e.g.*, unusual bacteria and fungi, many of which would not cause infection in immunocompetent patients.

Epidemiology

• Pneumonia occurs at all ages but is most frequent in very young and very old patients.

• Primary care physicians see on average 10 cases annually.

• One patient in every five seen needs hospital admission.

• Most cases occur in the winter months.

• Mycoplasma infection affects mainly teenagers and young adults.

• Legionella infection may occur in epidemics related to water systems in buildings.

• Psittacosis is often acquired from birds, especially parrots.

• Q fever is usually acquired from sheep.

Classification

Community-acquired pneumonia.

Nosocomial pneumonia.

Aspiration pneumonia: caused by inhalation of oropharyngeal secretions, during vomiting, or when consciousness is depressed.

Immunocompromised pneumonia: *e.g.*, with HIV infection, organ transplantation, cytotoxic chemotherapy.

Treatment

Diet and lifestyle

• Smoking and smoking-related diseases are a major risk factor for pneumonia; smoking education is therefore important.

Pharmacological treatment [4,5]

General guidelines

Oxygen: to maintain partial oxygen pressure in arterial blood >60 mm Hg; may cause hypercapnia in patients with chronic obstructive pulmonary disease, so arterial blood gases should be monitored.

Oral or parenteral fluids: to correct dehydration.

Nonsedative analgesia: for pleuritic chest pain.

Physical therapy: only if large sputum volumes are difficult to expectorate.

Intensive care, including assisted ventilation: valuable for patients in whom respiratory failure worsens despite treatment.

Antibiotics

• Initial treatment must be empirical; this can be modified later if indicated by microbiological results.

• Oral antibiotics are appropriate in mild infection, parenteral if infection is severe or accompanied by vomiting.

• Treatment should be for at least 7 days; severely ill patients need treatment for up to 3 weeks.

For mild community-acquired disease: azithromycin, penicillin, cephalosporin, or erythromycin.

For severe community-acquired disease: 2nd or 3rd generation cephalosporin (*e.g.*, cefuroxime), possibly with erythromycin.

For nosocomial infection: 2nd or 3rd generation cephalosporin, possibly with aminoglycoside; usually requires 2–3 weeks of therapy.

For aspiration: amoxicillin-clavulanate or clindamycin.

For immunocompromised disease: individually determined by causative pathogen.

Standard dosage	Amoxicillin, 500 mg 3 times daily. Erythromycin, 500 mg 4 times daily. Cefuroxime, 750 mg 3 times daily. Aminoglycoside guided by blood level. Clindamycin, 300 mg 3 times daily.
Contraindications	Hypersensitivity.
Main drug interactions	Warfarin.
Main side effects	Diarrhea.

Prophylaxis

Annual influenza vaccination: for patients over age 65 or those with chronic heart or lung disease, renal failure, or diabetes mellitus and for immunosuppressed patients.

Pneumococcal vaccination: for patients who are over 65 years old; asplenic; or have sickle cell disease, chronic renal failure, or chronic lung, heart, or liver disease; and those with diabetes mellitus or who are immunocompromised.

Treatment aims

To improve oxygenation.

To achieve rapid resolution of pneumonia and return to normal activities.

To prevent death or sepsis.

To relieve symptoms.

Prognosis

• Pyrexia usually settles within 48 h of starting treatment.

• Lethargy after pneumonia often lasts weeks or months.

• Radiographic shadowing is slow to clear and lags behind clinical recovery.

• Death is unusual in patients managed at home.

• 5%–10% of patients admitted to hospital die.

• Up to 50% reaching intensive care die.

• The mortality in nosocomial pneumonia is up to 30% and may be higher in immunocompromised patients.

Follow-up and management

• Patients should be seen 6 weeks after presentation, and chest radiography repeated to confirm recovery and exclude underlying lung disease, especially lung cancer.

Key references

1. Fine M, Smith D, Singer D: Hospitalization decision in patients with community-acquired pneumonia: a prospective study. *Am J Med* 1990, **89**:713–721.
2. Fang G, *et al.*: New and emerging etiologies for community-acquired pneumonia with implications for therapy. A prospective multicenter study of 359 cases. *Medicine* 1990, **69**:307–316.
3. Farr B, *et al.*: Prediction of microbial aetiology at admission to hospital for pneumonia from the presenting clinical features. *Thorax* 1989, **44**:1031–1035.
4. Niederman MS, *et al.*: American Thoracic Society guidelines for the initial management of adults with community-acquired pneumonia: diagnosis, assessment of severity, and initial antimicrobial therapy. *Am Rev Respir Dis* 1993, **148**:1418–1426.
5. Fein A, *et al.*: When the pneumonia doesn't get better. *Clin Chest Med* 1987, **8**:529–541.

Polycystic kidney disease, autosomal-dominant

Diagnosis

Definition

• Autosomal-dominant polycystic kidney disease is a subset of renal cystic disorders in which cysts are distributed throughout the cortex and medulla of both kidneys, and the kidneys are enlarged.

Symptoms and signs

• Although the process is usually not clinically apparent until the third or fourth decade, it has been found in infants and aborted fetuses, and all carriers show evidence of disease by the eighth or ninth decade.

Abdominal pain.

Hematuria.

Polyuria or nocturia.

Hypertension.

Abdominal distension.

Nephromegaly.

Investigations

Palpation: very enlarged cystic kidneys are easily palpable.

CT: most sensitive; shows multiple cysts in kidneys and occasionally in liver, pancreas, and spleen.

Ultrasonography: only cysts >1 cm are detectable.

Intravenous urography: shows stretched calyces.

Radioisotope scanning: shows multiple cystic defects in isotope image.

Complications

Chronic renal failure.

Hypertension: in 50% of patients.

Cyst rupture: pain, hematuria, and intrarenal hemorrhage.

Nephrolithiasis and nephrocalcinosis: in 10%–18% of patients.

Infection: within renal cysts or above obstructed ureter (gallium scan useful).

Malignant tumors: occasional.

Obstruction: clot or stone (acute on chronic renal failure).

Polycythemia: occasionally.

Distal renal tubular acidosis.

Differential diagnosis

Autosomal-recessive polycystic kidney disease.

Tuberous sclerosis.

Cystic dysplasia of kidneys.

Benign noninherited cysts.

Etiology

Genetics

• The disease is autosomal dominant, with almost complete penetrance and variable expression.

• The spontaneous mutation rate is relatively high (20% no family history).

• 85% of cases are linked to abnormal gene on chromosome 16 (ADPKD1 locus).

Pathogenesis

• The disease probably begins *in utero*.

• Cysts are formed from proximal or distal tubules, only 1% of which are affected.

• Renal damage is caused by compression of normal kidney tissue.

Epidemiology

• The autosomal-dominant form is the most common polycystic kidney disease.

• Affects 1 in 1000 world wide.

• The male:female ratio is equal.

• 10% of patients on dialysis suffer from the disease.

Associated extrarenal conditions

Aneurysms: berry, intracranial, abdominal aortic, dissecting thoracic, aortic root, and annulus aneurysms; 6% of patients with subarachnoid hemorrhage have autosomal dominant polycystic kidney disease; 10%–36% of patients with autosomal dominant polycystic kidney disease have intracranial aneurysms.

Liver cysts (in 20%–50% of patients): can cause obstructive jaundice and portal hypertension (rare); do not communicate with biliary tree; occasionally origin of cholangiocarcinoma.

Pancreatic cysts (in 5%–10%).

Cysts in other organs: ovary, uterus, spleen, thyroid, seminal vesicles, epididymis.

Valvular heart lesions: mitral incompetence, mitral valve prolapse (in 30%), tricuspid incompetence, pulmonary valve incompetence.

Diverticulosis (in 80%).

Hernia.

Treatment

Diet and lifestyle

• No special precautions are necessary in most patients; some are unusually susceptible to physical trauma.

• Genetic counseling should be offered.

Pharmacological treatment

• No specific treatment is available for the disorder, but the following can be considered:

Bed rest and analgesia for pain when bleeding occurs.

Blood pressure control.

Treatment of acidosis if present.

Treatment of renal failure when needed.

Prolonged antibiotic treatment for upper urinary tract infection.

Nonpharmacological treatment

• Hemodialysis and peritoneal dialysis are both suitable in patients with autosomal-dominant polycystic kidney disease.

• Polycythemia and repeated clotting of fistulas occasionally occurs in the hemodialysis group.

• Survival rate for these patients on dialysis is better than for patients with other renal diseases.

• Infection after renal transplantation is common; patients may require nephrectomy.

See Dialysis *and* Renal transplantation *for details.*

Treatment aims

To treat complications as they arise.

To control blood pressure.

To prepare patient for renal replacement therapy.

Prognosis

• 50% of patients progress to end-stage renal failure by the age of 75 years.

Follow-up and management

• Annual monitoring of blood pressure and renal function is needed (more frequently in patients with impaired renal function) because when or whether renal failure will develop in an individual patient generally cannot be predicted.

General references

Chapman AB, Rubinstein D, Hughes R: Intracranial aneurysms in autosomal dominant polycystic kidney disease. *N Engl J Med* 1992, **327**:916–920.

Gabow PA: Autosomal dominant kidney polycystic kidney disease—more than a renal disease. *Am J Kidney Dis* 1990, **16**:403–413.

Gabow PA: Autosomal dominant polycystic kidney disease. *N Engl J Med* 1993, **329**:332–342.

Gabow PA: Polycystic kidney disease: clues to pathogenesis. *Kidney Int* 1991, **40**:989–996.

Milutinovic J, Rust PF, Fialkow PJ: Intrafamilial phenotypic expression of autosomal dominant polycystic kidney disease. *Am J Kidney Dis* 1992, **19**:465–472.

Diagnosis

Symptoms

Heavy menstruation, oligomenorrhea or amenorrhea: endometrium remains estrogenized, in contrast with other causes of anovulation.

Infertility: anovulatory.

Recurrent miscarriage: associated with hypersecretion of luteinizing hormone.

Mild androgenism: hirsutism, acne, seborrhea [1].

Severe virilization: alopecia, voice change, clitoromegaly.

Signs

• The syndrome associated with polycystic ovaries is extremely variable; in most women with polycystic ovaries, the endocrine disturbance is subtle and the disorder has no outward signs.

Obesity.

Central adiposity.

Mild hypertension.

Hirsutism: documented by photography or Ferriman–Gallway score [1].

Acanthosis nigricans and pseudoacromegaly: features of severe insulin resistance.

• Abdominal and pelvic examinations are rarely helpful but should be done to exclude ovarian masses.

Investigations [2,3]

• The aims are to make a positive diagnosis, to exclude other causes of anovulation, infertility, recurrent miscarriage and virilization as appropriate, and to screen for features of insulin resistance (syndrome X).

• Diagnosis of polycystic ovarian disease should incorporate both an endocrine and a morphological assessment.

For the disorder [1]

Endocrine tests: nonraised follicle-stimulating hormone (<10 IU/L; all patients); raised luteinizing hormone (>10 IU/L; <30% on single sample); positive progestogen challenge.

Transvaginal ovarian ultrasonography: increased follicularity with expanded stromal compartment.

For other causes

Ultrasonography: to examine endometrium, possibly with endometrial biopsy (menstrual disorder); to diagnose small intraovarian tumors (virilization).

Full blood count: to rule out anemia (menstrual disorder).

Serum testosterone measurement: tumor more likely if concentration >2 ng/mL (virilization).

Serum ferritin measurement: low concentration contributes to alopecia (virilization).

For features of insulin resistance (risk factors for cardiovascular disease)

Blood pressure measurement.

Glucose tolerance test: especially during pregnancy and sex-steroid therapy.

Serum lipid measurement.

Complications

Endometrial cancer: despite anovulation, ovaries continue to secrete estradiol.

Diabetes mellitus, myocardial infarction, stroke: related to insulin resistance [4].

Differential diagnosis

Classic syndrome

Hypothyroidism.

Cushing's syndrome.

Acromegaly.

Androgen-secreting tumor.

Estrogenized amenorrhea

Granulosa cell tumor.

Etiology [3]

• Causes include the following:

Insulin receptor dysfunction.

Adrenal hyperandrogenemia.

Epidemiology [3]

• 10%–20% of apparently normal women are found to have polycystic ovaries on ultrasonography.

• 1% of young women (15–40 years) have clinically evident disease.

• Family studies show the prevalence of polycystic ovaries to be high among asymptomatic close relatives (80%).

• 50%–60% of women with anovulation are found to have polycystic ovaries on ultrasonography (30% in amenorrhea, 90% in oligomenorrhea).

• The disease is a factor in ~10% of couples with infertility and ~50% of cases of recurrent abortion.

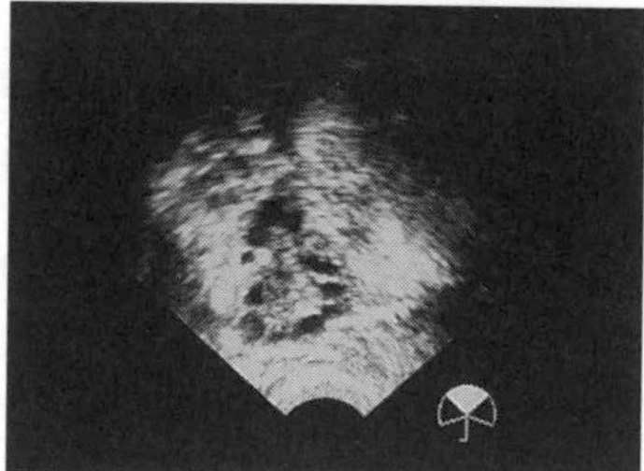

Transvaginal ultrasound scan of polycystic ovary showing multiple small follicles and echodense stroma.

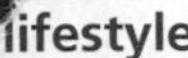

...t

...lifestyle

...e increased risk of cardiovascular disease, advice should be given about diet, ...xercise.

...estricted diet may help by improving ovarian function.

...ith oligo- or amenorrhea not wishing to conceive should be warned of the ...of conception.

Pharmacological treatment [3,5]

- Pregnancy must be ruled out before treatment begins.

For menstrual disorder

Combined oral contraceptive to improve regularity or reduce flow.

Cyclical progestogen or combined oral contraceptive to prevent endometrial neoplasia in women with oligo- or amenorrhea.

- Treatment is contraindicated in patients with undiagnosed abnormal menstruation.

For anovulatory infertility

- Each treatment should be tried in turn, starting with the simplest.
- After ovulation has been established, an adequate trial of treatment is needed (9 months).

Antiestrogen treatment (clomiphene): acts through the hypothalamus.

Laparoscopic ovarian surgery.

Exogenous gonadotropin treatment involves direct ovarian stimulation with human menopausal gonadotropin (hMG) or human follicle-stimulating hormone (hFSH), with human chorionic gonadotropin (hCG) to trigger ovulation.

Standard dosage *Antiestrogen:* clomiphene, 100 mg orally daily on days 2–6 of cycle for up to 3 cycles.
Exogenous gonadotropin: hMG or hFSH, 75 units s.c. daily.

Contraindications Pregnancy, hormone-dependent tumors, undiagnosed abnormal menstruation.

Special points *Antiestrogen:* near-normal conception rates expected; low risk of high-order multiple pregnancy (8% twin rate) and ovarian hyperstimulation; minimal monitoring needed (midluteal serum progesterone measurement).
Gonadotropin: risk of multiple pregnancy and ovarian hyperstimulation; detailed monitoring mandatory (serial follicle scanning and estradiol measurement); no clear benefit of pure hFSH over hMG.

Main drug interactions None.

Main side effects *Antiestrogen:* hot flushes, mild abdominal discomfort, visual disturbance (rare).
Gonadotropin: nausea, abdominal discomfort, allergy.

For recurrent miscarriage

Luteinizing hormone–releasing hormone agonist, with superovulation (hMG/hCG); risks of multiple pregnancy and ovarian hyperstimulation.

Laparoscopic ovarian surgery.

For virilization

Combined oral contraceptive: reduces libido; liver function must be checked; feminization of male fetus.

Flutamide: gastric upset common; possible feminization of male fetus.

Cimetidine: modest effect only.

Low-dose nocturnal corticosteroids: relatively ineffective, promote weight gain.

Spironolactone.

Ferrous sulfate: may improve alopecia if ferritin level is low.

Treatment aims

To prevent long-term health risks (syndrome X).

To alleviate symptoms.

To restore fertility.

Other treatments

Shaving, bleaching, electrolysis: for hirsutism.

Laparoscopic ovarian surgery: electrodiathermy or laser drilling; 80% ovulation rate; near-normal conception rate; normal twin rate and low miscarriage rate; effect lasts about 9 months on average.

Prognosis

- Acne and seborrhea respond within a few weeks, but the duration of the hair cycle means that improvement in hair growth may take many months.
- Symptoms generally return quickly after withdrawal of treatment.

Follow-up and management

- Follow up varies according to the disorder.

Key references

1. Fox R, *et al.*: Oestrogen and androgen states in oligo-amenorrhoeic women with polycystic ovaries. *Br J Obstet Gynaecol* 1991, **98**:294–299.
2. Fox R, *et al.*: Polycystic ovarian disease: diagnostic methods. *Contemp Rev Obstet Gynaecol* 1992, **4**:84–89.
3. Frank S: Polycystic ovary syndrome. *N Engl J Med* 1995, **333**:853–861.
4. Conway GS, *et al.*: Risk factors for coronary artery disease in lean and obese women with polycystic ovary syndrome. *Clin Endocrinol* 1992, **37**:119–125.
5. Jacobs HS: Polycystic ovary syndrome: aetiology and management. *Curr Opin Obstet Gynecol* 1995, **7**:203–208.

Diagnosis

Symptoms

Polymyalgia rheumatica

Pain and stiffness: bilateral and symmetrical, affecting neck, shoulder, and pelvic girdles; stiffness usually predominant, particularly severe after rest, and may prevent patient getting out of bed [1].

Giant-cell arteritis

Headache: in two-thirds or more of patients; severe pain, usually localized in the temple but may be occipital or be less defined and precipitated by brushing the hair [2,3].

Pain on chewing: due to claudication of muscles of mastication, in up to two-thirds of patients.

Visual disturbances: in 25%; visual loss evident in <10%.

Signs

Polymyalgia rheumatica

Unimpaired muscle strength: although pain makes interpretation of muscle testing difficult.

Tenderness of involved structures: with restriction of shoulder movement, if diagnosis delayed [1].

Peripheral synovitis: uncommon and transient.

Giant-cell arteritis

Scalp tenderness: particularly around temporal and occipital arteries; may disturb sleep [2].

Thickened, tender, and nodular arteries: with absent or reduced pulsation.

Partial or complete visual loss: due to anterior ischemic optic neuropathy [2,3].

Investigations

Baseline clinical investigations

- These are used to make the diagnosis and exclude other diagnoses.

ESR measurement: rate usually greatly raised, but can be normal [4].

Acute-phase protein (*e.g.*, CRP) measurement: concentration usually raised.

Full blood count.

Biochemical profile.

Rheumatoid factor test.

Serum protein electrophoresis (SPEP).

Thyroid function test.

Chest radiography.

Specific investigations

Temporal artery biopsy: for suspected giant-cell arteritis, not for polymyalgia rheumatica; findings can be focal, may be normal [2].

Complications

Visual loss: in up to 10% of patients, permanent blindness in giant-cell arteritis [5].

Differential diagnosis

Neoplastic disease.

Joint disease: osteoarthritis (particularly of cervical spine), rheumatoid arthritis, connective tissue disease.

Multiple myeloma.

Leukemia.

Lymphoma.

Muscle disease: polymyositis, myopathy.

Infections: *e.g.*, bacterial endocarditis.

Bone disease: particularly osteomyelitis.

Hypothyroidism.

Parkinsonism.

Depression.

Etiology

- A distinct prodromal event is often noted, resembling influenza, although viral studies are negative.
- HLA-DR4 is increased in both polymyalgia rheumatica and giant-cell arteritis.
- Lymphocytes in arteritic lesions express the T-cell phenotype, and the CD4+ subset predominates.

Epidemiology

- The peak age is 60–75 years.
- The female : male ratio is 3 : 1.
- The annual incidence of biopsy-positive disease is 6.7 in 100 000 people (16.8 in 100 000 >55years).
- The disease occurs predominantly in northern Europe and northern United States.

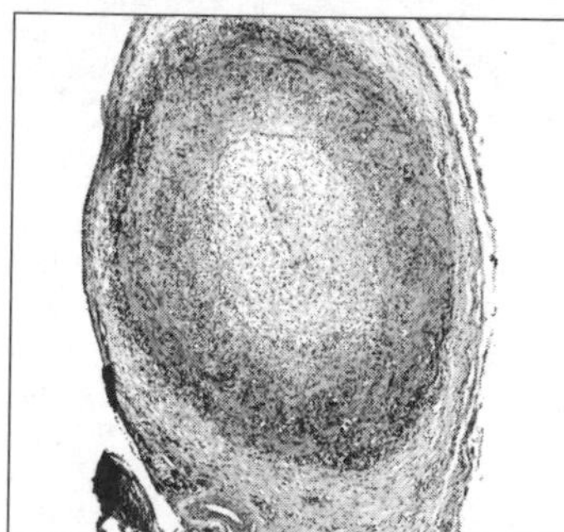

Occlusion of lumen due to intimal proliferation and inflammation of the media.

Treatment

Diet and lifestyle

• No special precautions are necessary.

Pharmacological treatment

• Patients with giant-cell arteritis should be referred as an emergency to a specialist to arrange a biopsy and to initiate treatment.

• Treatment by a systemic corticosteroid has long been recognized as mandatory in patients with giant-cell arteritis in order to prevent serious vascular complications, particularly blindness.

• Corticosteroids are usually also needed for patients with polymyalgia rheumatica.

• Many patients remain on treatment for years.

For polymyalgia rheumatica

Standard dosage	Prednisolone, 10–20 mg initially for 1 month, reduced by 2.5 mg every 2 weeks to 10 mg daily, then 1 mg daily every 2–4 weeks; maintenance dose 5–7 mg daily for 6–12 months; final reduction, 1 mg every 4 weeks [6].
Contraindications	Systemic infections; caution in pregnancy, hypertension, diabetes mellitus, osteoporosis, glaucoma, epilepsy, peptic ulceration.
Special points	In patients whose prednisolone dosage cannot be reduced because of recurring symptoms or who develop serious steroid-related side effects, azathioprine has been shown to have a modest steroid-sparing effect, and methotrexate may be more effective [7].
Main drug interactions	Rifampin and phenytoin reduce corticosteroid concentrations; anticoagulant dosage may need adjustment; reduced effect of NSAIDs.
Main side effects	Weight gain, edema, increased intraocular pressure, cataracts, glaucoma, gastrointestinal disturbances, peptic ulceration, diabetes, osteoporosis, skin atrophy [8].

For giant-cell arteritis without visual symptoms

Prednisolone, 40–60 mg daily initially for 8 weeks, reduced by 5 mg every 2 weeks to 10 mg daily; then as for polymyalgia rheumatica [9].

For giant-cell arteritis with possible or definite ocular involvement

Prednisolone, 60–80 mg daily initially for 8 weeks, reduced to 20 mg daily over next 4 weeks; then as for uncomplicated giant-cell arteritis [9].

Treatment aims

To relieve pain and symptoms.

To reduce the incidence of complications.

Prognosis

• Untreated, patients have prolonged ill health, and up to 20% of those with giant-cell arteritis go blind or develop vascular complications.

• Treated, between one-third and one-half of patients can discontinue treatment after 2 years.

Follow-up and management

• Treatment is monitored clinically and by acute-phase response (ESR, CRP).

• Long-term low-dose maintenance prednisolone ≤3 mg, is sometimes needed.

Key references

1. Lestico MR, *et al.*: Polymyalgia rheumatica. *Clin Pharmacol* 1993, **12**:571–580.
2. Chmelewski WL, *et al.*: Presenting features and outcomes in patients undergoing temporal artery biopsy: a review of 98 patients. *Arch Intern Med* 1992, **152**:1690–1695.
3. Reech KA, *et al.*: Neurologic manifestations of giant cell arteritis. *Am J Med* 1990, **89**:67–72.
4. Kyle V, Cawston TE, Hazleman BL: Erythrocyte sedimentation rate and c reactive protein in the assessment of polymyalgia rheumatica/giant cell arteritis on presentation and during follow-up. *Ann Rheum Dis* 1989, **48**:667–671.
5. Wilke WS, Hoffman GS: Treatment of corticosteroid resistant giant cell arteritis. *Rheum Dis Clin North Am* 1995, **21**:59–71.
6. Kyle V, Hazleman BL: Treatment of polymyalgia rheumatica and giant cell arteritis. I. Steroid regimens in the first two months. *Ann Rheum Dis* 1989, **48**:658–661.
7. Krall PL, Mazanec DJ, Wilke WS: Methotrexate for corticosteroid-resistant polymyalgia rheumatica and giant-cell arteritis. Cleve *Clin J Med* 1989, **56**:253–277.
8. Kyle V, Hazleman BL: Treatment of polymyalgia rheumatica and giant cell arteritis. II. Relation between steroid dose and steroid associated side effects. *Ann Rheum Dis* 1989, **48**:662–666.
9. Behn AR, Perera T, Myles AB: Polymyalgia rheumatica and corticosteroids: how much for how long? *Ann Rheum Dis* 1983, **42**:374–378.

Diagnosis

Symptoms

Weakness of proximal limb muscles: evolving over weeks or months, with difficulty in lifting, running, climbing stairs, getting up from a squatting position or low chair.

Dysphagia: due to weakness of pharyngeal muscles.

Muscle pain and tenderness, fleeting arthralgia, inability to raise head, Raynaud's phenomenon, dyspnea and cough.

Signs

Weakness of neck flexors and proximal limb muscles, with retained, hyperactive, or absent tendon reflexes: muscle wasting minimal or absent in early stages.

Investigations [1]

General

Full blood count, autoantibody screen, thyroid function tests: to identify overlap myositis and autoimmune thyroid disease.

Chest radiography, pulmonary function tests, ventilation perfusion studies: in patients with respiratory-muscle involvement or interstitial lung disease.

Video barium swallow: can be useful in patients with dysphagia.

ECG: to identify cardiac conduction defects and arrhythmias.

Special

Analysis of autoantibodies to aminoacyl transfer RNA synthetases: *e.g.*, Jo-1 antibody in patients with interstitial lung disease (positive in 70%).

Estimation of muscle creatine kinase activity in serum: activity usually increased 3–30-fold; serum creatine kinase concentration tends to reflect disease activity and is useful in monitoring treatment.

Needle electromyography: increased insertional activity with fibrillation potentials, positive sharp waves, and repetitive discharges; short and long duration, low amplitude, polyphasic motor unit action potentials.

Muscle biopsy: essential to establish diagnosis; samples from mildly to moderately affected proximal limb muscle (biceps or triceps brachii, vastus lateralis) that has not been needled for electromyography.

Light microscopy (cryostat sections): endomysial collections of inflammatory cells (lymphocytes, plasma cells, histiocytes) surrounding necrotic and nonnecrotic muscle fibers; regenerating muscle fibers with basophilic cytoplasm and prominent nucleoli; variable increase in endomysial connective tissue; necrotic fibers may be invaded by macrophages and lymphocytes.

Complications

Aspiration.

Interstitial lung disease.

Respiratory failure.

Raynaud's phenomenon: more common in dermatomyositis.

Cardiac conduction defects and dysrhythmias: rare.

Differential diagnosis

General

Dermatomyositis, paraneoplastic myositis.

Eosinophilic polymyositis.

Inclusion body myositis, sarcoid myopathy, mixed connective tissue disease, SLE, rheumatoid arthritis, Sjögren's syndrome, systemic sclerosis.

Myositides from other causes

HIV, influenza A and B virus, coxsackie virus, echovirus, adenovirus.

Spirochetes: *Borrelia burgdorferi* (Lyme disease).

Protozoa: toxoplasma.

Helminths: *Trichinella* spp., cysticerci.

Genetic disorders

Limb girdle dystrophies, late-onset nemaline myopathy, late-onset acid maltase deficiency, spinal muscular atrophy, lipid storage myopathies.

Drug-induced myopathies

Corticosteroids, penicillamine, lovastatin, cholestyramine, zidovudine, procainamide, chloroquine, colchicine, pancuronium with corticosteroids.

Other

Lambert–Eaton myasthenic syndrome.

Polymyalgia rheumatica.

Etiology

- The cause of idiopathic polymyositis is unknown; the increased incidence of HLA haplotype B8, DR3 suggests genetic susceptibility.

Epidemiology

- Idiopathic polymyositis affects all age groups but occurs most often in the 5th and 6th decades.
- The annual incidence is ~3 in one million population.
- It is slightly more common in women.

Pathogenesis

- Idiopathic polymyositis is a major histocompatibility complex class 1 restricted T-cell-mediated myotoxicity [2].
- $CD8^+$ cytotoxic T-lymphocytes expressing common alpha-beta receptor invade and destroy initially nonnecrotic muscle fibers.
- In a rare polymyositis variant, nonnecrotic fibers are invaded by $CD4^-$, $CD8^-$ T lymphocytes expressing the gamma-delta receptor, which interacts with heat-shock proteins.

Treatment

Diet and lifestyle

• Alcohol consumption should be restricted.

Pharmacological treatment [2]

First line

Standard dosage
Prednisone, 30–60 mg orally single daily dose for 4–6 weeks initially, tapered by 2.5–5 mg every 2–4 weeks depending on response and serum creatine kinase concentration to maintenance dose 10–15 mg daily.
Azathioprine, 25–50 mg orally daily initially, increased to 2.5–3 mg/kg daily over 4 weeks; maintenance 1–2 mg/kg daily.

Contraindications
Prednisone: caution in hypertension, peptic ulcer, diabetes mellitus, osteoporosis, glaucoma, psychosis, previous tuberculosis.
Azathioprine: rare hypersensitivity, pregnancy and breast feeding.

Special points
Prednisone: calcium and potassium supplements may be needed on long-term treatment.
Azathioprine: full blood count, platelet count, liver and renal function monitoring weekly for first 2 months, monthly for next 6 months, at least 3-monthly thereafter.

Main drug interactions
Prednisone: phenytoin, phenobarbital, oral anticoagulants, NSAIDs.
Azathioprine: allopurinol, neuromuscular blocking agents, cytostatics.

Main side effects
Prednisone: dyspepsia, peptic ulcer, weight gain, hypertension, cushingoid changes, potassium loss, glucose intolerance, cataract, osteoporosis, vertebral fractures, avascular osteonecrosis, euphoria, psychosis, muscle weakness.
Azathioprine: nausea, vomiting, diarrhea, bone-marrow suppression, disturbed liver function.

Second line

Pulsed methylprednisone, 0.5–1 g i.v. daily for 5 days.

Human immunoglobulin, 0.4 g/kg i.v. daily for 5 days [3,4].

Third line

• The following agents are indicated in refractory cases, usually with maintenance dose of oral steroids:

Methotrexate, 7.5–30 mg orally or 0.4–0.8 mg/kg i.v. weekly (adults).

Cyclophosphamide, 1–4 mg/kg orally daily.

Cyclosporin, 2–6 mg/kg orally daily (adults).

• All are contraindicated in hypersensitivity, pregnancy, and lactation.

• Monitoring of full blood count, platelet count, liver and kidney function is needed.

• Side effects include nausea, vomiting, diarrhea, alopecia, bone-marrow suppression, and hepatic and renal toxicity.

Treatment aims

To halt progression of disease and improve muscle strength.

Prognosis

• Remission is usually achieved and maintained in 50%–60% of patients with first-line treatment.

• Second-, third-, and fourth-line treatments have provided encouraging results in small uncontrolled trials, but their respective merits in cases refractory to first-line drugs have not yet been clearly established.

• Death is rarely due to muscle weakness and usually results from cardiopulmonary complications.

Follow-up and management

• Most patients need maintenance treatment for at least 1–2 years after remission has been achieved.

Key references

1. Dalakas MC: Clinical, immunopathologic, and therapeutic considerations of inflammatory myopathies. *Clin Neuropharmacol* 1992, **15**:327–351.
2. Hohlfeld R, Engel AG: The role of gamma-delta T-lymphocytes in inflammatory muscle disease. In *Heat Shock Proteins and Gamma-Delta T-cells*, vol 3. Edited by Brosnan CF. Basel: Karger; 1992:75–85.
3. Cherin P, *et al.*: Efficacy of intravenous gammaglobulin therapy in chronic refractory polymyositis and dermatomyositis: an open study with 20 adult patients. *Am J Med* 1991, **91**:162–168.
4. Soueidan SA, Dalakas MC: Treatment of inclusion-body myositis with high-dose intravenous immunoglobulin. *Neurology* 1993, **43**:876–879.

General reference

Mastaglia FL, Walton JN (eds): Inflammatory myopathies. In *Skeletal Muscle Pathology*. Edinburgh: Churchill Livingstone; 1992:453–491.

Diagnosis

Definition

• Postpartum mental illness is defined as a new episode of mental illness in a woman who has been well for at least the previous 6 months, with onset in the first 90 days post partum.

• The illness may be manifest later in the puerperium.

Symptoms and signs [1,2]

Puerperal psychosis (bipolar or manic-depressive psychosis)

• Onset is abrupt and occurs between days 3 and 16 in most women.

• Within a week, the picture settles to become clearly that of an acute severe affective psychosis.

Variable acute undifferentiated psychosis, with lucid intervals, perplexity, agitation, confusion: for first few days.

Hallucinations and delusions, emotional and behavioral disturbance, disrupted sleep and appetite.

Overactivity, elation, pressure of speech, flight of ideas: in one-third of patients.

Agitation, psychomotor retardation, self-neglect, depressive delusions about baby: in two-thirds; such patients may become catatonic and stop eating and drinking.

Severe depressive illness (unipolar depressive illness)

• Onset is early, with more gradual deterioration.

• One-third of patients, the most severely ill, verging on psychotic, present early (within first 6 weeks); two-thirds, those most likely to be missed, present later (between 10 and 20 weeks).

Disrupted sleep and early morning wakening, diurnal variation of mood.

Marked slowing of psychomotor functioning, impaired concentration, indecisiveness.

Prominent loss of pleasure and spontaneity: everything is an effort, particularly the baby.

Overvalued ideas or delusions of unworthiness, incompetence, and guilt.

Frequent intrusive, obsessional thoughts of failure as mother or harm coming to child.

See Depression and mania *for details.*

Investigations

• No special clinical investigation is needed beyond the normal physical postpartum investigations.

Complications

Delayed detection and treatment of severe mental illness, physical morbidity.

Suicide and infanticide: rare but tragic and often avoidable.

Prolonged morbidity.

Failure to establish relationship with child.

Removal of child by family or social services.

Lasting problems in child's social, emotional, and cognitive development and physical health.

Marital difficulties.

Differential diagnosis

The blues: tearfulness between days 3 and 5; spontaneous resolution within a few days.

Acute confusional state (delirium, organic brain syndrome): rare, caused by infection, eclampsia, or other neurological disorder.

Distress: caused by social, marital, or relationship problems.

• Severe depressive illness may follow major life stresses.

Etiology [3]

• Both biological and psychological factors are important.

• No current evidence suggests that the hormonal profile of mentally ill mothers differs from that of normal women; the postpartum drop to low progesterone concentrations is probably responsible for "the blues"; puerperal psychosis may be related to a predetermined hypersensitivity of dopamine receptors to the postpartum fall in estrogen.

• Manic depressive illness in a first-degree relative indicates a 1 in 3 risk for puerperal psychosis.

• Previous manic depressive illness (whether post partum or not) indicates a 1 in 2 risk after every delivery; previous postpartum depression indicates a 1 in 3 risk after subsequent deliveries; previous non-postpartum depression indicates a 1 in 5 risk or higher.

• Emergency cesarian section increases the risk of puerperal psychosis in primiparus women; infertility, assisted reproduction, previous obstetric loss, or traumatic delivery may contribute to severe depressive illness.

• Marital conflict, social adversity, lack of confidante, single status, and previous episode of depression all increase the risk of a mild depressive episode.

Epidemiology

• 10% of all women delivered suffer from postpartum mood changes.

• 3% of all women delivered suffer from a major depressive illness.

• 2 in 1000 women delivered are admitted to a psychiatric hospital suffering from a puerperal psychosis.

• Similar rates have been found in many cultures throughout the world.

Treatment

Diet and lifestyle

• No special precautions are necessary apart from providing social support while the patient is recovering.

Pharmacological treatment

• Women with puerperal psychosis or suffering from severe depression, with active suicidal ideation should be treated at an inpatient psychiatric unit.

• Most postnatal depressive illnesses can be managed at home if patient is not suicidal or infanticidal.

For puerperal psychosis

• The immediate priority is to sedate the patient with neuroleptics to a level that makes her safe, allows adequate nutrition, and reduces her agitation, confusion, and fear.

• Treatment often requires both antipsychotic and antidepressant medication.

Standard dosage Haloperidol, 5–20 mg daily orally for acute psychosis; alternatively risperidone. *See* Schizophrenia *for details.*

Contraindications *Neuroleptics:* hypersensitivity; caution in cardiovascular disease, hepatic impairment, epilepsy.

Special points If no response occurs within 7 days, electroconvulsive therapy or lithium carbonate can be tried (lithium serum concentration ~0.8–1.0 mg/L within 1 week; normal thyroid and renal function must be established first).
Neuroleptics: postpartum women are very sensitive to extrapyramidal side effects, so monitoring needed.
Tricyclic antidepressants: effect takes 10–14 days; should be started at same time as electroconvulsive therapy (may be sufficient alone for less severe illness).

Main drug interactions *Neuroleptics:* antagonize anticonvulsants.

Main side effects *Neuroleptics:* sedation, extrapyramidal effects, acute dystonias, akasthisia, parkinsonism.

For severe depressive illness

• Most women respond satisfactorily to antidepressants; 60% respond to tricyclic or selective serotonin reuptake inhibitor (SSRI) antidepressant.

• Excessive sedation should be avoided because of childcare responsibilities.

• Women should always be referred to a psychiatrist if they are severely distressed, in a state of hopeless despair, or suicidal.

See Depression and mania *for details.*

Drugs and breast feeding

• No psychotropic drug is of proven safety.

Treatment aims

To provide early detection and prompt treatment in the setting most appropriate for safe recovery.

To give priority to the needs of the baby.

To avoid unnecessary separation of mother and baby.

To provide social and psychological support.

Other treatments

• Psychosocial treatment includes:

Adjunctive psychotherapy and specific counseling for all patients.

Nondirective or cognitive therapy (6 sessions at weekly intervals) effective for mild depressive illness.

Practical social support and addressing of concurrent problems is essential.

• Psychosocial treatment is as effective as antidepressants for mild depressive illness.

Prognosis

• With early intervention and effective treatment, the prognosis is excellent; improvement beginning within 2 weeks and recovery within 6–8 weeks.

• Without treatment, the illness may be prolonged, although 60% of patients recover spontaneously within 6 months.

Follow-up and management

• Treatment should continue for at least 6 months after the patient has recovered, longer in the case of a relapse.

• Patients with previous manic-depressive episodes should take lithium.

The next baby

• For serious mental illness, the risk follows every childbirth.

Puerperal psychosis, 1 in 2 risk.

Postpartum depression, 1 in 3–5 risk.

Key references

1. Kumar R, *et al.*: Clinical survey of a psychiatric mother and baby unit: characteristics of 100 consecutive admissions. *J Affect Disord* 1995, **33**:11–22.
2. Wisner KL, Peindl K, Hanusa BH: Symptomatology of affective and psychotic illness related to childbearing. *J Affect Disord* 1994, **30**:77–87.
3. O'Hara MW: Social support, life events and depression during pregnancy and the puerperium. *Arch Gen Psychiatry* 1986, **43**:569–573.

Diagnosis

Symptoms

Symptoms of venous or arterial thrombosis.

Signs

• Patients to investigate include those with the following:

Venous thromboembolism before the age of 40–45 years.

Recurrent venous thrombosis or thrombophlebitis.

Thrombosis in an unusual site: *e.g.*, mesenteric vein, cerebral vein.

Unexplained neonatal thrombosis.

Skin necrosis.

Arterial thrombosis before the age of 30 years.

Relatives with a specific defect.

Unexplained prolonged coagulation screening tests.

Recurrent fetal loss, idiopathic thrombocytopenic purpura, SLE.

Investigations

• Functional and immunological assays are needed for a precise diagnosis.

• Screening tests and functional assays should be performed on fresh citrated blood samples collected with minimal venous stasis on all patients being investigated for a prothrombotic state.

Full blood count and film.

Measurement of prothrombin, activated partial thromboplastin, and thrombin time; fibrinogen.

Platelet aggregation studies.

Assays for antithrombin III, protein C, protein S, activated protein C resistance (factor V Leiden), plasminogen, heparin cofactor II, anticardiolipin antibodies, lupus anticoagulant, factor XII, dysfibrinogenemia, and homocystinuria.

Fibrinolytic tests: before and after stimulation (*i.e.*, venous occlusion or DDAVP).

Fibrin plate, tissue-type plasminogen activator, and PA1-1 assays.

Platelet activation markers analysis: *i.e.*, GMP-140 expression, plasma β-thromboglobulin.

Complications

Arterial and venous thrombosis and embolism.

Differential diagnosis

Hyperviscosity.

Etiology

Common acquired causes of thrombosis

Diabetes mellitus, hyperlipidemia, malignancy, myeloproliferative disorders, chronic liver disease, SLE, paraproteinemias, nephrotic syndrome.

• These disorders cause predisposition to thrombosis in a multifactorial way; specific homeostatic assays are generally unhelpful in the investigation and management of individual patients.

Inherited defects with increased tendency to thrombosis

Antithrombin III, protein C, protein S, factor V Leiden, plasminogen, heparin cofactor II, factor XII, dysfibrinogenemia, homocystinuria.

• Most of these disorders represent autosomal dominant traits with variable penetrance.

• Deficiency in the heterozygous state predisposes to thrombosis either spontaneously or in association with other high risk factors.

Pathophysiology

• The balance of the hemostatic mechanism can be shifted in favor of thrombosis in the following circumstances:

Increased coagulation system activity.

Increased platelet activity.

Decreased fibrinolytic activity.

Damaged vascular endothelial activity.

Epidemiology

• Epidemiological studies have shown an increased incidence of thrombotic events associated with raised concentrations particularly of fibrinogen, factor VII, and factor VIII:C, with a frequency of 1 in 2000–5000.

High risk factors for thrombosis

Surgical and nonsurgical trauma.

Age.

Immobilization.

Heart failure.

Prior venous thrombosis and varicose veins.

Paralysis of lower limbs.

Obesity.

Estrogen treatment.

Pregnancy and puerperium.

Smoking.

Raised blood viscosity.

Treatment

Diet and lifestyle

• No special precautions are necessary.

Pharmacological treatment

Prophylaxis for venous thromboembolism [1]

• The degree of risk must be assessed depending on the predisposing factors.

Low risk: early ambulation, graduated compression stocking.
Moderate risk: standard unfractionated heparin, 5000 units s.c. every 8–12 h.
High risk: low molecular weight heparin, s.c. every 12–24 h, dose depending on type of heparin.

• The degree of risk for surgical prophylaxis may be defined as follows:

Low risk: <40 years, minor surgery lasting <1 h.
Moderate risk: >40 years, abdominal or thoracic surgery lasting >1 h.
High risk: >40 years, knee and hip orthopedic surgery, obesity, and malignancy.

Heparin

Standard dosage Unfractionated heparin, 5000 units i.v. bolus, followed by 1000–2000 units/h i.v. for 5–7 days.
Low molecular weight heparin s.c. once daily [2].

Contraindications Rare hypersensitivity, risk of bleeding complications.

Special points Activated partial thromboplastin time must be monitored 6 h after start of treatment, then at least every 24 h, with dose adjustment to maintain ratio at 1.5–2.5 times control.

Main drug interactions Drugs that interfere with platelet aggregation or coagulation.

Main side effects Bleeding, thrombocytopenia, rebound thrombosis, osteoporosis (if treatment lasts >3 months), rare alopecia, skin rash.

• Heparinization can be reversed by administering protamine sulfate, 1 mg, which neutralizes ~100 units heparin; maximum dose, 40 mg i.v. in 10 min.

Warfarin [3]

Standard dosage Warfarin, 10 mg orally on days 1 and 2; 5 mg orally on day 3; then adjusted daily according to prothrombin time, maintained at 1–20 mg daily.

Contraindications Pregnancy.

Special points Prothrombin time must be monitored, with results expressed as INR with therapeutic range of 2.0–4.5.

Main drug interactions Many medications potentiate or antagonize effect; for any new medication, prothrombin time should be checked.

Main side effects Bleeding, skin necrosis after first few days of treatment in the case of protein C or S deficiency.

• Anticoagulant effects can be reversed by an infusion of fresh frozen plasma or factor II, IX, and X concentrate if bleed is life-threatening; vitamin K_1, 1–2 mg i.v., takes 6–24 h to reverse warfarin effect.

Antiplatelet agents

• These are indicated for prophylaxis and prevention of further arterial thrombotic events when platelet activation has been shown to be a primary pathological factor, particularly myocardial ischemia and cerebrovascular thrombotic strokes, including transient ischemic attack, for secondary thrombocytosis (>800 × 10^9/L), and for essential thrombocythemia.

Aspirin, 75 mg orally daily or 300 mg twice weekly, or dipyridamole, up to 100 mg orally 3 times daily (dipyridamole may cause severe headaches).

Treatment aims

To prevent thrombosis.

Prognosis

• Prognosis depends on the underlying cause and the degree of risk of arterial or venous thrombosis or embolism.

Follow-up and management

• Lifelong expert management is needed.

Therapeutic ranges for oral anticoagulation

INR 2.0–2.5: prophylaxis of deep-vein thrombosis.

INR 2.0–3.0: treatment of deep-vein thrombosis, pulmonary embolism, systemic embolism, prevention of venous thrombo-embolism in myocardial infarction, mitral stenosis with embolism, transient ischemic attacks, atrial fibrillation.

INR 3.0–4.5: recurrent deep-vein thrombosis and pulmonary embolism, arterial disease including myocardial infarction, mechanical prosthetic heart valves (tissue prosthetic values can be controlled at 2.0–3.0).

Key references

1. Lowe GDO: Risk of and prophylaxis for venous thromboembolism in hospital patients. *BMJ* 1992, **305**:567–574.
2. Hirsh J: Low molecular weight heparin. *Thromb Haemost* 1993, **70**:204–207.
3. Poller L: Oral anticoagulation. *J Clin Pathol* 1990, **43**:177–183.

Diagnosis

Symptoms

Pruritis: in 20% of patients.

Unpleasant odor: in severe cases.

Joint pain, tenderness, and morning stiffness: in cases with psoriatic arthritis.

Chills: secondary to loss of body heat in patients with generalized psoriasis.

Signs

Scalp

Scaling.

Skin

Psoriatic plaques: especially on extensor surfaces and areas of trauma; some patients have pustules (pustular psoriasis) [1].

Oral mucosa

Glossitis or geographic tongue: in 10% of patients.

Nails

• 50% of patients have nail involvement.

Pitting.

Subungual keratotic debris.

Onycholysis.

Discoloration: yellow-brown ("oil spots").

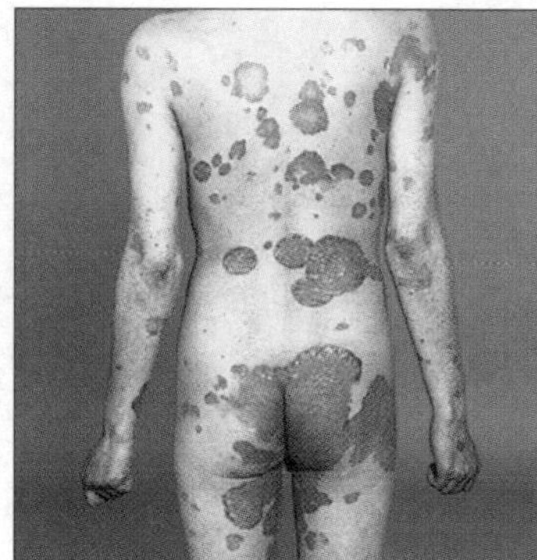

Chronic plaque psoriasis.

Musculoskeletal system

Sausage digits.

Periarticular swelling: especially small joints of fingers and toes.

Asymmetrical oligoarticular arthritis: most common.

Investigations

HIV test: if there is a history of sudden onset of severe psoriasis with no family history and no previous personal history [2].

Antistreptolysin O (ASO) titer: if guttate flare from recent streptococcal infection is suspected.

Complications

Exfoliative erythroderma.

Ankylosing spondylitis.

Psoriatic arthropathy.

Generalized pustular psoriasis: sheets of sterile pustules occurring in patients with psoriasis and associated fever, arthralgias, skin tenderness, and malaise.

Differential diagnosis

Lichen planus.

Tinea corporis.

Seborrheic dermatitis.

Reiter's disease.

Pityriasis rosea.

Secondary syphilis.

Subacute cutaneous lupus erythematosus.

Premycosis fungoides (parapsoriasis).

Drug reaction.

Atopic eczema: especially patients with advanced lichenification.

Etiology

•Psoriasis is a multifactorial disease with a definite genetic predisposition.

Positive family history in 30% of cases.

Histocompatibility antigen HLA-Cw6 strongly associated (relative risk of 24).

The presence of HLA-B17 or B27 is associated with more severe disease or associated arthritis.

•Although immunologic abnormalities of humoral and cell-mediated immunity have been described, no specific circulatory immune abnormalities have been identified.

•Epidermal transit time is rapidly increased (six- to ninefold).

Precipitating factors

Streptococcal infections.

Trauma: Koebner's phenomenon.

Drugs: beta-blockers, antimalarials, lithium, oral corticosteroid withdrawal.

Stress.

Sunlight: a small subset of patients actually worsen with sun exposure especially sunburn.

Alcoholism: may be related to decreased compliance in alcoholic patients.

Epidemiology

Incidence 1%–3% of world population [3].

Affects 2–8 million people in the US.

Peak onset is in the second decade of life, but it may appear at any age.

Treatment

Diet and lifestyle

- No specific precautions appear necessary.

Pharmacological treatment

- Cases of generalized pustular psoriasis of exfoliative erythroderma should be referred to a specialist immediately.

Topical treatment

Coal tar: safe and effective in plaque psoriasis; messy to apply (limiting compliance).

Steroids: effective and cosmetically acceptable; long-term use needs close supervision.

Vitamin D3 analogues: calcipotriene appears safe and effective in mild-to-moderate psoriasis; may be irritating [4].

Phototherapy: ultraviolet B useful for chronic plaque and guttate psoriasis, alone or with other treatments such as topical applications.

Systemic therapy

- Treatment should be given under supervision of a specialist [5].
- Methotrexate is used in widespread plaque, acute generalized pustular psoriasis, and erythrodermic psoriatic arthropathy as short-term or maintenance treatment.
- Retinoids are effective particularly in acral or generalized pustular psoriasis.
- Cyclosporin is effective for severe refractory psoriasis and psoriatic arthropathy.
- Long-term photochemotherapy (oral or topical psoralens with ultraviolet A) is complicated by increased risk of cutaneous squamous cell carcinoma.

Standard dosage This should be decided by a specialist who has experience with systemic therapy.

Contraindications History of previous hypersensitivity to drug.
Methotrexate: hepatic disease, alcohol abuse, malignancy [6].
Retinoids: hepatic and renal damage, pregnancy.
Cyclosporin: renal disease, uncontrolled hypertension, infection, malignancy.

Special points *Methotrexate*: pregnancy must be avoided.
Retinoids: pregnancy must be avoided during treatment and for up to 2 years afterwards.
Cyclosporin: sudden withdrawal may lead to relapse within a few weeks but not to the severe rebound seen with systemic steroids; monitoring should include blood pressure, serum creatinine, and glomerular filtration rate.

Main drug interactions *Methotrexate*: alcohol, salicylates, NSAIDs, probenecid, phenytoin, retinoids, pyrimethamine, furosemide.
Retinoids: reduce effect of warfarin.
Cyclosporin: NSAIDS may potentiate nephrotoxicity.
The following drugs increase cyclosporin levels (inhibit P450): diltiazem, danazol, ketoconazole, nicardipine, bromocriptine, fluconazole, verapamil, metoclopramide, itraconazole.

Main side effects *Methotrexate*: hepatic fibrosis (liver biopsy every 1.5 g cumulative dose), acute bone-marrow suppression.
Retinoids: raised serum lipids, elevated liver enzymes (abnormalities return to normal on cessation of treatment), spinal changes after prolonged treatment (diffuse idiopathic skeletal hyperostosis).
Cyclosporin: dose-related hypertension and nephrotoxicity (plasma creatinine should be monitored at baseline, then monthly).

Treatment aims

To control and prevent severe disease.

Prognosis

- Psoriasis is usually a chronic disease characterized by flares and remissions.

Follow-up and management

Individualized for each patient.

Key references

1. Zelickson BD, Muller SA: Generalized pustular psoriasis: a review of 63 cases. *Arch Dermatol* 1991, **127**:1339–1345.
2. Zalla MJ, Sue WP, Franesway AF: Dermatologist manifestations of human immunodeficiency virus infection. *Mayo Clin Proc* 1992, **67**:1089–1108.
3. Farber EM, Nall ML: The natural history of psoriasis in 5600 patients. *Dermatologica* 1974, **148**:1–18.
4. Highton A, Quell J: Calcipotreine ointment 0.005% for psoriasis: a safety and efficacy study. Calcipotreine study group. *J Am Acad Dermatol* 1995, **32**:67–72.
5. Greaves MW, Weinstein GD: Treatment of psoriasis. *N Engl J Med* 1995, **332**:581–588.
6. Petrazzuoli M, *et al*.: Monitoring patients taking methotrexate for hepatotoxicity: does the standard of care match published guidelines? *J Am Acad Dermatol* 1994, **31**:969–977.

Diagnosis

Symptoms

Precocious puberty

Pubertal development <8 years in girls, <9 years in boys.

Rapid growth.

Menstruation in girls.

Advanced skeletal maturation.

Behavioral disturbance.

Delayed puberty

Lack of pubertal development >14 years in girls, >15 years in boys.

Lack of pubertal growth spurt.

Small external genitalia in boys.

Possible anosmia.

Emotional disturbance, lack of confidence.

Signs

Precocious puberty

Secondary isosexual sexual development.

Tall stature.

Gynecomastia in boys.

Cutaneous pigmentation: McCune–Albright syndrome.

Acne, clitoromegaly: indicating virilization in girls.

Delayed puberty

Lack of secondary sexual development.

Short stature.

Signs of Turner's syndrome in girls.

Chronic pediatric illness: *e.g.*, Crohn's disease, thalassemia.

Family history of delayed puberty.

Investigations [1,2]

Precocious puberty

Hormone measurement: for gonadotropin and sex steroid concentrations.

CT of hypothalamic–pituitary region: to exclude structural lesion.

Ovarian ultrasonography: to assess ovarian development.

Adrenal CT: for gonadotropin-independent precocious puberty.

Delayed puberty

Full blood count, ESR and electrolytes analysis, liver function tests: to exclude chronic disease.

Hormone measurement: for gonadotropin and sex steroid concentrations.

Karyotyping: in girls.

Clomiphene test: in older patients, to exclude gonadotropin-releasing hormone deficiency.

Ovarian ultrasonography: to assess ovarian development.

Test of smell: to exclude Kallmann's syndrome.

CT of hypothalamic–pituitary region: to exclude structural lesion.

Complications

Precocious puberty

Progression of pubertal development.

Menstruation.

Advance of skeletal maturation.

Adult tall stature.

Delayed puberty

No secondary sexual development.

Absent pubertal growth.

Adult short stature.

Emotional, physical immaturity.

Psychological disturbance.

Infertility.

Differential diagnosis

Not applicable.

Etiology [1,2]

• Causes include the following:

True precocious puberty (gonadotropin-dependent)

Idiopathic (principally girls).
Structural lesions of hypothalamic region (tumors).
Postcranial irradiation.
Hydrocephalus.
Hypothyroidism.

Pseudoprecocious puberty (gonadotropin-independent)

McCune–Albright syndrome.
Adrenal tumors.
Congenital adrenal hyperplasia.
Gonadal tumors.
Human chorionic gonadotropin–secreting tumors.
Exogenous sex steroids.

Delayed puberty

Constitutional.
Chronic pediatric illness.
Malnutrition.
Hypopituitarism (idiopathic, tumors).
Isolated gonadotropin-releasing hormone deficiency and anosmia (Kallmann's syndrome).
Hyperprolactinemia.
Exercise (gymnasts).
Turner's or Klinefelter's syndromes.
Radiotherapy, surgery, chemotherapy, autoimmunity.

Epidemiology

• No data have been published.

Treatment

Diet and lifestyle

• No special precautions are necessary.

Pharmacological treatment [1,2]

For true precocious puberty

• Primary CNS lesions, *e.g.*, tumors, must be treated.

Gonadotropin-releasing hormone analogue fixed dose s.c. injection monthly or cyproterone acetate, 50–100 mg daily; treatment continued until appropriate age for puberty to progress.

• Long-term cyproterone treatment may induce adrenal insufficiency.

For pseudoprecocious puberty

• The primary cause or congenital adrenal hyperplasia must be treated.

Testolactone, up to 40 mg/kg/day for McCune–Albright syndrome.

For delayed puberty

• The primary cause must be treated, *e.g.*, chronic illness, pituitary tumor, hyperprolactinemia.

For boys: testosterone, from 50 mg every 2 weeks to 300 mg every 3 weeks i.m. depending on age.

For girls: ethinyl estradiol, 2–10 µg daily, increasing to 30 µg daily with norethindrome or medroxyprogesterone acetate, 5 mg daily on days 1–14 of each calendar month.

Treatment aims

To replace hormones.

Prognosis

• Prognosis is always good unless the disorder is caused by a tumor.

Follow-up and management

• Patients should be checked every 3–6 months to ensure that treatment is effective.

Key references

1. Bridges NA, Brook CDG: Premature sexual development. In *Clinical Endocrinology*. Edited by Grossman A. Oxford: Blackwell Scientific Publications; 1992:837–846.
2. Stanhope R, Albanese A, Shalet S: Delayed puberty. *BMJ* 1992, **305**:790.

Diagnosis

Symptoms

• Symptoms may be minimal.

Dyspnea, cough, sputum production, hemoptysis, chest pain, weight loss, fever.

• Hemoptysis with chest pain suggests Kaposi's sarcoma in those with AIDS but pneumonia in those with other forms of immunosuppression.

Signs

Tachypnea.

Cyanosis: indicating respiratory failure.

Consolidation: suggesting bacterial infection.

Collapse: suggesting infection or neoplasia.

Pleural effusion: suggesting mycobacterial infection or neoplasia.

Investigations

• The choice of investigation depends on the physical signs and symptoms and the degree of immunosuppression.

To assess degree of immunosuppression

Full blood count, differential leukocyte count: in patients with acquired immunosuppression, *e.g.*, to assess neutropenia, after organ transplantation.

Immunoglobulin measurement, CD4 count: in patients with acquired immunosuppression; normal CD4 count in early stages of HIV infection, bacterial infection common; low CD4 count in late stages of HIV infection, opportunistic infection or neoplasia more likely.

To assess pulmonary complications of immunosuppression

Chest radiography: to identify focal or generalized abnormality.

CT: to assess pulmonary abnormalities in more detail (*e.g.*, intrathoracic lymph nodes).

Oximetry or arterial blood gas measurement: at rest or exercise, essential for early detection of respiratory failure.

Sputum for special stains and cytology: in patients with nonproductive coughs, sputum may be induced by inhalation of 3% nebulized saline solution.

Bronchoscopy, bronchoalveolar lavage, transbronchial biopsy, open lung biopsy: for tissue diagnosis.

Mediastinoscopy: if mediastinal lymph-node disease has been identified.

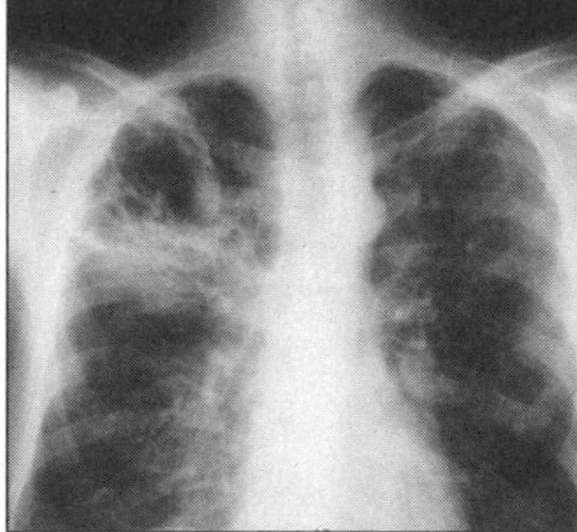

Chest radiograph showing cavitating aspergilloma.

Complications

Respiratory failure.

Disseminated infection.

Disseminated secondary malignancy.

Differential diagnosis

• The diagnosis depends on the course, stage, and degree of immunosuppression, in addition to local pathogenic load, which may differ in community, hospital, or geographical location.

Pneumocystis carinii pneumonia (*see Pneumocystis carinii* pneumonia in AIDS *for details*).

Bacterial infection (including mycobacteria).

Viral infection (*e.g.*, cytomegalovirus).

Fungal infection (*e.g.*, aspergillus, candida).

Parasitic infection (*e.g.*, *Strongyloides*).

Kaposi's sarcoma.

Secondary B cell lymphoma.

Secondary carcinoma.

Lymphocytic interstitial pneumonitis.

Graft-versus-host disease or rejection episodes in transplant recipients.

Etiology

Congenital causes

Genetically determined absence or reduction in immune response, *e.g.*, X-linked infantile hypogammaglobulinemia (Bruton type).

Acquired causes

HIV infection.

Organ transplantation.

Drug treatment, *e.g.*, steroids, azathiaprine, cyclosporin A (used in rheumatoid arthritis, asthma, ulcerative colitis).

Causes of relative immunosuppression

Diabetes.

Old age.

Epidemiology

• 1 in 100 000 people suffers from congenital immunosuppression.

• The incidence of acquired immunosuppression is increasing with the use of immunosuppressive drugs, organ transplantation, and HIV infection.

Treatment

Diet and lifestyle

• Excessive alcohol consumption should be avoided.

• Cigarette smoking should be stopped because of the increased incidence of pulmonary complications in immunosuppressed patients who smoke.

Pharmacological treatment

• Treatment depends on diagnosis, which should be as accurate as possible.

• In deteriorating patients, treatment must be started empirically, depending on the most probable cause or agent; this is determined by the combination of symptoms, signs, degree of immunocompromise, stage of immunocompromise, and local pathogenic load.

Antibiotics

• If a specific organism is not detected and the patient is deteriorating, broad-spectrum cover should be used when there is purulence on the Gram stain.

Antituberculous drugs

• Four-drug treatment (ethambutol, rifampin, pyrazinamide, isoniazid) is recommended until sensitivity is available.

Antiviral agents

• Treatment should be initiated only if diagnosis is established.

Ganciclovir, 6 mg/kg twice daily initially, then maintenance dose depending on response.

Foscarnet, 90 mg/kg continuous infusion over 90 min twice daily depending on renal function.

• Renal function and leukocyte count must be monitored.

Antifungal agents

• Treatment should be initiated only if diagnosis is established.

Amphotericin B, 0.5 mg/kg daily i.v., increasing to 1 mg/kg daily, depending on renal function.

Itraconazole, 200 mg daily.

Antiparasitic agents

Trimethoprim, 15 mg/kg, may be used for *Pneumocystis* spp. infection.

Chemotherapy

• Chemotherapy may be used in certain patients with Kaposi's sarcoma or secondary B cell lymphoma or carcinoma.

• The choice of treatment is determined locally, and the use of chemotherapy combined with radiotherapy for symptomatic treatment must be considered.

Treatment aims

To eradicate infection and to prevent recurrence.

To relieve symptoms of secondary neoplasia or Kaposi's sarcoma.

Other treatments

Controlled oxygen therapy.

Continuous positive airways pressure.

Mechanical ventilation: needs careful consideration, ideally with the patient or a relative, before initiation.

Prognosis

• Prognosis depends on the cause of immunosuppression and the form of pulmonary complication.

• Mortality is 10%–20% in transiently neutropenic patients with bacterial infection.

• If the immunosuppression is reversible, recurrence is unlikely after the patient has recovered from an acute event.

Follow-up and management

• In continuing immunosuppression, follow-up and management depend on the specific diagnosis: for example, HIV-infected patients may need prolonged prophylactic treatment against recurrence of *Pneumocystis carinii* infection.

General references

Dichter JR, Levine SJ, Shelhamer JH: Approach to the immunocompromised host with pulmonary symptoms. *Hematol Oncol Clin North Am* 1993, **7**:887–912.

Murray JF, Mills J: Pulmonary infectious complications of human immunodeficiency virus infection. Part I and Part II. *Am Rev Respir Dis* 1990, **141**:1356–1372; 1582–1589.

Verra F, *et al.*: Bronchoalveolar lavage in immunocompromised patients: clinical and functional consequences. *Chest* 1992, **101**:1215–1220.

Diagnosis

Symptoms

Pleuritic chest pain, dyspnea, hemoptysis: indicating acute minor pulmonary embolism.

Acute-onset dyspnea, syncope, central chest pain: indicating acute massive pulmonary embolism.

Gradual-onset dyspnea, pleuritic chest pain, decreasing exercise tolerance: indicating subacute massive pulmonary embolism.

Increasing dyspnea, effort syncope: indicating chronic pulmonary embolism.

Signs

• Pulmonary embolism is manifest in several ways, depending on the extent of pulmonary vascular obstruction, the time during which the obstruction accumulates, and the presence or absence of pre-existing heart or lung disease [1].

Shortness of breath, pleural rub, signs associated with pleural effusion: indicating pulmonary infarction.

Tachypnea or hyperventilation, reduced cardiac output, right heart failure: indicating massive pulmonary embolism.

Pulmonary hypertension: indicating chronic pulmonary embolism.

Investigations

• The diagnosis of pulmonary embolism needs a high index of clinical suspicion, combined with the results of investigations that may confirm or refute these suspicions.

Pulmonary angiography: allows definitive diagnosis but is invasive and needs specialized facilities; emboli seen as filling defects within contrast-filled pulmonary arteries [2].

Chest radiography: helps to exclude other conditions; may show vascular markings or large pulmonary artery shadow in massive embolism; may also show linear basal atelectasis in pulmonary infarction; but this is a nonspecific sign.

ECG: the classic S_1, Q_3, T_3 pattern is nonspecific and unusual. Sinus tachycardia is usual, although atrial fibrillation or flutter may occur.

Ventilation perfusion scanning: easily performed, low-risk procedure; normal scan virtually excludes pulmonary embolus; nondiagnostic scans need investigation for presence of peripheral venous thrombosis to support diagnosis of pulmonary embolism (if negative, untreated patient has <3% chance of subsequent pulmonary embolism) or pulmonary angiography; high-probability scan usually diagnostic, with 98% specificity, 91% positive predictive value (74% in patients with previous pulmonary embolism), but low sensitivity (41%); investigation must not be delayed because 14% of high-probability scans and 45% of indeterminate scans become normal by day 7 of treatment [3].

Echocardiography: primarily useful in differential diagnosis of dyspnea; thrombus seen within right heart or proximal pulmonary artery and high index of clinical suspicion may be considered diagnostic. Demonstration of right ventricular enlargement may lead to initial consideration of the diagnosis.

Doppler ultrasonography, phlebography, impedance phlethysmography: indirect investigations for proximal leg vein thrombosis; if positive, they may provide a useful alternative to pulmonary angiography in patients with suspected minor pulmonary embolism but indeterminate lung scan.

Complications

Death.

Pulmonary infarction, infection, cavitation, or hypertension.

Differential diagnosis

• Pulmonary embolism has a wide differential diagnosis and hence its reputation as "The Great Masquerader."

Acute minor pulmonary embolism
Pneumonia.

Acute massive pulmonary embolism
Septicemia.
Myocardial infarction.
Hypovolemia.
Pericardial tamponade.

Subacute massive pulmonary embolism
Pulmonary edema
Pneumonia
Hyperventilation.

Chronic pulmonary embolism
Primary pulmonary hypertension.

Etiology

• >90% of pulmonary emboli originate as deep venous thrombosis of the lower extremities.

• Common causes include the following:
Surgery within past 1 month.
Medical illness (*e.g.*, myocardial infarction or stroke).
Immobility, cancer, obesity, or oral contraception.
Pregnancy or estrogen therapy.
Indwelling central venous lines.
Hypercoagulable states, which may be acquired (*e.g.*, lupus anticoagulant, anti-cardiolipin antibodies) or inherited (*e.g.*, antithrombin III deficiency, protein C deficiency).

Epidemiology

• At necropsy, pulmonary embolism has been found in 9–26% of all patients; it was suspected before death in only ~16%.

• Deaths are more common in women and increase with age.

Treatment

Diet and lifestyle

• Patients should avoid periods of sustained immobility, *e.g.*, during longhaul flights.

Pharmacological treatment

Anticoagulant treatment: heparin

• Heparin is used for acute treatment of hemodynamicallly stable patients; it prevents further fibrin deposition and thrombus extension.

• Treatment must be commenced immediately if clinical suspicion is high.

Standard dosage	Heparin bolus, 5000–8000 units, then i.v. infusion to maintain activated partial thromboplastin time at 1.5–2.5 times control.
Contraindications	Active bleeding, recent cerebral hemorrhage or brain, eye, or spinal-cord surgery, malignant hypertension.
Special points	High-dose s.c. heparin reduces need for i.v. infusion and increases patient mobility.
Main drug interactions	Oral anticoagulants or drugs that interfere with platelet function, *e.g.*, aspirin or dextran solutions.
Main side effects	Bleeding, heparin-induced thrombocytopenia.

Anticoagulant treatment: warfarin

• Warfarin has no role in immediate treatment but prevents recurrence; it impairs coagulation, thus reducing thrombus formation.

Standard dosage	Warfarin, 10 mg daily for 2 days (average-sized adult); maintenance dose adjusted to obtain INR 2.0–3.0
Contraindications	As for heparin; avoided in pregnancy.
Special points	Should be started at same time as heparin treatment.
Main drug interactions	Many drugs may enhance or reduce the activity of warfarin; manufacturer's prescribing information should be consulted.
Main side effects	Bleeding.

Thrombolytic treatment

• This is indicated for hemodynamically compromised patients with proven pulmonary embolism (*i.e.*, high clinical suspicion and high-probability lung scan or pulmonary artery thrombus seen on echocardiography or angiography).

• Treatment promotes the dissolution of recently formed thrombus. It produces a more rapid resolution of emboli and improvement in cardiopulmonary status than heparin therapy alone does. No reduction in mortality, however, has been shown.

Standard dosage	Streptokinase, 250 000 units for 30 min followed by 100 000 units/h for 24 h. Urokinase, 4400 units/kg for 10 min followed by 4400 units/kg/h for 12–24 h. rt-PA, 100 mg by continuous infusion for 2 h.
Contraindications	Active bleeding, recent cerebrovascular accident, recent trauma, major surgery, or organ biopsy.
Special points	Local administration is no more effective and is not safer than peripheral administration, which is simpler. All thrombolytic agents appear equally effective. Should be followed by heparin treatment.
Main drug interactions	None.
Main side effects	Bleeding (the risk of major hemorrhage is twice that with heparin), allergic reactions to streptokinase.

Prophylactic treatment

• Most deaths from pulmonary emboli are sudden or occur in patients in whom the diagnosis was not suspected; therefore a significant reduction in mortality is only achieved by adequate prevention.

Physical measures: early mobilization, pneumatic calf compression, and graduated compression stockings.

Drugs: conventional heparin, 5000 units s.c. every 8–12 h; low molecular weight heparin, 3500–5000 units once daily depending on type used, or low-dose warfarin.

• Percutaneous or surgical placement of inferior vena cava filter may prevent subsequent embolism in patients with recurrent pulmonary embolism despite effective anticoagulation [4].

Treatment aims

To reduce morbidity of acute episode.

To prevent recurrence of pulmonary embolism or chronic pulmonary hypertension.

Other treatments

Inferior vena cava filters: used when anticoagulation is contraindicated or fails.

Pulmonary embolectomy.

Prognosis

• One-third of acute or subacute pulmonary emboli result in sudden death or are undiagnosed during life.

• Patients with untreated clinically apparent pulmonary emboli have a 30% mortality from recurrent emboli; this is reduced to 8% with effective treatment.

• Survivors of the acute or subacute episode usually have no clinical sequelae.

• Chronic pulmonary embolism carries a grave prognosis and pharmacological treatment is generally ineffective; elective thromboendarterectomy may produce long-term improvement in some patients.

• Patients who have had pulmonary emboli are at increased risk of further thromboembolic episodes when exposed to situations in which thrombosis might occur.

Follow-up and management

• Oral anticoagulant treatment and monitoring are continued for at least 3–6 months but may be continued indefinitely if underlying risk factors cannot be controlled.

Key references

1. Goldhaber SZ, Morpurgo M, WHO/ISFC Task Force on Pulmonary Embolism: Diagnosis, treatment, and prevention of pulmonary embolism. *JAMA* 1992, **268**:1727–1733.
2. Stein PD, *et al.*: Complications and validity of pulmonary angiography in acute pulmonary embolism. *Circulation* 1992, **85**:462–468.
3. PIOPED Investigators: Value of the ventilation/perfusion scan in acute pulmonary embolism. *JAMA* 1990, **263**:2753–2759.
4. Becker DM, Philbrick JT, Selby JB: Inferior vena cava filters indications, safety, effectiveness. *Arch Intern Med* 1992, **152**:1985–1994.

Diagnosis

Symptoms

Symptoms of hypertension.

Symptoms of associated coronary, cerebral, and peripheral vascular disease: in atherosclerotic disease.

Acute dyspnea: in "flash" pulmonary edema.

Signs

Hypertension.

Epigastric or renal angle bruits.

Femoral bruits and absent leg pulses: in atherosclerotic disease.

Investigations

Plasma creatinine measurement.

Renal ultrasonography: to measure kidney size (kidneys <8 cm long seldom worth revascularization).

Nuclear medicine scanning: paired pre- and postcaptopril scans may increase sensitivity and specificity.

Renal angiography.

• Other examinations are those for atherosclerotic disease elsewhere.

Magnetic resonance angiography.

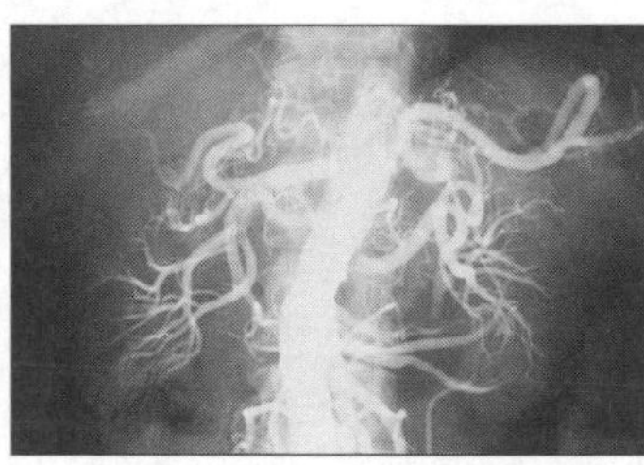

Widespread atherosclerotic disease in presence of renovascular disease, shown on angiography.

Complications

Hypertension, renal failure: in both fibromuscular and atherosclerotic forms (rare in fibromuscular dysplasia).

Differential diagnosis

Other causes of hypertension.

Other causes of renal failure.

Left ventricular dysfunction.

Etiology

• Causes include the following:

Fibromuscular disease: medial muscular hyperplasia.

Atherosclerotic disease: as for atherosclerosis elsewhere.

Large-vessel vasculitis, *e.g.*, Takayasu's arteritis.

Epidemiology

• Fibromuscular disease is rare (more common in younger female patients).

• Atherosclerotic disease occurs in 30% of patients with abnormal coronary angiograms and 42% with abnormal peripheral angiograms.

Treatment

Diet and lifestyle

• Patients should take measures to alleviate risk factors for atherosclerotic disease, *e.g.*, stopping smoking, losing weight, and reducing lipids.

Pharmacological treatment

• Hypertension is treated by the usual agents (*see* Hypertension *for details*), except in the following cases:

Fibromuscular dysplasia: angiotensin-converting enzyme (ACE) inhibitors should be avoided because they may reduce renal function in kidneys with renal artery stenosis.

Atherosclerotic disease: ACE inhibitors and beta blockers should be avoided because most patients have peripheral vascular disease.

Treatment aims

To control hypertension.

To preserve renal function.

To prevent "flash" pulmonary edema.

Other treatments

Percutaneous angioplasty: for fibromuscular disease, with surgery if not successful.

Angioplasty or surgery: for atherosclerotic disease, depending on patient (ostial lesions usually need surgical treatment).

Prognosis

• The 5-year survival rate is 92% for fibromuscular disease and 67% for atherosclerotic disease; age is a major factor.

• Renal artery stenosis may recur, especially after angioplasty.

Follow-up and management

• Blood pressure and plasma creatinine measurement and nuclear medicine scans should be repeated, with re-angiography, if restenosis is possible.

General references

Conolly JO, *et al.*: Presentation, clinical features and outcome in different patterns of atherosclerotic renovascular disease. *Am J Med* 1994, **87**:413–421.

Stansby G, Hamilton G, Scoble JE: Atherosclerotic renal artery stenosis. *Br J Hosp Med* 1993, **49**:388–395.

Diagnosis

Symptoms

• The clinical features are usually dominated by those of the primary condition.

Nausea, vomiting, pruritus, malaise, lethargy, myoclonus: features of uremia develop if diagnosis unduly delayed.

Seizures and coma: in severe cases.

Signs

Oliguria: <400 mL urine daily; classic but not universal sign.

Edema.

Investigations

• Priorities are the detection and documentation of possibly life-threatening complications, exclusion of prerenal and postrenal factors, diagnosis of intrinsic renal disease, distinction of acute from chronic renal failure, and monitoring of response to treatment.

Central venous pressure monitoring and pulmonary capillary wedge pressure measurement: using Swan-Ganz catheter, if in any doubt about prerenal factors.

Chest radiography: for fluid overload.

ECG, echocardiography: to exclude prerenal factors or pericardial changes.

Ultrasonography, plain abdominal radiography: to exclude postrenal factors.

Urine sodium and osmolality: can identify prerenal acute renal failure.

Urinalysis: proteinuria, dysmorphic erythrocytes, erythrocyte casts, other features of intrinsic renal disease.

Serology: for glomerulonephritis and vasculitis.

Creatine kinase and hydroxybutyrate dehydrogenase measurement: for rhabdomyolysis and hemolysis.

Calcium measurement: for metastatic bone deposits, iatrogenic, hypercalcemia.

Blood film: for fragments and platelet count, to detect microangiopathic hemolytic anemia.

Blood cultures: for sepsis.

Coagulation tests, fibrinogen and fibrin degradation products analysis: for disseminated intravascular coagulation.

Liver function tests: for hepatorenal syndrome.

Renal biopsy: possibly indicated in patients with acute renal failure when intrinsic renal disease is suspected and may require specific therapy.

Ultrasonography, alkaline phosphatase measurement, bone radiography: for kidney size, evidence of metabolic bone disease, and anemia, respectively, to distinguish acute from chronic renal failure.

Immunoglobulin and protein electrophoresis: for myeloma in elderly patients.

Complications

Sepsis, adult respiratory distress syndrome (noncardiogenic pulmonary edema): usually seen in patients with multiple organ failure.

Gastrointestinal hemorrhage: caused by gastric stress ulceration.

Bleeding: uremic platelet–endothelial dysfunction and sepsis lead to a bleeding diathesis.

Opportunistic infections, poor wound healing, muscle wasting: due to hypercatabolic state associated with uremia and infection.

Hypertension: often related to fluid overload, sometimes to primary renal disease.

Hypotension: often related to sepsis, occasionally to occult myocardial ischemia.

Hyperkalemia: especially in presence of acidosis and tissue breakdown.

Differential diagnosis

Prerenal: inadequate perfusion of otherwise normal kidneys.

Intrinsic renal disease: *e.g.*, acute or rapidly progressive glomerulonephritis.

Postrenal: blockage to flow of urine from otherwise normal kidneys.

Etiology

• Etiology is often complex, with more than one mechanism at play. Causes include the following:

Prerenal

Shock (hypovolemia, inadequate cardiac output, lack of peripheral resistance – sepsis, anaphylaxis).
Hepatorenal syndrome.
Angiotensin-converting enzyme inhibitors.

Renal

Acute tubular necrosis: ischemia, toxins (*e.g.*, aminoglycosides, paracetamol, hypercalcemia).
Acute glomerulonephritis.
Acute interstitial nephritis: *e.g.*, NSAIDs, antibiotics (sulfonamides, penicillins)
Infection (leptospirosis, Legionnaires' disease).
Thrombotic microangiopathies: *e.g.*, hemolytic uremic syndrome, thrombotic thrombocytopenic purpura, related conditions (*e.g.*, scleroderma renal crisis, accelerated-phase hypertension, pre-eclampsia, acute fatty liver of pregnancy, postpartum acute renal failure).
Vascular catastrophes: renal-vein thrombosis, renal-artery embolus or thrombosis, dissection of aorta, cholesterol emboli.
Pigment nephropathy: rhabdomyolysis, intravascular hemolysis.
Multiple myeloma: light-chain nephropathy.
Infection: bilateral pyelonephritis.

Postrenal

Intrarenal obstruction: urate, drugs, hemoglobin, myoglobin, light chains.
Extrarenal obstruction: stones, tumors, blood clots, bladder outflow, retroperitoneal fibrosis.

Epidemiology

• ~50 people in one million annually develop acute renal failure needing dialysis.

• Most acute renal failure develops in the context of other acute illnesses.

Treatment

Diet and lifestyle

• Acute renal failure is a medical emergency, usually occurring in hospital; diet is modified to supply sufficient energy while minimizing accumulation of toxins (protein 40–60 g, sodium 40–60 mEq, potassium 40–60 mEq daily).

• In the maintenance support of acute renal failure, more rigorous protein (>1.0 g/kg/d) and calorie (>25 kcal/kg/d) nutrition is recommended, with appropriate control for fluid balance.

Pharmacological treatment

For acute tubular necrosis

Optimization of vascular and extracellular fluid volume.

Maximization of perfusion of vital organs and exclusion of urinary obstruction.

Diuretics only after restoration of euvolemia and maximization of cardiac output: escalating doses of a loop diuretic (bumetanide, 2–5 mg i.v. every 4–6 h depending on urine flow rate) and dopamine (2.5–5 μg/kg/min) may restore urine flow; contraindicated in presence of obstruction, before hypovolemia is corrected, or if risk of cardiac arrhythmia.

Prompt identification and vigorous treatment of infection: culture of available body fluids, repeated frequently; regular change of venous lines; CRP monitoring and leukocyte count.

Control of acidosis and hyperkalemia.

Enteral feeding, total parenteral nutrition if necessary; fluid balance must be controlled before feeding.

Hematological support: hemoglobin should be kept at ~10 g/dL and albumin maintained by i.v. human albumin solutions.

H_2 blockers to prevent gastric stress ulceration.

For focal necrotizing and crescentic glomerulonephritis

Steroids, cyclophosphamide, and possibly plasma exchange only after biopsy confirmation if possible.

For acute interstitial nephritis

Withdrawal of offending drugs, possibly steroid therapy.

For infection

High-dose prolonged course of appropriate antibiotic (at least 4–6 weeks).

For hemolytic uremic syndrome and thrombotic thrombocytopenic purpura

Plasma exchange with fresh frozen plasma and possible prostacyclin infusion *(see* Hemolytic uremic syndrome *for details)*.

For pigment nephropathy, myeloma kidney

Forced alkaline diuresis: 0.9% saline, 500 mL alternating with 1.26% sodium bicarbonate solution, 500 mL every 4 h; bumetanide, 1–5 mg i.v. 8-hourly to maintain urine flow rate ≥100 mL/h; contraindicated in oliguria unresponsive to volume repletion and diuretics.

Treatment aims

To prevent development of acute tubular necrosis.

To relieve obstruction and prevent progressive renal damage.

To identify primary treatable renal disease.

To replace renal function.

Other treatments

• Acute tubular necrosis can be treated by renal replacement therapy, as follows:

Continuous arteriovenous or pumped continuous venovenous hemodiafiltration: preferred for immobile or intensive-care patients with hemodynamic instability.

Intermittent hemodialysis (alternate-day): for mobile or general-ward patients.

Prognosis

• In acute tubular necrosis, the prognosis depends roughly on the number of additional organs that are failing, as follows:
no other organs, survival is >80%;
+1 organ (*e.g.*, ventilation), 40%–50%;
+2 organs (*e.g.*, ventilation, inotropes), <20%;
+3 organs (*e.g.*, ventilation, inotropes, total parenteral nutrition), <10%;
+4 organs (*e.g.*, ventilation, inotropes, total parenteral nutrition, liver), <5%.

• Many patients with acute tubular necrosis have near-complete recovery of renal function and do not develop chronic renal disease.

• Some patients make only a partial recovery, which may indicate that the original injury was more severe; these patients may recover renal function for some months or years before developing hypertension and progressive chronic renal failure.

Follow-up and management

• Long-term follow-up is recommended in patients with persistent hypertension, impaired renal function, hematuria, or proteinuria.

General references

Bihari D, Neild G, eds: *Acute Renal Failure in the Intensive Therapy Unit.* Berlin: Springer-Verlag; 1990.

Rainford D, Sweny P, eds: *Acute Renal Failure.* London: Farrand Press; 1990.

Sweny P: Haemofiltration and haemodiafiltration: theoretical and practical aspects. *Curr Anaesth Crit Care* 1991, **2**:37–43.

Diagnosis

Definition

• Irreversible renal impairment is most often recognized by persistently high urea (BUN) and creatinine concentrations; it often progresses to end-stage renal failure.

Mild: glomerular filtration rate (GFR) 20–50 mL/min; creatinine 1.5–3.0 mg/dL.

Moderate: GFR 10–20 mL/min; creatinine 3.0–7.0 mg/dL.

Severe: GFR <10 mL/min; creatinine >7.0 mg/dL.

Symptoms

Puritus, malaise, nausea, anorexia: early nonspecific constitutional symptoms.

Drowsiness, twitching, blunting of intellect, diarrhea: late seizures and coma.

Symptoms of underlying disease.

Signs

Anemia.

Hypertension.

Brown line at distal end of nail.

Pallor and pigmentation.

Pruritis and scratch marks.

Red eyes: high calcium X phosphate product.

Edema.

Peripheral neuropathy: sensory, usually motor.

Proximal myopathy: severe metabolic bone disease.

Kussmaul's respiration: when acidosis is severe.

Pericarditis: causing tamponade when renal failure severe.

Investigations

Serum electrolytes, urea (BUN), creatinine, creatinine clearance, 24-h urinary protein, calcium and phosphate measurement.

Plain radiography of abdomen: to detect calculi and nephrocalcinosis.

Ultrasonography of kidneys: to measure size and exclude obstruction.

Kidney biopsy: for changes specific to underlying disease; contraindicated for small kidneys or very late chronic disease.

Immunoglobulin electrophoresis, Bence–Jones protein measurement: to diagnose multiple myeloma in elderly patients.

Radioisotope studies: captopril renography if renal artery stenosis suspected.

Complications

Anemia.

Renal osteodystrophy.

Hypertension.

Pruritus.

Peripheral neuropathy.

Pericarditis.

Acute or chronic renal failure: precipitated by hypovolemia, hypertension, infection, toxic agents, overzealous control of blood pressure.

Accelerated atherosclerosis: increased risk of stroke, heart attack, and peripheral vascular disease.

Differential diagnosis

Acute renal failure: short history, examination shows features of underlying disease, normal hemoglobin, no evidence of renal osteodystrophy, normal or enlarged kidneys.

Etiology

• The cause varies depending on the patient's age; the following may have a role:

Chronic glomerulonephritis in 20%–30% of patients.

Diabetes mellitus in 20%–30%.

Hypertension in 20%–30%.

Chronic interstitial disease in 10%–20%.

Polycystic kidney disease in 10%.

Renovascular disease in about 10%.

Drugs in 2.5%.

Hypertension in 20%–30%.

Hereditary nephritis in affected families.

In elderly patients: multiple myeloma, atherosclerotic renal artery stenosis, obstruction, and amyloid.

In children: congenital absence or dysplasia, obstruction: posterior urethral valves, juvenile nephronophthisis (cystic disease).

Family or previous history of renal disease (*e.g.*, childhood urinary tract infection).

Epidemiology

• The incidence of chronic renal failure is difficult to estimate accurately.

• In the US, >1 in 10 000 population each year develop end-stage chronic renal failure.

Progression

• Although chronic renal failure often progresses to end-stage renal failure, function may not deteriorate quickly and, in some patients, remains stable, although significantly impaired, for several years.

• Measurement of serum creatinine is the most useful clinical test in assessing progression (serum creatinine is related to muscle mass and renal function).

• Serum creatinine rises exponentially with deteriorating renal function.

• A mild increase in serum creatinine signals serious early loss of function.

• Plotting reciprocal serum creatinine values against time is a useful indicator of progression of renal failure.

Treatment

Diet and lifestyle

• Patients should eat a high-energy diet, with potassium restriction and protein intake restricted to 0.5–0.75 g/kg body weight daily; in later stages of chronic renal failure, decreased protein intake can help to control symptoms of nausea, vomiting, and anorexia.

• Phosphate intake should be restricted, and absorption reduced by phosphate binders (calcium carbonate or aluminium hydroxide).

• Vitamin D supplementation is sometimes needed, using 1-hydroxylated preparations.

Pharmacological treatment

• Specific treatment is directed at the underlying cause.

• Nephrotoxic drugs and NSAIDs must be avoided, and doses of other drugs must be adjusted for the degree of renal failure.

• Angiotensin-converting enzyme inhibitors may help to control blood pressure, particularly in diabetic patients; diastolic pressure should be <90 mm Hg. Care is needed with these agents when renal artery stenosis is suspected or when serum creatinine is chronically elevated to levels more than 4.0 mg/dL.

• Erythropoietin can be used to treat anemia and improve well-being.

• Progression to end-stage chronic renal failure can be slowed by some or all of the following:

Control of systemic hypertension.

Reduction of glomerular blood pressure, using angiotensin-converting enzyme inhibitors or calcium channel blockers.

Low-protein diets (in some patients).

Addressing the risk factors for accelerated atherosclerosis.

Nonpharmacological treatment

• Hemodialysis or peritoneal dialysis can be used *(see* Dialysis *for details).*

Treatment aims

To delay progression to end-stage renal failure.

To prevent renal bone disease.

To control hypertension.

To prevent acute on chronic renal failure (*e.g.*, by avoiding urinary tract infection, correcting obstruction).

Prognosis

• Timely dialysis or transplantation prolongs life.

• Comorbidity of multisystem diseases may limit survival.

Follow-up and management

• After chronic renal failure has been diagnosed, progress must be monitored at regular intervals ; important parameters include the following:

Weight (for nutrition and fluid status).

Blood pressure (control may retard progression).

Urea/blood urea nitrogen (may alter with increased catabolism or protein intake).

Creatinine.

Hemoglobin.

Serum calcium (iatrogenic hypercalcemia must be avoided: calcium is nephrotoxic).

Serum phosphate.

Serum alkaline phosphatase.

Albumin (particularly helpful in assessing nutrition).

General references

El Nahas M, Mallick NP, Anderson S: *Prevention of Progressive Chronic Renal Failure.* Oxford: Oxford University Press; 1993.

Knan IH, *et al.*: Chronic renal failure: factors influencing nephrology referral. *Q J Med* 1994, **87**:559–564.

Mogensen CE: Captopril delays progression to overt renal disease in insulin-dependent diabetes mellitus patients with microalbuminuria. *J Am Soc Nephrol* 1992, **3**:336.

Perneger TV, Whetton PK, Klag MJ: Risk of kidney failure associated with the use of acetaminophen, aspirin, and non-steroidal antiinflammatory drugs. *N Engl J Med* 1994, **331**:1675–1679.

Selection

Patient criteria

• Factors to check for include the following:

Age: biological age more important than chronological age, usual upper limit is 65–75 years.

Cancer: must be excluded.

Infection: *i.e.*, Staghorn calculi, tuberculosis, bronchiectasis, HIV must be excluded.

Cardiovascular status: angina detected by stress test or coronary angiography; intermittent claudication detected by duplex Doppler or digital vascular imaging; myocardial infarction remains the most common cause of death after transplantation; presence of peripheral vascular disease may compromise leg perfusion after transplantation.

Bladder function: positive urological history obtained by flow rate and residual bladder ultrasonography or video cystometrography, possibly with cystoscopy; bladder outflow tract obstruction may compromise graft function.

Donor criteria

• The criteria have been relaxed over the past 10 years because of a shortage of donors. Sepsis is no longer a contraindication if the organism is cultured. Diabetic donors may be considered, but frozen section of the kidney is needed before transplantation.

Age 2–75 years.

Absence of chronic renal disease.

Hepatitis B virus, HIV, and hepatitis C virus negative.

No malignancies: except primary brain tumors.

• Live-related donors should always be sought: parents can only be a haplotype match (50%), but siblings can be HLA-identical (100%), a haplotype match (50%), or a complete mismatch (0%).

Matching

Tissue typing

HLA on chromosome 6. Class I = A and B, class II = DR.

• 1A, 1B, 1DR antigen is inherited from each parent.

• For matching, the importance is as follows: DR > B > A; *i.e.*, 1A, 2B, 2DR match is better than 2A, 1B, 2DR match.

Direct cross match

• If donor lymphocytes combined with the patient's serum cause lymphocyte death, a positive cross match is implied, and the kidney is unsuitable.

• Highly sensitized patients have high levels of anti-HLA antibodies; this may be secondary to previous transplantation, blood transfusion, or pregnancies; the incidence of positive cross matches is increased.

Epidemiology

• 50%of patients on renal failure programs are unsuitable for transplantation because of age or coexisting diseases (*i.e.*, severe cardiovascular disease, cancer).

• >22 000 patients are on waiting lists in the US.

• >10 000 kidney transplantations are done each year in the US.

• Only 25% of transplants are taken from live-related donors in the US.

Transplantation or dialysis?

Advantages of transplantation

Improved quality of life.

No dialysis.

Correction of anemia.

Normal diet and fluid allowance.

Improved bone metabolism (however, increased osteoporosis from steroids).

Increased ease of travel.

Women of child-bearing age able to have children.

Cheaper.

Disadvantages of transplantation

Emotional stress.

Surgical and anesthetic donor risks.

Approximate costs

Hemodialysis: $35 000/year.

Transplantation: $50 000 in the first year, $5000–$10 000 in subsequent years.

Advantages of live-related donors

Improved graft survival.

Planned operation.

Shorter wait.

Lower incidence of postoperative acute tubular necrosis.

Usually, less rejection.

Treatment

Acute rejection

Clinical findings

Tenderness over graft.

Pyrexia.

Decreased urine output.

Fluid retention.

Hypertension.

Occasionally silent.

Investigation of graft dysfunction

Urine analysis: midstream urine, proteinuria, cytology.

Blood analysis: increased blood urea nitrogen, creatinine, potassium, leukocyte count, interleukin 2R, cyclosporin A concentration, blood cultures.

Ultrasonography: to exclude obstruction, possibly to diagnose rejection.

Renal isotope scans: show decreased perfusion.

Renal biopsy: open or needle biopsy.

Differential diagnosis

Acute tubular necrosis: 20%–50% of grafts have primary nonfunction lasting 1–2 weeks.

Cyclosporin A toxicity.

Graft pyelonephritis.

Ureteric obstruction.

Renal artery stenosis.

Cytomegalovirus.

Histological features

Acute cellular rejection: lymphocyte infiltrate, macrophages, natural killer cells.

Acute vascular rejection: as above, with fibrinoid necrosis and infiltration of vessel walls.

Chronic rejection: fibrosis, chronic vascular changes (intimal proliferation) leading to vascular occlusion.

Treatment

Hyperacute rejection: extremely rare, usually due to circulating preformed antibody.

Simple acute cellular rejection: pulse corticosteroid.

Steroid-resistant cellular rejection and vascular rejection: antithymocyte globulin, antilymphocyte globulin, OKT3.

Chronic rejection: no effective treatment.

Immunosuppression

Agents

Combinations of corticosteroid, azathioprine, cyclosporin A, and monoclonal and polyclonal antibodies.

New immunosuppressive drugs: tacrolimus, mycophenolate mofetil.

Side effects

All immunosuppressants: increased incidence of tumors (skin, reticuloendothelial system) and infection (*e.g.*, opportunistic infections, cytomegalovirus).

Azathioprine: bone-marrow suppression (leukocytes, hemoglobin, platelets), hepatotoxicity.

Steroids: cushingoid facies, buffalo hump, central obesity, striae, thinning of skin, bruising, proximal myopathy, acne vulgaris, hirsuitism, osteoporosis, aseptic necrosis of the hips, diabetes, hyperlipidemia.

Cyclosporin A: hirsuitism, tremor, gum hyperplasia, nephro-, neuro-, or hepatotoxicity.

Tacrolimus: kidney and liver toxicity; neurotoxicity.

OKT3 (anti-T-cell monoclonal antibody): first-dose effect (acute pulmonary edema), increased incidence of lymphoproliferative disorders.

Cadaveric kidney storage

- The kidney should be perfused with buffered ice-cold fluid of high osmolarity.
- It should then be wrapped in two sterile bags and stored on crushed ice for up to 48 h.
- Prolonged storage times can be achieved using perfusion machines (expensive and rarely used in the US).

Blood transfusion and transplantation

- Transfusion increases patient sensitization, but patients who have received transfusion have better success when they do receive a transplant.
- The beneficial effect on transplantation outcome is less clear since the introduction of cyclosporin A.

Surgical complications

Early

Hemorrhage, renal vein and renal artery thrombosis, urinary leak.

Late

Renal artery stenosis, ureteric stenosis, ureteric reflux.

Prognosis

- 1-year kidney graft survival rates are 90% (live) and 70%–90% (cadaveric).
- Graft loss is highest in the first 3 months.
- After the first year, ~4% of grafts are lost annually (mainly due to chronic rejection).

Follow-up and management

- Regular monitoring of immunosuppression and renal function (monthly or bimonthly).
- Regular outpatient visits are needed (3 times weekly initially, decreasing to once every 2 weeks, and eventually once every 4 months).
- A 20% rise in creatinine is investigated initially with ultrasonography and biopsy.

General references

Braun WE, Marwick TH: Coronary artery disease in renal transplant recipients. *Cleve Clin J Med* 1994, **61**:370–385.

Suthanthiran M, Strom TB: Renal transplantation. *N Engl J Med* 1994, **331**:365–376.

Diagnosis

Definition

• Renal tubular acidosis is a disorder of renal hydrogen secretion or bicarbonate reabsorption.

• The following subtypes of renal tubular acidosis have been defined:

Type 1 (distal): defect in distal hydrogen secretion, probably related to defect in hydrogen ATPase.

Type 2 (proximal): decreased proximal bicarbonate reabsorption, probably a defect in brush border sodium–hydrogen exchanger.

Type 3: described in older textbooks but does not exist.

Type 4 (*e.g.*, hyporeninemic hypoaldosteronism): decreased distal acidification due to aldosterone lack and decreased distal sodium reabsorption.

Symptoms

• Renal tubular acidosis has no specific symptoms.

Weakness, musculoskeletal pains, low back pain: in type 1 disease.

Failure to thrive: in children in type 2 disease; often associated with Fanconi's syndrome or other chronic renal disease and symptoms including bone pain from osteomalacia.

Symptoms of diabetes mellitus: in type 4 disease (frequent association).

Signs

• These are rare.

Weakness leading to paralysis: in type 1 disease.

Signs of diabetes mellitus: in type 4 disease.

Investigations

• The diagnosis of renal tubular acidosis is indicated by a hyperchloremic metabolic acidosis defined from blood gas analysis with a normal plasma anion gap (*see box*), defined by $(Na^+ + K^+) - (Cl^- + HCO_3^-)$; this differentiates it from an increased anion gap acidosis such as in lactic acidosis.

Plasma potassium analysis: to detect hypokalemia in patients with type 1 or type 2 disease.

Short ammonium chloride loading test: if urine pH >6.0 to diagnose type 1 disease.

Sodium bicarbonate loading test: if urine pH <6.0 to diagnose type 2 disease.

Plain abdominal radiography: in type 1 disease, to look for nephrocalcinosis.

Parathyroid hormone measurement: to detect primary hyperparathyroidism (associated with type 2 disease).

Complications

• These can be renal as in type 1 disease or general complications of the underlying disease as in type 4 disease.

Nephrocalcinosis and nephrolithiasis: in type 1 disease.

Diabetes mellitus leading to renal failure from diabetic nephropathy: most common condition associated with type 4 disease.

Hypokalemia in type 1 and type 2 disease.

Hyperkalemia in type 4 disease.

Differential diagnosis

Type 1 with nephrocalcinosis

Medullary sponge kidney, idiopathic hypercalciuria, hyperparathyroidism.

• Purgative abuse or chronic diarrhea can lead to a hyperchloremic acidosis with an abnormal short ammonium chloride loading test; this can be differentiated by the urinary ammonium excretion, which is normal in with patients with diarrhea but low in patients with type 1 disease.

Etiology

Causes of type 1 disease

Idiopathic, Sjögren's syndrome, SLE, primary biliary cirrhosis, amphotericin.

Causes of type 2 disease

Idiopathic, cystinosis, Fanconi's syndrome, Wilson's disease, primary hyperparathyroidism, acetazolamide.

Causes of type 4 disease

Diabetes mellitus (most important in clinical practice), urinary obstruction, sickle cell disease; mimicked by potassium-sparing diuretics.

Epidemiology

• Types 1 and 2 are rare; type 4 occurs relatively frequently.

Causes of normal anion gap acidosis

Failure of renal acidification due to renal tubular acidosis or acetazolamide.

Gastrointestinal loss of bicarbonate due to diarrhea, purgative abuse, pancreatic fistula, ureteric diversion (*e.g.*, ureterosigmoidostomy).

Ingestion of acid (*e.g.*, hydrochloric).

Parenteral nutrition.

Treatment

Diet and lifestyle

• No special precautions are necessary.

Pharmacological treatment

For types 1 and 2 disease

• Patients should be given oral sodium bicarbonate up to 1–2 mEq/kg (type 1) or 3–5 mEq/kg (type 2) daily, titrated to improve acidosis.

• Potassium and, in type 2 disease, vitamin D supplements may also be needed.

• Acidosis can never be completely corrected by oral supplements.

For type 4 disease

• Fludrocortisone or diuretics (loop or thiazide) with sodium bicarbonate are indicated.

• Potassium-sparing diuretics, NSAIDS, or angiotensin-converting enzyme inhibitors, which worsen hyperkalemia, must be avoided.

Standard dosage Fludrocortisone, 100–400 μg daily.
Bumetanide, 1–5 mg, and sodium bicarbonate up to 4 g daily.

Contraindications *Fludrocortisone*: volume overload.
Bumetanide: volume depletion.
Sodium bicarbonate: volume overload.

Main drug interactions None.

Main side effects Fluid overload if inadequate diuretic given with sodium bicarbonate.

Treatment aims

To prevent nephrocalcinosis and nephrolithiasis in type 1 disease.

To treat bone disease with vitamin D if deficiency present in type 2 disease.

To avoid life-threatening hyperkalemia caused by concomitant medication in type 4 disease.

Prognosis

• Type 1 disease can progress to renal failure (not usual).

• The prognosis for types 2 and 4 disease depends on the associated conditions.

Follow up and management

• Acidosis and, in type 1 disease, nephrocalcinosis and nephrolithiasis must be monitored.

General references

Battle DC, *et al.*: The use of the urinary anion gap in the diagnosis of hyperchloremic acidosis. *N Engl J Med* 1988, **318**:594–599.

Kurtzman NA: Disorders of distal acidification. *Kidney Int* 1990, **38**:720–727.

Maher ER, Scoble JE: Renal tubular acidosis. *Br J Hosp Med* 1989, **42**:116–119.

Restrictive cardiomyopathy and constrictive pericarditis

Diagnosis

Symptoms

Dyspnea.

Fatigue.

Ankle or abdominal swelling.

Signs

Restrictive cardiomyopathy

Raised jugular venous pressure.

Inspiratory increase in jugular venous pressure: Kussmaul's sign.

Palpable apex beat.

Mild or moderate cardiomegaly.

Third or fourth heart sounds.

Peripheral edema.

Ascites.

Constrictive pericarditis

Raised jugular venous pressure, with rapid diastolic "y" descent.

Kussmaul's sign.

Diffuse or impalpable apex beat.

Intercostal indrawing of apex in systole: Broadbent's sign.

Early diastolic pericardial "knock."

Widened splitting of second heart sound.

Investigations

• The two conditions overlap considerably, and separating them on clinical findings and investigations may be impossible; thoracotomy may be needed to exclude or confirm the diagnosis.

Chest radiography: *restrictive cardiomyopathy*, shows mild or moderate cardiomegaly; *constrictive pericarditis,* show normal heart size and pericardial calcification.

ECG: *restrictive cardiomyopathy*, shows T-wave changes or bundle branch block, and atrial arrhythmias; *constrictive pericarditis*, shows nonspecific T-wave flattening and atrial fibrillation; *both,* shows low voltage complexes.

Echocardiography: *restrictive cardiomyopathy,* shows myocardial thickening and characteristic "ground-glass" appearance (in amyloid); *constrictive pericarditis*, shows normal myocardial thickness and thickened pericardium; *both,* show normal ventricular dimensions with enlarged atria and good systolic and poor diastolic function.

CT or MRI: *restrictive cardiomyopathy,* shows myocardial thickening and normal pericardium; *constrictive pericarditis,* shows normal myocardial thickness and pericardial calcification.

Cardiac catheterization: *restrictive cardiomyopathy,* shows left ventricular filling pressure exceeding right ventricular filling pressure and pulmonary artery systolic pressure often >45 mm Hg, with myocardial biopsy possibly diagnostic; *constrictive pericarditis,* shows identical left and right ventricular filling pressures and pulmonary artery systolic pressure usually <45 mm Hg, with normal myocardial biopsy; *both,* show rapid "y" descent in atrial pressure and early dip in diastolic pressure, with pressure rise to plateau in mid or late diastole.

Complications

Symptomatic hypotension.

Atrial and ventricular arrhythmias.

Progressive "heart failure": in constrictive pericarditis, the "heart" itself is not failing, but the resulting clinical features are similar to those of restrictive cardiomyopathy.

Hepatic failure: resulting from chronic hepatic venous congestion.

Nephrotic syndrome.

Conduction abnormalities: in restrictive cardiomyopathy.

Differential diagnosis

Biventricular heart failure: myocardial infarction, myocardial ischemia, dilated cardiomyopathy.

Myocardial thickening: hypertension, aortic stenosis, hypertrophic cardiomyopathy.

Cardiac tamponade.

Nephrotic syndrome (other causes).

Etiology

Causes of restrictive cardiomyopathy

Amyloidosis.

Glycogen storage disorders.

Hemochromatosis.

Endomyocardial fibrosis.

Eosinophilia.

Neoplastic infiltration.

Collagen vascular disorders.

Pseudoxanthoma elasticum.

Myocardial fibrosis of any origin.

Causes of constrictive pericarditis

• Most causes are unknown.

Tuberculosis (<15% of patients).

Chronic renal failure.

Connective tissue disorders.

Neoplastic infiltration.

Irradiation (often years earlier).

Postpurulent pericarditis.

Hemopericardium after surgery (rare).

Epidemiology

• Both conditions are rare.

• All age groups are affected.

• Glycogen storage disorders are incompatible with progression to adult life.

Treatment

Diet and lifestyle

- Patients' daily activities are restricted by fatigue, breathlessness, and fluid retention.

Pharmacological treatment

Restrictive cardiomyopathy

- Specific measures are generally unsatisfactory.
- Amyloid has no known pharmacological treatment; however, avoidance of digitalis and cacium channel blockers is recommended.
- Patients with hemochromatosis should be given iron-chelating agents, *e.g.*, desferrioxamine.
- Corticosteroids are only effective during the acute myocardial phase of eosinophilia.

Constrictive pericarditis

- The only satisfactory treatment is surgical.
- Patients with tuberculous pericarditis should be pretreated by antituberculous therapy; if the diagnosis is confirmed after pericardial resection, full antituberculous therapy should be continued for 6–12 months after resection. *See* Tuberculosis, extrapulmonary *for details.*

Nonpharmacological treatment

Restrictive cardiomyopathy

Permanent pacing for conduction abnormalities in amyloid.

Bimonthly phlebotomy often for 2–3 years to reduce iron storage in hemachromatosis.

Endocardial resection after fibrosis is established in eosinophilia.

Transplantation occasionally.

Constrictive pericarditis

Complete surgical resection of the pericardium (myocardial inflammation or fibrosis may delay symptomatic response).

Treatment aims

To relieve symptoms.

To remove underlying causes.

Prognosis

- Prognosis is good after resection for constrictive pericarditis.
- Restrictive cardiomyopathy has poor prognosis, particularly due to amyloidosis or malignancy.

Follow-up and management

- Management is purely palliative.

Key references

1. Maisch B: Pericardial diseases, with a focus on etiology, pathogenesis, pathophysiology new diagnostic imaging methods, and treatment. *Curr Opin Cardiol* 1994, **9**:379–388.
2. Spyrou N, Foale R: Restrictive cardiomyopathies. *Curr Opin Cardiol* 1994, **9**:344–348.
3. Ward D: Pericardial and myocardial disease. *Practitioner* 1993, **237**:929–932.

Diagnosis

Symptoms

• Acute rheumatic fever is a multisystem disorder occurring 1–5 weeks after group A streptococcal infection.

• Its manifestation is variable, involving any of the following:

Joint pain (migratory polyarthropathy): ranging from simple pain to disabling arthritis; classically involves large joints in succession, with "overlapping" involvement.

Breathlessness and chest pain (pancarditis): cardiac failure with occasional clinical pericardial involvement.

Rapid purposeless involuntary movements (Sydenham's chorea): including slurred speech, jerky movements, facial tics and grimacing, emotional lability; manifest only during wakefulness; may occur as late isolated feature of disease.

Subcutaneous nodules: painless firm lesions (up to 2 cm diameter) over bony prominences and tendons; tend to appear late and last 1–2 weeks.

Erythema marginatum: red rash extending circumferentially on trunk and proximal limbs; changes rapidly over minutes.

Signs

Joint involvement: joints may be exquisitely tender, red, swollen; refusal to bear weight (especially in children).

Signs of cardiac failure, tachycardia, cardiomegaly, pericardial rub, mitral regurgitation, Carey–Coombs aortic regurgitation, first-, second-, or third-degree atrioventricular block.

Chorea: "bag of worms" tongue of chorea (fasciculation on protrusion), "Milkmaid's grip" (squeezing and relaxing motion on gripping the hand), pendular knee jerks.

Skin rash and nodules.

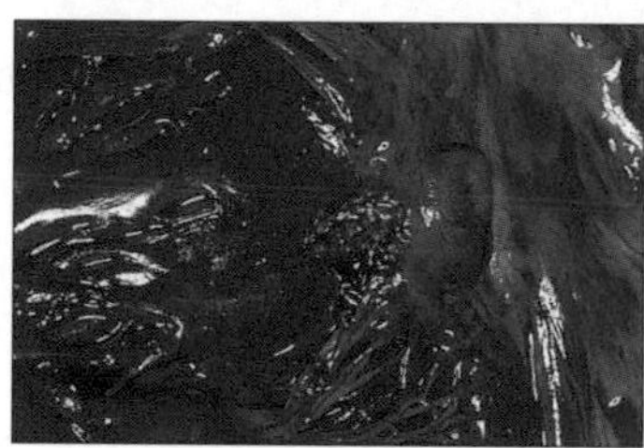

Vegetation on mitral valve, the major reason for continued prophylaxis after rheumatic heart disease.

Investigations

• No single test is diagnostic; the diagnosis is simplified by application of the Duckett-Jones criteria.

• The most important laboratory contribution is evidence of antecedent streptococcal infection.

• No significant laboratory abnormality may be seen in pure chorea.

Throat swab: usually negative, but positive result indicates increased disease activity.

Antistreptolysin O, anti-DNAse B, antihyaluronidase titers: if all three done, 95% chance of positive result.

Full blood count: leukocytosis common; moderate normochromic, normocytic anemia often seen.

ESR, CRP measurement: usually raised.

Liver function tests: aspartate transaminase possibly raised.

Urinalysis: sediment positive for leukocytes and erythrocytes (not pathognomonic of glomerulonephritis).

ECG: shows tachycardia and first-, second-, or, rarely, third-degree heart block.

Echocardiography: shows myocardial thickening and dysfunction, pericardial effusion, and valvular dysfunction.

Complications

Recurrent episodes: with continuing evidence of inflammatory activity.

Rheumatic heart disease: major long-term sequela.

Differential diagnosis

Other causes of polyarthropathy, fever, and cardiac involvement.

Viral arthritides, *e.g.*, rubella, hepatitis B.

Septic arthritis *e.g.*, *Neisseria* spp. infection.

Infective endocarditis.

Acute rheumatoid arthritis.

Stills' disease.

Serum sickness, *e.g.*, after penicillin.

SLE.

Prepurpuric phase Henoch–Schönlein purpura.

Etiology

• Acute rheumatic fever is an exudative, proliferative inflammation of connective tissues, especially heart, joints, and subcutaneous tissues.

• It only occurs after group A streptococcal infection of the upper respiratory tract.

• Particular serotypes, *e.g.*, types 5 and 18, are often implicated, whereas others, *e.g.*, type 12, are not.

Epidemiology

• The incidence of acute rheumatic fever mirrors that of acute streptococcal pharyngitis in a population.

• The peak incidence is at 5–15 years; it is rare in children <4 years but well described in adults.

• The overall male:female ratio is equal; women, however, are more likely to develop Sydenham's chorea and mitral stenosis.

Duckett-Jones criteria for diagnosing acute rheumatic fever

Modified by the American Heart Association.

• Acute rheumatic fever is indicated by two major or one major and two minor criteria if supported by evidence of preceding streptococcal infection.

Major manifestations

Carditis.

Polyarthritis.

Chorea.

Erythema marginatum.

Subcutaneous nodules.

Minor manifestations

Previous rheumatic fever or rheumatic heart disease.

Arthralgia.

Fever.

Raised ESR and CRP concentration, leukocytosis, prolonged PR interval.

Treatment

Diet and lifestyle

• Strict bed or chair rest is advised with mobilization according to clinical status.

Pharmacological treatment

Antibiotics

• Antibiotics do not modify an acute attack or influence the development of carditis.

• They are used to eradicate streptococci from the pharynx and tonsils to prevent recurrence and further valve damage, as prophylaxis for all rheumatic carditis patients, or to cover dental extractions and other surgical interventions (long-term penicillin G benzathine, i.m. 4-weekly).

Standard dosage	Penicillin V, 500 mg 4 times daily for 10 days (adult; *see manufacurer's current prescribing information for children*). Erythromycin, 250 mg 4 times daily for 10 days (adults; *see manufacurer's current prescribing information for children*).
Contraindications	Hypersensitivity.
Special points	Shorter courses may not eradicate streptococci from pharynx.
Main drug interactions	Oral anticoagulants, theophylline preparations (erythromycin).
Main side effects	Hypersensitivity and rash (penicillin), gastrointestinal intolerance.

Antiinflammatory agents

• These do not cure or prevent subsequent development of rheumatic disease.

• Early indiscriminate use may obscure diagnosis in mild cases.

Standard dosage	Aspirin, 80–100 mg/kg daily (children), 6–8 g daily (adults); reduced after 2 weeks and continued for 6–8 weeks. *For more severe carditis or patients intolerant of high-dose salicylates:* prednisolone, 40–60 mg daily for 2 weeks, reduced over next 3–4 weeks, followed by aspirin.
Contraindications	*Aspirin:* breast feeding, gastrointestinal ulceration, hemophilia. *Prednisolone:* current acute gastrointestinal blood loss.
Special points	*Aspirin:* one of the few indications for aspirin treatment in childhood. *Prednisolone:* possible adrenal suppression on sudden withdrawal.
Main drug interactions	*Aspirin:* anticoagulants. *Prednisolone:* danger of gastrointestinal hemorrhage if combined with NSAIDs.
Main side effects	*Aspirin:* hypersensitivity, gastrointestinal bleeding. *Prednisolone:* glucose intolerance, Cushing's syndrome, growth retardation.

Other options

Diuretics, possibly with angiotensin-converting enzyme inhibitors.

Digoxin.

Anticoagulants.

• Use is determined by the degree of carditis or cardiac failure and the stage of illness.

Treatment aims

To eradicate current streptococcal infection and prevent reinfection.

To prevent further episodes of acute disease.

To relieve acute arthritic symptoms.

To prevent infective endocarditis on valves already damaged by carditis.

Prognosis

• Untreated acute rheumatic fever usually lasts up to 3 months.

• Severe carditis extends acute illness to 6 months.

• Most patients with valvular disease develop cardiological complications needing intervention by middle age.

• 6% of patients free of carditis during an acute attack have rheumatic heart disease at 10 years.

• 30% of patients with mild carditis and no pre-existing disease have murmurs at 10 years.

• 40% of patients with apical or basal murmurs in an acute attack have residual disease at 10 years.

• 70% of patients with cardiac failure or pericarditis in an acute attack have residual disease at 10 years.

• Exceptions are patients with "pure" chorea, who frequently develop rheumatic heart disease despite absence of signs of carditis at outset.

Follow-up and management

• Patients must be kept under strict supervision until signs of acute inflammation have subsided.

• Penicillin or alternative prophylaxis is needed at least until the age of 18 years (some clinicians advocate life-long prophylaxis).

• Adequate prophylaxis is needed for minor surgical interventions, *e.g.*, dental treatment.

General references

Homer C, *et al.*: Clinical aspects of acute rheumatic fever. *J Rheumatol* 1991, **18 (suppl 29)**:2–12.

Simmons NA: Recommendations for endocarditis prophylaxis. *J Antimicrob Chemother* 1993, **31**:437–438.

Diagnosis

Symptoms

• Symptoms are mostly trivial; patients are systemically well.

Mild fever.

Rash: in ~50% of infected patients.

Signs

Rash: fine, erythematous pink macules, almost confluent on trunk on second day, rarely lasts >3 days.

Reddened throat: sometimes with tonsillar exudates.

Enlarged lymph nodes: notably occipital, sometimes splenomegaly.

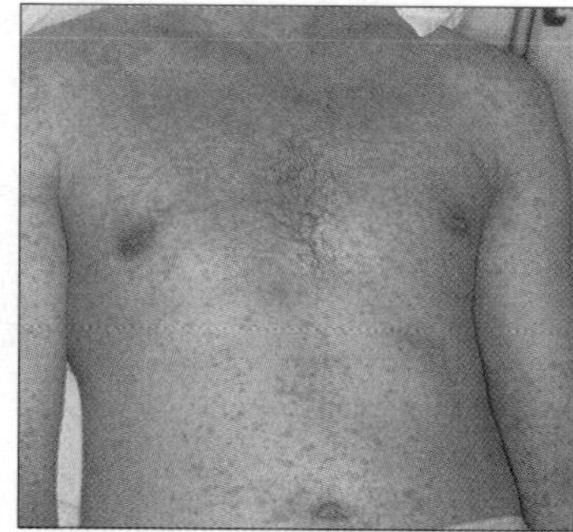

Fine nonblotchy rash of rubella.

Investigations

• The diagnosis of rubella is established serologically.

• A patient's unconfirmed history of rubella should be discounted.

Serology: IgM detectable in serum within 1–2 days of rash; hemagglutination-inhibiting antibodies rise within 1–2 days of rash, peak in 6–12 days, and thereafter fade but remain detectable at lower levels.

Complications

General

Arthralgia or arthritis of fingers, wrists, and knees: usually in young women.

Encephalitis.

Thrombocytopenia.

Neuritis.

Congenital rubella

Cataract, retinopathy, microphthalmos, glaucoma.

Patent ductus arteriosus, ventricular septal defect, pulmonary stenosis.

Deafness.

Thrombocytopenic purpura, hepatosplenomegaly, hepatitis, CNS defects, bone lesions.

Differential diagnosis

• Patients with rubella are usually well and the rash is not blotchy.

Measles: marked prodrome, malaise, dusky-red maculopapular erythematous rash that travels down body over 3 days.

Adenovirus or enterovirus infections, mild scarlet fever, cytomegalovirus or Epstein–Barr virus infection, toxoplasmosis.

Etiology

• Infection is by rubella virus, an RNA virus.

• Transmission is by respiratory droplets.

• Fetal infection occurs secondary to maternal viremia; the incidence and type of defect are related to the age of the fetus at the time of infection.

• Significant defects are found with early infection.

Epidemiology

• Rubella occurs worldwide.

Infectivity

• ~16% of affected infants have major defects at birth after maternal rubella in the first trimester.

• Rubella is moderately infectious: patients are infectious during the rash and probably for ~7 days before and up to 5 days after illness, although the virus is detectable in throat secretions up to 10 days before and until 16 days after the rash.

• Babies with congenital rubella excrete the virus in throat and urine for prolonged periods.

Mean incubation period

~18 days.

Treatment

Diet and lifestyle

- No special diet is necessary.
- Affected patients should keep away from pregnant women.

Pharmacological treatment

Symptomatic

Analgesics, *e.g.*, acetaminophen.

Prophylactic

- Vaccination is by live attenuated virus: this may produce a mild rubella-like illness; women should not be pregnant or become so within 8–12 weeks of vaccination.
- It is routinely recommended in the second year of life as part of MMR, for 10–14-year-old girls at present, and any identified susceptible adult women of childbearing potential.
- Prompt serological testing of pregnant contacts of a patient with rubella is essential to assess susceptibility.
- The use of hyperimmune globulin should be considered if the risk is significant and if therapeutic abortion would not be considered should rubella develop later.

Treatment aims

To relieve symptoms.

To prevent congenital rubella.

Prognosis

- The prognosis in rubella is excellent.
- Deaths are rare and usually associated with encephalitis.

Follow-up and management

- Follow-up and management is not needed except in pregnancy, when risks and discussion of termination should be considered.

General references

Anonymous: *Immunization against Infectious Diseases.* London: HMSO; 1992

Miller E, *et al.*: Rubella surveillance to June 1994. *Comm Dis Rep* 1994, **4**:R146–R152.

Morgan-Capner P. Diagnosing rubella. *BMJ* 1989; **229**:338–339.

Diagnosis

Symptoms

• Patients may have no respiratory symptoms.

Dyspnea: on exertion.

Cough: usually unproductive.

Chest discomfort: vague intermittent ache.

Fatigue, malaise, weight loss, fever, anorexia.

Symptoms of the complications of sarcoidosis.

Signs

Fine inspiratory crackles and wheezes: rarely.

Lymphadenopathy.

Uveitis, keratoconjunctivitis sicca, retinopathy.

Erythema nodosum, skin nodules, maculopapular rash, lupus pernio.

Nasopharyngitis.

Hepatomegaly, splenomegaly, portal hypertension.

Bone cysts, polyarthralgia, myopathy.

Investigations [1]

Chest radiography: 90% of patients have abnormal radiographs, which show a wide variety of appearances (*see* Clinical staging).

Pulmonary function tests: may be entirely within normal limits, despite extensive radiographic shadows, or may show significant physiological dysfunction with clear radiographical lung fields. A restrictive defect is most common.

Tuberculin skin test: negative in two-thirds of patients.

Blood tests: leukocyte count may show lymphopenia; ESR may be raised; serum immunoglobulins and electrophoresis may show panhyperglobulinemia; serum angiotensin-converting enzyme increased in two-thirds of acute patients; hypercalcemia in ~18% of patients; liver function indices in a few may show intrahepatic cholestasis.

24-h urine collection: hypercalciuria may be present despite normal serum calcium concentration.

ECG: arrhythmias, bundle branch block pattern in some patients.

Biopsy of lymph node, lung tissue, skin, liver, or other tissue: shows noncaseating epithelioid granulomata.

Fiberoptic bronchoscopy with transbronchial biopsy: the procedure of choice in patients with suspected pulmonary involvement.

Bronchoalveolar lavage: may be helpful adjunct to diagnosis; many patients with "active" sarcoidosis show increased percentage of lymphocytes, predominantly of the "helper" T-cell type; as fibrosis develops, an increase in neutrophils occurs.

• Special situations may call for the following: ^{67}Ga scans (often positive in sarcoidosis); radioactive ^{201}Tl (taken by sarcoid tissue and by ischaemic myocardium); high resolution CT scan (with MRI, may be particularly useful in unusual or difficult diagnostic circumstances such as neurosarcoidosis); ophthalmological assessment, including slit lamp examination and fluorescein angiography (needed in patients with associated occular symptoms).

Complications

Peripheral neuropathy, facial-nerve palsy, other cranial-nerve palsies, papilledema, meningitis, space-occupying lesions, epilepsy, cerebellar ataxia, hypopituitarism, diabetes insipidus.

Bundle branch block, arrhythmias, congestive cardiac failure, pericarditis, cardiomyopathy, cor pulmonale.

Disordered calcium metabolism, hypercalcemia, hypercalciuria, nephrocalcinosis.

Enlarged parotid and lacrimal glands.

Glaucoma, cataract: complication of chronic uveitis.

Differential diagnosis

Hilar lymphadenopathy

Tuberculosis, Hodgkin's lymphoma, infectious mononucleosis, leukemia, metastases, enlarged pulmonary arteries.

Hilar lymphadenopathy with pulmonary infiltration

Tuberculosis, pneumoconiosis, lymphangitic carcinoma, idiopathic hemosiderosis, pulmonary eosinophilia, alveolar-cell carcinoma, histiocytosis X.

Diffuse pulmonary infiltration

The above and also chronic beryllium disease, honeycomb lung, rheumatoid lung, Sjögren's syndrome, interstitial lung disease, cystic fibrosis, hypersensitivity pneumonitis.

Noncaseating granulomata

Tuberculosis and other mycobacterial infections, fungal infections, leprosy, syphillis, cat-scratch disease, berylliosis, hypersensitivity pneumonitis, foreign-body reactions, lymphoma, carcinoma, biliary cirrhosis, Crohn's disease, hypogammaglobulinemia, granulomatous vasculitides, parasitic infection.

Etiology [2,3]

• The cause is unknown, but the following may have a role:

Transmittable agents.

An atypical reaction to tuberculosis or other mycobacteria.

Genetic predisposition.

Epidemiology

• Sarcoidosis is usually manifest in the 20–40-year age group.

• It is more usual in temperate than in tropical climates.

• The prevalence rates are difficult to establish because the disease is often asymptomatic; in the US, the incidence is 40 in 100 000 population.

• Sarcoidosis is more prevalent and tends to be more chronic in blacks, who have higher risk of nonrespiratory manifestations.

Clinical staging

Stage 0: normal chest (5%–10% of patients).

Stage I: bilateral hilar adenopathy (50%).

Stage II: bilateral hilar adenopathy and peripheral pulmonary infiltration; paratracheal nodes may also be enlarged (25%).

Stage III: parenchymal infiltration only (15%).

Treatment

Diet and lifestyle

• No special precautions are necessary.

Pharmacological treatment

• Treatment is not needed in many patients because the disability is mild and remission is usual.

Corticosteroids

• These can suppress the manifestations of acute sarcoidosis, with rapid clearing of radiographic lesions; whether they alter the long-term outcome or prevent development of late fibrosis if started early remains unproven.

Standard dosage Prednisone, 30–60 mg daily for 4–6 weeks; with rapid tapering to 15 mg daily for 3 months.

Contraindications Uncontrolled hypertension, diabetes mellitus, infection, severe osteoporosis.

Special points Relapses treated by increased dose; some patients with objective evidence of relapse on >3 occasions may need long-term low-dose maintenance prednisone.

Main drug interactions Antihypertensive drugs.

Main side effects Weight gain, edema, bruising, purple striae in skin (particularly abdomen), moon face, osteoporosis, collapse of vertebrae, diabetes mellitus, hypertension, myopathy (especially proximal girdle muscles), hirsutism, menstrual disturbances, psychotic reactions, cataracts, withdrawal phenomena.

Immunosuppressants

• Treatment should be given under specialist supervision.

• In resistant cases, immunosuppressants are sometimes partially effective (*e.g.*, chloroquine, methotrexate).

Standard dosage Chloroquine, 200 mg on alternate days for up to 9 months.
Methotrexate, 10 mg once weekly for 3 months; repeated courses every 6 months, possibly with oral steroids or chloroquine, may be necessary in some patients.

Contraindications Hepatic and renal impairment.

Special points Chloroquine usually given with low-dose steroids.

Main drug interactions Alcohol, NSAIDs, antacids.

Main side effects *Chloroquine:* visual disturbances, irreversible retinal damage, corneal opacities.
Methotrexate: hepatic fibrosis, acute bone-marrow suppression.

NSAIDs

• Anti-inflammatory agents are usually used in acute "exudative" sarcoidosis, *e.g.*, in patients with acute uveitis, phlyctenular conjunctivitis, polyarthritis, and erythema nodosum.

Standard dosage Indomethacin, 50–200 mg daily in divided doses, with food.

Contraindications Active peptic ulceration; severe renal, cardiac, and hepatic failure.

Main drug interactions Angiotensin-converting enzyme inhibitors, anticoagulants, antidiabetics, antidepressants, 4-quinolones.

Main side effects Gastrointestinal disturbances, ulceration, and bleeding, blood disorders (thrombocytopenia), headache, dizziness.

Treatment aims

To prevent development of irreversible pulmonary fibrosis.

Prognosis [4,5]

• 50% of patients remit spontaneously.

• Accompanying hilar adenopathy usually regresses within ~1 year.

• ~10% of patients develop parenchymal lesions, of which many resolve within 1 year.

• ~40% of patients resolve spontaneously within 1 year; the rest may progress with varying speed to irreversible fibrosis, which, in severely ill patients, may be complicated by upper-zone bullous disease and aspergillomas, with recurrent infection and haemoptysis.

Follow-up and management

• Regular clinical review is needed for patients being treated by steroids or immunosuppressants.

Key references

1. Winterbauer R, Belic N, Moores K: A clinical interpretation of bilateral hilar adenopathy. *Ann Intern Med* 1973, **78**:65–71.
2. Mitchell IC, Turk JL, Mitchell DN: Detection of mycobacterial rRNA in sarcoidosis with liquid-phase hybridisation. *Lancet* 1992, **339**:1015–1017.
3. Nakata K, *et al.*: Gamma-delta T-cells in sarcoidosis. Correlation with clinical features. *Am J Respir Crit Care Med* 1994, **149**:981–988.
4. Spiteri MA, Clarke SW, Poulter LW: Alveolar macrophages that suppress T-cell responsiveness may be crucial to pathogenic outcome of pulmonary sarcoidosis. *Eur Respir J* 1992, **5**:394–403.
5. Hunninghake G, *et al.*: Outcome of the treatment for sarcoidosis. *Am J Respir Crit Care Med* 1994, **149**:893–898.

Diagnosis

Symptoms and signs

Prodromal

Not always obvious.
Deteriorating social and occupational function.
Odd behavior.
Depressed mood.
Schizotypal, schizoid, or paranoid personality traits.

Positive symptoms

Hallucinations: auditory or visual are most common, but any modality may occur.
Delusions: may include paranoid, jealous, grandiose, somatic, erotomanic, and religious types; ideas of reference are frequent; though control, reading, broadcasting, echoing, insertion, and withdrawal are common.
Disorganized, loose, or incoherent speech.
Grossly disorganized behavior.
Catatonic behavior.

Negative symptoms

Flat or blunted affect.
Paucity of speech; poverty of content of speech.
Poor hygiene and grooming.
Loss of interest, goals, motivation, and drive.
Anhedonia.
Loss of social interest.
Inability to experience intimacy and closeness.
Loss of sexual interest.
Poor attention and concentration.

Residual symptoms

Odd beliefs and behaviors.
Deterioration in social and occupational function.
Persistent negative symptoms.

Investigations

• No laboratory test is diagnostic, and no single clinical feature is pathognomonic; the diagnosis requires a pattern of both positive and negative symptoms, after medical and affective causes of psychosis have been systematically eliminated [1,2].

• Known medical causes of psychosis must be ruled out by the following tests:

For all patients

Comprehensive history and physical examination.
Toxicology screen.
Chemistry panel.
Complete blood count (CBC).
CT or MRI: of brain.
Thyroid function tests.
Syphilis serology: fluorescent treponemal antibody (FTA) or rapid plasma reagin (RPR).

If clinically indicated

Cerebrospinal fluid studies: glucose, cell count, protein, and VDRL.
HIV antibody screen.
Antinuclear antibody (ANA).
Heavy metals screen.
EEG.
B_{12} and folate levels.
ESR, ceruloplasmin, blood copper, and 24-h urine copper.
Tuberculin skin test.
Polysomnography.
24-hour urine porphyrin screen.
Lyme antibody.
Psychological testing.

Complications

Suicide: 10% of deaths.
Depression: occurs in 50% of cases, most often after an acute episode.
Homelessness.
Crime: unclear if there is an increased incidence of violent crime perpetrated by schizophrenic patients; these patients are more often the victims than the perpetrators of both violent and nonviolent crimes.
Substance abuse.

Differential diagnosis

Drug-induced psychoses.
Affective disorders.
Delusional disorders.
Personality disorders.
Seizure disorder.
Other neurological disorders.
Other metabolic and autoimmune disorders.
Toxic exposures.
Malingering and factitious disorders.

Etiology

• The cause of schizophrenia is unclear, but the following are considered to have a role:
Genetics: 50% concordance for monozygotic twins.
In utero and perinatal complications.
Increased ventricle-to-brain ratio [1].
Increased subcortical dopamine activity.
Decreased prefrontal dopamine activity.

Epidemiology

• The lifetime risk of schizophrenia is 1%.
• Age of onset is 17–30 for men, and 20–40 for women [1].
• Annual incidence is 15–20 in 100 000.

Clinical course

• Prodromal symptoms typically predate the diagnosis by months or years.
• Positive symptoms tend to occur episodically, in acute episodes, which are the most common cause of hospitalization.
• Negative symptoms tend to be chronic and progressive and are correlated with social and occupational deterioration.
• Residual symptoms tend to remain even when other symptoms are well controlled [1].

Treatment

Diet and lifestyle

Not relevant.

Pharmacological treatment

• Antipsychotic (neuroleptic) medications are generally required for acute and maintenance treatment.

Haloperidol

Useful for control of psychotic symptoms and acute agitation; available in pill, concentrate, injectable, and depot forms.

Standard dosage	Haloperidol, 5-20 mg/d orally for acute psychosis and maintenance; 2-5 mg i.m. for acute agitation.
Contraindications	Coma, bone-marrow depression, closed-angle glaucoma.
Main drug interactions	Enhanced sedative effect with other CNS depressants.
Main side effects	Extrapyramidal symptoms (muscle rigidity, bradykinesia, dystonic reactions, restlessness, and tremor), anticholinergic effects (dry mouth, constipation, blurred vision, urinary hesitancy), sedation, tardive dyskinesia.
Special considerations	Neuroleptic malignant syndrome is a rare (1%) but potentially lethal complication.

Risperidone

Good for first-episode and long-term treatment of psychosis in compliant patients [3].

Standard dosage	2-6 mg/d, usually given twice daily.
Contraindications	None.
Main drug interactions	Enhanced sedative effect with other CNS depressants.
Main side effects	Hypotension, sedation, extrapyrimidal symptoms at higher doses (restlessness, tremor, muscle rigidity, bradykinesia, and dystonic reactions), tardive dyskinesia.
Special considerations	High cost relative to typical neuroleptics; available only in pill form.

Other drugs

• Depot neuroleptics: haloperidol and fluphenazine decanoate are available for i.m. injection every 1-4 weeks. Good option for noncompliant patients.

• Clozapine: For patients who have not responded to, or cannot tolerate, at least two conventional antipsychotics. Because of the 1%-2% risk of agranulocytosis, weekly complete blood count monitoring is required throughout treatment [4].

• Anticholinergic drugs: benztropine, 2-8 mg/d given 2 or 4 times daily, is effective for extrapyramidal side effects.

• Propranolol, 20-160 mg/d given 2 or 4 times daily, may be effective for akathisia (restlessness).

• Lorazepam, 1-6 mg/d given 4 times daily, may be used for akathisia or agitation. For violent patients, 1-2 mg i.m. may be administered alone or with haloperidol.

• Lithium: Particularly useful when affective symptoms are present; doses of 600-1800 mg/d given 2 or 3 times daily, are typically required to maintain the optimal serum level of 0.8-1.2 mEq/L.

Nonpharmacologic treatment

• Social skills training may reduce deficits related to negative symptoms [5].

• Vocational rehabilitation is often useful to maintain some level of employment.

• Behavioral therapy may reduce unacceptable behavior.

• Family psychoeducation is valuable to increase participation in, tolerance of, and understanding of the patient's symptoms and treatments.

• Civil commitment may be sought when involuntary hospitalization and treatment are required.

• Electroconvulsive therapy may be useful for catatonia or very severe psychosis.

Treatment aims

Acute: to ensure safety and to resolve psychotic symptoms.

Long-term: to prevent relapse and deterioration and to provide psychosocial rehabilitation.

Prognosis

• 75%–80% of untreated patients relapse within 2 years.

• 20%–25% of patients treated with conventional neuroleptics relapse within 2 years.

• 25%–30% of patients do not respond to conventional neuroleptics.

• 10%–15% of patients respond only to clozapine, not to other antipsychotics.

Follow-up and management

• Lifelong treatment is usually required.

• Maintenance neuroleptic is essential in most cases to prevent relapse.

• Medication noncompliance is the major reason for relapse.

• The risk of suicide and aggression must be monitored.

• Interdisciplinary, community-based treatment is preferred as follows:
The case manager monitors treatment compliance; availability of treatment resources; and provision of food , clothing, and shelter.
The social worker handles financial and legal issues; a payee may be required.
The psychiatric nurse or technician may administer medication and help monitor treatment response and side effects.

Key references

1. Carpenter WT Jr, Buchanan RW: Schizophrenia. *N Engl J Med* 1994, **330**:681–690.
2. Johnstone EC: Schizophrenia: problems in clinical practice. *Lancet* 1993, **341**:536–538.
3. Marder SR, Meibach RC: Risperidone in the treatment of schizophrenia. *Am J Psychiatry* 1994, **151**:825–835.
4. Baldessarini R, Frankenberg F: Clozapine: a novel antipsychotic agent. *N Engl J Med* 1991, **324**:746–754.
5. McGlashan TH, *et al.*: Psychosocial treatment of negative symptoms in schizophrenia. In *Modern Problems in Pharmacopsychiatry*. Edited by Andreason NC. New York: Karger; 1990:175–200.

Diagnosis

Symptoms

• Symptoms of hypotensive shock are nonspecific; they include the following:

Restlessness.

Confusion or stupor.

Breathlessness.

Chest pain.

• Symptoms of the underlying cause may predominate.

Signs

Hypotension: a useful definition is systolic blood pressure <90 mm Hg.

Oliguria: <30 mL/h.

Cyanosis.

Confusion.

Peripheral vasoconstriction or vasodilatation: may indicate high or low systemic vascular resistance, respectively.

Tachycardia and third heart sound.

Investigations

Initial investigations

Full blood count, hematocrit, U&E, toxicology screen, and creatinine analysis.

Cardiac enzyme analysis: if myocardial injury suspected.

Blood culture: if any infective process known or suspected.

Arterial blood gas analysis: to assess hypoxemia and acidosis.

ECG and chest radiography: mandatory.

Circulatory assessment

• This should ideally be done in an intensive care unit.

Central venous cannulation: to measure central venous pressure.

Arterial cannulation: sphygmomanometry may be unreliable in shock.

Pulmonary artery catheterization: for pulmonary artery pressure, pulmonary capillary wedge pressure, and thermodilution cardiac output.

Echocardiography: for left ventricular function or if valve lesion, ventricular septal defect, or tamponade suspected.

Complications

Myocardial ischemia or infarction.

Acute renal failure.

Ischemic stroke.

Hepatic dysfunction.

Paralytic ileus.

Lactic acidosis: an indicator of severe tissue hypoxia.

Differential diagnosis

Not applicable.

Etiology

Central venous pressure < –3 cm H_2O*
Indicates hypovolemia.
Warm peripheries (low systemic vascular resistance): vasodilatation due to septicemia or drug overdose.
Cool peripheries (high systemic resistance): normal hemoglobin or hematocrit indicates hemorrhage; high hemoglobin indicates salt and water loss, *e.g.*, from peritonitis, pancreatitis, diabetic ketoacidosis, burns, polyuric phase of acute tubular necrosis.

Central venous pressure > +1 cm H_2O*
Indicates "pump failure."
Tension pneumothorax.
Pulmonary embolism.
Impaired myocardial contractility due to acute myocardial infarction or ischemia, sepsis, acidemia, electrolyte disturbance, negatively inotropic agents (*e.g.*, beta antagonists, antiarrhythmic agents).
Arrhythmia.
Cardiac tamponade.
Ruptured interventricular septum.
Acute mitral or aortic valve regurgitation.
Aortic stenosis.

*Measured from the sternal angle.

Epidemiology

Not applicable.

Septicemia and hypotensive shock

• The circulatory hallmark of sepsis is an unpredictable derangement of regional blood flow. Inappropriate vasodilatation of muscle and skin arterioles may coexist with profound vasoconstriction of the renal and splanchnic vascular beds.
• The hypotension has many causes, *e.g.*, a fall in systemic vascular resistance to <25% of normal, depression of myocardial contractility by hypoxemia and acidemia, dilatation of venous capacitance vessels resulting in low central venous pressure, and disruption of capillary function causing leakage of intravascular fluid and plasma proteins into alveoli, gastrointestinal tract, peritoneal cavity, and other tissues.
• The combination of myocardial impairment and damage to alveolar capillary basement membranes means that attempts to restore the blood pressure by rapid intravenous infusion of fluid will probably result in pulmonary edema.

Treatment

Diet and lifestyle

Not applicable.

Pharmacological treatment

- Whenever possible, the underlying cause should be treated.
- Immediate measures include the following:

Provision of oxygen: hypoxemia contributes to lactic acid production.
Treatment of arrhythmias: cardioversion preferable to negatively inotropic antiarrhythmic drugs.
Plasma expander administration, if central venous pressure < –3 cm H_2O.
Correction of any electrolyte disturbance.
Broad-spectrum antibiotic treatment, if sepsis suspected.
Inotropic support for hypotension without hypovolemia, as follows:

For oliguria

- Dopamine is the first choice in oliguria; it enhances renal blood flow at a low dose, inotropic and vasoconstrictor at doses >5 µg/kg/min (beta$_1$, alpha agonism). It must be administered centrally.

Standard dosage	Dopamine, 3–5 µg/kg/min.
Contraindications	Pheochromocytoma.
Main drug interactions	Monoamine oxidase inhibitors.
Main side effects	Vomiting, tachycardia, angina, headache.

After myocardial infarction

- Dobutamine is the first choice after myocardial infarction; it is predominantly a beta$_1$ agonist; it improves myocardial oxygen supply : demand ratio and causes peripheral vasodilatation (hence its use if the systemic vascular resistance is high).

Standard dosage	Dobutamine, 5–20 µg/kg/min.
Contraindications	Outflow tract obstruction, proarrhythmic tendencies.
Main drug interactions	Hypotension with other vasodilators.
Main side effects	Tachycardia, local phlebitis, hypokalemia.

For severe hypotension

- Epinephrine is the most positively inotropic catecholamine; it acts as a beta agonist at low dose, and an alpha agonist at doses >10 µg/min and causes peripheral vasoconstriction (hence its use if systemic vascular resistance is low).

Standard dosage	Epinephrine, 2–40 µg/min.
Contraindications	Hypertension, tachyarrhythmias.
Main drug interactions	Inhalational anesthetics, tricyclic antidepressants.
Main side effects	Tachycardia, arrhythmias.

For bradycardia, atrioventricular block, and right heart failure

- Isoproterenol is used in bradycardia, atrioventricular block, and right heart failure; it causes pulmonary and systemic vasodilatation; it worsens myocardial supply : demand ratio and ventilation/perfusion mismatch.

Standard dosage	Isoproterenol, 1–10 µg/min.
Contraindications	Cardiac ischemia, hyperthyroidism.
Main drug interactions	Inhalational anesthetics, tricyclic antidepressants.
Main side effects	Atrial and ventricular tachyarrhythmias.

If systemic vascular resistance is profoundly low

- Norepinephrine is used if the systemic vascular resistance is profoundly low; its alpha agonism causes vasoconstriction; a rise in blood pressure occurs at the expense of a fall in cardiac output.

Standard dosage	Norepinephrine, 1–10 µg/min.
Contraindications	Myocardial dysfunction.
Main drug interactions	Tricyclic antidepressants.
Main side effects	Digit necrosis, myocardial ischemia.

Treatment aims

To increase cardiac output, blood pressure, and tissue oxygen delivery to a level that avoids the detrimental end-organ effects of anaerobic metabolism and lactic acid production [1].

Other treatments

Mechanical ventilation

- This allows effective correction of hypoxemia and eliminates the work of breathing (most useful in acute left ventricular failure).

Intra-aortic balloon pump

- This is a temporary measure (24–48 h) while spontaneous improvement or definitive treatment (*e.g.*, valve or ventricular septal defect repair) is awaited.
- It is useful in cardiac surgery and refractory unstable angina.
- Complications, in 20% of patients, include leg ischemia, aortic dissection, hemolysis, thrombocytopenia, infection.

Surgery

- Surgery is indicated early in rupture of interventricular septum or papillary muscle, aortic dissection, and subacute myocardial rupture causing tamponade.

Prognosis

- The main determinant of outcome is the underlying disorder: for example, hypotension due to diabetic ketoacidosis in a young person has a favorable prognosis, whereas cardiogenic shock resulting from acute anterior myocardial infarction has a mortality of 80%–90%.

Follow-up and management

- No follow-up is needed.

Key reference

1. Weil MH, *et al.*: Acute Circulatory Failure. In *Heart Disease* edn 4. Edited by Braunwald E. Philadelphia: WB Saunders; 1992:569–587.

Sickle cell disease

Diagnosis

Symptoms

• Patients with SS and Sβ° thalassemia are generally more severely affected than those with SC, Sβ⁺ being the mildest disorder.

Acute painful vaso-occlusive crisis: causes >90% of hospital admissions affecting bones, joints, and muscles; initial presentation in one-third is the "hand foot" syndrome from age of 4 months; limb pain in older children, more central pain distribution in adolescents and adults.

Chronic pain: in hip or shoulders, caused by avascular necrosis.

Signs

• Often patients present with no signs in mild crisis.

Constitutional upset mimicking septicemia: in severe crisis (infection can precipitate crisis).

Localized swelling, tenderness, and redness of bone, joint, or muscle.

Abdominal pain mimicking more severe disease.

Limited range of hip or shoulder movement: with active avascular necrosis.

Investigations

For diagnosis

• Investigations should be made preferably when the patient is in an unstable state.

Full blood count: to establish degree of anemia.

Reticulocyte count: to establish degree of hemolysis.

Hemoglobin electrophoresis: to determine variant hemoglobins.

"Sickle test": to confirm presence of hemoglobin S.

Hemoglobin F estimation: high concentrations diminish severity.

Extended erythrocyte grouping: to ensure appropriate erythrocytes for transfusion.

Plasma blood urea nitrogen, creatinine, electrolytes analysis: to monitor renal function.

Liver function tests: to monitor hemolysis and exclude hepatitis.

In crisis

• The results should be compared with those from the stable state.

Full blood count: hemoglobin raised with dehydration; falls in sequestration and aplasia.

Blood urea nitrogen, creatinine, electrolytes analysis: to detect dehydration.

Liver function tests: to measure dysfunction.

Cultures and viral screening: urine, blood, sputum, throat swab; to exclude infection (before antibiotic treatment); screening for parvovirus (not routine unless severely anemic).

Reticulocyte count.

Viral screen, chest radiography, blood gas and arterial oxygen saturation measurement: if patient has chest pain or signs.

Complications

Stroke: in 8% of patients, median age 7 years.

Sequestration syndromes: common cause of death; erythrocytes pooled in the organ, causing hemoglobin to fall by ≤2 g/dL, leading to dysfunction of the following organs: spleen (in infants; high risk of recurrence), liver (in children and adults), chest (a medical emergency, exchange transfusion if partial arterial oxygen pressure <60 mm Hg), splanchnic circulation (in adults, clinical picture of paralytic ileus that resolves spontaneously).

Infection: common and serious or life-threatening because of autosplenectomy, therefore susceptible to encapsulated bacteria, especially *Streptococcus pneumoniae* and *Salmonella* spp., aplastic crisis due to parvovirus B19.

Priapism, proliferative retinopathy, cholecystitis and cholelithiasis secondary to hemolysis.

Differential diagnosis

• It can be difficult to distinguish simple vaso-occlusive crisis from that associated with infection.

• Other diseases may also manifest (*e.g.*, appendicitis) or coexist.

Etiology

• Sickle cell disease is inherited in a Mendelian recessive manner.

• Clinical problems also occur when hemoglobin S interacts with other variant hemoglobins (*e.g.*, SC) and with a β-thalassemia gene (β° or β⁺).

Epidemiology

• It is rarely manifest before the age of 4–6 months because of the continued production of fetal hemoglobin due to the late switching off of the fetal hemoglobin gene.

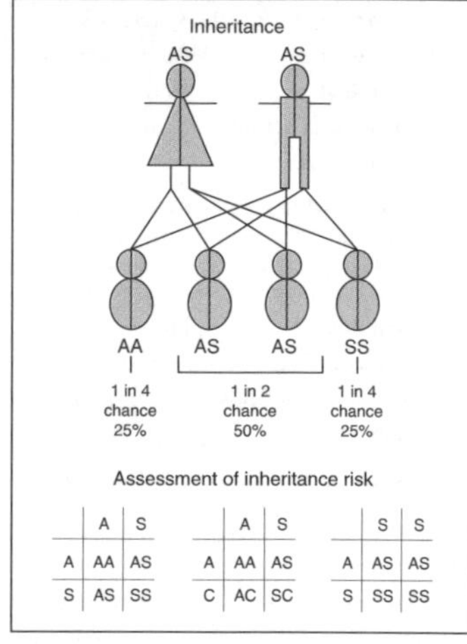

Assessment of inheritance risk. Among Jamaican and American sickle cell patients of African heritage, 50%–70% are Benin, 15%–30% are Bantu-CAR, and 5%–15% are Senegal haplotypes.

Treatment

Diet and lifestyle

• Patients should avoid factors that precipitate painful crisis, *e.g.*, infection, dehydration, exhaustion, cold, marked temperature changes, smoking, high altitude, and unpressurized aircraft; in some patients, stress is reported to be a precipitant.

Pharmacological treatment [2,3]

Analgesia

Standard dosage *For mild to moderate pain*: acetaminophen, 12–15 mg/kg 8-hourly, codeine phosphate, 1–2 mg/kg 6-hourly (up to 3 mg/kg in 24 h), or NSAIDs, all orally.
For severe pain: morphine, 0.1 mg/kg i.v. loading dose, then 1–2 mg/kg i.v. infusion over 24 h using patient-controlled analgesia system, or meperidine, 50–150 mg i.m. every 1–4 h in adults.

Contraindications *Oral drugs*: hepatic and renal impairment, peptic ulceration, asthma.
Parenteral drugs: raised intracranial pressure.

Special points *Meperidine*: respiratory rate must be monitored hourly.

Main drug interactions *Codeine and morphine:* alcohol, anxiolytics and hypnotics, domperidone and metoclopramide, cimetidine.
Diclofenac: caution with other analgesics, anticoagulants, antihypertensives, beta-blockers, and cardiac glycosides.

Main side effects *Oral drugs*: rashes, blood dyscrasias, acute pancreatitis, constipation, respiratory depression.
Morphine: respiratory depression, nausea, bronchospasm, severe pruritus.
Meperidine: seizures.

Antibiotics

• Antibiotics are indicated for patients in severe crisis or when infection is suspected.

Standard dosage Amoxicillin, 500 mg 3 times daily.

Contraindications Penicillin allergy.

Special points If pneumococcal infection is suspected, penicillin should be added.

Main drug interactions Anticoagulants, antacids, oral contraceptives.

Main side effects Nausea, diarrhea, rashes, pseudomembranous colitis.

Nonpharmacological treatment

Rehydration

Oral fluids increased in patients with mild pain; i.v. clear fluids in patients with severe pain at 80 mL/kg/24 h.

Oxygen treatment

60% oxygen if partial arterial oxygen pressure on air is <60 mm Hg; 35% if 60–70 mm Hg; 28% if 70–80 mm Hg.

Blood transfusion

See Transfusion medicine *for further details.*

Additive: when hemoglobin <5 g/dL and patient symptomatic from anemia; for aplastic crisis, sequestration, bleeding (*e.g.*, renal papillary necrosis).

Exchange: when hemoglobin >5 g/dL but improved oxygen transport needed.
overall aim: hemoglobin S <20%, total hemoglobin 11–14.5 g/dL (possibly 3–4 procedures); for chest syndrome (if partial arterial oxygen pressure <60 mm Hg), priapism (if >4 h), acute neurological deficit or splanchnic sequestration, severe or protracted crisis (occasionally), preoperatively in selected patients.

Long-term transfusion: to maintain hemoglobin at 11–14.5 g/dL, with hemoglobin S <25%; for neurological deficit, sickle chronic lung disease, prevention of pain (occasionally), pregnant women (selected).

Treatment aims

To provide early and effective relief of pain.
To treat infection.
To maintain hydration.
To maintain tissue oxygenation.

Prognosis

• All types of sickle cell disease are variable in clinical manifestations; no markers exist to predict severity for a particular patient.
• 87% of patients are alive at 20 years, 50% at 50 years.
• Deaths in childhood are most commonly due to infection.
• Deaths in adolescents and young adults are most commonly due to neurological and lung complications.
• Deaths in middle age are most commonly due to chronic organ failure.
• Successful outcome after bone-marrow transplantation has now been recorded and drugs that raise hemoglobin F levels look promising.

Follow-up and management

• Full education and counseling must be ensured, with family screening and genetic advice.
• Penicillin prophylaxis must be ensured for children, and antipneumococcal and hemophilus B vaccination should be considered.
• Children should be checked for upper airways obstruction.

Key references

1. Davies SC: Bone marrow transplant for sickle cell disease. *Blood Reviews* 1992, 7:4–9.
2. Davies SC, Wonke B: The management of haemoglobinopathies. *Baillière's Clin Haematol* 1991, 4:361–389.
3. Embury SH, *et al.*: *Sickle Cell Disease: Basic Principles and Clinical Practice.* New York: Raven Press; 1994.

Diagnosis

Symptoms and signs

Impetigo

Isolated lesions or multiple small areas of golden yellow crusts, weeping areas, blisters: ruptured lesions leave raw areas.

Erysipelas

Inflammation substantially limited to skin, erythema with well defined and palpable margins, swelling, local heat, mild superficial pain, fever and malaise.

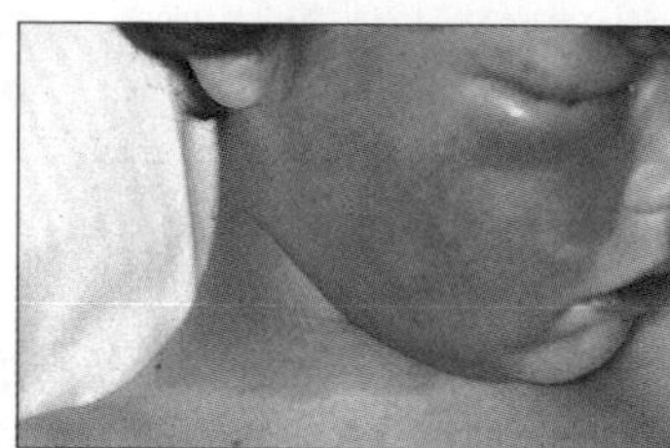

Erysipelas.

Deep infections

More swelling, deeper pain, less well defined edges than in erysipelas, perhaps crepitus on palpation, and overlying skin necrosis: indicating cellulitis.

Boils or abscesses: focal areas of pus formation, often painful, abscesses may be enlarged and pointing.

Severe boil with central necrosis and multiple discharging sinuses: carbuncle.

Methicillin-resistant *Staphylococcus aureus* infections

• Patients are usually asymptomatic, *i.e.*, colonized, but some may have local or generalized life-threatening sepsis.

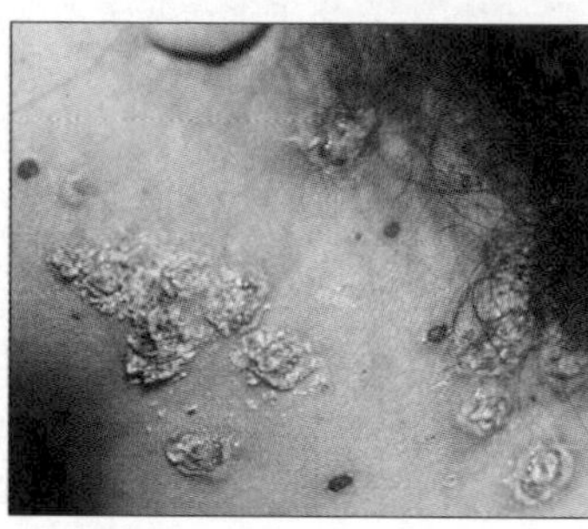

Impetigo.

Investigations

Microbiology: areas of impetigo should be swabbed; methicillin-resistant *Staphylococcus aureus* infection cannot be diagnosed clinically; swabs should be taken from nose, throat, perineum, eczematous areas, axillae, sputum, urine (if catheter present), any site of possible infection (including surgical wounds), intravenous access points; often not needed for classic erysipelas; if confirmation of causative organism of erysipelas or cellulitis desired, a few milliliters of saline solution can be injected into involved area and immediately aspirated (using same needle, which should not be withdrawn); site of entry of infection should be swabbed; abscess pus should be sent for microscopy and culture.

Blood culture: if skin is intact over areas of cellulitis.

Complications

Lymphangitis, scarlet fever, septicemia, poststreptococcal rheumatic fever: rare complications of erysipelas.

Spread of infection to contiguous tissue, septicemia: complications of cellulitis.

Rupture, septicemia: complications of boils.

Differential diagnosis

Not applicable.

Etiology

• Impetigo is usually caused by *Staphylococcus aureus*, especially when bullous, occasionally by *Streptococcus pyogenes*.

• Erysipelas is caused by *Strep. pyogenes*.

• Cellulitis is usually caused by *Strep. pyogenes* but also by a wide range of anaerobes, *e.g.*, *Clostridium perfringens*, and facultative anaerobes; often several pathogens are isolated.

• Boils and carbuncles are caused by *Staph. aureus*.

Epidemiology

• Up to 40% of the population are nasal carriers of *Staphylococcus aureus*.

• Where antibiotic use is intense, *e.g.*, hospitals, most staphylococci are resistant to penicillin but retain sensitivity to methicillin, cloxacillin, and floxacillin.

• Outbreaks of methicillin-resistant *S. aureus*, usually in hospitals, have been reported since 1960; some strains are virulent, whereas others are harmless unless they infect vulnerable patients.

• Most strains of methicillin-resistant *S. aureus* are resistant to other frequently used antibiotics, and some strains are highly transmissible ("epidemic strains").

• Pharyngeal carriage of *Streptococcus pyogenes* is more common in younger age groups and can reach 15%–20% in crowded conditions, especially in winter.

• Impetigo is most common in children aged 2–5 years in warm climates and with poor hygiene; the incidence increases in summer.

• The frequency and severity of invasive streptococcal disease has been increasing in the USA and Europe since the late 1980s.

Treatment

Diet and lifestyle

• No special precautions are necessary.

Pharmacological treatment

For erysipelas

• Erysipelas usually responds to penicillin parenterally if the illness is severe.

Standard dosage Penicillin G, 300–600 mg i.v. 6-hourly
Penicillin V, 500 mg orally 6-hourly.

Contraindications Hypersensitivity.

Special points Dicloxacillin or new macrolides are other options.

Main drug interactions None.

Main side effects Gastrointestinal disturbances, sensitivity reactions.

For cellulitis

• Usually dicloxacillin.

Standard dosage Dicloxacillin, 500 mg 4 times daily.

Contraindications Hypersensitivity.

Special points Erythromycin is an alternative.

Main drug interactions None.

Main side effects Gastrointestinal disturbances, sensitivity reactions.

For boils and abscesses

• No antibiotics are needed in the case of free drainage, with no surrounding inflammation.

• Otherwise, floxacillin or erythromycin should be used.

For methicillin-resistant *Staphylococcus aureus* (MRSA) infection

• If the patient is widely colonized, topical antiseptics can be tried (including triclosan, hexachlorophene, chlorhedixine, povidone-iodine), although success is uncertain.

• If the carriage is limited, particularly to the nose, topical mupirocin can be used.

• If the patient has an invasive infection or if eradication of MRSA is necessary to allow more appropriate treatment for underlying conditions, treatment with antibiotics under specialist supervision may be appropriate.

• MRSA strains are often sensitive to vancomycin or teicoplanin; fusidic acid, rifampin, or ciprofloxacin may also have a role.

Standard dosage Hexachlorophene applied sparingly every 4–6 h after washing.
Mupirocin applied to nares 3 times daily for up to 10 days.
Vancomycin, 1 g 2 times daily.

Contraindications *Hexachlorophene:* damaged skin, pregnancy, breast-feeding, children <2 years.
Mupirocin, vancomycin: hypersensitivity.

Main drug interactions *Vancomycin:* cholestyramine, aminoglycosides, loop diuretics.

Main side effects *Hexachlorophene:* redness (overgenerous application).
Mupirocin: minor burning, stinging, itching.
Vancomycin: hypotension, nephrotoxicity, ototoxicity, bone-marrow suppression, sensitivity reactions, phlebitis, muscle spasm.

• Clearance is accepted if weekly sets of screening swabs are negative over 3 weeks.

• Patients must initially be isolated on further admission, and continued carriage must be assessed.

Treatment aims

To eradicate infection.

To avoid spread of methicillin-resistant *Staphylococcus aureus* infection.

Other treatments

Surgical exploration to define the extent and nature of anaerobic cellulitis and to treat it.

Incision of pointing abscesses.

Prognosis

• Further attacks of erysipelas are common at the same site; patients should report promptly for antibiotic treatment.

Follow-up and management

• No follow-up is needed.

Prevention of spread of methicillin-resistant *Staphylococcus aureus* (MRSA)

• The patient must be isolated.
• The Infection Control Team must be contacted immediately.
• The source of the MRSA must be sought.
• The risk to other patients must be assessed.
• The patient's notes must be marked "MRSA infected."
• Infected staff must be identified and controlled.
• Hands must be washed after any patient contact.
• Gloves must be worn when infected tissue or dressings are being handled.
• Facemasks must be worn if exposure to infected aerosols is possible.
• "Infection Control" disposal of soiled material is vital.
• Rooms must be terminally disinfected.
• The patient can be discharged unless contacts are vulnerable; if discharge is not possible, infected individuals must be isolated (even if asymptomatic).
• Unnecessary staff–patient contact must be minimized (barrier nursing).
• The use of staff not familiar with the involved ward must be minimized.

General reference

Duckworth DJ: Diagnosis and management of methicillin resistant *Staphylococcus aureus* infection. *BMJ* 1993, **307**:1049–1052.

Diagnosis

Definition

• Central sleep apnea is a clinical syndrome with a range of causes, which can be loosely divided into two groups:

Neuromuscular weakness or chest-wall disease: the primary problem is inefficiency of the respiratory pump; patients may develop daytime ventilatory failure.

Periodic respiration (Cheyne–Stokes breathing): the primary problem is disordered respiratory feedback control; patients do not develop daytime ventilatory failure.

Symptoms

Daytime sleepiness, restless sleep, transient breathlessness: during the arousal and tachypnea that follow an apnea; symptoms of sleep disturbance.

Morning headache and nausea, poor exercise tolerance, ankle swelling, daytime breathlessness: only with neuromuscular or chest-wall disease; symptoms of respiratory failure.

Symptoms of primary causative disease.

Signs

Cyanosis, peripheral edema, raised venous pressure, signs of pulmonary hypertension or right ventricular hypertrophy: signs of ventilatory failure and cor pulmonale.

Raised venous pressure and edema: signs of heart failure.

Muscle fasciculation, weakness, loss of tendon reflex: signs of myopathy, dystrophy, motor neuron disease, postpoliomyelitis syndrome.

Supine breathlessness and paradoxical abdominal movement on sniffing: signs of diaphragm weakness due to bilateral phrenic palsy, acid maltase deficiency, or other muscular disease.

Upper motor neuron and brain stem signs: signs of stroke.

Chest-wall deformity: signs of scoliosis, thoracoplasty.

Investigations

Initial

Awake arterial oxygen saturation and blood gas analysis: for possible hypercapnia; alveolar–arterial oxygen gradient often normal.

Spirometry: to exclude chronic obstructive pulmonary disease and assess lung volume; daytime ventilatory failure with central sleep apnea rare if vital capacity >1.5 L standing; supine fall in forced vital capacity of >20% suggests marked diaphragm weakness.

Hemoglobin analysis: for polycythemia.

Nerve physiology, muscle biopsy, ECG, echocardiography: can also be considered.

Sleep studies [1]

• These are used to exclude obstructive sleep apnea, show characteristic apneas without continuing respiratory effort, show worsening hypoventilation during rapid eye movement sleep, and quantify the severity of the abnormality present.

• Interpretation can be difficult because some patients with apnea due to pharyngeal collapse make little respiratory effort and some patients with a primary failure of respiratory drive have secondary airway collapse.

Complications

Ventilatory failure, cor pulmonale, pneumonia: in patients with neuromuscular or chest-wall disease.

Accidents: particularly motor accidents, due to poor daytime vigilance.

Differential diagnosis

Daytime sleepiness

Obstructive sleep apnea.

Narcolepsy.

Idiopathic hypersomnolence.

Periodic movements of legs during sleep.

Inadequate sleep.

Respiratory failure

Chronic obstructive lung disease.

Obstructive sleep apnea.

Etiology [2]

Neuromuscular or chest-wall disease

• Patients just able to sustain normal ventilation while awake hypoventilate as respiratory drive falls at onset of sleep.

• This worsens further with the muscle atonia of rapid eye movement sleep.

• How this contributes to the daytime ventilatory failure is not clear.

• The sleeping hypoxemia probably accelerates blunting of ventilatory drive, which allows further daytime ventilatory deterioration.

• Thoracic wall stiffness and respiratory muscle fatigue are probably also important.

Periodic respiration

• This develops when the feedback loop controlling respiration has an excessive feedback gain or delay.

• Contributing factors include excessive central drive levels (CNS disease), circulatory delay (heart failure), hypoxemia, hypocapnia, and arousal from sleep (high altitude).

Epidemiology [3]

• Neuromuscular causes of central sleep apnea are unusual.

• Sleeping periodic respiration affects >50% of patients with severe chronic heart failure and >20% of inpatients with neurological disease.

Treatment

Diet and lifestyle

• Changing diet and lifestyle do not alter central sleep apnea.

• Patients should not smoke: concurrent lung disease worsens respiratory failure.

Pharmacological treatment

• Patients with hypoventilation syndromes should be cautioned against the use of sedative medications, which may induce acute respiratory failure.

For neuromuscular or chest-wall disease [4]

• The mainstay of treatment for these conditions is nocturnal ventilatory support.

• Respiratory stimulants may be tried (*e.g.*, theophylline, acetazolamide, medroxyprogesterone), but their long-term efficacy has been disappointing..

For periodic respiration

• Many patients with periodic respiration are asymptomatic and need no treatment; treatment of symptomatic periodic respiration remains experimental.

• Underlying heart failure should be controlled.

• Oxygen, low-dose carbon dioxide, positive airway pressure, or acetazolamide may have a role.

Nonpharmacological treatment [5,6]

Nocturnal ventilatory support

• This is indicated for patients with central sleep apnea, daytime ventilatory failure and an otherwise good quality of life.

• It improves daytime symptoms, respiratory failure, and cor pulmonale, thereby improving prognosis.

• Techniques include nasal positive pressure ventilation, the rocking bed, tank and cuirass ventilators.

Advantages: corrects sleep disruption, daytime sleepiness, and respiratory failure.

Disadvantages: need for specialist care to acclimatize patient to ventilator and for follow-up.

Causes of treatment failure: ventilator or mask failure due to mechanical failure or air leaks, poor compliance due to mouth air leak, nasal obstruction, claustrophobia, inadequate patient education, or poor mask fit, upper airway collapse secondary to extrathoracic negative-pressure (tank or cuirass) ventilation, incorrect diagnosis (respiratory failure due to obstructive lung disease).

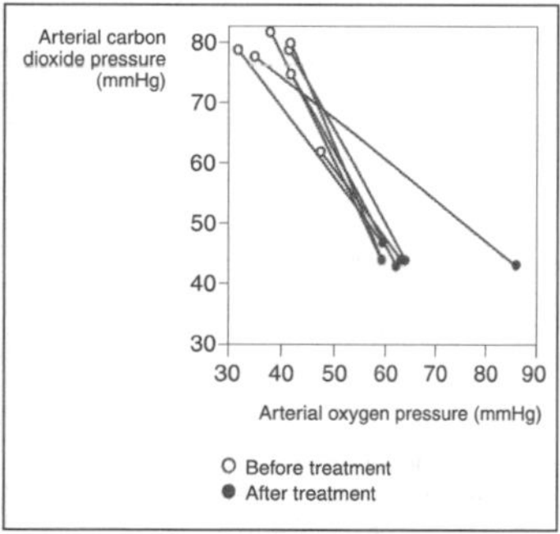

Improvements in awake arterial blood gases in seven patients with neuromuscular or chest wall disease and ventilatory failure after overnight support ventilation.

Oxygen

• Overnight oxygen (24%–28%) may improve symptoms of patients in whom ventilatory support is not appropriate; it has not been shown to improve prognosis in this group and may worsen daytime ventilatory failure.

Treatment aims

Neuromuscular or chest-wall disease

To improve symptoms and quality of life.

To correct respiratory failure and cor pulmonale.

To improve mortality and morbidity.

Periodic respiration

To improve sleep disturbance symptoms.

Prognosis

Neuromuscular or chest-wall disease

• Untreated patients with significant daytime respiratory failure and central sleep apnea have a limited life expectancy (usually only a few months).

• With successful nocturnal ventilatory support, the prognosis approaches that of the underlying condition.

Periodic respiration

• Cheyne–Stokes breathing is not now thought to predict mortality independently of the severity of the underlying disease.

Follow-up and management

• Patients with neuromuscular or chest-wall disease and an otherwise good prognosis, but not in daytime ventilatory failure, need review so that overnight ventilation can be started with onset of daytime hypercapnia.

• Patients on domiciliary nocturnal ventilation need long-term support.

Key references

1. Bradley TD, Phillipson EA: Central sleep apnea. *Clin Chest Med* 1992, **13**:493–505.
2. Khoo MCK, Gottschalk A, Pack AI: Sleep-induced periodic breathing and apnea: a theoretical study. *J Appl Physiol* 1991, **70**:2014–2024.
3. Phillipson EA: Control of breathing during sleep. *Am Rev Respir Dis* 1978, **118**:909–939.
4. Goldstein RS: Hypoventilation: neuromuscular and chest wall disorders. *Clin Chest Med* 1992, **13**:507–521.
5. Hill NS: Noninvasive ventilation. *Am Rev Respir Dis* 1993, **147**:1050–1055.
6. Meyer TJ, Hill NS: Noninvasive positive pressure ventilation to treat respiratory failure. *Ann Intern Med* 1994, **120**:760–770.

Diagnosis

Definition

• Obstructive sleep apnea is a recurrent obstruction to breathing due to upper-airway narrowing or collapse during sleep.

Symptoms [1]

• Symptoms are often manifest for several years before diagnosis.

Daytime sleepiness, snoring, restless sleep: usual adult presentation, often with history of witnessed apneas from partner.

Nocturnal choking or panic attacks, irritability, nocturia, enuresis, impotence, cognitive dysfunction, memory loss, social disharmony, emotional disturbances: less common.

Behavioral disturbance, failure to thrive: nonspecific features in children, in addition to adult symptoms.

Signs

Obesity: particularly neck; characteristic but not invariable.

Small crowded pharynx with mucosal edema.

Retrognathia.

Tonsil hypertrophy: usual cause of obstructive sleep apnea in children.

Nasal obstruction.

Respiratory failure or cor pulmonale: in 10% of patients.

Features of hypothyroidism or acromegaly: rare.

Investigations

Initial

Awake arterial oxygen saturation or blood gas analysis, spirometry, hemoglobin analysis: for ventilatory failure (arterial oxygen and blood gases), obstructive pulmonary disease (spirometry), and polycythemia (hemoglobin).

Thyroid or growth hormone estimations: can be considered.

Sleep studies

• Sleep studies are needed to establish the diagnosis by showing upper-airway obstruction with continuing respiratory efforts; no ideal combination of physiological signals exists, but markers of respiratory effort, apnea, and sleep disturbances are all needed.

Polysomnography: gold standard; includes EEG sleep staging, oronasal airflow assessment, and measurement of thoracoabdominal movement or esophageal pressure; accurately identifies obstructive apneas but time-consuming and expensive and disturbs patient's sleep [2].

Complications

Respiratory failure, cor pulmonale: usually in patients with peripheral airways obstruction (often mild).

Accidents: particularly motor accidents, due to poor daytime vigilance.

Cardiovascular disease: increased vascular mortality (improves with effective treatment).

Differential diagnosis

Daytime sleepiness

Narcolepsy.

Idiopathic hypersomnolence.

Central sleep apnea.

Periodic breathing.

Periodic movements of legs during sleep.

Inadequate sleep.

Respiratory failure

Chronic obstructive pulmonary disease.

Neuromuscular weakness.

Scoliosis.

Etiology [3]

• Causes include the following:

Pharyngeal narrowing due to obesity, endopharyngeal masses (including tonsils), retrognathia, micrognathia, hypothyroidism, acromegaly.

Reduced pharyngeal muscle activity due to alcohol, sedative drugs, neuromuscular disorders.

Nasal obstruction.

Epidemiology

• The peak age of presentation is 40–60 years.

• The male:female ratio is 4–10:1.

• The sleep apnea/hypopnea syndrome may affect 1%–4% of men over age 40 years.

Variants of obstructive sleep apnea

Simple snoring: in 20% of men.

Snoring with arousals from sleep: severe sleep fragmentation and daytime sleepiness after heavy snoring without apneas or hypoxemia.

Obstructive sleep hypopnea: airflow does not entirely cease.

Central variant: patients do not make efforts to breathe during the apneas, particularly while lying supine; snoring or typical obstructive sleep apnea usually occurs in other postures.

Laryngeal sleep apnea: sleeping stridor due to laryngeal disease or denervation or Shy–Drager syndrome.

Treatment

Diet and lifestyle

• Weight loss can correct obstructive sleep apnea, but most patients also need other treatment.

• Reduced alcohol intake helps simple snoring and mild obstructive sleep apnea.

• Obstructive sleep apnea present only when patient is supine is improved by avoiding this posture.

Pharmacological treatment [4]

• Avoidance of alcohol and sedatives before bedtime is an important part of therapy.

• Drug treatment is secondary to continuous airways pressure.

Nasal steroids and decongestants

• These reduce simple snoring but have little effect on obstructive sleep apnea; they may be needed during continuous positive airway pressure therapy.

Standard dosage	Beclomethasone, 42–84 μg; or budesonide, 64 μg, twice daily in each nostril.
Contraindications	None.
Special points	Vasoconstrictor decongestants worsen nasal obstruction with sustained use and should be avoided.
Main drug interactions	None.
Main side effects	Nasal dryness.

Tricyclic antidepressants

• Antidepressants have a minor role in mild obstructive sleep apnea by suppressing rapid eye movement sleep, when sleep apnea often worsens.

Standard dosage	Protriptyline, 10–20 mg orally at night.
Contraindications	Cardiac disease, epilepsy, mania, liver disease, glaucoma.
Main drug interactions	Alcohol, monoamine oxidase inhibitors, antihistamines, anticonvulsants.
Main side effects	Anticholinergic effects, arrhythmias, impotence, urinary retention.

Nonpharmacological treatment [5]

Nasal continuous positive airways pressure

• This is the main treatment in most patients with substantial daytime sleepiness.

Advantages: dramatic correction of sleep disruption, daytime sleepiness, snoring, and apneas.

Disadvantages: unsightly, mask may be claustrophobic or cause nasal ulceration if badly fitted.

Causes of treatment failure: machine or mask failure; poor compliance due to nasal obstruction, claustrophobia, inadequate patient education, poor mask fit (air leaks or nasal ulceration), mouth air leak; incorrect diagnosis (central sleep apnea, narcolepsy, respiratory failure from another cause).

Surgery

• Surgery is indicated for patients with the following:

Structural nasal obstruction (*e.g.*, polyps, deviated septum).

Tonsil hypertrophy.

Facial maldevelopment.

Severe obstructive sleep apnea with continuous positive airways pressure failure.

• Tracheostomy is rarely indicated.

• Surgery should be attempted only in established centers.

• Soft-palette resection is not consistently curative.

Treatment aims

To relieve symptoms.

To correct respiratory failure.

To reduce excess vascular mortality.

Prognosis

• After effective treatment, patients are symptom-free and have a similar prognosis to weight-matched controls.

• Few patients reduce their weight sufficiently to stop continuous positive airway pressure treatment (CPAP).

Follow-up and management

• Patients on CPAP treatment need review including maintenance of their equipment, replacement of masks and consideration of reducing their airway pressure or stopping treatment after weight loss.

Key references

1. Findley LJ, Weiss J, Jabour EP: Drivers with untreated sleep apnoea. *Arch Intern Med* 1991, **151**:1451–1452.
2. Douglas NJ, Thomas S, Jan MA: Clinical value of polysomnography. *Lancet* 1992, **339**:347–350.
3. McNamara SG, Grunstein RR, Sullivan CE: Obstructive sleep apnoea. *Thorax* 1993, **48**:754–764.
4. Kryger MH: Management of obstructive sleep apnea. *Clin Chest Med* 1992, **13**:481–492.
5. Sanders M, Kern N: Obstructive sleep apnea treated by independently adjusted inspiratory and expiratory positive airway pressures via nasal mask. Physiologic and clinical implications. *Chest* 1990, **98**:317–324.

Diagnosis

Symptoms

Insomnia

Daytime fatigue, sleepiness.

Depression.

Obstructive sleep apnea [1]

Obstructive snoring, gasping.

Breath holding.

Partial arousal.

Excessive daytime sleepiness.

Narcoleptic syndrome

Excessive daytime sleepiness.

Sudden weakness: with laughter or expectation of sudden event (cataplexy).

Short night sleep latency.

Insomnia.

Excessive motor activity during sleep: leg kicking and sleep-walking.

Sleep paralysis (loss of muscle tone).

Hypnopompic or hyponagogic hallucinations.

Parasomnias

Hypnic jerks: at sleep onset.

Sleep-walking and night terrors: 60–90 min after sleep onset, during non-rapid eye movement sleep.

Cluster headache, painful erections, nightmares: during rapid eye movement (REM) sleep; accompanied by dreaming.

Enuresis, sleep-talking, leg-kicking: common.

Bruxism, head-banging: less common.

Circadian sleep disorders

Sleep phase disturbance (lag or lead).

Signs

• No abnormal physical signs are manifest in most sleep disorders, although obstructive apneas are associated with retrognathia, micrognathia, macroglossia, or enlarged tonsils or soft palate.

Investigations

Polysomnography: necessary in most sleep–wake disorders, including the narcoleptic syndrome; allows detailed scientific sleep study and may occasionally clarify diagnosis of sleep disorder, particularly when combined with video monitoring [2].

Sleep oximetry: useful in evaluation of sleep apnea and review of treatment.

Multiple sleep latency test: in narcoleptic syndrome and other forms of daytime sleepiness; in narcolepsy, sleep latency is short and REM often begins within 15 min of sleep onset; ≥2/5 naps containing REM sleep is suggestive of narcolepsy.

Plasma and urinary screen: for hypnotic or CNS stimulant drugs, occasionally useful in suspected drug abuse or poor drug compliance.

Complications

• Sleep disorders may be as disabling as epilepsy.

Daytime sleepiness, depression.

Work and social problems: major cause of traffic accidents.

Differential diagnosis

Not applicable.

Etiology

• Insomnia is often multifactorial, with abnormal lifestyle, physical and psychological factors and sometimes hypnotic-stimulant drug or alcohol misuse.

• Familial insomnia is not uncommon.

• The narcoleptic syndrome has 99% association with HLA DR2 and DQw1; only 1 in 500 HLA DR2 positive patients, however, has the narcoleptic syndrome.

• Circadian sleep disorders are due to shift work or psychological factors (*e.g.*, avoiding school).

Epidemiology

• Chronic insomnia occurs in up to 20% of adults; it is more common in women than in men.

• Persistent excessive daytime sleepiness is usually caused by obstructive sleep apnea, the narcoleptic syndrome, or periodic leg movements with frequent arousals.

• Parasomnias including bed wetting and sleep walking are common, most frequently in childhood.

• Circadian sleep disorders caused by shift work occur in one-third of the workforce; shift work is tolerated better by younger people.

• The delayed sleep phase syndrome has an incidence of 1 in 10 000 people.

Treatment

Diet and lifestyle

• Regular bedtime, a comfortable quiet bed, presleep relaxation, a warm drink, and avoidance of rumination may improve insomnia.

• In the narcoleptic syndrome, 2–3 planned short naps during the day may improve alertness.

• Sleep regularity with fixed stable bedtime and wake-time is useful in the management of many parasomnias and insomnia.

Pharmacological treatment

For insomnia

Standard dosage Short-term (2–3 months) benzodiazepine or nonbenzodiazepine hypnotic, *e.g.*, temazepam, 2–3 times weekly, can be considered.

Contraindications Pregnancy, psychiatric illness, sleep apnea.

Special points Long-term nightly use to be avoided; can be combined with psychological support, although hypnotics not main-line treatment for most forms of chronic insomnia.

Main drug interactions Enhanced sedative effect with many other drugs; metabolic interactions.

Main side effects Waking sedation, tolerance.

For narcoleptic syndrome: daytime sleepiness [3]

Standard dosage Methylphenidate, maximum 60 mg daily, pemoline, mazindol, dextroamphetamine; exact dose titration and timing essential.

Contraindications Vascular disease, hypertension, pregnancy, prostatism, breast-feeding.

Special points Stimulants ineffective for cataplexy.
Regular monitoring of patients on long-term treatment needed.

Main drug interactions Sympathomimetics, monoamine oxidase inhibitors.

Main side effects Talkativeness, euphoria, gastrointestinal irritation, sweating, constipation.

For narcoleptic syndrome: cataplexy

Standard dosage Clomipramine or imipramine, 10–50 mg once daily.

Contraindications Recent myocardial infarction, heart block.

Special points Cataplexy does not respond to stimulants, but these can be used in combination with clomipramine.

Main drug interactions As for tricyclic antidepressants.

Main side effects Appetite changes, sexual malfunction, or orthostasis.

Treatment aims

To restore normal waking alertness and mood.

To prevent sleep hypoxia, arousal, and cor pulmonale.

To alleviate symptoms of narcolepsy.

Other treatments

Continuous positive airways pressure: effective in patients with obstructive sleep apnea.

Consideration of surgery.

Prognosis

• The prognosis varies widely among the different sleep disorders.

• The narcoleptic syndrome does not remit.

• In many forms of insomnia, the prognosis is poor.

Follow-up and management

• Assessment of insomnia requires medical, psychiatric, and psychological review; a written treatment plan should be drawn up with the patient, aiming for sustained benefit in 3–6 months of treatment

• In patients with the narcoleptic syndrome, progress should be monitored using a sleep–wake diary; drug compliance should be ensured by monitoring plasma and urine concentrations.

Patient support

American Sleep Disorders Association,
1610 14th St NW, Suite 300,
Rochester, MN 55901-2205;
phone (507) 287-6006.

Driving regulations

• The general guideline is that driving ability with excessive daytime sleepiness depends on the success of and degree of compliance with treatment.

Key references

1. Hill NS: Noninvasive ventilation. *Am Rev Respir Dis* 1993, **147**:1050–1055.
2. Douglas NJ, Thomas S, Jan MA: Clinical value of polysomnography. *Lancet* 1992, **339**:347–350.
3. Thorpy MJ: *Handbook of Sleep Disorders*. New York: Marcel Dekker; 1990.

Diagnosis

Symptoms

• The neurological symptoms are progressive.

Localized back pain.

Radicular pain.

Numbness or paresthesia, weakness: below level of lesion; may be asymmetrical.

Loss of control of sphincters.

Signs

At level of lesion

Spinal tenderness or deformity: depending on the disease.

Weakness, wasting, reflex loss: root lesion.

Below level of lesion

• Signs may be asymmetrical, *e.g.*, Brown–Sequard's syndrome.

• With spinal cord lesions, sacral sensation may be relatively "spared."

Weakness.

Sensory loss.

Spasticity, clonus, hyperreflexia, extensor plantars: if above L1, *i.e.*, spinal cord.

Flaccidity, areflexia: if below L1, *i.e.*, cauda equina.

Investigations

• Laboratory investigations may indicate cause, suggest alternative diagnosis, or help in preparation for surgery.

Full blood count and ESR measurement: may identify anemia or suggest infection.

Serum vitamin B_{12}, syphilis serology, serum acid phosphatase measurement, plasma protein electrophoresis: may be helpful in some patients.

Chest radiography: may show mass or infection.

Plain radiography of spine: may show loss of pedicle or vertebral collapse.

Myelography, CT myelography, MRI: may be needed urgently; CSF should always be saved, particularly if a compressive lesion is not identified.

Plain CT: in some patients.

Complications

Irreversible neurological damage: due to infarction of cord or roots.

Urinary infection: due to neurogenic bladder.

Deep venous thrombosis and pressure sores: from immobility.

Differential diagnosis

Spastic paraparesis

Inflammatory myelopathies: acute transverse myelitis, multiple sclerosis, HIV infection, tropical spastic paraparesis, sarcoidosis (human T-cell leukemic virus I).

Vascular myelopathies: spinal stroke (anterior spinal artery distribution), vascular malformation.

Malformations: Arnold Chiari (possible lower brain stem or cerebellar signs), syringomyelia (absent arm reflexes and suspended sensory loss).

Cerebral lesions: bilateral strokes, parasagittal tumor.

Flaccid paraparesis

Flaccidity and absent reflexes (spinal shock) caused by acute spinal cord lesions; rare in compression.

Acute Guillain–Barré syndrome: symmetrical, distal sensory loss, areflexia.

Etiology

• Causes include the following:

Extradural tumors: secondary carcinoma, lymphoma, myeloma [1].

Intradural–extramedullary tumors: meningioma, neurofibroma.

Intramedullary tumors: glioma, ependymoma, lipoma.

Disc protrusions: usually cervical or lumbar, usually spontaneous, often sudden onset.

Osteophytic ridges: may combine with narrow spinal canal, *i.e.*, cervical or lumbar canal stenosis.

Infection: pyogenic epidural abscess, tuberculosis.

Trauma: fractures or dislocations of vertebrae.

Hematomas: epidural and subdural (rare).

Epidemiology

Occurs in 5% of patients with systemic malignancy.

Treatment

Diet and lifestyle

Not relevant.

Pharmacological treatment

Chemotherapy or radiotherapy: after decompression or biopsy of malignant lesion.

Steroids: before and after surgery to minimize spinal-cord edema (*e.g.*, dexamethasone, 16 mg daily in divided doses).

Nonpharmacological treatment

• If acute spinal cord compression is suspected, the patient must be referred to a neurosurgical unit immediately.

• Any delay may lessen the chance of recovery.

Decompression

• Lesions lying posterior to the spinal cord or within the dura mater should be removed from behind through a laminectomy.

• Lesions lying anterior to the dura mater, with the exception of lumbar disc protrusions, should be removed from the front.

Spinal stabilization

• Lesions that cause collapse of the vertebral bodies cause forward angulation; stabilization should be by insertion of a graft from the front or instrumental stabilization attached to laminae in extension, *e.g.*, Hartshill rectangle.

Radiotherapy

• Radiotherapy is useful after surgery for metastatic lesions or as primary therapy in selected cases.

Treatment aims

To establish the diagnosis.

To reverse neurological deficit while preserving spinal stability, if lesion removable.

To prevent progression or recurrence, if lesion not removable.

Prognosis

• The prognosis depends on the underlying cause, the rate rather than degree of compression, and the delay in decompression.

• Patients with long-established myelopathy due to hard disc material or osteophytic bars have poor prognosis; those with soft disc protrusions do well.

• Myelopathies due to prostatic metastases have a relatively good prognosis.

• Metastases from breast or bronchus have a poor prognosis; direct invasion from bronchus has a very poor prognosis.

• Good recovery even from severe neurological deficit may follow successful surgical removal of benign tumors.

• Prognosis is good if decompression occurs before the onset of severe paraparesis.

Follow-up and management

• Patients need subsequent physical therapy, rehabilitation, surgical appliances (*e.g.*, walking aids, orthoses, wheelchair), occupational therapy, and home assessment.

• Patients should be referred to a spinal unit if the residual deficit is severe.

• Complications can be prevented by anti-embolism stockings, low-dose s.c. heparin, prevention of pressure sores, bladder care, and early treatment of intercurrent infection.

Key reference

1. Portenoy RK, *et al.*: Back pain in the cancer patient: an algorithm for evaluation and management. *Neurology* 1987, **37**:134–138.

Diagnosis

Definition

• Stroke is defined as rapidly developing (usually over minutes) clinical symptoms or signs of focal and, at times, global loss of cerebral function, with symptoms lasting >24 h, with no apparent cause other than that of vascular origin.

Symptoms

• Symptoms depend on the vascular territory involved.

Anterior (carotid) circulation

Speech, visuospatial, motor, or sensory loss: indicating cortical lesions.

Isolated contralateral sensory or motor loss: indicating deeper hemispheric lesions.

• Extensive hemispheric involvement may lead to altered consciousness due to cerebral edema.

Posterior circulation

Homonymous hemianopia or brain stem disturbance: *e.g.*, diplopia, vertigo, imbalance, altered consciousness.

• Headache, loss of consciousness, and seizures are more common presenting features in subarachnoid or primary intracerebral hemorrhage than in cerebral infarction.

Signs

• Signs range from none or very subtle (*e.g.*, subjective sensory disturbance) to brain death.

Investigations

• Diagnosis of stroke remains clinical, based predominantly on the history.

• Primary investigations are aimed at identifying abnormalities that may further compromise cerebral function (in patients admitted to hospital) or provide etiological clues.

• Secondary investigations are aimed at detecting the cause of stroke, which influences early management.

• Tertiary investigations are aimed at preventing recurrence and excluding unusual causes (*see* Transient ischemic attacks).

Primary investigations

Full blood count, ESR, glucose measurement, coagulation studies, ECG, chest radiography.

Secondary investigations

CT: sensitive at differentiating hemorrhage from infarction immediately; may appear normal early in infarction; final topographical distribution of any infarction best seen at days 7–10.

MRI: useful early in the course and for brain stem or posterior fossa stroke.

Lumbar puncture: for suspected subarachnoid hemorrhage if CT normal.

• Other specific tests indicated by clinical setting (*e.g.*, blood cultures).

Complications

Infections (*e.g.*, aspiration pneumonia, urinary tract infection).

Venous thromboembolism.

Cardiac arrhythmias, cardiac failure, myocardial infarction.

Fluid imbalance.

Pressure sores.

Spasticity, contractures.

Mood disorders.

Seizures.

Falls, fractures.

Differential diagnosis

Intracranial tumor.

Subdural hematoma.

Etiology

Causes of cerebral infarction

As for transient ischemic attacks (*see separate entry*).

Causes of intracranial hemorrhage

Hypertension.

Aneurysm or arteriovenous malformation.

Hypercoagulability.

Cerebral vasculitis.

Epidemiology

• Stroke is the third most common cause of death in industrialized countries.

• It is the largest single cause of severe disability in people living at home.

Classification

• Stroke can be classified as follows:

Cerebral infarction: in 80% of patients.

Primary intracerebral hemorrhage: in 10%.

Subarachnoid hemorrhage: in 5%.

Uncertain: in 5%.

• Cerebral infarction may be further classified on clinical criteria, as follows:

Total anterior circulation infarction: hemiplegia, hemianopia, new cortical deficit.

Partial anterior circulation infarction: two of the above three, new cortical deficit alone, or motor or sensory deficit more restricted than lacunar infarction.

Lacunar infarction: pure motor or sensory stroke, sensorimotor stroke, or ataxic hemiparesis; thought to be caused by intrinsic disease of single perforating artery.

Posterior circulation infarction: evidence of brain stem lesion or homonymous hemianopia.

Treatment

Diet and lifestyle

• Attention to control hypertension, hyperlipidemia, and cessation of smoking are very important preventive measures.

Pharmacological treatment

• Heparinization is currently indicated for posterior circulation ischemic stroke, cardiogenic emboli, and in many cases, for crescendo transient ischemic attacks (TIAs) and stoke in progression.

• Aspirin has been proved to be beneficial in reducing long-term risk after TIAs in undifferentiated groups at risk.

• Coumadin may be useful for some patients with embolic sources or nonoperable critical stenosis; broader use is under investigation.

• Ticlopidine, 500 mg daily, is useful in some patients with small vessel or posterior circulation disease but is associated with occasional neutropenia and requires close monitoring [1].

• The role of acute thrombolytic therapy is currently under investigation.

Nonpharmacological treatment

Surgery [2]

• Some patients with intracerebral hematomas may benefit from surgical drainage, although no universally acceptable selection criteria exist.

• Patients with subarachnoid hemorrhages should be managed in an intensive care unit and may require aneurysm repair.

• Carotid endarterectomy is indicated in symptomatic patients with stenosis >70% and in selected asymptomatic patients.

• Embolectomy is currently under investigation.

Rehabilitation

• Stroke units combining physical, occupational, and speech therapy save lives.

• Immobilized patients should wear antiembolism stockings.

• Support from the social services is an important but often neglected element in a patient's recovery.

• Physical, speech, and occupational therapy are vital to recovery.

Treatment aims

To prevent further cerebral damage or secondary complications.

To treat the cause of the stroke, where possible.

To enable survivors to achieve independence.

Prognosis

• For cerebral infarction, the overall 30-day case fatality is 10%.

• ~50% of survivors remain dependent.

• Important prognostic indicators include type and extent of stroke, age, and presenting level of consciousness.

• Intracranial hemorrhage carries a notably worse prognosis.

Follow-up and management

• The key aim is to identify and modify treatable risk factors (*e.g.*, hypertension, smoking).

• Starting 1–2 weeks after cerebral infarction, lifelong antiplatelet treatment is indicated (aspirin, 75–150 mg daily).

• Anticoagulation is effective as primary and secondary prophylaxis for cerebral infarction when atrial fibrillation is present.

• For patients who recover well from a carotid distribution stroke, endarterectomy may be indicated.

Key references

1. Hass WK, *et al.*: A randomized trial comparing ticlopidine with aspirin. *N Engl J Med* 1989, **321**:501–507.
2. ACAS Group: Endarterectomy for asymptomatic carotid artery stenosis. *JAMA* 1995, **273**:1421–1459.

General references

Caplan LR: *Stroke: A Clinical Approach*, edn 2. Oxford: Butterworth Heinemann; 1993.

Barnett HJM, *et al.*: *Stroke*, edn 2. New York: Churchill Livingstone; 1992.

Diagnosis

Symptoms

• Mild chronic hyponatremia (serum sodium concentration 125–135 mEq/L) may be asymptomatic.

• More profound hyponatremia (serum sodium concentration <120 mEq/L) can cause the following:

Headache.*	**Confusion.**	**Seizures.**
Malaise.	**Depression.**	**Coma.**
Nausea and vomiting.	**Cramps.**	**Death.**
Irritability.	**Drowsiness.**	

*The severity of the symptoms depends on the rate of fall of serum sodium as much as on the absolute value.

Signs [1]

• Mild chronic hyponatremia usually has no specific signs.

• Severe hyponatremia may cause the following:

Diminished reflexes.

Extensor plantar responses.

Cardinal features

Dilutional hyponatremia: plasma osmolality appropriately low for serum sodium.

Urine osmolality greater than plasma osmolality.

Persistent renal sodium excretion.

Absence of hypotension, hypovolemia, or edema-forming states.

Normal thyroid, renal, and adrenal function.

Investigations [1]

• Laboratory tests are not specific for the diagnosis but help to exclude other causes of hyponatremia and to identify underlying causes.

Chest radiography: to check for lung cancer.

Serum sodium measurement: low concentration.

Plasma osmolality measurement: <270 mOsm/kg.

Blood glucose measurement: to exclude spurious hyponatremia in hyperglycemia.

Serum protein and lipoprotein measurement: to exclude pseudohyponatremia.

Serum uric acid measurement: low concentration.

Urine osmolality measurement: usually >300 mOsm/kg.

Renal function tests: creatinine clearance rate or serum creatinine concentration.

Thyroid function tests: thyroxine, thyroid-stimulating hormone; to exclude hypothyroidism.

Adrenocortical tests: short cosyntropin test; to exclude cortisol deficiency.

Plasma vasopressin measurement.

Pituitary function tests: to exclude corticotropic hormone deficiency.

Pituitary fossa radiography.

Complications

Permanent neurological deficit, high neurological morbidity and mortality: caused by prolonged profound hyponatremia or aggressive treatment leading to rapid rise in serum sodium concentration..

Differential diagnosis [2]

Hyponatremia associated with hypervolemia

Cardiac failure.

Cirrhosis.

Nephrotic syndrome.

Renal failure.

Hyponatremia associated with hypovolemia

Gastrointestinal fluid loss.

Severe burns.

Mineralocorticoid deficiency (*i.e.*, Addison's disease).

Salt-losing nephritis.

Etiology [2–4]

• Causes include the following:

Neoplastic disease: *e.g.*, lung cancer, pancreatic cancer, lymphoma.

Chest disorders: *e.g.*, pneumonia, tuberculosis, abscess.

Neurological disorders: *e.g.*, head injury, infections, hemorrhage.

Drugs: *e.g.*, thiazides, cytotoxic agents, carbamazepine.

Epidemiology

• Hyponatremia is the most common electrolyte disturbance seen in hospitals (~10% of patients have serum sodium concentrations of <130 mEq/L).

• ~50% of all hyponatremia is due to the syndrome of inappropriate diuresis.

Treatment

Diet and lifestyle

- Fluid should be restricted to 0.5–1.0 L daily.
- Patients must eat a well balanced diet.

Pharmacological treatment [1,5]

- The underlying cause of the syndrome should be treated (*e.g.*, cancer of the bronchus).
- Specific V_2-receptor antagonists to block the antidiuretic effect of vasopressin are awaited.

Induction of partial nephrogenic diabetes insipidus

Standard dosage Demeclocycline, 1.2 g in divided doses.
Lithium carbonate 0.4–1.2 g daily.

Contraindications *Demeclocycline*: renal failure, pregnancy, children.
Lithium carbonate: renal and cardiac disease.

Special points *Demeclocycline:* full effect may need up to 3 weeks of treatment.
Lithium carbonate: plasma concentrations must be measured.

Main drug interactions *Demeclocycline:* warfarin.
Lithium carbonate: diuretics, antibiotics, antihypertensives, sumatriptan.

Main side effects *Demeclocycline:* nausea, diarrhea, photosensitivity.
Lithium carbonate: gastrointestinal disturbances, goiter, CNS dysfunction.

Inhibition of neurohypophysial vasopressin secretion

Standard dosage Phenytoin, 300 mg daily.

Contraindications Renal and hepatic dysfunction, porphyria.

Main drug interactions Antibacterials, anxiolytics, hypnotics, calcium antagonists.

Main side effects Drowsiness, ataxia.

Induction of diuresis and natriuresis

Standard dosage Furosemide, 40–80 mg daily, and slow sodium chloride, 3 g orally daily.

Contraindications Decompensated liver cirrhosis; caution in prostatism.

Main drug interactions Antifungals, potassium-losing drugs.

Main side effects Hypokalemia, gastrointestinal disturbances.

Treatment aims

To relieve symptoms of hyponatremia.

To increase serum sodium concentration to 125–140 mEq/L.

Prognosis

- This depends on the underlying cause.
- Patients with serum sodium concentrations <110 mEq/L have high morbidity and mortality (~50%).
- Development of osmotic demyelination syndrome indicates poor prognosis (~50% mortality).

Follow-up and management [1]

- Depending on the underlying condition, fluid restriction or drug treatment may be needed indefinitely.
- Serum sodium concentrations must be checked monthly.

Osmotic demyelination syndrome [6]

- This occurs after rapid correction of chronic severe hyponatremia, irrespective of the means of increasing serum sodium concentrations.
- It is found in central pontine and intracerebral structures.
- It is clinically evident 2–4 days after correction of serum sodium concentrations.
- It can be avoided by increasing serum sodium by <0.5 mEq/L/h.

Key references

1. Robertson GL: Syndrome of inappropriate antidiuresis. *N Engl J Med* 1989, **321**:538–539.
2. Ayus JC, Arieff AI: Pathogenesis and prevention of hyponatremic encephalopathy. *Endocrinol Metab Clin North Am* 1993, **22**:425–446.
3. Baylis PH, Thompson CJ: Osmoregulation of vasopressin and thirst in health and disease. *Clin Endocrinol* 1988, **29**:549–576.
4. Berl T, *et al.*: Clinical disorders of water metabolism. *Kidney Int* 1976, **10**:117–132.
5. Arieff AI: Management of hyponatraemia. *BMJ* 1993, **307**:307–308.
6. Sterns RH, Riggs, J, Achochet SS: Osmotic demyelination syndrome following correction of hyponatremia. *N Engl J Med* 1986, **314**:1535–1542.

Diagnosis

Symptoms and signs

Tiredness: indicating anemia.

Polyarthralgias and nonerosive symmetric arthritis: involving predominantly small joints (rarely deforming) [1,2].

Rashes: photosensitive, discoid, and, less often, classic facial butterfly rash [1].

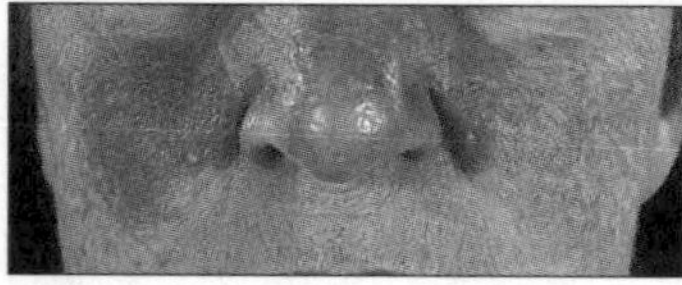

Classic butterfly rash.

Vasculitic lesions of extremities: leading to gangrene of digits.

Oral or pharyngeal ulcers.

Myalgia.

Pleuritic or pericardial pain: indicating serositis.

Epistaxis, bleeding gums, menorrhagia, purpura: symptoms of thrombocytopenia.

Visual and auditory hallucinations or epilepsy.

Edema or hypertension: *e.g.*, nephrotic syndrome or acute nephritic illness.

Alopecia [1].

Raynaud's phenomenon.

Lymphadenopathy.

Fever.

Livedo reticularis.

Investigations

Laboratory tests

• These are useful in the diagnosis of SLE, but no single diagnostic test is available [1].

Complete blood count: may reveal anemia, leukopenia, neutropenia, lymphopenia, or thrombocytopenia; raised ESR common in active disease; evidence of hemolytic anemia requires further investigation, *e.g.*, a Coombs' test [1].

Antinuclear antibody analysis: antibodies found in at least 95% of SLE patients but not disease-specific; antibodies to double-stranded DNA and Sm are relatively disease-specific but do not occur in all patients (~50% and ~5%, respectively); antibodies to Ro, La, and U1 ribonucleoprotein helpful in defining disease subsets and overlap syndromes; positive antiphospholipid antibodies and lupus anticoagulant define patients at risk from major arterial and venous thromboses [1].

For markers of disease activity or organ involvement

ESR measurement: raised ESR with normal CRP usual except when bacterial infection coexists [1,3].

Plasma-complement analysis: low C3, C4, and CH50 indicate activity.

Anti–double-stranded DNA antibody analysis: antibodies can rise with disease flares, especially those involving the kidney.

Dipstick testing of urine: for proteinuria and hematuria.

Microscopic examination: for red cell casts, leukocyte casts.

Measurements of renal function and 24-h urine protein loss.

Complications

Severe renal involvement [3].

Cerebral involvement: infarcts or neuropsychiatric disease [3].

Infections secondary to immunosuppression.

Major thrombotic events: especially when high-titer antiphospholipid antibodies are present [4].

Differential diagnosis

Other connective tissue diseases: *e.g.*, rheumatoid arthritis, progressive systemic sclerosis.

Infection.

Malignancy.

Etiology

• Causes include the following:

Genetic factors and inherited defects of the early components of the classic complement pathway.

Environmental factors: *e.g.*, sunlight.

Drugs: *e.g.*, hydralazine, procainamide, phenytoin.

Epidemiology

• The prevalence of SLE in the US is 45 in 100 000 women, 3.7 in 100 000 men [5].

• The highest incidence is in the 20–40 year age group.

• SLE is unusual in children.

Treatment

Diet and lifestyle

• Patients, especially those with photosensitivity, should avoid sunlight and should use high-factor sun screen (ultraviolet A and B).

Pharmacological treatment

Indications

Discoid lupus erythematosus rashes: topical steroids.

Joint and skin involvement: hydroxychloroquine.

Systemic involvement: acute treatment by corticosteriods, introduction of cytotoxic agents, *e.g.*, azathioprine, chlorambucil, methotrexate.

Severe vasculitis (including cerebral and renal involvement): pulse cyclophosphamide and methylprednisolone [6].

Systemic treatment

Standard dosage

Hydroxychloroquine, 200 mg once or twice daily.
Prednisone, 10–40 mg daily and azathioprine, 1–2.5 mg/kg daily to allow subsequent steroid reduction.
Pulse methylprednisolone, 1 g i.v. daily for 3 days and pulse cyclophosphamide, 500–750 mg/m^2, adjusted downward for creatinine clearance <35 mL/min or myelosuppression.
Cyclophosphamide is given i.v. monthly or 6 months, then i.v. every 3 months until clinical improvement or toxicity occurs.
Cyclophosphamide dosing is complex and should be supervised by a specialist (*e.g.*, rheumatologist, nephrologist, pulmonologist).

Contraindications

Known hypersensitivity, systemic infections.

Special points

Cyclophosphamide: infusions must be preceded by a full blood count to check for bone-marrow toxicity, in particular evidence of neutropenia.

Main drug interactions

Cyclophosphamide: concurrent allopurinol should be avoided because of enhanced toxicity.

Main side effects

Hydroxychloroquine: retinopathy, skin rashes.
Azathioprine: bone-marrow suppression, gastrointestinal disturbances, liver toxicity.
Cyclophosphamide: nausea and vomiting, hair loss, hemorrhagic cystitis, premature menopause [6].
All cytotoxic agents: teratogenicity (adequate contraception essential) [6].

Treatment aims

To alleviate disease flares.

Prognosis

• Renal and cerebral involvement and the complications of treatment, especially infection, are the major contributors to mortality.

• The survival rate has improved in the past 2 decades and is now ~95% at 5 years.

Follow-up and management

• Prompt treatment of lupus flares is mandatory.

• The use of oral cytotoxic drugs requires monthly blood counts to check for bone-marrow suppression and liver function tests with methotrexate.

Key references

1. Tan E, *et al.*: The 1982 revised criteria for the classification of systemic lupus erythematosus. *Arthritis Rheum* 1982, **25**:1271–1277.
2. Mills JA: Systemic lupus erythematosus. *N Engl J Med* 1994, **330**:1871–1879.
3. Boumpas DT, *et al.*: Systemic lupus erythematosus: emerging concepts. Part 1. Renal, neuropsychiatric, cardiovascular, pulmonary and hematologic disease. *Ann Intern Med* 1995, **122**:940–950.
4. Petri M: Systemic lupus erythematosus and pregnancy. *Rheum Dis Clin North Am* 1994, **20**:87–118.
5. Rothfield NF: Clinical features of SLE. In *Textbook of Rheumatology*. Edited by Kelley NN, *et al.* Philadelphia: W.B. Saunders; 1988.
6. Fox DA, McCune WJ: Immunosuppressive drug therapy of systemic lupus erythematosus. *Rheum Dis Clin North Am* 1994, **20**:265–291.

Diagnosis

Symptoms

• Scleroderma is unlikely in the absence of Raynaud's phenomenon.

• It has two major subgroups of prognostic and therapeutic importance, as follows:

Limited cutaneous disease

• This occurs in 60% of patients.

• It was previously called CREST syndrome [1].

Swollen painful fingers: ulcers possible.

Thick skin on hands.

Calcium deposits.

Swallowing difficulty.

Diffuse cutaneous disease

• This occurs in 40% of patients.

Puffy hands, feet, arms, legs, tight skin.

Weight loss, fatigue.

Muscle and joint pain.

Breathlessness, dry cough, palpitations.

Indigestion, bloating, diarrhea [2,3].

Signs

Limited cutaneous disease

Early (<10 years)

• Distribution is limited to hands, feet, and face.

Sclerodactyly, swollen fingers, microstomia.

Pitting scars, pulp atrophy.

Digital ulcers.

Telangiectasia.

Calcinosis.

Late (>10 years)

Loud pulmonary second sound.

Right heart failure.

Abdominal bloating.

Wasting and other signs of malabsorption.

Diffuse cutaneous disease

Early (<5 years)

Diffusely puffy or sclerosed skin, including truncal changes.

Friction rubs.

Joint contractures.

Muscle weakness.

Digital pits and ulcers.

Basal crepitations, pericardial rub, arrhythmia.

Late (>5 years)

Dry, shiny skin.

Ulcers: atrophic, on fingers or elbows.

Muscle wasting.

Joint contractures.

Cardiac or respiratory failure.

Investigations

Full blood count: to detect anemia of chronic disease.

Creatinine clearance measurement: to assess renal function.

Autoantibody tests: antinuclear antibodies are positive in 90% of patients; full screen useful to mark subsets of systemic sclerosis or overlap with other disorders.

Nailfold capillary tests (ophthalmoscope or microscopic): useful in "prescleroderma" and early disease; abnormal pattern of vessel drop-out and distortion.

Esophageal scintiscanning: to detect dysmotility (other "gut" tests as indicated).

ECG, echocardiography, Doppler ultrasonography: to detect cardiac involvement and to estimate pulmonary artery pressure.

Chest radiography, pulmonary function tests, high-resolution CT: to detect lung involvement; CT best test for presence and extent of early fibrosis.

Electromyography, biopsy: to diagnose muscle disease.

Joint radiography: to detect acro-osteolysis, calcinosis.

Skin biopsy: usually not needed in established disease, best used in early puffy stage for diagnosis or to differentiate systemic sclerosis from fasciitis.

Complications

Hypertensive renal crisis: in diffuse cutaneous disease, usually within first 5 years of disease; in 7%–10% of patients.

Pseudo-obstruction: late complication often of limited cutaneous disease; in <5%.

Carcinoma of lung: associated with pulmonary fibrosis.

Differential diagnosis

Eosinophilic fasciitis.

Mixed connective tissue disease.

Overlap syndromes.

Chronic graft-versus-host disease.

Eosinophilic myalgic syndrome.

Vinyl chloride disease.

Toxic-oil syndrome.

Scleromyxedema.

Scleredema of Buschke.

Carcinoid syndrome.

Insulin-dependent diabetes mellitus skin changes.

Chronic reflex sympathetic dystrophy.

Idiopathic pulmonary fibrosis.

Primary pulmonary hypertension.

Cardiomyopathies.

Intestinal hypomotility syndromes.

Etiology

• In most cases, the cause is unknown, but the following may play a role:

Genetic: HLA classes II and III genes (weak association).

Environmental: organic chemicals (*e.g.*, vinyl chloride), epoxy resins, silica, rapeseed oil, drugs (*e.g.*, bleomycin).

Epidemiology

• Systemic sclerosis occurs world wide.

• 12–20 in one million people are affected annually.

• The female : male ratio is 3 : 1 overall and 10 : 1 in people of child-bearing age.

• The disease is more severe in nonwhites.

• 30–60 years is the usual age of onset.

Treatment

Diet and lifestyle

• Patients should avoid cold and sudden drops in temperature.

• Patients should stop smoking.

• Skin care involves protection and moisturizers (cosmetic cover for telangiectasia).

• Patients should follow a daily exercise program to prevent, reduce, or delay contractures and to maintain strength and function.

Pharmacological treatment

For Raynaud's phenomenon and vascular insufficiency [4]

• Response can be variable, so more than one drug within a class is worth trying.

Standard dosage *Calcium antagonists: e.g.*, nifedipine, 10–40 mg slow release twice daily.
Angiotensin-converting enzyme (ACE) inhibitors: captopril, 6.25–18.75 mg daily; enalapril, 5–15 mg daily.

Contraindications *Calcium antagonists:* pregnancy; caution in hepatic or renal disease
ACE inhibitors: pregnancy.

Special points *ACE inhibitors:* may cause rapid fall in blood pressure.

Main drug interactions *Calcium antagonists:* antiepileptics, antiarrhythmics.
ACE inhibitors: must not be given with potassium-sparing diuretics.

Main side effects *Calcium antagonists:* flushing, headache, edema.
ACE inhibitors: dry cough, voice change, rashes.

For early diffuse disease

• No drug is of proven efficacy [5–8].

Standard dosage D-Penicillamine, 750–1000 mg daily; methotrexate, 7.5–15 mg orally weekly; cyclosporin A, 2.5–5 mg/kg orally daily; prednisolone, 20 mg on alternate days.

Contraindications Pregnancy, existing liver and renal disease.

Main drug interactions Cyclophosphamide with allopurinol, cyclosporin with ACE inhibitors.

Main side effects Bone-marrow toxicity, renal and liver impairment, alopecia, rashes.

For esophageal involvement [5–8]

Standard dosage *Proton-pump inhibitor:* omeprazole, 20 mg daily.
Prokinetic drug: cisapride, 10 mg 3–4 times daily for 12 weeks, taken 30 min before meal or at bedtime.

Contraindications Pregnancy, breast-feeding.

Special points *Omeprazole:* can increase bowel colonization.

Main drug interactions Oral anticoagulants, phenytoin, theophylline.

Main side effects *Omeprazole:* constipation, headache, diarrhea.
Cisapride: abdominal cramps, diarrhea.

For mid-gut involvement: bacterial overgrowth

• Rotation antibiotics can be used in various combinations, *e.g.*, metronidazole, 400–600 mg twice daily, tetracycline, 250 mg 3 times daily; erythromycin, 250 mg 4 times daily, or ciprofloxacin, 500 mg twice daily.

• These should be given for short periods, *e.g.*, 3–4 weeks, with "holidays" of 1–2 weeks.

Pharmacological treatment

Lumbar or digital sympathectomy for severe Raynaud's phenomenon with critical ischemia.

Selective removal of calcinosis.

Treatment aims

To reduce symptoms.
To halt disease.
To treat complications.

• Systemic sclerosis has no cure.

Prognosis

5-year cumulative survival rate is 34%–73%.

Factors adversely affecting outcome: increasing age; male sex; extent of skin involvement; lung, heart, and kidney disease.

• For patients with diffuse cutaneous disease, the first 5 years are the most dangerous; with limited cutaneous disease, the most dangerous period is after 10 years, with a risk of pulmonary hypertension and widespread gut disease.

Follow-up and management

• Diffuse disease needs frequent follow-up in the first 4 years, *i.e.*, 3-monthly or more frequently if necessary; hypertensive renal crisis is the greatest risk.

• Limited disease needs yearly follow-up, with attention to late disease complications, *i.e.*, pulmonary hypertension, malabsorption.

• Attention to vascular insufficiency, possible superimposed infections, and changing internal organ involvement permits therapeutic adjustments that can improve quality of life for patients.

Key references

1. Medsger TA Jr: Systemic sclerosis (scleroderma), localized forms of scleroderma and calcinosis. *Arthritis and Allied Conditions* 1993, **2**:1253–1292.
2. LeRoy EC: Pathogenesis of systemic sclerosis. *Arthritis and Allied Conditions* 1993, **2**:1293–1299.
3. Penez M, Kohn SR: Systemic sclerosis. *J Am Acad Dermatol* 1993, **28**:525–547.
4. Kahaleh MB: Raynaud's phenomenon and vascular disease and scleroderma. *Curr Opin Rheumatol* 1994, **6**:621–627.
5. Torres MA, Furst DE: Treatment of generalized systemic sclerosis. *Rheum Dis Clin North Am* 1990, **16**:217–241.
6. Pope J: Treatment of systemic sclerosis. *Curr Opin Rheumatol* 1993, **5**:792–801.
7. Medsger TA Jr: Treatment of systemic sclerosis. *Ann Rheum Dis* 1991, **50**(suppl):877–886.
8. Van-den Hoogen FH, *et al.*: Treatment of systemic sclerosis. *Curr Opin Rheumatol* 1994, **6**:637–641.

Tachycardia, supraventricular

Diagnosis

Definition

• Supraventricular tachycardias include the following:

Sinus tachycardia.

Atrial fibrillation.

Atrial flutter.

Atrial tachycardia.

Atrioventricular re-entrant tachycardia.

Atrioventricular nodal re-entrant tachycardia.

• Atrioventricular re-entrant and nodal re-entrant tachycardias, the two common supraventricular tachycardias arising from the atrioventricular junction, are discussed here.

Symptoms

Palpitation: paroxysms of regular palpitation at 140–240 beats/min, with sudden onset and offset [1].

Syncope: palpitation may be associated with syncope or presyncope at onset of attack, when blood pressure is probably at its lowest.

Chest pain: unusual but may occur during attacks, particularly in presence of ischemic heart disease.

Paroxysmal attacks: occasionally precipitated by postural changes or may be associated with particular times in menstrual cycle.

Signs

Fast, regular pulse.

Signs of left ventricular failure: unusual unless structural heart disease is coexistent.

• Atrioventricular dissociation is not evident (no cannon waves in neck).

• Blood pressure is usually well maintained after the first few seconds of an attack.

Investigations

ECG: regular rhythm present, usually with narrow QRS complexes; occasionally, pre-existing or rate-related bundle branch block leads to broad QRS complexes [2].

Chest radiography: usually normal unless structural heart disease coexistent.

Electrophysiology: indicated if catheter ablation contemplated or for risk assessment in symptomatic patients with Wolff–Parkinson–White syndrome.

Complications

Left ventricular failure: caused by coexistent structural heart disease; supraventricular tachycardia may cause ventricular failure in the absence of pre-existing structural heart disease only if tachycardia is incessant and has continued uninterrupted for many months or years.

Differential diagnosis

Atrial tachycardia or atrial flutter.

Ventricular tachycardia: if atrioventricular re-entrant tachycardia is conducted with bundle branch block.

• When the history is being taken, establishing the presence or absence of structural heart disease, *e.g.*, cardiomyopathy or previous myocardial infarction, is important. A history or known diagnosis of either of these conditions makes a diagnosis of ventricular tachycardia much more probable than atrioventricular re-entrant or nodal re-entrant tachycardia. If the QRS complex is broad and has a pattern unlike that of classic left or right bundle branch block, then diagnosis is probably ventricular tachycardia.

Etiology

Atrioventricular re-entrant tachycardia

• The structural substrate is a congenital abnormality of the conducting system of the heart, whereby an extra electrical connection exists between the atria and the ventricles.

• Tachycardia arises when an electrical impulse passes from the atrium to the ventricle through the normal atrioventricular node but returns to the atria by the accessory pathway.

Atrioventricular nodal re-entrant tachycardia

• Patients have two functionally separate pathways within or close to the atrioventricular node.

• Tachycardia arises in a similar way to that arising in patients with atrioventricular re-entrant tachycardia.

Epidemiology

• These arrhythmias occur frequently and form most of the tachycardias in patients with structurally normal hearts.

• Men are more likely to have atrioventricular re-entrant tachycardia, and women atrioventricular nodal re-entrant tachycardia.

• Paroxysms of palpitation may start in infancy but more usually in teenage years or twenties.

Treatment

Diet and lifestyle

• If the tachycardias are initiated by atrial premature beats, abstinence from caffeine may help.

• Otherwise, no special precautions are necessary.

Pharmacological treatment

Acute treatment

Standard dosage Adenosine, i.v. bolus dose followed by saline flush, starting at 3 mg, with a second dose of 6 mg if tachycardia does not terminate after 60 s; a further dose of 12 mg is given if tachycardia does not terminate after another 60 s [3].
Verapamil, 5 mg i.v slowly (30 s); if tachycardia has not terminated after 5 min, a second 5-mg dose may be given, if hypotension has not occurred.

Contraindications *Adenosine:* asthma.
Verapamil: poor ventricular function.

Special points *Adenosine:* although 12 mg is maximum adult dose recommended in product license, bolus doses of 18 mg may occasionally be need to terminate tachycardia; may exacerbate bronchoconstriction.
Verapamil: negatively inotropic and should not be given to patients with known abnormal ventricular function or with signs of cardiomegaly on chest radiography; best not given to patients with a broad complex tachycardia because it may cause cardiovascular collapse if erroneously given to patients with ventricular tachycardia; i.v. verapamil should not be given to patient taking oral beta blockers because sinus arrest or dramatic hypotension may occur.

Main drug interactions *Adenosine:* increased effect with dipyridamole; decreased effect with theophylline.

Main side effects *Adenosine:* flushing and chest tightness (transient).

Prophylaxis

• Beta blockade (*e.g.*, atenolol, 50–100 mg) is often effective in this role, particularly if the attacks are exercise-induced.

• Digoxin, 0.125 mg, and verapamil, 120 mg 3 times daily, may be effective but are contraindicated in the presence of a delta wave because they may increase the ventricular rate if atrial fibrillation complicates the Wolff-Parkinson-White syndrome.

Treatment aims

To terminate an acute paroxysm of tachycardia.

To suppress tachycardia.

To cure tachycardia.

Other treatments

Vagal maneuvers

• Deep breathing or the Valsalva maneuver (best done with patient lying down), with straining for at least 15 s, should terminate tachycardia a few seconds after strain release.

Radiofrequency catheter ablation [4]

• This is the treatment of choice for patients with recurrent symptomatic junctional tachycardias that do not respond to prophylactic drug treatment or as an alternative to chronic pharmacologic therapy.

Prognosis

• Prognosis is generally excellent, and life expectancy does not differ from that of the normal population.

• Symptomatic patients with the Wolff–Parkinson–White pattern on the ECG during sinus rhythm have a small risk of sudden death, associated with the development of atrial fibrillation.

Follow-up and management

• Oral aspirin is advisable for 6 weeks after catheter ablation because the damaged endothelium may provide a focus for thrombus formation.

• Patients should be assessed for recurrence of symptoms or re-emergence of the Wolff–Parkinson–White pattern on the ECG.

Key references

1. Bennett DH: Cardiac Arrhythmias. Oxford: Butterworth Heinemann, 1993.
2. Nathan AW: Cardiac Arrhythmias. In *Essentials of Cardiology.* Edited by Timmis AD, Nathan AW. Oxford: Blackwell, 1993.
3. Camm AJ, Garratt CJ: Drug therapy: adenosine and supraventricular tachycardia. *N Engl J Med* 1991, **325**.1621–1629.
4. Jackman WM, *et al.*: Treatment of supraventricular tachycardia due to atrioventricular nodal reentry by radiofrequency catheter ablation of slow pathway conduction. *N Engl J Med* 1992, **327**:313–318.

Tachycardia, ventricular

Diagnosis

Symptoms

• Symptoms are not always manifest.

Palpitations.

Sudden shortness of breath.

Dizzy spell.

Blackouts.

Cardiac arrest.

Sudden death.

Signs

• Signs are not always manifest.

Tachycardia: 100–300 beats/min.

Hypotension and associated signs.

Cannon waves in jugular venous pressure, variable blood pressure, variation in intensity of first heart sound: signs of atrioventricular dissociation.

Investigations

12-lead ECG: initially, to confirm diagnosis, after treatment, for comparison of sinus rhythm; reveals tachycardia with QRS complexes 140 ms duration, evidence of atrioventricular dissociation (independent P waves, fusion beats, capture beats, second- degree ventriculo-atrial block), marked left or right axis deviation during tachycardia, absence of RS complexes in chest leads during tachycardia [1].

Adenosine test: initially, to distinguish from junctional or atrial tachycardia; if patient presents with stable tachycardia and if 12-lead ECG cannot be interpreted as showing ventricular tachycardia, incremental boluses of adenosine 0.05–0.20 mg/kg i.v. should be given, which terminates almost all junctional tachycardias, slows most atrial tachycardias, but affects almost no ventricular tachycardias except those arising in the right ventricular outflow tract.

Cardiac enzyme analysis: after treatment, if history suggests infarction.

Cardiac ultrasound: to determine whether there is underlying cardiomyopathic or valvular abnormality.

Exercise test: under supervision of arrhythmia specialist to look for coronary disease, to provoke arrhythmia, and to assess drug efficacy.

24-h ambulatory ECG recording: to quantify frequency of ventricular arrhythmia and associated arrhythmias (*e.g.*, ventricular premature beat).

Echocardiography: to assess left and right ventricular function.

Left ventricular and coronary angiography.

Programmed electrophysiologic testing: to determine inducibility, morphology, and suppressibility of arrhythmia.

Complications

Cardiac arrest.

Sudden death.

Cardiogenic shock.

Pulmonary edema.

Differential diagnosis

Supraventricular tachycardia: either atrial or junctional, with either right or left bundle branch block.

• All wide-complex tachycardias should be considered ventricular in origin until proved otherwise.

Etiology

• Causes include the following:

Acute ischemia: coronary obstruction by thrombus.

Large scar old infarction: previous surgery, dysplasias.

Microscopic scar infiltration: fibrosis.

No clinical disease: *e.g.*, right ventricular outflow tachycardia.

Right ventricular dysplasia.

Hypertrophic cardiomyopathy.

Viral myocarditis.

Functional disease: "fascicular" tachycardia.

Tumors, malformations, other causes (rare).

Epidemiology

• 2–10% of patients suffering a myocardial infarction have a sustained ventricular tachycardia or cardiac arrest within 12 months.

Treatment

Diet and lifestyle

• Patients should avoid strenuous exercise and eat a normal diet unless they have evidence of coronary disease.

Pharmacological treatment

• The underlying disease process (*e.g.*, coronary artery disease) or associated cardiogenic fluid retention must be treated.

Emergency

Cardiopulmonary resuscitation if necessary.

Lidocaine, 50 mg i.v., in stable patients.

Direct-current cardioversion in unstable patients (synchronized) or if drug treatment fails.

• A succession of drugs is unwise, especially in patients with coronary disease and impaired ventricular function.

• Verapamil must not be given: it may cause profound collapse and even death.

Long-term

• Drug treatment should be supervised by a cardiologist with a special interest in arrhythmias.

• All antiarrhythmic drugs have arrhythmogenic properties, especially when used in combination with other antiarrhythmic drugs [2].

• Whether long-term drug treatment improves prognosis is not known.

Standard dosage	Disopyramide, 250 mg slow release twice daily; alternatively, procainamide or quinidine. Flecainide, 100 mg twice daily; alternatively encainide or propafenone. Sotalol, 80 mg twice daily; alternatively amiodarone.
Contraindications	*Disopyramide:* very poor left ventricular function. *Flecainide:* previous myocardial infarction; caution in patients with coronary disease [2]. *Sotalol:* as for beta blockers generally.
Special points	*Flecainide:* increases pacing threshold [2]. *Sotalol:* prolongs action potential duration (unlike other beta blockers). *Amiodarone:* high incidence of toxic effects, long elimination half-life; should be considered only if less toxic agents have failed.
Main drug interactions	*Disopyramide:* antihistamines, antiepileptics. *Flecainide:* antidepressant, fluoxetine, antimalarial agents. *Sotalol:* as for beta blockers generally.
Main side effects	*Disopyramide:* vagolytic effects (dry mouth, slow stream). *Flecainide:* dizziness, arrhythmias. *Sotalol:* as for beta blockers generally.

Treatment aims

To suppress recurrence of tachycardia (drug treatment).

To terminate recurrence of tachycardia (device treatment).

To destroy the arrhythmia "substrate," possibly offering a cure (ablation).

To correct mechanical heart disease and refractory arrhythmias (transplantation).

Other treatments

• Alternative long-term treatments include:

Implantation of automatic defibrillator device to terminate tachycardia: this also treats ventricular tachycardia by rapid pacing.

Ablation of localized focus or circuit causing tachycardia: radiofrequency energy and low-energy direct current are most popular sources; success rate <50%.

Electrophysiologically guided surgery.

Transplantation in selected patients with severe ventricular impairment.

Prognosis

• Prognosis depends on the underlying disease process and presentation.

• 1-year mortality in patients resuscitated from cardiac arrest occurring out of hospital is up to 50%.

• Long-term prognosis is excellent for ventricular tachycardia associated with a normal heart.

Follow-up and management

• Patients should be referred to a center specializing in ventricular tachycardia to allow the correct treatment to be selected.

• Long-term drug treatment can be assessed by ambulatory monitoring (in patients with frequent ventricular premature contractions) or electrophysiological studies (in patients with inducible tachycardia).

• Ventricular tachycardia is not a curable disease and needs long-term follow-up.

Key references

1. Shenasa M, *et al.*: Ventricular tachycardia. *Lancet* 1993, **341**:1512–1518.

2. Echt DS, *et al.*: Mortality and morbidity of patients receiving encainide, flecainide, or placebo. *N Engl J Med* 1991, **324**:781–788.

Diagnosis

Symptoms and signs [1,2]

Delayed puberty and hypogonadism [3]

Failure to gain sufficient weight: in children (picky eating or anorexia).
Severe weight loss and malnutrition: in adults.
Poor virilization, tall stature with long limbs, gynecomastia, failure to develop sex drive, nocturnal emissions or masturbation; small firm testes, partial puberty, azoospermia: indicating Klinefelter's syndrome.
Hypergonadotropic gonadism, progressive decline in sperm count: azoospermia within months, with later progressive decline in Leydig cell function; after testicular irradiation or chemotherapy.
Failure of puberty, and eunuchoidism: indicating isolated gonadotropin deficiency.
Anosmia: indicating Kallmann's syndrome.
Evidence of pituitary tumor or past damage, hormonal deficiencies, absence of secondary sexual hair: indicating pituitary failure.
Mild hypogonadism with Turner's features, pulmonary stenosis: indicating Noonan's syndrome.
Obesity, micropenis, hypotonia, mental retardation, moderate hypogonadism: indicating Prader–Willi syndrome.

Adult male infertility [4]

Diminished sperm count, defective sperm motility.
Absent or obstructed epididymis or vas deferens, postepididymitis or seminal vesiculitis: indicating obstruction.
Postorchitis, torsion, incomplete testicular descent: indicating tubular damage.
Swelling: sometimes painful; empties on lying down; indicating varicocele.
Dystrophia myotonica-myotonia, cataracts, frontal alopecia, mental impairment, testicular atrophy with generally normal virilization, peritubular fibrosis.
Mental retardation, mild dysmorphic features, large testes as adults: indicating fragile X syndrome.

Male pseudohermaphroditism

Normal female genitalia, primary amenorrhea: indicating failure of testis to develop.
Inguinal testes, female external genitalia with short, blind vagina, female breasts at puberty, scant secondary sexual hair: indicating defective androgen receptor.

Investigations [1]

Hormone tests: single clotted blood for serum luteinizing hormone, follicle-stimulating hormone, prolactin and testosterone; 17-hydroxyprogesterone in well virilized patients possibly with early puberty with small testes and suppressed gonadotropins (congenital adrenal hyperplasia); raised follicle-stimulating hormone with oligo- or azoospermia indicates almost certain irreversible primary testicular damage; dynamic tests add little more.
Serum oestradiol measurement: for gynecomastia.
Karyotyping: for Klinefelter's syndrome in hypergonadotropic hypogonadism.
Semen morphology, count, motility, and postcoital test.
Immunology: mixed agglutination reaction, to detect antisperm antibodies.
Testicular biopsy: not often indicated.
Ultrasonography: for testicular masses or prostatic disease.
Pituitary CT or nuclear MRI: for possible tumors.

Complications

Delayed puberty and hypogonadism

Major psychological damage: if untreated at puberty.
Long-term increased risk of fracture: especially vertebral and hip.

Infertility

Androgen deficiency: in severe disorders or spermatogenesis.
Psychosocial problems.

Male pseudohermaphroditism

Psychological damage: without effective and sympathetic handling at outset.
Malignancy: in XY patients with streak gonads.

Differential diagnosis

Delayed puberty and hypogonadism
Growth-hormone deficiency.

Male pseudohermaphroditism
Female pseudohermaphroditism.

Etiology [1,2,4]

- Causes include the following:

Genetic factors: X-linked in testicular feminization, microdeletion, chromosome 15 abnormality in Prader–Willi syndrome.
Hormone or enzyme deficiencies.
Testicular irradiation or chemotherapy.

Epidemiology [1,2]

- Male pseudohermaphroditism is rare.
- Testicular feminization occurs in 1 in 60 000 males.
- Kallmann's syndrome occurs in 1 in 10 000 males.
- Prader–Willi syndrome occurs in 1 in 10 000–20 000 births.
- Congenital adrenal hyperplasia occurs in 1 in 7000 people.
- All other enzyme deficiencies are much rarer.
- Delayed puberty, oligospermia, and azoospermia are all common.
- Gynecomastia occurs in one-third of boys in puberty; it is common later in life.

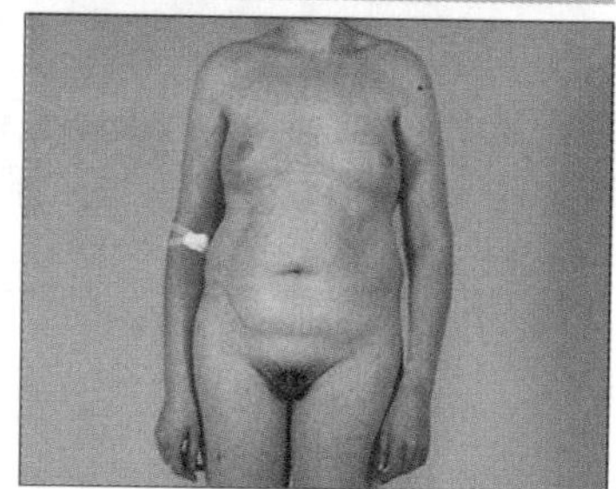

26-year-old man with untreated Kallmann's syndrome.

Treatment

Diet and lifestyle

• Most phenotypic female patients with androgen-receptor disorders (male pseudohermaphroditism, testicular feminization, pure XY gonadal dysgenesis) are raised as females.
• Patients with 5α-reductase deficiency generally identify as male.

Pharmacological treatment [1,2]

• For each patient, the relative importance of androgen deficiency and infertility and practicability of treatment must be defined clearly.

For androgen deficiency

Standard dosage Testosterone enanthate or cypionate, 200–300 mg every 2–3 weeks; transferase testosterone patch daily.
For gonadotropin deficiency, when fertility is desired: pulsatile gonadotropin-releasing hormone, 15 μg s.c. every 90 min by pump, or human chorionic gonadotropin, 2000 IU s.c. twice weekly or 5000 IU s.c. weekly, with subsequent menotropin, 225 IU 3 times weekly.

Contraindications Caution if history of violent behavior.

Special points *Gonadotropin replacement:* sperm count should rise for 6 months; sperm may be stored in sperm bank for future use; menotropin very expensive.

Main drug interactions None.

Main side effects Secondary sexual characteristics, balding, stimulation of prostatic hyperplasia; gynecomastia with human chorionic gonadotrophin therapy.

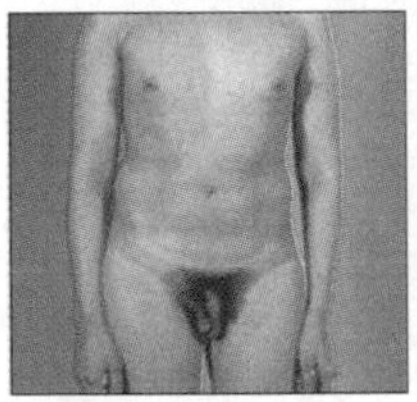

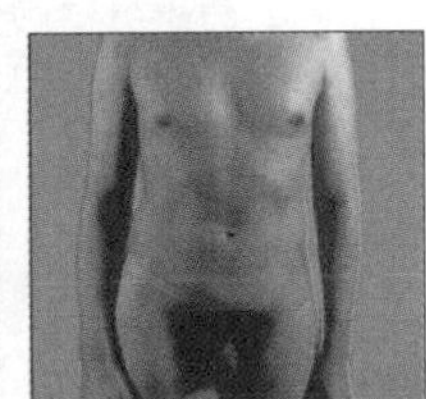

Hypogonadal patient with partial gonadotrophin deficiency (fertile eunuch syndrome) before (*left*) and after (*right*) 1 year's treatment with twice-weekly human chorionic gonadotropin.

For male congenital adrenal hyperplasia

Standard dosage Glucocorticosteroid, *e.g.*, hydrocortisone, 15–30 mg daily in divided doses.
For salt-losers: mineralocorticosteroid replacement (fludrocortisone, 0.1 mg orally twice daily).

Contraindications None.

Special points Corticotropic hormone suppression should restore normal gonadotropins and spermatogenesis.

Main drug interactions With hepatic enzyme inducers (*e.g.*, rifampicin), more glucocorticosteroid and mineralocorticosteroid are needed.

Main side effects Hypercortisolism with excessive glucocorticosteroid.

For 5α-reductase deficiency

• Patients should be treated by high-dose testosterone, up to 200 mg weekly.

For gynecomastia

• The cause should be removed if possible.
• Danazol in low doses is worth a therapeutic trial.
• Surgery (mastectomy through periareolar incision) is indicated for severe cases.

Treatment aims

To restore virilization and normal sex drive and potency.

To prevent long-term risk of osteoporotic fracture.

Prognosis

• Androgen deficiency itself does not adversely affect life expectancy.
• Prader–Willi syndrome and dystrophia myotonica do adversely affect life expectancy.

Follow-up and management

• Regular attendance is necessary for testosterone treatment.
• Patients with germ-cell damage should have annual measurement of serum luteinizing hormone, follicle-stimulating hormone, and testosterone, with onset of androgen replacement early rather than late.

Key references

1. Griffen JE, Wilson JD: Disorders of the testes and male reproductive tract. In *Williams Textbook of Endocrinology*, edn 8. Edited by Wilson JD, Foster DW. Philadelphia: WB Saunders; 1992:799–852.
2. Grumbach MM, Conte FA: Disorders of sex differentiation. In *Williams Textbook of Endocrinology*, edn 8. Edited by Wilson JD, Foster DW. Philadelphia: WB Saunders; 1992:853–951.
3. Anderson DC: Endocrine diseases. In *Textbook of Medicine*, edn 2. Edited by Souhami RL, Moxham J. London: Churchill Livingstone; 1994:706–718.
4. Anderson DC, Large DM: Endocrine function of the testis: normal and abnormal. In *Scientific Foundation of Urology*, edn 3. Edited by Chisholm GD, Fair WR. Oxford: Heinemann; 1990:379–390.

Diagnosis

Symptoms

• β-Thalassemia is manifest during the first year of life in 90% of patients; a few present at 3–4 years (late-onset β-thalassemia major).

• 10% of patients with β-thalassemia major have a mild course (not dependent on transfusion).

• Patients may be asymptomatic; detection is from antenatal screening and diagnosis.

Poor weight gain.

Failure to thrive.

Fever.

Diarrhea.

Increasing pallor.

Distended abdomen.

Signs

Pallor.

Heart failure.

Splenomegaly.

Jaundice.

Investigations

Blood tests: low hemoglobin, mean corpuscular hemoglobin, mean cell volume; absent or reduced hemoglobin A (β° or β^{+} thalassemia), variable hemoglobin F and A_2 (using electrophoresis).

Genetic analysis: defines specific mutations, may help to predict disease severity and prognosis and facilitate first-trimester diagnosis.

Complications

Splenomegaly leading to hypersplenism (neutropenia, thrombocytopenia, anemia).

Anemia causing severe bone changes, short stature, and heart failure.

Differential diagnosis

Iron deficiency.

Etiology

• Thalassemia is caused by defective synthesis of the α- or β-globin chain (α- and β-thalassemia, respectively).

• The disorder is inherited (Mendelian recessive).

• It occurs in Mediterranean, Asian, Arabic, and Chinese groups because of a selective advantage against *Plasmodium falciparum*.

Epidemiology [1]

• Thalassemia is one of the most common inherited disorders throughout the world

• Among African Americans, approximately 30% of the population is either heterozygous or homozygous for the α-thalassemia-2 deletion.

• In southwest Europe, it is declining because of prevention programs; in consanguineous marriages, the birth rate of β-thalassemia increases by 30%

Treatment

Diet and lifestyle

• Patients must avoid red meat and liver, and they should be encouraged to lead a normal active lifestyle.

Pharmacological treatment

Treatment of transfusional iron overload

• Desferrioxamine is infused s.c. over 8–12 h from a portable syringe driver pump 5–6 nights/week.

• Chelation therapy is started when ferritin is 1000 µg/L (after 12–24 transfusions).

• Initial dose of 20 mg/kg desferrioxamine is diluted in 5–10 mL water for injection. Vitamin C, 100–200 mg orally (increases urinary iron excretion), is added when the patient is on desferrioxamine.

• In iron-overloaded patients, the desferrioxamine dose is 50 mg/kg daily.

• For cardiomyopathy, continuous desferrioxamine is given through an i.v. delivery device (Hickman Line, Port-a-Cath).

Complications of treatment

Alloimmunization to blood group antigens (in 25% of patients), febrile and urticarial transfusion reactions (in 75% of patients), cytomegalovirus infection and immunosuppression, transfusion-transmitted hepatitis B and C viruses: due to chronic transfusion (risk of HIV, 1 in 65 000).

Cardiomyopathy (most common cause of death), reduced growth, hypoparathyroidism, diabetes, failure of puberty: due to inadequate chelation.

Short stature, bone changes (pseudorickets), visual disturbances, hypersensitivity, hearing problems, pulmonary edema: due to desferrioxamine toxicity (overchelation).

Treatment aims

To provide good quality of life.

To provide a long life.

Other treatments

Bone-marrow transplantation: 94% success rate if patient compliant with desferrioxamine and has no liver fibrosis or enlargement; success rate affected by age and liver status.

Splenectomy for hypersplenism.

Prognosis

• Maintenance transfusion and regular iron chelation preserve excellent health, and the prognosis is now open-ended.

• Early death is generally the result of intractable heart failure secondary to iron overload and infections.

Follow-up and management [3]

• The patient's ferritin, liver function, and bone metabolism must be monitored 3 times yearly, with annual anti-hepatitis C virus, anti-HIV, and hepatitis B surface antigen checks.

• Oral glucose tolerance tests must be done yearly from the age of 10 years in patients with a family history of diabetes or from the age of 16 years in those without.

• Other endocrine and cardiac investigations should be made if clinically indicated.

• Patients should have yearly audiometry and twice-yearly eye tests.

•Splenectomized patients have higher risk of infection and may need vaccinations.

Key references

1. Davies SC, Modell B, Wonke B: *Access to Healthcare for People from Black and Ethnic Minorities*. London: Royal College of Physicians; 1993:147–168.
2. World Health Organization: *The Haemoglobinopathies in Europe*. Geneva: World Health Organization, 1988.
3. Davies SC, Wonke B: The management of haemoglobinopathies. *Baillières Clin Haematol* 1991, 4:361–389.

Diagnosis

Symptoms

• Patients can be asymptomatic (thyroid swelling is noted by someone else).

Neck swelling: rapid increase in size (particularly important symptom if patient is taking thyroid hormone).

Pain in neck, radiating to jaw or ear.

Dysphagia.

Dyspnea.

Dysphonia.

Symptoms of thyrotoxicosis: rare.

Bone pain, hemoptysis, abdominal discomfort: indicating metastases.

Signs

Thyroid swelling (goiter): single nodule, multinodular, diffuse.

Cancer: most common in single nodules, least in diffuse goiter.

Fixation of thyroid swelling to local structures.

Cervical lymphadenopathy.

Spinal-cord compression, spastic paraparesis.

Hepatomegaly, bone swellings, tenderness: indicating metastases.

Investigations [1]

• No laboratory test distinguishes malignant from benign lesions of the thyroid.

Thyroid function tests: serum free thyroxine and thyroid-stimulating hormone to exclude hyperthyroidism and hypothyroidism.

Thyroid autoantibody tests.

Serum calcitonin measurement: raised concentration (basal or stimulated) in medullary thyroid cancer.

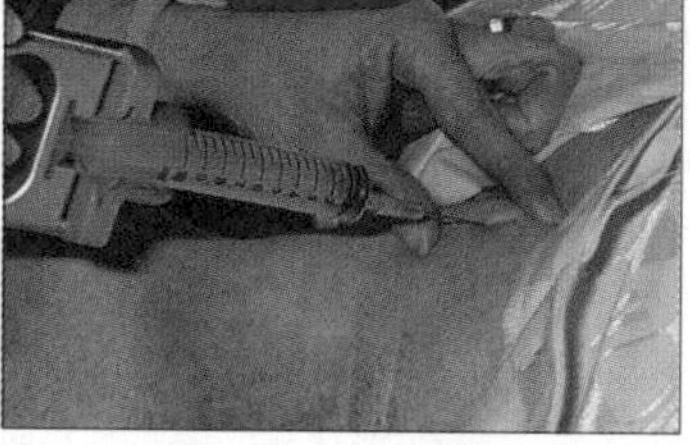

Fine-needle aspiration of a thyroid nodule, allowing rapid cytological examination of aspirated material.

Fine-needle aspiration cytology: routine preoperative evaluation of most patients with thyroid nodules.

Ultrasonography: to detect solid, solitary nodules (with greater risk of malignancy).

Isotope scanning: to detect hypofunctioning, solitary nodules (with greater risk of malignancy).

Serum thyroglobulin evaluation: of no use for diagnosis; great value in monitoring treated patients.

Complications

Local infiltration of trachea, esophagus, nerves.

Metastases of bone, liver, lung.

Differential diagnosis

Benign thyroid disease: diffuse goiter, single or multiple nodules.

Hashimoto's disease.

Other causes of lymphadenopathy.

Etiology [2]

• Causes include the following:

External irradiation of head and neck.

Iodine deficiency.

Proto-oncogene expression (ret oncogene unique to papillary thyroid cancer).

Genetic: medullary cancer in multiple endocrine neoplasia syndrome.

Epidemiology [2]

• Thyroid cancer accounts for <0.5% of new malignancies and <0.5% of cancer deaths.

• Goiter, including thyroid nodules, is present in up to 10% of the population.

• The female : male ratio is 3 : 1.

• The risk of malignancy is increased when nodules develop in people aged >60 years.

Tumor pathology

• Papillary thyroid cancer is the most frequently diagnosed malignant thyroid tumor.

• Follicular thyroid cancer is a relatively unusual malignancy (~15% of all thyroid cancers).

• Hürthle cell cancer occurs in 3%–6% of patients.

• Anaplastic cancer accounts for <10% of patients.

Treatment

Diet and lifestyle

• No evidence indicates that environmental factors affect the prognosis of established thyroid cancer.

• An iodine-replete diet and avoidance of external irradiation to head and neck reduces the risk of developing thyroid cancer.

Pharmacological treatment [1–3]

• After surgery, patients can be considered for radioiodine treatment.

• No consensus has been reached on ^{131}I ablation of the thyroid in patients with small solitary papillary lesions.

• Routine ablation of thyroid remnant is indicated in patients with follicular thyroid cancer.

• Ablation has a clear role in the management of residual disease or established metastases.

• All patients with differentiated thyroid cancer need suppressive thyroxine treatment after definitive treatment; thyroxine is necessary in all patients rendered hypothyroid after treatment.

Nonpharmacological treatment

• The extent of surgery (simple lobectomy, near-total thyroidectomy, total thyroidectomy) depends on pathology and surgical preference.

• Anaplastic thyroid cancer is resistant to treatment; best results are achieved with a combination of surgery, external irradiation, and chemotherapy.

• Surgery is the primary mode of treatment for papillary, follicular, and medullary thyroid cancers.

• Surgical removal of involved lymph nodes is indicated.

Treatment aims

To minimize morbidity and mortality of disease.

To minimize morbidity of diagnostic and therapeutic interventions.

Prognosis [1,2]

• Prolonged survival is usual.

• Patients with localized papillary or follicular thyroid cancers have an excellent prognosis, (10–20-year recurrence rates of 5%–10% and death rates of 2%–5%).

• Adverse prognostic factors include older age, greater degree of invasiveness, distant metastases, and abnormal chromosomal number within tumor tissue.

• Anaplastic cancer is very aggressive, with a 5-year survival rate of 7%.

Follow-up and management [1,2]

• After radioablation of the thyroid, total-body radioiodine scans can detect recurrent or metastatic disease and may be performed at 12-monthly intervals.

• Serum thyroglobulin is a valuable tumor marker; patients with differentiated papillary or follicular thyroid cancers have normal or undetectable concentrations in the absence of tumor but raised concentrations in the presence of residual, recurrent, or metastatic disease.

Key references

1. Kaplan MM, ed: Thyroid Carcinoma. *Endocrinol Metab Clin North Am* 1990, vol. 19, No. 3.
2. DeGroot LJ, *et al.*: Natural history, treatment, and course of papillary thyroid carcinoma. *J Clin Endocrinol Metabol* 1990, **71**:414–424.
3. Samaan NA, *et al.*: The results of different modalities of treatment of well differentiated thyroid carcinoma: a retrospective review of 1599 patients. *J Clin Endocrinol Metab* 1992, **75**:714–720.

Diagnosis

Definition

• Definition criteria require fever, rash, hypotension, clinical or test evidence of involvement of three systems, negative results from blood (except in the case of *Staphylococcus aureus*), CSF, and throat culture, and exclusion of measles, leptospirosis, and Rocky Mountain spotted fever.

• Mild or near-miss toxic shock syndrome that does not reach the clinical severity of the full definition is almost certainly more prevalent and poorly recognized. It may resolve because of general antibiotic use or end of menstruation.

Symptoms

High temperature: often to 40°C.

Vomiting and diarrhea: usually watery.

Faintness: especially on standing.

Aching muscles.

Rash.

Signs

Hypotension: systolic blood pressure <90 mm Hg or postural drop of >15 mm Hg; below fifth percentile for age in children <16 years.

Rash: patchy erythema, likened to sunburn, especially on trunk, thighs, palms, soles.

Tender muscles.

Reddened mucosal surfaces: conjunctival, oral, vaginal.

"Red strawberry" tongue.

Confusion: without focal neurological signs.

Puffy hands and feet.

Investigations

Hematology: thrombocytopenia usual.

Biochemistry: to assess renal function and liver inflammation; creatine kinase concentration often high.

Bacteriology: cultures of blood, stool, urine, vagina, cervix, wounds; *Staphylococcus aureus* isolates to be forwarded for toxin production and phage typing.

Complications

Renal failure, coma, peripheral gangrene, adult respiratory distress: in varying combinations due to hypotension.

Marked desquamation: especially of palms, soles, and digits, 1–2 weeks after onset.

Hair loss, occasional nail loss: after 2–3 months.

Differential diagnosis

Infective gastroenteritis.
Septicemia, especially gram-negative.
Scarlatina.
Kawasaki syndrome.

Etiology

• Toxins are produced by *Staphylococcus aureus*, mostly toxic shock syndrome toxin-1, but also enterotoxin A, B, or C. (Streptococcal toxins can produce a similar illness.)

• They are absorbed into the body during menstruation (especially with tampons) or at sites of infection (wound or burn, sinusitis, empyema, postinfluenzal bronchopneumonia, conjunctivitis).

Epidemiology

• In the US, where illness fulfilling diagnostic criteria has been notifiable, for the past 7 years, only 50% of the notifications have been menstrually related.

• Menstrual toxic shock syndrome occurs most often in high-absorbency tampon users aged 15–25 years.

• The incidence of menstrual toxic shock syndrome has declined since the early 1980s in the US, probably as a result of increased health education, reduced tampon absorbency, and removal of acrylate fibers from tampons.

• Toxic shock syndrome has also been associated with the use of contraceptive diaphragms and sponges.

• Nonmenstrual toxic shock syndrome develops in both sexes and at any age.

• ~80% of adults have toxic shock syndrome toxin-1 antibodies, suggesting that mild or subclinical immunizing events happen frequently.

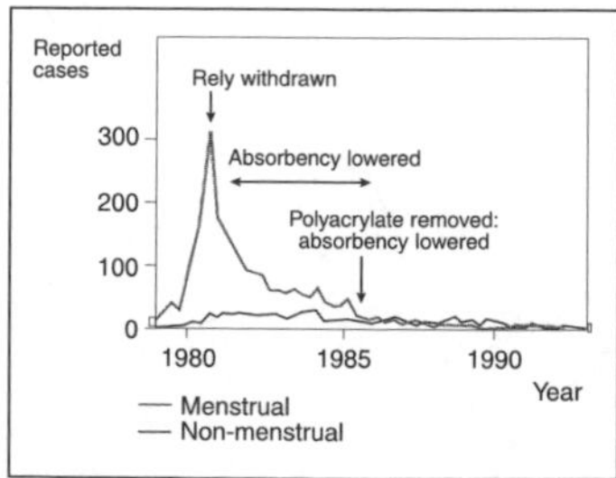

Incidence of toxic shock syndrome in the US 1979–1993.

Treatment

Diet and lifestyle

• To reduce the likelihood of menstrually related toxic shock syndrome, women must wash hands before and after inserting tampons, use the lowest absorbency tampons that cope with their needs, change tampons regularly (at least every 4–6 h), use pads overnight, remove and stop using tampons if acute symptoms develop during menstruation, and inform their physician of symptoms of current menstruation. Details of toxic shock syndrome are given on leaflets within tampon cartons, and a health warning is printed on the outside.

Pharmacological treatment

General resuscitation

• Severely ill patients need management and monitoring in intensive care units.

• Crystalloid solutions should be used, initially with inotropic support.

• Other modalities, *e.g.*, dialysis, ventilation, should be used when indicated.

Antibiotics

• Although nafcillin does not appear to speed resolution of toxic shock syndrome, it is used empirically in case of septicemia and for localized infections at other sites.

Standard dosage Nafcillin, 1 g i.v. 6-hourly.

Contraindications Hypersensitivity, porphyria.

Special points Reduces recurrence rate in future menstrual periods. Third-generation cephalosporin can be used instead.

Main drug interactions None.

Main side effects Sensitivity reactions, jaundice.

Antitoxin

• The therapeutic usefulness of toxic shock syndrome toxin-1 antibodies (found in normal immunoglobulin or plasma) has not been determined.

Treatment aims

To limit hypoxic damage (prompt resuscitation).

To stop further toxin production and absorption (removal of tampons, drainage of pus, i.v. floxacillin).

To prevent subsequent relapses (floxacillin, advice on future tampon use).

Prognosis

• Mortality is 3%.

• Chronic morbidity varies and is related to acute ischemic damage to vital organs.

• The risk of recurrence during the next menstrual period is small, and symptoms tend to be milder.

• Recurrences may also follow nonmenstrual toxic shock syndrome, especially if anti-staphylococcal antibiotics are not used, and often follow subsequent skin or mucous membrane infection.

Follow-up and management

• Women should be advised against using tampons for the first few periods but can then reintroduce low-absorbency tampons, with frequent changing, and gradual return to advised standard routine thereafter.

• If further menstrual symptoms develop, tampon use must be stopped, and the patient should be given floxacillin and resuscitative measures in relation to symptoms.

General references

Centers for Disease Control: Reduced incidence of menstrual toxic shock syndrome—United States 1980–1990. *MMWR Morb Mortal Wkly Rep* 1990, **39**:421–423.

Communicable Diseases Surveillance Centre: Toxic shock syndrome and related conditions in the United Kingdom: 1992 and 1993. *Commun Dis Rep CDR Rev* 1994, **4**:65.

Kain KC, Schulzer M, Chow AW: Clinical spectrum of nonmenstrual toxic shock syndrome. *Clin Infect Dis* 1993, **16**:100–106.

Diagnosis

Symptoms

Primary infection

Fever, lymphadenopathy, glandular fever-like illness.

Secondary infection

Reactivation of tachyzoites: in cysts in any tissue, particularly brain, also eye, heart, and lung; symptoms are due to focal brain abscess, possibly with diffuse meningoencephalitis.

Focal symptoms

- These occur in 70% of patients with cerebral abscess.
- Initially, they may be subtle or transient, evolving to persistent focal neurological deficits, including the following:

Hemiparesis, hemisensory loss, movement disorders, ataxia, visual field deficits, cranial nerve palsies, aphasia.

Severe localized headaches: in 45% of patients.

Focal and secondarily generalized seizures: in 38%.

Nonfocal symptoms

- These may predominate in up to 40% of patients.

Fever and malaise (variable), disorientation, psychosis, neck stiffness (in 5%), increasing confusion and coma.

Signs

- Focal signs, *e.g.*, cerebellar tremor, extrapyramidal signs, and hemiplegia, are common; they indicate multiple or focal CNS lesions.
- Signs of infection (fever, meningism) are unreliable and inconsistent.

Investigations

Toxoplasma serology: initial investigation; IgG reflects chronic infection; IgM, acute seroconversion; negative test does not exclude diagnosis.

CT of brain with contrast: urgent; in 70%–80% of patients, shows single or multiple ring-enhancing lesions with edema (mainly in basal ganglia and bilaterally at corticomedullary junction).

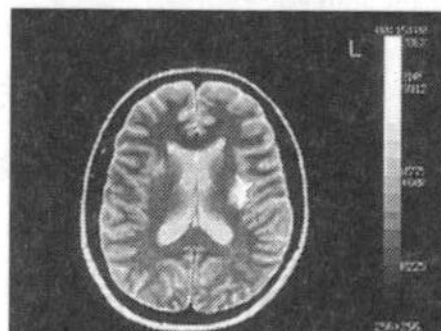
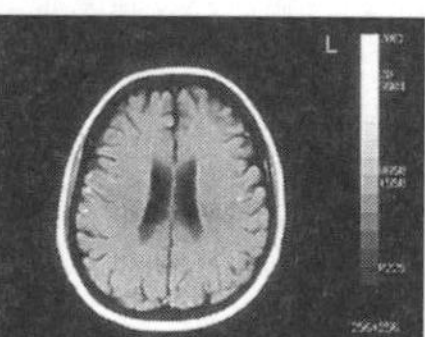
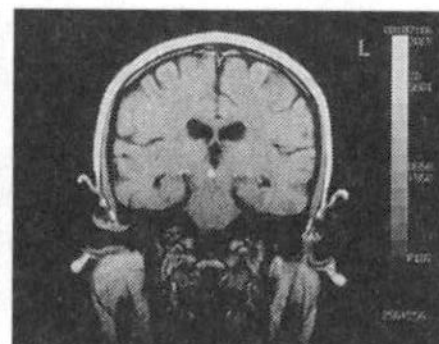

MRI of a patient with cerebral toxoplasmosis. Transverse section before (*left*) and after contrast (*middle*) shows multiple lesions; coronal section (*right*) shows several cortical lesions and one brain stem lesion.

MRI of brain: as alternative to CT scanning or for patients with single or no lesions on CT (20%–30%); increases sensitivity for multiple lesions and may reveal lesions accessible to biopsy; demonstration of single lesion strongly suggests cause other than toxoplasmosis.

Lumbar puncture: in absence of cerebral edema on brain scan; to detect intrathecal toxoplasma antibody production; CSF cellularity, protein, and glucose nonspecific in HIV.

Brain biopsy: indicated for single lesions on MRI or for nonresponders to treatment.

Complications

Fitting, coning, or hydrocephalus.

Panhypopituitarism, inappropriate antidiuretic hormone secretion.

Diffuse encephalitis, death.

Differential diagnosis

Focal neurological dysfunction

Primary CNS lymphoma, metastatic non-Hodgkin's lymphoma, progressive multifocal leukodystrophy (common).

Cytomegalovirus, herpes simplex virus, herpes zoster virus, cryptococcal meningitis, abcesses (*Tuberculosis, Nocardia, Candida* spp.), cerebrovascular disease (rare).

Diffuse encephalitis

AIDS encephalitis, AIDS dementia syndrome, cytomegalovirus or herpes simplex encephalitis.

Etiology

- Toxoplasmosis is caused by infection with *Toxoplasma gondii*; spread is by the feco-oral route.
- Silent chronic infection is characterized by tachyzoites in tissue cysts throughout the body.
- Acute reactivation involves cyst rupture, causing an encephalitis and a focal necrotizing vasculitic process.

Epidemiology

- Toxoplasmosis is ubiquitous in human populations.
- The incidence reflects the background seroprevalence in a given group: 10%–40% of adults in the US are seropositive (90% in France).
- Up to 30% of HIV-infected people who are seropositive for *Toxoplasma gondii* develop cerebral toxoplasmosis, usually with CD4 counts $<100 \times 10^6$/L.
- Overall, toxoplasma accounts for 40% of known CNS infection and 33% of intracerebral lesions in AIDS patients.

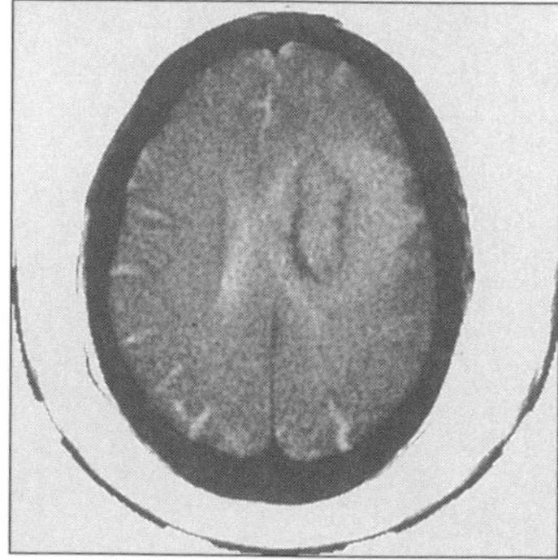

Contrast-enhanced CT of the same patient shows a single lesion in the left temporal lobe.

Treatment

Diet and lifestyle

• No special precautions are necessary.

Pharmacological treatment

• Treatment is begun empirically for a presumptive diagnosis of toxoplasma encephalitis based on clinical presentation and CT or MRI evidence (usually) of multifocal rung-enhancing lesions in a person who has positive serology to *Toxoplasma gondii*.

• The main regimen is pyrimethamine and folinic acid with sulfadiazine. Clindamycin or atovaquone is used in sulfa-intolerant patients.

Standard dosage
Pyrimethamine, 75 mg to load (or 100–200 mg), then 50 mg orally daily.
Folinic acid, 15 mg daily to prevent myelosuppression.
Sulfadiazine, 4–6 g daily in divided doses.
Clindamycin, 2400 mg daily in divided doses, if sulfa-intolerant.
Atovaquone, 750 mg 4 times daily.

Contraindications
Pyrimethamine: hepatic or renal impairment.
Sulfadiazine: pregnancy, renal or hepatic failure, jaundice, porphyria.
Clindamycin: diarrheal states.

Special points
Careful monitoring of neurological condition and repeat CT or MRI to check for improvement in the first 14 days of treatment are imperative.
With clinical and radiographic improvement, treatment is normally continued for 4–6 weeks; if no improvement occurs in the first 14–21 days, stereotactic brain biopsy should be considered.
Pyrimethamine, sulfadiazine: disrupt folic acid metabolism; blood count must be monitored weekly.
Clindamycin: liver function and blood count must be monitored.

Main drug interactions
Pyrimethamine: increased antifolate effect with phenytoin and trimethoprim.
Sulfadiazine: warfarin, phenytoin, pyrimethamine, cyclosporin.
Clindamycin: neostigmine, tubocurarine.

Main side effects
Pyrimethamine: nausea, vomiting, myelosuppression (folate).
Folinic acid: pyrexia.
Sulfadiazine: nausea, vomiting, rashes, blood dyscrasias (treatment must be stopped immediately), nephrotoxicity, headache, hepatitis (rare); adverse reaction rate 40%.
Clindamycin: nausea, vomiting, rash, diarrhea (rare but serious pseudomembranous colitis; treatment must be stopped immediately).
Atovaquone: diarrhea, rash.

• In patients with significant mass effect or decreased consciousness level, steroids are indicated, *e.g.*, high-dose dexamethasone, 8 mg orally or i.v. 4 times daily.

• Steroids may complicate the interpretation of clinical improvement and CT or MRI resolution during empirical antitoxoplasma treatment.

• They should be reduced and withdrawn as soon as is reasonable and repeat scans performed to check for exacerbation.

Treatment aims

To cure acute illness.

To prevent relapse.

Prognosis

• 90% of patients, including those in coma, respond to antitoxoplasma chemotherapy in 14–21 days, often sooner, but one-third have residual neurological defect.

• The relapse rate is up to 50%.

Follow-up and management

• Maintenance treatment must be lifelong because of the presence of cysts, against which chemotherapy is ineffective.

• Pyrimethamine, 25–50 mg daily, sulfadiazine, 2–4 g daily (or clindamycin), and folinic acid, 10 mg on alternate days, must be continued indefinitely.

General references

Mariuz P, Luft BJ: Toxoplasmic encephalitis. In *AIDS Clinical Review*. Edited by Volberding and Jacobson, 1992.

Porter SB, Sande MA: Toxoplasmosis of the central nervous system in the acquired immune deficiency syndrome. *N Eng J Med* 1992, **327**:1643–1647.

Indications

Erythrocytes

• A low hemoglobin level *per se* is not an indication for transfusion. Factors such as the patient's condition, the rate of fall of hemoglobin, and the cause of anemia must be considered to determine the correct treatment.

Whole blood

For acute massive blood loss.

Erythrocyte concentrates

For chronic blood loss or anemia.

For blood loss <1 blood volume in elective surgery (in additive solution).

Filtered blood

To prevent or delay nonhemolytic febrile transfusion reactions in patients who are erythrocyte dependent.

For newly diagnosed patients with aplastic anemia who are potential bone-marrow transplant recipients.

When cytomegalovirus-antibody negative blood is indicated but not readily available.

For intrauterine transfusion.

Washed cells

For patients with proven hypersensitivity reactions to plasma proteins.

For neonates who have necrotizing enterocolitis.

Cryopreserved erythrocytes

For patients needing blood of rare phenotypes or blood compatible with multiple erythrocyte alloantibodies.

For patients with anti-IgA in the absence of IgA-negative blood.

Irradiated erythrocytes

For recipients at risk of graft-versus-host disease: in utero transfusion, after bone-marrow transplantation.

For rare cases of transfusions from relatives.

Platelets [2]

To prevent or treat bleeding in patients with thrombocytopenia and rarely to treat bleeding in patients with platelet function defects: the cause of thrombocytopenia and significance of hemorrhage influence the use of platelet transfusions.

For acute bone-marrow failure (*e.g.*, due to aplasia, chemotherapy): if platelet count $10–50 \times 10^9/L$, serious spontaneous bleeding is unlikely, although minor bleeding (purpura, epistaxis) may occur; prophylactic platelet transfusions to maintain count $>10 \times 10^9/L$ reduces risk of hemorrhage as effectively as keeping count higher and reduces morbidity but not mortality; patients with fever, infection, coagulopathy, or rapid fall in platelet count should be transfused to maintain platelets $>20 \times 10^9/L$.

For acute disseminated intravascular coagulation: when thrombocytopenia is associated with bleeding (not indicated in chronic disseminated intravascular coagulation without bleeding).

For massive blood loss: to maintain platelets $>50 \times 10^9/L$.

Prophylaxis for surgery: to maintain platelets $>50 \times 10^9/L$ or $>100 \times 10^9/L$ for surgery in a critical site, *e.g.*, brain or eye (not routinely with cardiopulmonary bypass).

For autoimmune thrombocytopenia: platelet transfusions rarely used..

Fresh frozen plasma [3]

To replace single coagulation factor deficiencies when a specific or combined factor concentrate is unavailable.

For immediate reversal of warfarin effect.

For acute disseminated intravascular coagulation.

For thrombotic thrombocytopenic purpura.

For bleeding or disturbed coagulation associated with massive transfusion, liver disease, or cardiopulmonary bypass surgery.

Autologous transfusion [1]

Advantages

• The possibilities of alloimmunization, immunosuppression, and transfusion-transmitted infection are avoided.

Disadvantages

• Not all patients are eligible.

• Predeposited blood may be unused, *e.g.*, if surgery is cancelled, or may be insufficient to meet the patient's needs.

• Collecting predeposited autologous blood is more expensive than using standard units.

Options

Autologous predeposit: up to 5 units of blood collected and stored during the weeks before surgery.

Acute normovolemic hemodilution: blood drawn from patient under anesthetic and replaced by crystalloid so that blood lost during surgery has a lower hematocrit; when blood loss starts or at end of procedure, patient's whole blood is returned.

Erythrocyte salvage: blood lost at operating site recovered and processed for transfusion.

Directed blood donations

• Blood donations from relatives or friends should be discouraged unless needed on medical grounds.

• Evidence suggests that "directed" donations are generally less safe than blood supplied by the American Red Cross.

Techniques

Erythrocytes

Whole blood: packed cell volume (PCV) 0.35–0.45, 1 unit = 510 mL ± 10%; if blood loss and replacement exceed twice the blood volume, thrombocytopenia and abnormalities of hemostasis may develop.

Fresh blood (<24 h): blood that has not been microbiologically tested must not be transfused.

Erythrocyte concentrates: PCV 0.55–0.75, 1 unit = 220–340 mL.

Erythrocyte concentrates in additive solution: PCV 0.5–0.7, 1 unit = 280–420 mL; not to be used for exchange or large-volume transfusion in neonates.

Filtered blood (leukodepleted $<5 \times 10^6$ leukocytes/unit): PCV and quantity variable; rigorous validation of blood processing and component preparation needed, quality assurance program shows bedside filtration to be unreliable [4].

Washed cells (residual protein <0.5 g/unit): must be used within 24 h of preparation.

Cryopreserved erythrocytes (thawed and washed): volume usually <200 mL; must be used within 24 h of preparation.

Irradiated erythrocytes (minimum dose, 25 Gy): must be used within 1 day if for intrauterine transfusion because of increased potassium.

Platelets [5]

Administration

- Platelets for transfusion should preferably be of the recipient ABO and RhD group.
- If RhD-positive platelets are transfused to a RhD-negative woman potentially capable of childbearing, 250 IU anti-D immunoglobulin should be given subcutaneously with each dose of platelets.

Dose and response

- A standard dose of 300×10^9 may be issued as pooled or single platelet concentrates derived from individual donations or as a single apheresis donation, respectively, to raise the platelet count (adult) by $\sim 40 \times 10^9$/L.
- Patient factors, including sepsis, certain drugs, disseminated intravascular coagulation, splenomegaly, uremia, and platelet antibodies, can reduce the expected platelet increment.
- Patients who are repeatedly transfused with platelets may develop immunological refractoriness due to HLA alloimmunization and should receive platelets from HLA-matched donors.
- In some cases, platelet-specific alloantibodies develop, requiring type-specific platelet transfusions.

Fresh frozen plasma [3]

Administration

- Fresh frozen plasma (FFP) should be ABO and RhD compatible, although compatibility testing is not required.
- Group O FFP should be transfused only to Group O recipients.
- If an RhD-negative woman potentially capable of childbearing is transfused with RhD-positive FFP, 50 IU anti-D immunoglobulin should be given per unit of FFP transfused.

Dose

- A generally accepted starting dose is 12–15 mL/kg.
- The clinical and laboratory responses should be monitored to assess response and plan further management.

Management of adverse effects of transfusion [1]

Hemolytic transfusion reactions
(ABO incompatibility most severe)
Safe documentation and checking of systems for compatibility testing and blood administration; treatment for acute renal failure and disseminated intravascular coagulation may be needed.

Febrile nonhemolytic transfusion reactions
Treatment by antipyretics and use of leuko-depleted cellular components if recurrent.

Allergic reactions to foreign proteins
Cessation of infusion; treatment of urticarial reactions by diphenhydramine; emergency treatment needed if anaphylaxis has developed; IgA-deficient patients who have anti-IgA should receive components from IgA-deficient donors.

Alloimmunization
Provision of antigen-negative units to transfusion-dependent patients.

Iron overload
Consideration of iron-chelation treatment in transfusion-dependent patients.

Transfusion-transmitted infection
Use of blood components from volunteer unpaid donors who have been screened by sensitive techniques for relevant viral markers; consideration of hepatitis A and B vaccination of transfusion-dependent patients.

Key references

1. Contreras M: *ABC of Transfusion*, edn 2. London: British Medical Association; 1992.
2. Murphy MF, *et al.*: Guidelines for platelet transfusion. *Transfusion Med* 1992, **2**:311–318.
3. Contreras M, *et al.*: Guidelines for the use of fresh frozen plasma. *Transfusion Med* 1992, **2**:57–63.
4. Anonymous: *Leucocyte Depletion of Blood and Blood Components: Consensus Conference*. Edinburgh: Royal College of Physicians of Edinburgh; 1993.
5. Mollision PL, Engelfriet CP, Contreras M: *Blood Transfusion in Clinical Medicine* edn 9. Oxford: Blackwell Scientific Publications; 1993.

Diagnosis

Definition

• A transient ischemic attack is abrupt loss of focal cerebral or monocular function with symptoms lasting <24 h, which, after adequate investigations, is presumed to be due to embolic or thrombotic vascular disease.

Symptoms

• Symptoms such as syncope, confusion, convulsions, incontinence, and isolated dizziness are not acceptable for transient ischemic attacks.

Carotid territory

• This is the site of 80% of transient ischemic attacks.

Unilateral paresis: weakness, heaviness, or clumsiness.
Unilateral sensory loss.
Aphasia.
Transient monocular visual loss: amaurosis fugax.

Vertebrobasilar territory

• This is the site of 20% of transient ischemic attacks.

Bilateral or alternating weakness or sensory symptoms.
Vertigo, diplopia, dysphagia, ataxia: patients must have two or more simultaneously.
Sudden bilateral blindness: in patients aged >40 years.

Uncertain arterial distribution

Hemianopia alone.
Dysarthria alone.

Investigations [1]

• Investigations are of little help in the recognition of transient ischemic attacks; they are directed at determining the cause of the attack.
• Baseline tests should be done in most cases; further investigations depend on the clinical situation, age of the patient, and results of the baseline tests.

Baseline tests

Full blood count: to detect anemia, polycythemia, leukemia, and thrombocythemia.
ESR measurement: to detect vasculitis, infective endocarditis, and hyperviscosity.
Plasma glucose measurement: to detect diabetes and hypoglycemia.
Plasma cholesterol measurement: to detect hypercholesterolemia.
Syphilis serology: to detect syphilis.
Urinalysis: to detect diabetes and renal disease.
ECG: to detect left ventricular hypertrophy, arrhythmia, and myocardial ischemia or infarction.
Coagulation studies.

Nonroutine investigations

Electrolytes analysis: in patients on diuretics, to detect hyponatremia and hypokalemia.
Urea analysis: in hypertensive patients, to detect renal impairment.
Thyroid function test: in patients in atrial fibrillation, to detect thyrotoxicosis.
Chest radiography: to detect enlarged heart, calcified valve, and pulmonary arteriovenous malformation.
Cranial CT or MRI: to detect infarct and structural lesion.
Carotid ultrasonography or angiography: to detect carotid stenosis, in patients with carotid transient ischemic attacks.
Temporal artery biopsy: to detect giant cell arteritis.
Blood culture: to detect infective endocarditis.
Cardiac enzyme analysis: to detect acute myocardial infarction.

Cholesterol emboli seen on fundoscopy in a patient with amaurosis fugax.

Complications

None, by definition.

Differential diagnosis

Migraine with aura.
Partial epileptic seizures.
Structural intracranial lesions: tumor, vascular malformation, chronic subdural hematoma, giant aneurysm.
Multiple sclerosis: in patients aged <40 years.
Labyrinthine disorders: *e.g.*, Meniere's disease, benign positional vertigo.
Peripheral nerve or root lesion.
Metabolic disorders: *e.g.*, hypoglycemia.
Psychological disorders: *e.g.*, hyperventilation.

Etiology

Causes

Embolism complicating atherosclerosis of arteries to brain (50% of attacks).
Intracranial small-vessel disease (lipohyalinosis) (20%).
Embolism from the heart (20%).
Inflammatory arterial disease (*e.g.*, giant-cell arteritis).
Arterial dissections.
Hematological disorders (*e.g.*, polycythemia).

Risk factors

• Factors that increase the risk of degenerative arterial disease in general include the following:
Age, hypertension, diabetes mellitus, cigarette smoking, plasma cholesterol, plasma fibrinogen.
• Markers for arterial disease include the following:
Ischemic heart disease, peripheral vascular disease, cervical arterial bruit, left ventricular hypertrophy.
• Evidence of cardiac embolic source includes the following:
Atrial fibrillation, recent myocardial infarction, valvular disease, prosthetic heart valves.

Epidemiology [2]

• 15% of patients suffering their first stroke have had preceding transient ischemic attacks; only half of these attacks will have been seen or recognized by a doctor.
• The annual incidence of patients with attacks who present for further investigation and treatment is about 0.5 in 1000.
• The incidence increases with age.
• More men are affected than women.

Treatment

Diet and lifestyle

• Treating raised blood pressure reduces the risk of stroke by 50%, even after only a few years; the effect on coronary events is less impressive. Targets should be a systolic and diastolic pressure of below about 180 mm Hg and 100 mm Hg, respectively.

• The effect of stopping smoking is most marked on reducing cardiac events, and all patients should be encouraged vigorously to stop.

• Reducing serum cholesterol leads to a reduced risk of cardiac events, but no reliable data for stroke are available. A diet low in saturated fats should be advised.

• Physical exercise should be encouraged and probably helps by facilitating weight, cholesterol, and blood pressure control.

Pharmacological treatment

Antiplatelet drugs

• Antiplatelet drugs have shown clear evidence of benefit in a meta-analysis of all trials: the risk of nonfatal myocardial infarction and stroke is reduced by one-third; the risk of all fatal vascular events is reduced by one sixth.

• Aspirin is the best agent currently available.

Standard dosage	Aspirin, 75–150 mg.
Contraindications	Active peptic ulceration.
Special points	As effective as higher doses, with a lower risk of gastro-intestinal toxicity.
Main drug interactions	Increased risk of bleeding with warfarin.
Main side effects	Gastrointestinal hemorrhage.

Anticoagulants

• Anticoagulants are indicated when a definite cardiac source of emboli has been identified (*e.g.*, mitral valve disease with atrial fibrillation, prosthetic heart valve, recent myocardial infarction, dilated cardiomyopathy).

• In nonrheumatic atrial fibrillation, warfarin is superior to aspirin.

• Short-term warfarin may be used empirically for symptomatic treatment of frequent attacks resistant to aspirin. Warfarin may also be useful for intracranial stenosis and posterior circulation disease.

• Possible benefits of warfarin must always be weighed against definite side effects in individual patients.

Standard dosage	Warfarin sufficient to maintain INR at 2–4.
Contraindications	Bleeding diathesis, active peptic ulceration.
Special points	Requires regular blood monitoring.
Main drug interactions	Alcohol, NSAIDs, antiepileptics, antidepressants.
Main side effects	Hemorrhage.

Treatment aims

To prevent stroke or other serious vascular events (secondary prevention).

Other treatments

Carotid endarterectomy: for symptomatic carotid stenoses >70% only [3].

Prognosis

• The risk of stroke in the first year after a transient ischemic attack is 12%.

• Thereafter, the risk is 7% each year (seven times the risk in the normal population).

• The greatest risk occurs in the first month after the attack.

• Cardiac death occurs more often than stroke death after an attack.

• The combined risk of all serious vascular events (stroke, myocardial infarction, other vascular death) is ~9% annually.

Follow-up and management

• Risk factors (*e.g.*, hypertension) must be adequately controlled and antiplatelet therapy maintained.

Key references

1. Hankey GJ, Warlow CP: *Transient Ischaemic Attacks of the Brain and Eye*. London: WB Saunders; 1994. [Major Problems in Neurology 27.]
2. Dennis M, *et al.*: The prognosis of transient ischemic attacks in the Oxfordshire community stroke project. *Stroke* 1990, **21**:848–853.
3. European Carotid Surgery Trialist's Collaborative Group: MRC European Carotid Surgery Trial: interim results for symptomatic patients with severe (70–99%) or with mild (0–29%) carotid stenosis. *Lancet* 1991, **337**:1235–1243.

Diagnosis

Definition

• Tremor is an involuntary, rhythmic, smooth, sinusoidal oscillation of a body part. Faster tremors (6–12 Hz) are usually of fine amplitude; slower tremors (2–5 Hz) are coarse and of large amplitude. Tremors may be described according to the following:
Cause or underlying diagnosis.
Clinical circumstances of occurrence: rest (limb supported), postural (limb outstretched), kinetic (during voluntary movement), task-specific action (*e.g.*, during writing), intention (in terminal stages of movement).
Affected body part: *e.g.*, head, voice, hand, leg.
Frequency (cycles/s or Hz, considerable overlap).

Symptoms

Rhythmic shaking of hands, legs, trunk, or head: often resulting in clumsiness and loss of manual dexterity.
Slow voluntary movement (with rest tremor): suggesting Parkinson's disease.
Unsteadiness when standing (shaking legs), relieved by walking or sitting: suggesting primary orthostatic tremor.

Signs [1]

Parkinsonian

Rest ("pill-rolling"), possibly with postural tremor: 4–5 and 5–6 Hz, respectively; arms affected more than legs, which are affected more than jaws or lips.

Midbrain (rubral)

Rest, postural, intention tremor: 2–5 Hz; particularly affecting proximal arms.

Cerebellar

Postural, intention, kinetic tremor: 3–6 Hz; arms and trunk more than legs; titubation (head and truncal tremor).

Essential

Postural, kinetic tremor: 5–8 Hz; arms more than head more than legs; isolated.

Neuropathic

Postural, kinetic tremor: 4–6 Hz; arms more than legs.

Dystonic

Postural, kinetic tremor: 2–6 Hz; arms more than legs; exacerbated in certain postures.

Primary orthostatic

Tremor of legs and trunk when standing: 14–16 Hz.

Physiological

Postural tremor: 8–12 Hz; affecting arms; normal finding.

Exaggerated physiological

Postural tremor: 8–12 Hz; affecting arms; larger amplitude than physiological tremor.

Focal

Postural tremor: 4–8 Hz; affecting head, face, jaw, chin, tongue, voice, trunk (alone).

Task-specific action

Kinetic tremor during specific tasks: ~6 Hz; affecting arms, lips, and head.

Investigations

• Investigations are needed to exclude symptomatic tremor or identify the cause.
Serum ceruloplasmin, thyroid function, blood glucose measurement: for Wilson's disease, thyrotoxicosis, and hypoglycemia, respectively.
Nerve conduction studies, electromyography, serum immunoglobulin measurement: in patients with suspected neuropathy.
Brain imaging: if clinical suspicion of structural lesion, *e.g.*, hemitremor, focal neurological signs, midbrain or cerebellar tremor.

Complications

Clumsiness, loss of manual dexterity, difficulty writing, embarrassment.

Differential diagnosis

Repetitive myoclonus: brisk, abrupt jerks.
Chorea: flowing random variable movements.
Dystonia: intermittent fixed postures.

Etiology [2]

Hereditary
Essential tremor (50% of cases inherited autosomal-dominant).

Idiopathic
Physiological tremor.
Primary orthostatic tremor.
Task-specific action tremors.

Symptomatic
Parkinson's disease.
Akinetic rigid syndromes.
Dystonic tremor.
Thyrotoxicosis.
Cerebellar disease: multiple sclerosis, degenerative ataxias.
Midbrain lesions: multiple sclerosis, vascular.
Wilson's disease.
Peripheral neuropathy (especially demyelinating).
Exaggerated physiological tremor.
Drug-induced tremor.
Toxins.

Epidemiology

• Essential tremor occurs in 300 in 100 000 population.
• Parkinson's disease occurs in 200 in 100 000 population (increasing with age).

Diagnostic difficulties [3]

Drug-induced tremor
Beta-2 agonists, caffeine, theophylline, tricyclic antidepressants, 5-HT reuptake inhibitors, lithium, neuroleptics, amphetamines, valproate, steroids, thyroxine.

Toxin-induced tremor
MPTP (1-methyl-4-phenyl-1,2,3,6-tetrahydropyridine), mercury.

Drug-withdrawal tremor
Alcohol, barbiturates, benzodiazepines, opiates.

Exaggerated physiological tremor
Drugs (as above), drug withdrawal (as above), metabolic disease: thyrotoxicosis, hypoglycemia, pheochromocytoma, anxiety, fatigue.

Treatment

Diet and lifestyle

- Caffeine and fatigue may exacerbate tremor.
- Alcohol may help essential tremor, but addiction is a possibility.
- Aids for stability when standing (*e.g.*, shooting stick) help orthostatic tremor.

Pharmacological treatment

For essential tremor

Standard dosage	Propranolol, 60–180 mg long-acting preparation daily. Primidone up to 50 mg 2 times daily.
Contraindications	*Propranolol:* obstructive airways disease, heart failure.
Main drug interactions	None.
Main side effects	*Propranolol:* hypotension, bradycardia, bronchospasm. *Primidone:* fatigue.

For parkinsonian tremor

L-Dopa, anticholinergic, amantadine, dopamine agonists in doses as for Parkinson's disease *(see* Parkinson's disease *for details).*

Treatment aims

To identify and remove causes of exaggerated physiological tremor.

To identify and treat causes of symptomatic tremor.

Other treatments

Thalamotomy or thalamic stimulation: in severe tremors refractory to drugs.

Prognosis

- The prognosis depends on the cause of the tremor.

Follow-up and management

- Follow-up depends on the cause of the tremor.

Key references

1. Weiner WJ, Land AE: *Movement Disorders.* New York: Futura Publishing Company; 1989:221–256.
2. Cleeves L, Findley LJ, Marsden CD: Odd tremors. In *Movement Disorders* 3. Edited by Marsden CD, Fahn S. Oxford: Butterworth Heinemann; 1994:434–498.
3. Findley LJ: Tremors: differential diagnosis and pharmacology. In *Parkinson's Disease and Movement Disorders.* Edited by Jankovic J, Tolosa E. Baltimore: Williams and Wilkins; 1993:293–313.

Tuberculosis, extrapulmonary

Diagnosis

Symptoms

• Disease may be focal, disseminated, or multifocal. Proportion by site: lymphatic ~35%; genitourinary, bone, joint ~15% each; disseminated, abdominal, cerebral <10% each; cutaneous, other sites <5% each.
• Systemic symptoms usually imply more widespread disease; focal disease may be acute or insidious (more usual).

Fever, malaise, fatigue, weight loss, night sweats.
Pain: in bone or joint, abdomen, gastrointestinal tract, or meninges.
Tissue swelling: in lymph node, joint, or peritoneum.
Frequency, dysuria, loin pain: in renal disease.
Cough, fever: in disseminated disease.
Headache, vomiting, confusion: in CNS disease.

Signs

Fever, wasting: due to tuberculous toxicity.
Erythema nodosum: a hypersensitivity reaction.
Choroidal tubercles: in miliary disease.
Nontender, fluctuant lymph node: perhaps discharging.
Hematuria.
Bone or joint deformity, cold abscess, spinal-cord signs.
Chest signs, hepatosplenomegaly: in dissemination.
Ascites, abdominal distension, bowel obstruction.
Nuchal rigidity, obtundation, focal signs: indicating meningitis.

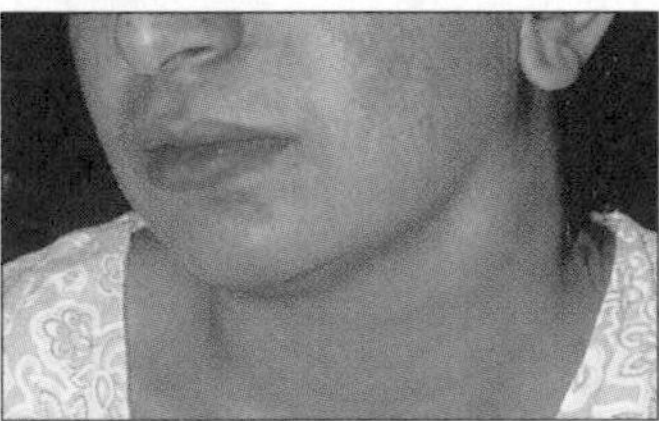

Asian woman with multiple tuberculous lymph nodes (most typical manifestation of extrapulmonary tuberculosis in Asian patients).

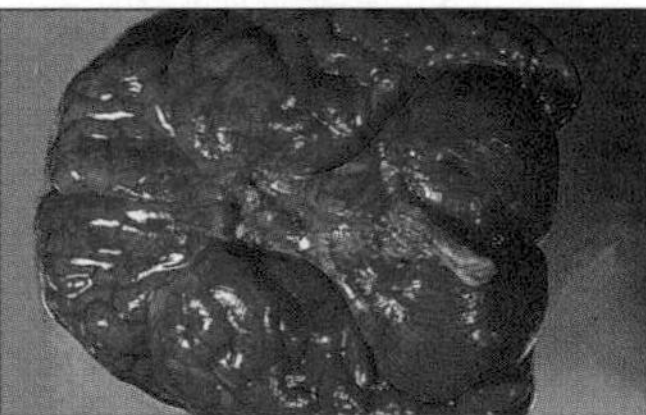

Massive cerebral edema typical of advanced tuberculous meningitis.

Investigations

• Tests may suggest the diagnosis (ESR, skin test, radiography), identify the site (CT or specialized radiography, intravenous pyelography, isotope renography), or confirm the diagnosis (culture in ~50%, microscopy in ~35%, histology in ~35%).

Chest radiography: to check for new or old changes.
Blood analysis: may show anemia, high ESR, pancytopenia, or leukemoid reaction.
Tuberculin skin test: possibly negative (especially in disseminated infection).
Sputum or urine culture.
Biopsy of bone marrow, liver, lymph node, joint, or bowel.

Complications

Cryptic disseminated tuberculosis, acute miliary disease, or meningitis: due to dissemination from a focal lesion.
Focal damage: from vasculitis, fibrosis, abscess, sinus formation, or caseation.
Hydrocephalus, spinal block, cerebral vasculitis.
Adult respiratory distress syndrome: in miliary disease.
Ureteric obstruction or renal destruction by caseation.
Spinal-cord involvement: in 20% of patients with vertebral disease.
Bone or joint deformity.
Gastrointestinal stenosis, adhesions, obstruction.

Differential diagnosis

Lymphoma, toxoplasmosis, atypical mycobacterioses.
Infection: *e.g.*, endocarditis, brucellosis, pneumocystosis.
Noninfective disease: *e.g.*, lymphoma, collagenoses.
Chronic pyelonephritis.
Other arthritides, osteomyelitis, neoplasm.
Crohn's disease, starch or sarcoid peritonitis.
Viral or fungal infections or CNS neoplasm.

Etiology

• Tuberculosis is caused by infection by *Mycobacterium tuberculosis* (now rarely *M. bovis*).
• Extrapulmonary disease may be due to lymphohematogenous, contiguous, or "down-stream" mucosal spread.
• Predisposing factors include genetics and race (rate in ethnic groups from Indian subcontinent 50 times European rate), immunocompromise (due to disease, drugs, alcohol), extremes of age, and HIV infection.

Epidemiology

• Extrapulmonary tuberculosis develops in ~25% of patients; pulmonary infection may coexist.
• The annual notification rate is 3–10 cases/100 000 in the US.

Tuberculosis and HIV infection

• ~3.5 million people world wide are co-infected.
• The infections may be mutually synergistic.
• Dissemination is much more probable.
• Many patients have extrapulmonary disease.
• Patients are more likely to be anergic on skin testing.
• Response to standard triple or quadruple treatment is usually good.

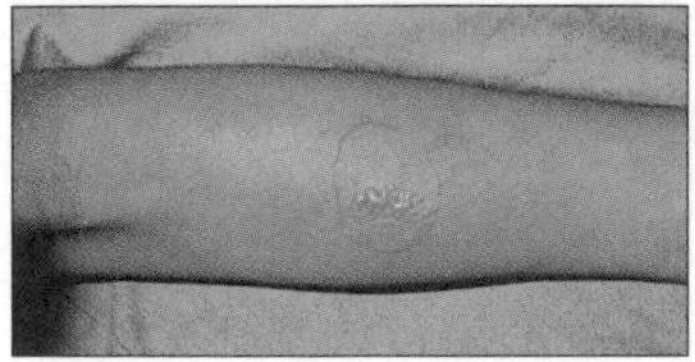

Strongly positive reaction to Mantoux test.

Treatment

Diet and lifestyle

- Weight loss and malnutrition must be reversed.
- Alcohol or drug addiction should be treated.
- Social circumstances, *e.g.*, homelessness, should be improved.

Pharmacological treatment

- The advice of a tuberculosis specialist must be sought and the case reported to state authorities.
- In a seriously ill patient, empirical treatment is justified even when the diagnosis is unconfirmed; treatment is invariably instituted before sensitivities are available.
- Efforts should be made to establish diagnosis, but procrastination may be dangerous.
- Patients must comply with the drug regimen for the duration of treatment.

Standard chemotherapy

Standard dosage — *Initial phase (2 months):* 4 drugs, usually isoniazid, with pyridoxine, rifampin, pyrazinamide, and ethambutol.
Continuation phase (4–12 months): two drugs, usually isoniazid and rifampin.

Contraindications — *Isoniazid:* drug-induced liver disease, porphyria.
Rifampin: jaundice, porphyria.
Pyrazinamide: liver damage, porphyria.
Ethambutol: optic neuritis.

Special points — For suspected resistance: addition of ethambutol.
For documented resistance: drugs as indicated by sensitivities.
For cerebral, bone and joint, and drug-resistant infections: longer treatment (9 months).
For unreliable compliance: intermittent, supervised treatment 2–3 times weekly.

Main drug interactions — *Rifampin:* oral contraceptive.

Main side effects — *Isoniazid:* neuropathy (pyridoxine prophylaxis), hepatitis, hypersensitivity reactions.
Rifampin: hepatitis, gastrointestinal upset, influenza symptoms, purpura.
Pyrazinamide: hepatitis, gastrointestinal upset.

Steroids

- Steroids should be considered when the host's inflammatory response contributes significantly to the disease process; they are indicated for the following:

Severely ill patients who are moribund due to overwhelming infection or who have miliary disease with alveolar-capillary block or cerebral disease.

Patients with peritonitis, pericarditis, spinal block, renal infection (to reduce adhesions, effusions, and fibrosis).

Patients with lymph-node or cerebral infection (to reduce swelling).

Patients with drug hypersensitivity reactions.

Treatment aims

To secure survival (especially in disseminated and cerebral disease).

To preserve organ function and prevent deformity.

To relieve symptoms.

To prevent relapse by eradicating infection.

To prevent drug resistance by ensuring compliance.

Other treatments

- Surgery is often done both before and after the diagnosis is confirmed.
- It is indicated for the following forms of tuberculosis:

All: for biopsy diagnosis (>35% of patients), relief of obstruction due to inflammatory response, and correction of deformity.
Lymphatic: for chronic sinus and unresponsive or marked node enlargement.
Renal: ureteric obstruction or stricture, obstinate symptoms (*e.g.*, pain).
CNS: for hydrocephalus, cerebral edema.
Spinal: for cord pressure, bone graft.
Joint: to minimize deformity.
Gut: for obstruction, adhesions, strictures.
Pericardial: to relieve constriction.
Female genital: for stricture, infertility.

Prognosis

- Prognosis is related to the precariousness of the organ involved, the stage of disease progression, and the vulnerability of host.
- Mortality is significant in cerebral disease (10%–30%) and disseminated disease (10%–25%).
- Survival can be expected in other forms, although chronic sequelae may develop.
- The prognosis in lymph-node and dermatological tuberculosis is excellent.

Follow-up and management

- Drug toxicities that may affect compliance must be identified.
- The patient must be monitored for complications and long-term sequelae.

General references

Langdale LA, *et al.*: Tuberculosis and the surgeon. *Am J Surg* 1992, **163**:505–509.

Shafer RW, *et al.*: Extrapulmonary tuberculosis in patients with human immunodeficiency virus infection. *Medicine* 1991, **70**:384–397.

Diagnosis

Symptoms

Primary infection

• 90% of patients have no symptoms; the following are seen rarely:

Malaise, fever, erythema nodosum, phlyctenular conjunctivitis.

Postprimary infection

• Often no symptoms are seen.

Malaise, weight loss, fever, night sweats.

Cough, mucoid or mucopurulent sputum, hemoptysis, dyspnea, dull chest ache, pleuritic chest pain.

Enlarged neck glands.

Hematuria, infertility.

Abdominal pain, chronic diarrhea, weight loss.

Meningism.

Progressive back pain, paraspinal swelling, swollen joints.

Malaise, weight loss, fever, meningism: symptoms of miliary tuberculosis; may be nonspecific, particularly in elderly patients.

Signs

• Physical examination is often unhelpful.

Evidence of weight loss, pyrexia, erythema nodosum: in primary infection.

Signs of pulmonary collapse, consolidation, or effusion, crackles (upper zones, increased after coughing), amphoric breath sounds over a large cavity.

Lymphadenopathy, palpable kidney, right iliac fossa mass, swollen joint, meningism.

Hepatosplenomegaly, choroid tubercles, meningism: signs of miliary tuberculosis.

Investigations

Chest radiography:
Primary: normal in 70% of patients; more often abnormal in children <5 years; typically shows unilateral hilar lymphadenopathy; bronchial compression can produce segmental or lobar collapse or hyperinflation, particularly in lower, lingula, and middle lobes; ulceration into bronchial tree, producing distal patchy consolidation, or into pleura, producing effusion.
Postprimary: classically shows bilateral upper-zone consolidation progressing to cavitation, fibrosis, and upper-lobe contraction; chronic tuberculosis lesions often calcified.

Tuberculin testing: positive test implies current or past infection or previous bacille Calmette–Guérin vaccination; positivity increases with age in US; useful in identifying primary disease in younger patients; strongly positive response (*e.g.*, Sterneedle tuberculin test grade 3 or 4) with previous vaccination suggests previous primary infection.

Bacteriology: samples stained (fluorescent auramine or Ziehl-Neelsen) and cultured (*e.g.*, in Löwenstein-Jensen medium); useful in establishing diagnosis in postprimary disease and in guiding management; sputum smear often positive in cavitating disease; examination of two good early-morning sputum samples allows identification of 90% of smear-positive cases; smear-positive sputum implies significant risk of infection; culture and sensitivity testing takes 4–8 weeks.

Complications

Lobar or segmental collapse or consolidation, pleural effusion, pericardial involvement, tuberculoma formation: in primary tuberculosis.

Postprimary or miliary tuberculosis, later infection at distant sites: caused by blood dissemination at time of primary infection.

Differential diagnosis

• Radiographic and some clinical features can be mimicked by the following:

Lung cancer.

Sarcoidosis.

Some bacterial pneumonias.

Allergic bronchopulmonary aspergillosis.

Pneumoconiosis.

Actinomycosis.

Etiology

• Causes include the following:

General disease
Inhalation of *Mycobacterium tuberculosis* either from the cough of a patient with sputum-positive disease or from infected droplets in a microbiology laboratory.

Postprimary disease
Reactivation of dormant *M. tuberculosis* disseminated at the time of primary infection; risk increased in patients with diseases causing depressed immunity (*e.g.*, malnutrition, alcoholism, diabetes, AIDS).

Epidemiology

• The estimated annual incidence in the US is 4–20/100 000 people.

• The annual incidence in Indian, Pakistani, and Bangladeshi ethnic groups is ~170 in 100 000.

• Recently, the overall incidence has increased slightly.

Atypical tuberculosis

• The frequency of atypical tuberculosis is increasing in elderly men with pre-existing lung disease.

• It is mostly caused by *Mycobacterium kansasaii, malmoense, xenopi, avium,* or *avium-intracellulare* (*M. avium-intracellulare* particularly in later stages of AIDS).

• Presentation is similar to that of *M. tuberculosis* infection: 10%–40% of patients may be asymptomatic.

• Management is complicated, involving prolonged multidrug treatment, including rifampin and ethambutol; expert advice is needed.

Treatment

Diet and lifestyle

• Smoking must be stopped, and nutrition improved.

Pharmacological treatment

• Treatment must be supervised by a physician experienced in all aspects of tuberculosis management.

• Patients must be educated about the disease and the importance of prolonged treatment.

• Sputum-positive patients must be advised that they remain infectious for the first 2 weeks of treatment.

Standard 6-month unsupervised regimen

Standard dosage Isoniazid, 300 mg daily (child, 10 mg/kg daily; maximum, 300 mg) for 6 months,
rifampin, 450–600 mg daily (child, 10 mg/kg daily) for 6 months,
pyrazinamide, 1.5–2 g daily (child, 35 mg/kg daily) for 2 months, and
ethambutol, 15 mg/kg daily for 2 months.

Contraindications *All:* previous severe adverse event.
Isoniazid: drug-induced liver disease, porphyria; caution in liver or renal disease.
Rifampin: jaundice, porphyria; caution in liver disease.
Pyrazinamide: liver disease, porphyria; caution in renal impairment, gout, or diabetes.

Special points *Isoniazid:* isoniazid-resistant *Mycobacterium tuberculosis* present in 4%–6% of patients.
Rifampin: colors urine and tears orange; may stain soft contact lenses.

Main drug interactions *Isoniazid:* binds to pyridoxine and may produce deficiency; inhibits phenytoin metabolism.
Rifampin: hepatic enzyme induction increases metabolism and reduces effect of anticonvulsants, oral contraceptive pill, steroids, and digoxin.
Pyrazinamide: interferes with renal testing for ketones; reduces renal excretion of uric acid.

Main side effects *Isoniazid:* gastrointestinal intolerance, exacerbation of acne, hepatotoxicity (in 1%–2% of patients; can be severe), peripheral neuropathy (in 2%; prevented by pyridoxine supplements 10 mg daily).
Rifampin: nausea, abnormal liver function tests (usually mild and reversible), influenza-like reaction.
Pyrazinamide: hepatotoxicity, arthralgia, precipitation of gout, urticaria.

• Ethambutol should be considered if resistance is suspected.

• Longer periods are needed for meningitis and with extensive disease.

• Pyridoxine, 10 mg daily, may be added when deficiency is a possibility.

Supervised regimen

Isoniazid, 15 mg/kg 3 times weekly (adult and child) for 6 months.

Rifampin, 600–900 mg (child, 15 mg/kg) 3 times weekly for 6 months.

Pyrazinamide, 2–2.5 g (child, 50 mg/kg) 3 times weekly for 2 months.

Other drugs

Corticosteroids: improve outcome in pericarditis and meningitis; of value in patients with severe infection, persistent pyrexia, or weight loss; higher doses needed if rifampin used.

Streptomycin, capreomycin, cycloserine, ethionamide for multiresistant or atypical infection: specialist advice must be sought.

Treatment aims

To achieve bacteriological and clinical cure.

To prevent resistance (with combination treatment).

To prevent or treat disease in contacts.

Prognosis

• ~6% of adults with pulmonary tuberculosis die of it before finishing chemotherapy.

• Only ~3% relapse if the full course of chemotherapy is taken; the rate is higher if compliance is poor.

Follow-up and management

• Close supervision is necessary throughout chemotherapy.

• Compliance must be checked; urine must be checked for rifampin.

• The patient must be checked for adverse effects.

• Response must be assessed: symptoms, weight gain, radiographic changes.

Prevention

• Notification of new cases to public health authorities for communicable disease control is a legal requirement.

• Care is needed in people with close contact with sputum-positive disease: 10% develop tuberculosis, mostly identified by initial tuberculin testing or chest radiography.

• Bacille Calmette–Guérin vaccination has a protective efficacy of ~70%.

General references

Joint Tuberculosis Committee of the British Thoracic Society: Chemotherapy and management of tuberculosis in the United Kingdom. *Thorax* 1990, **45**:403–408.

Subcommittee of the Joint Tuberculosis Committee of the British Thoracic Society: Control and prevention of tuberculosis in Britain: an updated code of practice. *BMJ* 1990, **300**:995–999.

Diagnosis

Symptoms

Persistent fever: developing after recent visit to endemic country.

Mounting fever, headache, malaise, anorexia, dry cough, constipation: in first week of illness.

Continuing fever, mental apathy: in second week.

Abdominal distension, "pea-soup" diarrhea: in third week.

Signs

Pyrexia: in first week.

Rose spots: 2–4 mm erythematous maculopapules in crops on lower chest and upper abdomen in 30% of patients in second week.

Vagueness and withdrawal, splenomegaly, relative bradycardia: in second week.

Delirium or stupor, distended tender abdomen, dehydration, poor-volume rapid pulse, signs of complications: in third week.

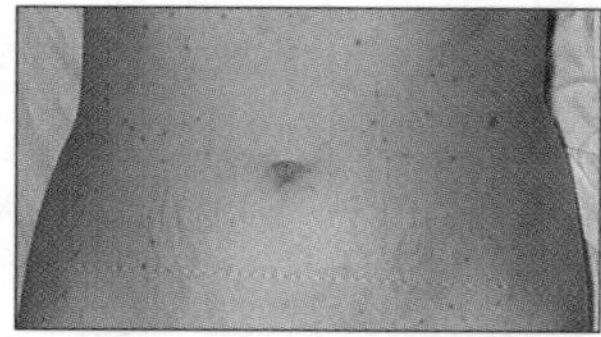

Rose spots in a patient with typhoid fever.

Investigations

• Definitive diagnosis needs positive blood or bone-marrow culture.

Blood culture: highest positivity during first week (80%), declining thereafter; often negative if patient has already been given antibiotic.

Bone-marrow culture: often remains positive despite antibiotic administration.

Stool and urine culture: often positive from third week onwards; diagnostic only if clinical picture is compatible.

Widal's test: unreliable and difficult to interpret, so rarely performed.

Full blood count: leukocyte count decreased, with relative lymphocytosis after first week.

Liver function tests: often mildly raised aspartate and alanine transaminase concentrations.

Complications

• Complications occur only in untreated patients after the second week.

Intestinal hemorrhage: indicated by sudden drop in temperature, rise in pulse rate, and rectal bleeding.

Intestinal perforation: signs of peritonitis may be difficult to detect in an already tender and distended abdomen; presence of gas under diaphragm and ascites may be the only signs.

Myocarditis: indicated by rapid, thready pulse and ECG abnormalities.

Jaundice: may be due to cholangitis, hepatitis, or hemolysis.

Typhoid abscesses: in different organs (rare).

Differential diagnosis

• Fever in a traveler returning from endemic areas may also be due to the following:

Malaria (most important).

Tropical viral infections.

Typhus.

Amebic liver abscess.

Trypanosomiasis and leishmaniasis.

Other causes of fever that are common world wide.

Etiology

• Causes include the following:

Infection by *Salmonella typhi* or *paratyphi* A, B, or C.

Prolonged bacteremia.

Gallbladder infection.

Inflamed Peyer's patches in small intestine (may ulcerate during third week, leading to bleeding or perforation).

Epidemiology

• The disease is endemic in the Indian subcontinent, southeast Asia, the Middle East, Africa, and Central and South America; paratyphoid B also occurs in southern and eastern Europe.

• Transmission is through food or water contaminated by feces or urine of a sufferer or carrier.

Treatment

Diet and lifestyle

• Adequate nutrition and fluid replacement must be ensured.

• Chronic carriers, especially those handling foods, must practice strict hygiene because of the fecal–oral transmission of the disease; in such patients, attempts should be made to clear carriage.

Pharmacological treatment

General and supportive care

• Nutritional and fluid-electrolyte deficiencies should be corrected in patients presenting late.

Specific treatment

• 4-quinolones are currently the drug of choice in adults.

• Defervescence occurs in 3–5 days.

• Treatment failure, relapse, and chronic carriage are rare.

• Other drugs include third-generation cephalosporins and corticosteroids (in severe toxemia).

Standard dosage	Ciprofloxacin, 500 mg orally twice daily for 14 days (200 mg i.v. with vomiting or diarrhea). *In children (but see* Special points): 10 mg/kg orally or i.v. daily in 2 divided doses. Ceftriaxone, 3–4 g i.v. daily as single dose or 75–100 mg/kg i.v. daily in 2 divided doses for 7–10 days (shorter duration may be equally effective). Adjunctive dexamethasone, 3 mg/kg i.v. initially, then 1 mg/kg 6-hourly for 48 h.
Contraindications	Hypersensitivity. *Dexamethasone:* caution in pregnancy, renal insufficiency, hypertension, and diabetes.
Special points	*Ciprofloxacin:* currently not recommended in pregnant women and children because of arthropathy in growing animals; this has not, however, been observed in children, and ciprofloxacin should not be withheld if benefits outweigh risks. *Ceftriaxone:* can be used in children and pregnant women but must be given intravenously.
Main drug interactions	*Ciprofloxacin:* NSAIDs, oral iron, anticoagulants. *Ceftriaxone:* probenecid. *Dexamethasone:* phenytoin, barbiturates, ephedrine or rifampin may increase the metabolic clearance of corticosteroids.
Main side effects	*Ciprofloxacin:* nausea, abdominal pain, diarrhea (all unusual). *Ceftriaxone:* headache, nausea, rash. *Dexamethasone:* fluid and electrolyte disturbances.

Treatment of chronic carriers

• Ciprofloxacin, 750 mg, or norfloxacin, 400 mg twice daily for 28 days, is highly effective.

Drug resistance

• Chloramphenicol, cotrimoxazole, and amoxicillin are highly effective if the infecting strains are sensitive to the above drugs.

Treatment aims

To achieve clinical cure.

To prevent complications and relapse.

To prevent chronic fecal carriage after recovery.

Other treatments

• Surgery is needed for intestinal perforation (hemorrhage managed conservatively).

• Cholecystectomy should be reserved for carriers with symptomatic gallbladder disease.

Prognosis

• Untreated, typhoid and paratyphoid fevers have a mortality of up to 20%, mostly from myocarditis and intestinal hemorrhage or perforation; these complications are rarely seen in the US.

• Recovery begins in the fourth week in the absence of complications.

Follow-up and management

• ~10% of patients relapse, and 3% become chronic fecal carriers after treatment with chloramphenicol, cotrimoxazole, or amoxicillin but rarely after ciprofloxacin treatment.

• After clinical recovery, six consecutive negative stool and urine cultures should be obtained over 3 weeks.

General references

Lassere R, Sangalang RP, Santiago L: Three day treatment of typhoid fever with two different doses of ceftriaxone, compared to 14 day therapy with chloramphenicol: a randomised trial. *J Antimicrob Chemother* 1991, **28**:765–772.

Mandal BK: Modern treatment of typhoid fever. *J Infect* 1991, **22**:1–4.

Diagnosis

Symptoms

General

Urgency to defecate.

Tenesmus: suggests proctitis; may be misinterpereted as constipation.

Mild attack

Diarrhea up to 4 times daily or passage of small amounts of macroscopic blood *per rectum*: without appreciable constitutional symptoms.

Moderate attack

Diarrhea >4 times daily: without severe bleeding or severe constitutional symptoms.

Severe attack

Diarrhea ≥6 times daily.

Blood mixed with feces.

Fever >37.5°C, abdominal pain, anorexia, or weight loss.

• Extracolonic symptoms (all rare) include pyoderma gangrenosum of the skin, erythema nodosum, episcleritis, arthritis, sclerosing cholangitis.

Signs

Mild or moderate attack

• Typically no signs are manifest.

Severe attack

Pallor.

Fever >37.5°C, tachycardia.

Hypoalbuminemia: <3.0 g/dL.

Diffuse abdominal tenderness.

• Any signs of severe disease warrant emergency admission, intensive therapy, and daily monitoring to exclude toxic dilatation.

Investigations

Stool culture: should always be done even in established ulcerative colitis, to exclude *Clostridium difficile*, *Entamoeba histolytica*.

Full blood count, ESR, liver chemistries.

Sigmoidoscopy and rectal biopsy.

Plain abdominal radiography: allows exclusion of dilatation and gives good guide to disease extent (bowel containing feces is probably not severely inflamed).

Colonoscopy: allows accurate assessment of extent of disease and histological confirmation of presence of disease or dysplasia.

Barium enema: less frequently used because of inability to obtain histology.

• Colonoscopy and barium enema should be avoided in an acute attack because they may cause exacerbation.

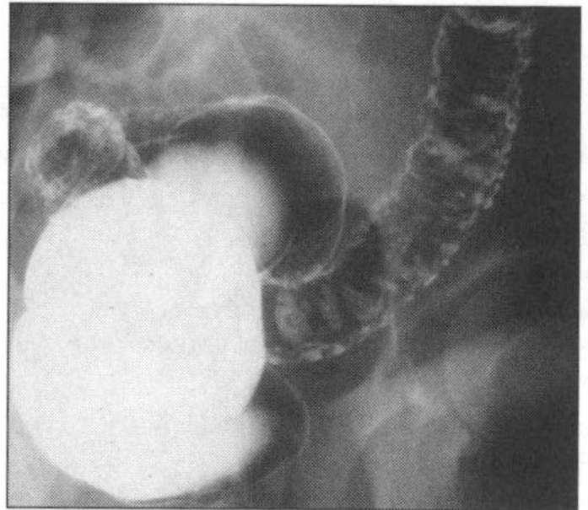

Double-contrast barium enema in severe ulcerative colitis, showing submucosal ulceration in sigmoid and descending colon.

Complications

Hemorrhage: chronic blood loss causing anemia common, severe acute bleeding rare.

Perforation: in 5%, often a sequela of toxic megacolon; 50% mortality; avoidable with careful management and surgical referral.

Strictures: (unusual) colonoscopy and biopsy needed to exclude malignancy.

Colon cancer.

Differential diagnosis

Microscopic (lymphocytic) colitis.

Collagenous colitis.

Drug-associated disorders: oral contraceptives have been associated with a Crohn's-like colitis; NSAIDs and purgatives may cause microscopic colitis.

Diversion colitis.

Crohn's colitis.

Irradiation proctitis: associated with vascular ectasia.

Ischemic colitis: rarely affects rectum.

Bacterial or amebic infection (dysentery).

Irritable bowel syndrome: should not cause bleeding or nocturnal diarrhea.

Cytomegalovirus, herpes simplex, cryptosporidia in immunosuppressed patients.

Colon cancer.

Acute self-limited colitis

Etiology

• The cause is unknown, but the following may have a role:

Autoimmunity.

Defective mucosal barrier.

Altered neutrophil function [1].

Epidemiology

• Patients present at any age; the highest prevalence is in the 2nd and 3rd decades, but a second peak in the 5th and 6th decades has been reported.

• The prevalence in northwestern Europe and the US is 1 in 1500; it is rarely diagnosed in developing countries.

• An unexplained association with nonsmoking exists (95% of sufferers are nonsmokers or exsmokers).

• No convincing association with diet or stress has been found.

• The risk in first-degree relatives increases 15-fold.

Clinical patterns

Acute fulminant.

Relapsing/remitting: in ~66% of patients.

Chronic continuous: more often in patients who are elderly at first presentation.

Single attack of colitis (stool culture negative): in <1%.

Rectum involved in >90%, extending proximally for variable length.

Treatment

Diet and lifestyle

• No special precautions are necessary.

Pharmacological treatment

For mild attacks

Standard dosage *Initially:* sulfasalazine, 1 g 4 times daily; mesalamine, 1.2–2.4 g daily; or olsalazine, 1.5–3 g daily. Proctitis may be managed with rectal corticosteroid as foam or rectal 5-aminosalicylic acid preparation.
Maintenance: sulfasalazine, 1.5–4 g daily, mesalamine, 1.2–2.4 g daily, or olsalazine, 1.5–3 g daily; or 5-aminosalicylic acid enemas for disease limited to the distal colon [2].

Contraindications Salicylate intolerance, renal failure.

Special points Regular full blood counts and urea measurement advised. Increasing dose gradually and taking with food may reduce gastrointestinal side effects.

Main drug interactions *Sulfasalazine:* warfarin, anticonvulsants.

Main side effects Occasional nephrotoxicity.
Sulfasalazine: nausea, headaches, malaise, dyspepsia, reversible male infertility.
Mesalamine: occasional nausea, diarrhea, interstitial nephritis.
Olsalazine: diarrhea in 10%–20% of patients.

For moderate attacks

Standard dosage Prednisone, 40 mg orally once daily, with oral 5-aminosalicylic acid preparation.

Contraindications Systemic infections, hypersensitivity.

Special points Weekly review essential; hospital admission if no improvement within 2 weeks.
Corticosteroids used in short courses; response should occur within 1–4 weeks then taper off drug over 6–8 weeks; if response poor, more severe attack should be assumed; corticosteroids of no value in maintaining remission.

Main drug interactions None.

Main side effects Occasional steroid-psychosis; hyperglycemia, asceptic necrosis; steroid-related side-effects uncommon if long-term treatment avoided.

For severe attacks

• Treatment includes admission to hospital for close observation, bed rest, high-dose i.v. corticosteroids (*e.g.*, solumedrol, 15 mg every 6 h), total parenteral nutrition if patient is vomiting or malnourished, deep venous thrombosis prophylaxis.

• The colonic diameter should be monitored by plain radiography daily.

For toxic dilatation

• Dilatation of the transverse colon to a diameter of >7 cm accompanied by signs of fever or tachycardia may be treated intensively for up to 48 h, but any clinical or radiographic deterioration during this period or failure to respond to treatment necessitates immediate surgery.

Treatment aims

To achieve and maintain remission, with good quality of life.

To avoid life-threatening complications by prompt, effective treatment.

Other treatments

• 20% of patients need colectomy at some time; surgery is indicated for the following:

Failed full medical treatment for severe colitis (after 1–2 weeks of hospitalization on i.v. steroids or a trial of cyclosporin A).

Toxic megacolon or perforation.

Chronic ill health due to persistent mild or moderate colitis, with poor quality of life.

Cancer or raised dysplastic lesion.

Progressive colonic dilatation in patients already on systemic prednisone >40 mg daily or who deteriorate or do not respond to medical treatment.

Prognosis

• Most patients have relapses interspersed with periods of prolonged remission; 90% are capable of full-time work.

• Life expectancy is normal.

• The risk of colon cancer is significantly increased beginning 10–15 years after onset of disease in patients with pancolitis.

Follow-up and management

• After a single mild attack, patients should continue taking 5-aminosalicylic acid preparations for 1 year or, for severe or multiple attacks, until they have been free of disease for at least 5 years.

• Patients should be screened by colonoscopy for dysplasia or early colon cancer on a yearly basis if disease present more than 10 years.

Patient support

Crohn's and Colitis Foundation of America, 386 Park Ave S., New York, NY 10016-7374.

Key references

1. Podolsky DK: Inflammatory bowel disease (parts 1 and 2). *N Engl J Med* 1991, **325**:928–937; 1008–1016.
2. Crotty B, Jewell DP: Drug therapy of ulcerative colitis. *Br J Clin Pharmacol* 1992, **34**:189–198.

Diagnosis

Symptoms and signs

Lower urinary tract infection

Dysuria, frequency, and suprapubic tenderness: indicating cystitis.

Dysuria, frequency, fever, perineal pain, obstructive voiding dysfunction, tenderness: indicating acute prostatitis.

Relapsing infection, voiding dysfunction, abdominal or back pain: indicating chronic prostatitis.

Upper urinary tract infection

Fever, chills, prostration, back or flank pain and tenderness, dysuria, and frequency: indicating acute pyelonephritis.

Fever and chills, flank pain and tenderness, flank or abdominal mass, dysuria, and frequency: indicating renal abscesses.

Symptomatic bacteremia of urinary tract origin: clinical features of bacteremia often overshadow those relating to urinary tract.

Investigations

To establish presence of infection

Urine culture: $>10^2$ colony-forming units (CFU) coliforms/mL or $>10^5$ CFU noncoliforms/mL in symptomatic women, 10^3 CFU bacteria/mL in symptomatic men, $>10^5$ CFU bacteria/mL in asymptomatic patients on two consecutive specimens, $>10^2$ CFU bacteria/mL in catheterized patients, any growth of bacteria from a suprapubic aspirate in symptomatic patients.

Urine microscopy: pyuria (>10 leukocytes/mL unspun urine) supportive evidence of urinary tract infection but not specific; pus cells in "sterile" urine (sterile pyuria) may indicate fastidious organisms or previous antibiotic treatment; microscopic hematuria in 50% of patients.

Dipstick testing of urine: combined leukocyte esterase and nitrite test useful screening procedure, with negative predictive value of 96%–97% at level of 10^5 CFU/mL.

To establish site of infection

• Whether infection is confined to the lower tract or has ascended to the upper tract has important treatment implications; the distinction is usually made clinically.

Radiography

• Radiography is used to identify structural abnormalities of urinary tract, including reflux nephropathy, obstruction, calculi, congenital abnormalities, and, in children, vesicoureteric reflux.

• It is indicated in children and men in first infection and in women with recurrent infections, upper urinary tract infection, unusual infecting organism, fever persisting >48 h after starting treatment, coexistent hypertension, or persistent microscopic hematuria.

Intravenous urography: investigation of choice in adults (usually delayed until after recovery); ultrasonography may be substituted or added in the case of renal impairment or when renal abscess or pelvic disease is suspected.

^{99m}Tc-DMSA scan and ultrasonography: with either voiding cystourethrography or radionuclide cystography; investigation of choice in children.

Complications

Reflux nephropathy: cortical scarring and clubbing of underlying calyces in infants with bacteriuria associated with vesicoureteric reflux.

Renal damage, perinephric abscess formation, septicemia: due to infection in presence of complicating factors (*e.g.*, obstruction, stones, vesicoureteric reflux).

Differential diagnosis

Urethritis: chlamydia, gonorrhea, herpesvirus.

Vaginitis: bacteria, trichomonas, yeasts.

Perineal lesions: herpesvirus, other sexually transmitted diseases, dermatological conditions, physical or chemical irritants.

Etiology

• The common uropathogens are normal constituents of the colonic flora.

• *Escherichia coli* accounts for 85% of community-acquired urinary tract infection.

• Catheterization, instrumentation, cross infection, and selection of resistant bowel and environmental flora account for the different microbiological spectrum of hospital-acquired urinary tract infection.

• Almost always, infection is due to ascent of microorganisms through the urethra from the colonized perineum.

Epidemiology

• 3.7% of boys and 2% of girls in the first year of life have bacteriuria.

• 4%–7% of pregnant women have bacteriuria, compared with 1%–3% of young, nonpregnant women.

• Urinary tract infection is rare in young men except in practicing homosexuals.

• 10%–20% of elderly people living at home and up to 50% of institutionalized elderly people have bacteriuria.

Complicated or uncomplicated infection

• This distinction is useful for directing treatment.

• The following suggest occult renal involvement in apparent lower urinary tract infection or the presence of complicated urinary tract infection:

Male sex.
History of childhood urinary tract infection.
Symptoms for >7 days at presentation.
Recent antibiotic use.
Pregnancy.
Institutionalization: in elderly patients.
Recent instrumentation.
Indwelling catheter.
Underlying urinary tract abnormality.
Diabetes.
Immunosuppression.

Treatment

Diet and lifestyle

• A high fluid intake may help to alleviate dysuria during an acute episode; in the long term, it may be useful prophylactically.
• In women, postcoital voiding may be helpful; those using diaphragms and spermicides may benefit from changing to alternative contraceptive methods.

Pharmacological treatment

Indications

For lower urinary tract infections (uncomplicated): 3–5 day courses of trimethoprim, co-trimoxazole, nitrofurantoin, or co-amoxiclav; as effective as 7–14 day course; result in fewer relapses than single-dose treatment.

For lower urinary tract infections (complicated): chemotherapy as above continued for 7–14 days; short courses not suitable.
In pregnant women: 7–10 day course of amoxicillin, cephalexin, or nitrofurantoin; early screening and treatment of asymptomatic bacteriuria.
In men with prostatitis: trimethoprim, co-trimoxazole, or a quinolone for 4 weeks (longer for chronic prostatitis); nonbacterial prostatitis may respond to doxycycline or erythromycin.

For upper urinary tract infections (uncomplicated): severity of constitutional upset determines need for hospitalization.
In patients treated at home: oral trimethoprim, co-trimoxazole, co-amoxiclav, or quinolone for 14 days.
In hospitalized patients: initially, i.v. cefuroxime, cefotaxime, ciprofloxacin, co-amoxiclav, or co-trimoxazole; when fever subsides, oral treatment dictated by culture, continued for 14 days; relapses treated for 6 weeks.

For upper urinary tract infection (complicated):
In previously instrumented or catheterized patients: initially i.v. ceftazidime or amoxicillin with ciprofloxacin or gentamicin.
In patients with obstructed, infected upper tract: chemotherapy as above, with prompt drainage by percutaneous nephrostomy pending definitive surgery.
In patients with renal abscess: chemotherapy as above, with i.v. flucloxacillin, then 4–6 week courses of antibiotics based on cultures; percutaneous drainage usually needed.

Selected regimens

Amoxicillin, 500 mg orally 3 times daily.
Cefotaxime, 1 g i.v. 3 times daily.
Ceftazidime, 1–2 g i.v. twice daily.
Cefuroxime, 750 mg i.v. 3 times daily.
Cephalexin, 500 mg orally 4 times daily.
Ciprofloxacin, 500 mg orally or 200 mg i.v. twice daily.
Co-amoxiclav, 750 mg orally or 1.2 g i.v. 3 times daily.
Co-trimoxazole, 960 mg orally or i.v. twice daily.
Flucloxacillin, 500 mg i.v. 4 times daily.
Gentamicin, 80 mg i.v. 3 times daily.
Nitrofurantoin, 100 mg orally 4 times daily.
Trimethoprim, 200 mg orally twice daily.

Antibiotics: contraindications and side effects

Chronic renal failure: nitrofurantoin ineffective, causes neuropathy; tetracyclines worsen uremia; aminoglycosides can be used but concentrations must be monitored to avoid nephrotoxicity and auditory/vestibular toxicity.

Pregnancy: tetracyclines cause bone or teeth dystrophy; trimethoprim possibly teratogenic; quinolones possibly cause arthropathy; aminoglycosides cause auditory/vestibular toxicity.

Infancy: tetracyclines cause bone or teeth dystrophy; sulfonamides cause hemolysis.

Prophylaxis

• Postcoital or nightly: trimethoprim, 100 mg, nitrofurantoin, 100 mg, or co-trimoxazole, 480 mg, reduces recurrence in women with normal urinary tracts.

• Prophylaxis is also useful after acute pyelonephritis in pregnancy.

Treatment aims

To relieve symptoms.
To prevent increase in prematurity and perinatal mortality.
To prevent and eradicate systemic sepsis.
To prevent progressive renal damage.

Prognosis

• Renal impairment in reflux nephropathy may progress without persisting infection and reflux.
• Adults with uncomplicated infection suffer minimal long-term sequelae if adequately treated.
• Complicated upper tract infections are potentially more damaging and may cause progressive renal scarring.

Follow-up and management

• Follow-up urine cultures are essential in pregnancy, after uncomplicated acute pyelonephritis, and after all complicated urinary tract infections.
• Any predisposing factors should be treated.
• Obstruction must be relieved by surgery or intermittent self-catheterization when indicated; calculi must be removed.

Recurrent infection

Relapse
• Relapse occurs soon after cessation of treatment.
• The same organism is involved.
• Relapse indicates inappropriate drug or duration of treatment, poor compliance, occult renal involvement, or underlying urinary tract abnormality.

Reinfection
• Reinfection occurs >6 weeks after cessation of treatment.
• A different organism is involved.
• Reinfection indicates failure of host defenses.

General references

Hooton TM, Stamm WE: Management of acute uncomplicated urinary tract infection in adults. *Med Clin North Am* 1991, **75**:339–357.

White RHR: Management of urinary tract infection and vesicoureteric reflux in children. *BMJ* 1990, **300**:1391–1392.

Wilkie ME, *et al.*: Diagnosis and management of urinary tract infection in adults. *BMJ* 1992, **305**:1137–1141.

Diagnosis

Symptoms

Itching and swelling of skin.

Arthralgia: in severe urticaria or urticarial vasculitis.

Painful or burning sensation of the skin: in urticarial vasculitis.

Signs

Evanescent, red, elevated nonpitting papules or plaques: often with blanched centers or annular configurations.

Angioedema of the lips and periorbital regions: not uncommon.

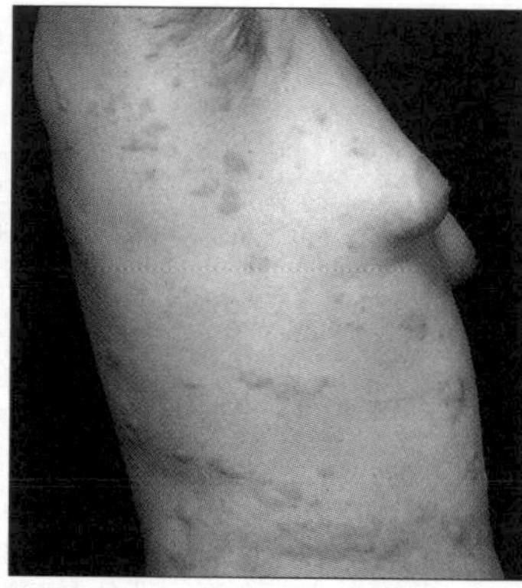

Scattered urticarial wheals on the trunk.

Investigations

Acute urticaria (<6 weeks) [1,2]

• Usually an elaborate work-up is not warranted; a standard history is taken and a physical examination is performed with a special emphasis on food and drug ingestion.

Chronic urticaria (>6 weeks) [1,2]

• Very challenging and costly tests are rarely helpful.

• In the initial work-up, care should be taken to look for intolerance to aspirin and tartrazine (FDA yellow dye no. 5) and benzoic acid derivatives used as food preservatives; also low-grade chronic infections should be ruled out.

• Chronic urticaria may be a presenting sign of underlying connective tissue disease or malignancy, especially in cases of urticarial vasculitis.

Complications

Underlying connective tissue disease or malignancy: can be missed in work-up of chronic urticaria [3].

Anaphylactic shock: in cases of IgE-mediated acute urticarial reactions.

Differential diagnosis

Urticarial vasculitis.

Urticarial component of bullous pemphigoid.

Erythema multiforme.

Herpes gestationis.

Erythema annulare centrifugum.

Erythema chronicum migrans.

Cutaneous larva migrans (creeping eruption).

Mycosis fungoides.

Erythema marginatum.

Erythema infectiosum (fifth disease).

Dermal contact dermatitis.

Cholinergic urticaria.

Solar urticaria.

Cold urticaria.

Pressure urticaria.

Hereditary angioedema: usually involves only mucous membranes with few urticarial skin lesions; life-threatening laryngeal spasm.

Etiology

•A cause is usually not identified except in cases of acute urticaria from food or drug ingestion.

•Chronic urticaria is most often idiopathic.

Epidemiology

Affects 20% of population at some point in their lives.

Treatment

Diet and lifestyle

• Known triggering agents such as food dyes and preservatives and aspirin must be identified and avoided.

Pharmacological treatment

• Topical steroids or antipruritic agents are often helpful.

H_1 and H_2 antagonists [4]

Standard dosage	Terfenadine, 60 mg orally twice daily. Astemizole, 10 mg orally daily. Hydroxyzine hydrochloride, 25 mg orally every 6–8 h. Doxepin, 10–50 mg orally 3 times daily. Cyproheptadine, 4 mg orally 3 times daily "used for cold urticaria." Loratadine, 10 mg orally 3 times daily.
Contraindications	Porphyrias.
Main drug interactions	*Terfenadine*, *astemizole* with concurrent erythromycin can cause fatal ventricular arrhythmias.
Main side effects	Drowsiness, anticholinergic effects, ventricular arrhythmias reported after concurrent use of terfenadine and astemizole with erythromycin.

Systemic corticosteroids

Often used in cases of acute urticaria.

Should be avoided as a first-line treatment in all but acute and severe cases of urticaria.

Standard dosage	Prednisone, 40–60 mg orally daily decreased over a 2- to 3-week period. Triamcinolone, i.m. 40–60 mg as a single dose.
Contraindications	History of peptic ulcer disease, tuberculosis, glaucoma, diabetes.
Main drug interactions	None.
Main side effects	Aseptic necrosis of bone, especially the femoral head; exacerbation of narrow-angle glaucoma; transient hyperglycemia.

Treatment aims

To relieve itching and reduce swelling.

Prognosis

Excellent for acute urticaria.

•50% of patients with chronic urticaria are symptom free after 1 year.

•75% of patients with chronic urticaria and angioedema still have attacks after 5 years.

Follow-up and management

Individualized for each patient.

Key references

1. Cooper KD: Urticaria and angioedema: diagnosis and evaluation. *J Am Acad Dermatol* 1991, **25**:166–174.
2. Huston DP, Bressler RB: Urticaria and angioedema. *Med Clin North Am* 1992, **76**:805–840.
3. Mehregan DR, *et al.*: Urticarial vasculitis: a histopathologic and clinical review of 72 cases. *J Am Acad Dermatol* 1992, **26**:441–448.
4. Ring J, Behrendt H: H_1 and H_2 antagonists in allergic and pseudoallergic diseases. *Clin Exp Allergy* 1990, **20**:43–49.

Diagnosis

Symptoms and signs

Major hematemesis or melena.

Chronic blood loss, with iron-deficiency anemia: indicating portal-hypertensive gastropathy.

• Sites of bleeding in patients with portal hypertension are esophageal (most frequent); fundal, lesser curve, antral, in hiatal hernia (gastric varices); ileostomy, colostomy, colonic, and rectal (ectopic varices). These may present with massive rectal bleeding [1].

Investigations

Esophagogastroduodenoscopy: to evaluate varices and gastric mucosa for portal gastropathy.

Doppler ultrasonography, angiography: to establish patency of portal vein.

Blood tests, CT, liver biopsy: to identify cause of underlying liver disease.

Measurement of portal venous, wedged hepatic venous, or intravariceal pressure: endoscopic needle, endoscopic pressure gauge; special investigations, mainly for research use in studies using pharmacologic agents.

Complications

Infection: in ~30% of patients during admission.

Renal failure: acute tubular necrosis, hepatorenal syndrome.

Delirium tremens, Wernicke–Korsakoff syndrome: related to alcohol withdrawal.

Ascites: precipitated by fluid overload.

Portal systemic encephalopathy: precipitated by blood in gut and liver hypoxia.

Aspiration pneumonia.

Spontaneous bacterial peritonitis.

Differential diagnosis

Bleeding caused by the following:
Peptic ulcer.
Mallory–Weiss tear.
Gastric erosions.
Gastric carcinoma.
Portal-hypertensive gastropathy.
Gastric vascular malformations.
Other sources of gastrointestinal bleeding.

Etiology

• Precipitants of variceal bleeding include the following:
Infection.
Drugs: *e.g.*, aspirin, NSAIDs.
Development of hepatocellular carcinoma or portal-vein thrombosis in cirrhotic patients.
Heavy alcohol binges in cirrhotic patients.

Epidemiology

• Varices develop in 90% of patients with cirrhosis; the risk of hemorrhage is highest in the first 2 years after identification.
• The risk of bleeding is highest in patients with large esophageal varices (>5 mm diameter), red signs on varices, and poor liver function.

Conditions complicated by variceal bleeding

Precirrhotic severe alcoholic hepatitis/ fatty liver.
Cirrhosis.
Schistosomiasis.
Splenic-vein thrombosis: usually causes gastric fundal varices, with no esophageal varices.
Budd–Chiari syndrome.
Congenital hepatic fibrosis.
Idiopathic portal hypertension.
Nodular regenerative hyperplasia of liver.
Partial nodular transformation of liver.

Pugh's modified grading of the severity of liver disease

Points	1	2	3
Encephalopathy	None	Grade 1–2	Grade 3–4
Ascites	Absent	Slight	Moderate
Bilirubin (mg/dL)	<2.0	2.0–3.0	>3.0
Albumin (g/L)	>35	28–35	<28
Prothrombin (secs, prolonged)	1–3	4–10	>10

Pugh's grade A, 5–6; B, 7–9; C, 10–15 points.

Treatment

Diet and lifestyle

• Patients must avoid NSAIDs or aspirin.

• Alcohol should be avoided if the liver disease is alcoholic cirrhosis.

• Patients should have ready access to aute care medical services.

Pharmacological treatment

Emergency drug treatment

• Octreotide is useful when emergency endoscopy is not available or is delayed; octreotide, 25–50 μg/h i.v. for 5 days [2].

Vasopressin: probably not effective and associated with significant complications.

Prophylaxis: primary and secondary

• Propranolol reduces the risk of first hemorrhage; the resting pulse rate should be reduced to 60 beats/min or by 25%. Treatment is recommended in cirrhotic patients with large varices and red signs. Beta blockade also reduces bleeding from portal gastropathy and possibly reduces the risk of recurrent variceal bleeding.

• For prevention of recurrent hemorrhage, endoscopic sclerotherapy or banding should be repeated until varices are obliterated.

Nonpharmacological treatment

Resuscitation

Airway protection to prevent aspiration.

Insertion of large i.v. line (cross-matching of at least 6 units blood).

Crystalloid and colloid infusion to maintain circulation while cross-matched blood is awaited.

Vasoconstriction.

Possible use of filters and blood warmers after transfusion of 4 units of blood.

Insertion of central venous line to guide further replacement therapy when systolic blood pressure >100 mm Hg.

Fresh frozen plasma to correct clotting abnormalities.

Platelet transfusion if thrombocytopenia exists.

Emergency treatment

Emergency endoscopy to confirm variceal bleeding.

Emergency endoscopic sclerotherapy or banding: treatment of choice; complications include fever, aspiration, esophageal perforation, and mediastinitis; gastric fundal varices respond poorly to sclerotherapy; complication rate of banding lower than that of sclerotherapy [3].

Balloon tamponade for temporary control of bleeding or bleeding refractory to sclerotherapy.

Other options

Transjugular intrahepatic portal-systemic stent shunt: if emergency endoscopic treatment fails; also under evaluation for prevention of recurrent hemorrhages, but high rate of shunt occlusion (30% at 1 year) and encephalopathy (10%–20%) [4].

Emergency shunt surgery.

Emergency esophageal transection.

Liver transplantation: can be considered for prevention of recurrent hemorrhage in patients with liver failure.

Treatment aims

• The aims of treatment, in order of importance, are as follows:

To resuscitate.

To control bleeding quickly.

To maintain liver function.

To identify and treat complications.

To prevent rebleeding.

Prognosis

• Sclerotherapy has high success rates, with bleeding controlled in 90% of patients after 2–3 sessions.

• 70% of patients rebleed after balloon tamponade, so definitive treatment must be arranged.

• Mortality is 30%–40% with the first variceal bleed, 15%–20% with subsequent bleeds.

• Prognosis depends on the underlying liver function.

• Approximately one-third of deaths in cirrhotic patients are related to bleeding.

Follow-up and management

• Patients should be followed-up every 3 months for the first year after the varices have been obliterated by sclerotherapy.

Key references

1. Burroughs A, Bosch J: Clinical manifestations and management of bleeding episodes in cirrhotics. In *Oxford Textbook of Clinical Hepatology*. Edited by McIntyre N, *et al.* Oxford: Oxford University Press; 1991:408–425.

2. Planas R: A prospective randomized trial comparing somatostatin and sclerotherapy in the treatment of acute variceal bleeding. *Hepatology* 1994, **20**:370–375.

3. Stiegman GV, *et al.*: Endoscopic sclerotherapy as compared with endoscopic ligation for bleeding oesophageal varices. *N Engl J Med* 1992, **326**:1527–1532.

4. Rossle M, *et al.*: The transjugular intrahepatic portosystemic stent-shunt procedure for variceal bleeding. *N Engl J Med* 1994, **330**:165–171.

Diagnosis

Symptoms

Crops of painful purple areas on skin.

Symptoms of the predisposing disease.

Signs

Painful, palpable purpura: the three "P's."

Crops of purple nodules: usually in dependent areas.

Lesions: tender; do not blanch; hemorrhagic blisters; black, necrotic, ulcerating in severe disease.

Finger pulp 2–3 mm lesions: indicating connective tissue disease, particularly rheumatoid arthritis.

Nail bed linear lesions: indicating trauma, connective tissue disease, or systemic infection.

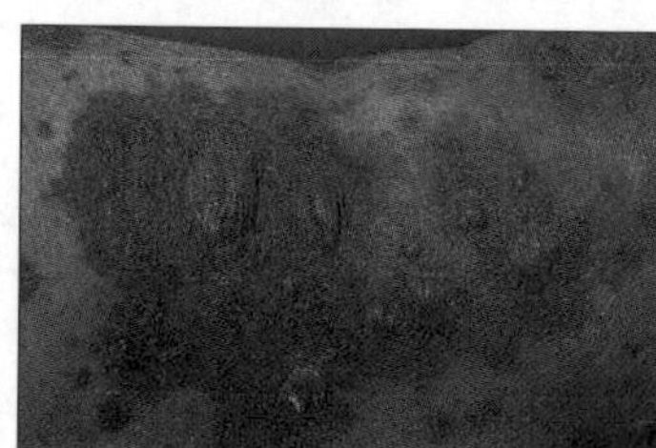

Cutaneous vasculitis on the legs, showing red/purple palpable painful lesions, some of which have overlying hemorrhagic blisters.

Net-like pattern (livedo reticularis): indicating connective tissue disease, cryoglobulinemia, antiphospholipid syndrome, or polyarteritis nodosa.

Subcutaneous nodules along arteries: indicating polyarteritis nodosa.

Investigations

Urinalysis, urine microscopy, serum creatinine measurement: to identify renal involvement.

Blood culture, culture of possible sites of infection: to identify infective cause.

Measurement of rheumatoid factor, antinuclear antibodies, antineutrophil cytoplasmic antibodies, anticardiolipin antibodies: to identify connective tissue disorders.

Cryoglobulin measurement: collected after fasting and taken to laboratory at 37°C.

Skin biopsy: not indicated if clinical picture is typical, because histology often shows nonspecific leukocytoclastic vasculitis, but may help in patients with drug-induced, infective, or inflammatory vasculitis; may also be helpful in identifying infiltrating inflammatory cells, type and size of blood vessels involved, and whether granulomatous changes are present.

Complications

Ulceration: particularly on lower limbs; may follow skin biopsy.

Secondary infection.

Renal involvement: in 30%–60% of patients.

Joint, gastrointestinal tract, CNS, or lung involvement.

Differential diagnosis

Purpura.

Thrombocytopenia.

Platelet dysfunction.

Corticosteroid treatment.

Old age.

Scurvy.

Trauma.

Nonaccidental injury in children.

Hemangioma.

Kaposi's sarcoma.

Bacillary angiomatosis.

Etiology

Causes include the following:

Environmental factors

Gravitational stasis.

Cold exposure.

Infection

Acute: meningococcal meningitis (1–3 weeks after throat infection), gonorrhea.

Chronic: urinary infections, dental abscess, leprosy, hepatitis B and C.

Drugs

Antibiotics: *e.g.*, sulfonamides.

Warfarin (rarely causes hemorrhagic skin infarction).

Inflammation

Immune complexes: *e.g.*, connective tissue disorders.

Cryoglobulins: *e.g.*, in malignancy.

Autoantibodies: *e.g.*, antineutrophil cytoplasmic antibody in Wegener's granulomatosis (may be secondary phenomenon).

Epidemiology

- Vasculitis is a common condition.
- The male:female ratio is equal.
- It can affect people at any age.

Treatment

Diet and lifestyle

• Patients must avoid cold, gravitational effects (with bed rest during acute episodes), and tight garments.

Pharmacological treatment

• Drugs that are probable causes of vasculitis should be discontinued.

• Precipitating infections should be treated by antibiotics.

Prednisone

• Prednisolone may be ineffective, and side effects limit use to patients with severe progressive systemic disease.

Standard dosage	Prednisone, 60–80 mg daily initially.
Contraindications	Untreated infection; caution in pregnancy because causes neonatal adrenal suppression.
Main drug interactions	Antihypertensives, antidiabetics, diuretics, antiepileptics.
Main side effects	Diabetes, osteoporosis, mental disturbance, peptic ulceration, infections, suppressed growth in children, proximal myopathy, cataracts, hypertension, acute adrenal insufficiency.

Dapsone

• Dapsone is often effective against chronic vasculitis, although this is not mentioned on the manufacturer's prescribing information.

Standard dosage	Dapsone, 50–100 mg daily.
Contraindications	Porphyrias, severe anemia, glucose-6-phosphate dehydrogenase.
Special points	Folate supplements needed in pregnancy (causes neonatal hemolysis and methemoglobinemia). Regular blood checks necessary.
Main drug interactions	Probenecid.
Main side effects	Agranulocytosis, hemolytic anemia, headaches, nausea, neuropathy, exfoliative dermatitis, hepatitis.

Indomethacin

• Indomethacin is sometimes effective in urticarial vasculitis, although this is not mentioned on the manufacturer's prescribing information.

Standard dosage	Indomethacin, 50–150 mg daily.
Contraindications	Active peptic ulceration; caution in renal impairment, epilepsy, parkinsonism, salicylate hypersensitivity.
Special points	Excreted in breast milk.
Main drug interactions	Warfarin, angiotensin-converting enzyme inhibitors, haloperidol, digoxin, diuretics, lithium, probenecid.
Main side effects	Gastrointestinal discomfort, nausea, ulceration and bleeding, asthma, tinnitus, headache, vertigo, drowsiness, convulsions, fluid retention, renal failure, hypertension, corneal deposits, thrombocytopenia, angioedema.

Treatment aims

To alleviate discomfort.

To prevent skin ulceration.

To detect systemic involvement early.

Other treatments

• Plasmapheresis: has been used to remove immune complexes in patients with SLE; no evidence of benefit has been shown in controlled studies.

Prognosis

• Individual episodes may clear after 3–6 weeks.

• Relapse and chronic disease are common.

• Patients with infective or drug-induced vasculitis usually recover fully on removal of the cause, although chronic vasculitis or, rarely, fatal systemic necrotizing vasculitis occur.

• The prognosis of inflammatory vasculitis depends on the cause: up to 25% of patients with renal involvement develop chronic renal problems in Henoch–Schönlein purpura.

Follow-up and management

• Renal involvement must be detected by weekly urinalysis and microscopy during an episode and serum creatinine and blood pressure measurement every 2 weeks.

• Cutaneous complications must be treated.

• Patients must be monitored for side effects of treatment.

General references

Berlit P: The spectrum of vasculopathies in the differential diagnosis of vasculitis. *Semin Neurol* 1994, **14**:370–379.

Somer T, Finegold SM: Vasculidities associated with infections, immunization, and antimicrobial drugs. *Clin Infect Dis* 1995, **20**:1010–1036.

Watts RA, Scott DG: ABC of rheumatology, rashes, and vasculitis. *BMJ* 1995, **310(6987)**:1128–1132.

Diagnosis

Symptoms

• Symptoms depend on the size and site of the vessel involved. The following concentrates particularly on primary systemic vasculitis involving small- and medium-sized arteries.

Malaise, weight loss, fever, diffuse myalgia, arthralgia.
Symptoms of any underlying disease or secondary vasculitis: *e.g.*, rheumatoid arthritis, SLE.
Rash.
Epistaxis, nasal crusting, sinusitis: especially in Wegener's granulomatosis.
Chest pain, hemoptysis, dyspnea, cough, late-onset asthma (normally precedes Churg-Strauss syndrome).
Mouth ulcers, abdominal pain, diarrhea.
Numbness, weakness.

Signs

Pyrexia, lymphadenopathy, muscle wasting, weakness.
Microscopic hematuria or proteinuria, or both.
Skin purpura, ulcer, infarction.
Nasal crusting or collapse, septal perforation: especially in Wegener's granulomatosis.
Crackles, wheeze, cardiomyopathy, pericarditis: especially in Churg-Strauss vasculitis.
Mononeuritis or mononeuritis multiplex, peripheral neuropathy.
Arthritis: usually of large joints.

Investigations

Urinalysis: most urgent investigation because renal involvement influences prognosis.
Plasma urea and creatinine, 24-hour urinary protein and creatinine clearance measurement: to assess renal function.
Full blood count: shows anemia, leukocytosis (leukocyte count normal or low in vasculitis secondary to rheumatoid arthritis or SLE), eosinophilia (especially in Churg-Strauss vasculitis), thrombocytosis.
ESR, CRP, and liver enzyme (*e.g.*, alkaline phosphatase) measurement: raised values.
Antineutrophil cytoplasmic autoantibody analysis: most useful for diagnosis; diffuse cytoplasmic staining (anti-proteinase III) in 80% of patients with systemic Wegener's granulomatosis, 50% limited Wegener's; perinuclear staining less specific (antimyeloperoxidase) but common in microscopic polyangiitis and idiopathic crescentic glomerulonephritis.
Other autoantibody tests: antinuclear antibody and rheumatoid factor nonspecific; may reflect underlying disease; C3 and C4 usually increased in primary vasculitis, low or normal in vasculitis associated with SLE and rheumatoid arthritis; high levels of cryoglobulins may indicate need for plasma exchange.
Von Willebrand's factor antigen test: measure of vascular damage; also increased in noninflammatory vascular injury (*e.g.*, thrombosis).
Viral studies: for hepatitis B, cytomegalovirus, Epstein-Barr virus.
Chest radiography: shows nodules, fibrosis, infiltrate.
Sinus radiography: shows sinusitis, bone destruction.
Angiography: shows microaneurysms in up to 70% of patients with polyarteritis nodosa; rarely with Wegener's granulomatosis and Churg-Strauss vasculitis.
Two-dimensional echocardiography: to exclude vegetations and atrial myxoma.
Biopsy: of kidney, skin, nose, muscle, sural nerve, rectum, or temporal artery.

Complications

Renal failure: acute, especially if diagnosis or treatment delayed, or chronic (<10% of patients dependent on dialysis).
Gangrene or infarction: can lead to amputation or chronic skin ulcer.
Neuropathy: possibly permanent (*e.g.*, footdrop), although 60% improve on treatment.
Subglottic stenosis: leading to tracheostomy.
Nasal collapse: permanent and may necessitate later plastic surgery.
Severe pulmonary hemorrhage: may cause breathlessness; and unexplained anemia.
Coronary arteritis: may cause myocardial infarction and heart failure.
Hypertension.

Differential diagnosis

Nonspecific systemic illness
Infection: subacute bacterial endocarditis, other chronic and atypical infections.
Connective tissue disease.
Malignancy: especially myeloproliferative, metastatic disease, multiple myeloma.
Sarcoid, HIV, Goodpasture's syndrome.

Vasculopathy and necrotizing granuloma
Lymphomatoid granulomatosis, idiopathic midline granuloma.
Cholesterol atheroembolism.
Cardiac myxoma, antiphospholipid antibody syndrome.

Etiology

• Causes include the following:
Autoimmune: autoantibodies, *e.g.*, antineutrophil cytoplasmic autoantibodies in Wegener's granulomatosis.
Immune complex: particularly secondary vasculitis associated with SLE and rheumatoid arthritis.
Viral infection: *e.g.*, hepatitis B, HIV, cytomegalovirus.
Neoplasms (especially hematological).

Epidemiology

• The annual incidence may be increasing, ~40 per million being affected each year.
• The male:female ratio is 1.5:1.
• The age range is wide, with an increasing incidence with age in women.

Classification

Large-artery
Giant-cell arteritis, Takayasu's arteritis.

Medium-artery
Polyarteritis nodosa, Kawasaki disease.

Medium- or small-artery
Wegener's granulomatosis, Churg–Strauss vasculitis, microscopic polyangiitis.

Small-vessel
Henoch–Schönlein purpura, essential mixed cryoglobulinemia, leukocytoclastic cutaneous vasculitis.

• Secondary vasculitis, *e.g.*, infection, drugs, rheumatoid arthritis, SLE, and Sjögren's syndrome, usually involves either medium or small arteries or pure small vessel.

Treatment

Diet and lifestyle

• Because they are often immunosuppressed, patients should take precautions against possible infections.

Pharmacological treatment

Steroids

• Steroids are only used alone in patients with small-vessel or large-artery disease (*see* Classification).

Standard dosage — *Continuous:* prednisolone, 15–60 mg orally depending on severity and type of vasculitis; usually reducing course.
Pulse: methylprednisolone, 1 g i.v. or 100 mg orally for 3 days; dose and frequency varied according to response.

Contraindications — Infection (*e.g.*, subacute bacterial endocarditis).

Special points — Adrenal suppression may be a problem with long-term treatment.

Main drug interactions — Drugs that induce liver enzymes promote steroid metabolism; prednisolone antagonizes antihypertensive treatment.

Main side effects — Diabetes, hypertension, osteoporosis, mood change, cushingoid appearance.

Immunosuppressants

• Immunosuppressants are indicated for more severe vasculitis, particularly of small or medium artery.

Standard dosage — *Continuous:* cyclophosphamide, 2 mg/kg orally daily.
Pulse: cyclophosphamide, 15 mg/kg i.v.; alternatively, 5 mg/kg orally daily for 3 days; dose and frequency vary according to response, renal function, and leukocyte count (measured at 7, 10, and 14 days).

Contraindications — Pregnancy (first trimester especially), uncontrolled infection.

Main drug interactions — None.

Main side effects — Bone-marrow suppression, hemorrhagic cystitis (rare with pulse treatment), nausea, alopecia, infertility.

Combination treatment

Pulse i.v. cyclophosphamide, 15 mg/kg, and methylprednisolone, 1 g 2-weekly for 6 courses (remission induction), then 3-weekly for 2 pulses, then monthly for 3 pulses (maintenance).

Pulse oral cyclophosphamide, 5 mg/kg daily, and prednisone, 100–200 mg daily for 3 consecutive days; interval between treatments as for pulse i.v. treatment.

Continuous oral cyclophosphamide, 2 mg/kg daily, and prednisone, 40–60 mg daily; prednisolone reduced to 20 mg daily by month 3, to 10 mg daily by month 6.

• Cyclophosphamide should be withdrawn at 9–12 months.

• Longer treatment or change to azathioprine, 2 mg/kg daily, is often needed in patients with Wegener's granulomatosis or rheumatoid vasculitis.

Other drugs

Azathioprine: steroid-sparing and immunosuppressive.

Plasmapheresis: for pulmonary hemorrhage and severe renal disease.

Treatment aims

To induce and maintain remission.

To recognize and treat relapses early.

To avoid toxicity and side effects.

Prognosis

• In patients with Wegener's granulomatosis or polyarteritis nodosa, 75% remit and 50% relapse with continuous oral treatment.

• The 2-year survival rate ranges from 10% with no treatment to 80% with cyclophosphamide treatment.

• For patients with small-vessel vasculitis, the prognosis is good.

Follow-up and management

• Long-term follow-up is essential, with regular clinical examination, full blood count, renal function tests (especially urinalysis), and immunology.

• Daily steroids are more often used for large- and small-vessel vasculitis, with reduction in dose when the patient is in remission, aiming for alternate-day treatment.

• Early recognition of relapse is essential.

Key references

1. Chakravarty K, Scott DGI: Management of systemic vasculitis. *Rheumatol Rev* 1992, **1**:81–99.
2. Gross WL, Schmitt WH, Caernok E: ANCA associated diseases: a rheumatologist's perspective. *Am J Kidney Dis* 1991, **2**:175–179.
3. Hoffman G: Wegener's granulomatosis: an analysis of 158 patients. *Ann Intern Med* 1992, **116**:488–498.

Diagnosis

Symptoms

• Most viral warts are asymptomatic, but occasionally they cause severe pain (especially plantar warts).

Signs

Common wart (verruca vulgaris)

Well-demarcated verrucous papule with "seeds" (*i.e.*, thrombosed capillaries).

Plantar wart (verruca plantaris)

Hyperkeratotic plaque: on the plantar surface of the feet, often painful to pressure.

Flat wart (verruca plana)

1–3 mm flat-topped papules: on face or legs (spread by shaving) or elsewhere.

Genital wart (condyloma acuminatum)

White moist cauliflower-like friable papules: occur anywhere on the anogenital skin or mucosa.

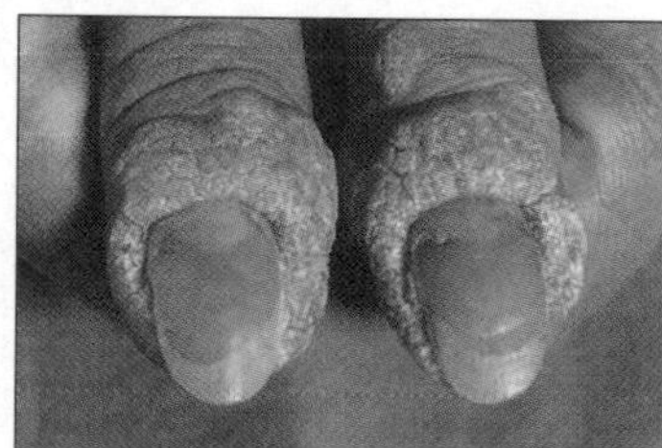

Periungual viral warts.

Investigations

• A viral wart is a clinical diagnosis.

Rapid plasma reagin (RPR) test: to rule out secondary syphilis in cases in which condyloma latum is considered.

Biopsy: in select cases to rule out verrucous carcinoma.

Colposcopy: in female patients with condyloma.

Proctoscopy and cytoscopy.

Complications

• Viral warts can have widespread involvement and spread in immunosuppressed patients (HIV-negative and HIV-positive).

Oncogenic potential: Bowens disease (viral induced) on glans penis.

Urogenital dysplasia and carcinoma: associated with anogenital and laryngeal warts and cervical condylomata.

Squamous cell carcinomas in situ: secondary to human papillomavirus subtypes 6, 11, 16, 18, 31, 33.

Obstruction of urethral meatus: by urethral condyloma, making treatment extremely difficult.

Laryngeal condyloma: can develop in the birth canal in children born to mothers with condyloma acuminatum, causing respiratory difficulty in the infant; laryngeal condyloma can also occur in surgeons after treating condyloma with carbon dioxide laser [1].

Squamous cell carcinoma: from verruca vulgaris following irradiation [2].

Differential diagnosis

Molluscum contagiosum.

Stucco keratosis (form of seborrheic keratosis resembling verruca planae).

Flegel's disease.

Acrokeratosis verruciformis.

Epidermodysplasia verruciformis.

Pitted keratolysis.

Punctate keratoderma.

Arsenical keratosis.

Condyloma latum.

Acquired digital fibrokeratoma.

Recurrent infantile digital fibroma.

Acrochordon (skin tag).

Etiology

Cause

Human papillomavirus infections; sensitive DNA hybridization techniques have identified more than 60 types of viral DNA.

Spread

• Spread of viral warts is by contact (*i.e.*, skin to skin in verruca vulgaris; sexual contact with condyloma acuminatum; maternal genital tract for neonates).

Epidemiology

• Anogenital warts occur most often in young sexually active patients.

Treatment [3]

Diet and lifestyle

Condyloma acuminatum: Close prenatal care and counseling in pregnant women.

Education, emphasizing importance of examination and treatment of sexual partners.

Use of condoms.

Pharmacological treatment

• Treatment should be individualized, as treatment is difficult and no one method can be used in all patients with equal success.

For cutaneous warts

Standard dosage	Salicylic acid as ointments, plasters, gels (concentration from 10%–50%) applied nightly for 3–4 months. Combination of salicylic acid and lactic acid applied nightly for 3–4 months.
Contraindications	Local hypersensitivity.
Special points	The main objective is to cause inflammation but not infection or scarring.
Main drug interactions	None.
Main side effects	Skin irritation and pain.

Second-line treatment

Liquid nitrogen: either applied or sprayed onto the wart in order to cause a blister; repeated at 2- to 4-week intervals.

Electrodesiccation and curettage: often results in scarring.

CO_2 laser.

Pulsed dye laser.

Interferon injections for condyloma [4].

For anogenital warts

Standard dosage	Podophyllin or 5-fluorouracil applied sparingly to affected areas once daily, increased to twice daily as tolerated.
Contraindications	Widespread areas of involvement due to possible systemic absorption.
Special points	Treatment is individual with respect to severity of disease.
Main drug interactions	None.
Main side effects	Local irritation, burning, ulceration, pain, and blistering.

Other treatment

Other treatment includes CO_2 laser.

Treatment aims

To clear clinical disease without causing scarring.

Other treatments

Hypnosis, particularly in children [5].

Contact sensitization.

Prognosis

• Warts spontaneously resolve in some patients.

Follow-up and management

• Routine cervical cytology in women with anogenital warts is warranted because of the oncogenic potential (colposcopy if indicated) [6].

Key references

1. Gloster HM Jr, Roenigk RK: Risk of acquiring human papillomavirus from the plume produced by the carbon dioxide laser in the treatment of warts. *J Am Acad Dermatol* 1995, **32**:436–441.
2. Kopelson PL, *et al.*: Verruca vulgaris and radiation exposure are associated with squamous cell carcinoma of the finger. *J Dermatol Surg Oncol* 1994, **20**:38–41.
3. Drake LA, *et al.*: Guidelines for care of warts: human papillomavirus. Committee on Guidelines of Care. *J Am Acad Dermatol* 1995, **32**:98–103.
4. Reichman RC, *et al.*: Treatment of condyloma acuminatum with three different interferon-alpha preparations administered parenterally: a double-blind placebo-controlled trial. *J Infect Dis* 1990, **162**:1270.
5. Ewin DM: Hypnotherapy for warts (verruca vulgaris): 41 consecutive cases with 33 cures. *Am J Clin Hypn* 1992, **35**:1–10.
6. Krays SJ, Stone KM: Management of genital infection caused by human papillomavirus. *Rev Infect Dis* 1990, **12**:S620–S632.

Diagnosis

Symptoms

Fatigue, weakness and weight loss: in >80% of patients.

Bleeding tendency: in 60%.

Sensorimotor peripheral neuropathy: in 15%.

Headache, dizziness, vertigo, confusion, stroke, drowsiness, breathlessness, dependent edema: features of hyperviscosity syndrome in 20%.

Epistaxis, gastrointestinal hemorrhage, dependent purpura.

Signs

Lymphadenopathy: in 40%.

Splenomegaly: in 30%.

Hepatomegaly: in 30%.

Peripheral neuropathy: in 15%.

Ataxia; nystagmus; hemiplegia; dementia; coma; signs of congestive cardiac failure; dependent purpura; hemorrhage; dilated, tortuous retinal veins with "sausage-like" segmentation; retinal hemorrhage; papilledema: signs of hyperviscosity syndrome.

Investigations

Full blood count: shows normocytic, normochromic anemia in 80% of patients; rouleaux, sometimes spuriously raised mean cell volume, neutropenia, thrombocytopenia; lymphocytes may be increased but seldom $>5 \times 10^9$/L.

Cell marker analysis: surface immunoglobulin of single light chain class (κ or λ); $CD19^+$, $CD20^+$, $CD37^+$, $CD38^+$, $CD5^-$, $CD10^-$.

Bone-marrow aspiration: increase in small lymphocytes and plasmacytoid lymphocytes, sometimes in plasma cells.

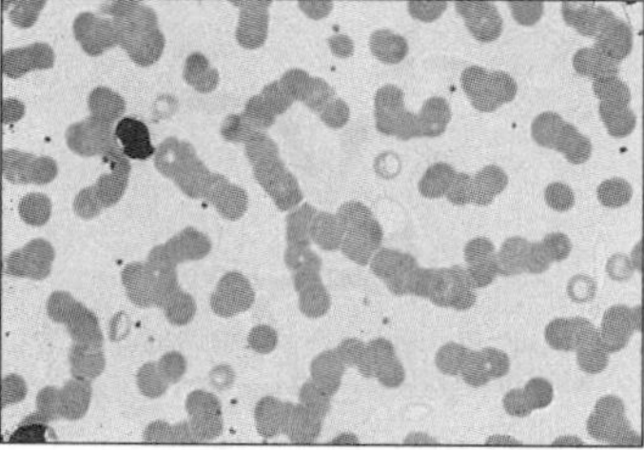

Rouleaux on Romanowsky-stained blood film.

Serum electrophoresis: monoclonal spike in beta or gamma globulins; identifiable as IgM by immunoelectrophoresis; serum IgG and IgA often reduced.

Plasma viscosity measurement: raised; hyperviscosity syndrome only if relative serum viscosity >4 times water.

Cryoglobulin analysis: proteins that precipitate at 4°C found in 15% of patients.

Cold agglutinin analysis: erythrocyte autoantibodies (anti-I or anti-i) agglutinate erythrocytes in the cold; idiopathic acquired variety monoclonal IgM.

• Clotting studies may indicate a pseudo von Willebrand's state with prolonged activated partial thromboplastin time, bleeding time, and abnormal platelet function.

Complications

Amyloid: in <10%.

IgM monoclonal protein autoantibody activity: occasionally.

Peripheral neuropathy, cold agglutination syndrome, acquired hemophilia: due, respectively, to antimyelin, antierythrocyte, and anti–factor VIII.

Differential diagnosis

Diseases associated with IgM monoclonal proteins:

Essential (benign) monoclonal macroglobulinemia (27%).

Cold agglutinin syndrome (3%).

Chronic lymphocytic leukemia (10%).

Other B-cell lymphomas (30%).

IgM myeloma (3%).

Extramedullary plasmacytoma (2%).

Waldenström's macroglobulinemia (25%).

Etiology

• Presumably, a mutation event occurs in a susceptible clone.

• Proliferation of antibody-producing cells in response to antigenic stimulation may become autonomous when a mutation leads to a lack of control of the cell cycle.

Epidemiology

• Waldenström's macroglobulinemia is predominantly a disease of the elderly; the median age at presentation being 65 years.

• The annual incidence is 1 in 200 000.

• It occurs more often in men than women.

• Familial incidence is slightly increased.

Bleeding abnormalities

• The IgM paraprotein interferes with the formation of the platelet plug.

• Platelet adhesiveness is reduced, as is the release of platelet factor 3.

• The paraprotein also interferes with the coagulation cascade and may be an antibody against factor VIII.

• Some paraproteins bind to fibrin and inhibit fibrin monomer aggregation, resulting in a bulky gelatinous clot with impaired clot retraction.

• Factor X deficiencies may be seen in patients who develop amyloidosis.

Treatment

Diet and lifestyle

• The patient should be encouraged to live as normal a life as possible.

Pharmacological treatment

• Chlorambucil, given under specialist supervision, is the mainstay of treatment, but only ~50% of patients respond.

• Other alkylating agents give similar responses and probably could be used interchangeably.

• Higher response rates have been reported using combination chemotherapy (*e.g.*, BCNU, vincristine, cyclophosphamide, melphalan, and prednisone), but such studies have been very small.

• Recent reports have suggested that fludarabine is a useful drug, but again, the number of patients treated has been small. Similarly, early reports indicate that interferon-α may be of value [1].

Standard dosage	Chlorambucil orally daily for 2 weeks every 4 weeks.
Contraindications	No absolute contraindications.
Special points	Full blood count essential because chlorambucil may cause bone-marrow suppression.
Main drug interactions	No major interactions known.
Main side effects	Bone-marrow suppression, nausea and vomiting, diarrhea, oral ulcers, hypersensitivity rashes, occasionally myelodysplasia, acute leukemia.

Treatment aims

To relieve symptoms.

To prolong life.

Other treatments

• Plasma exchange should be instituted urgently for hyperviscosity syndrome; one plasma volume exchanged at regular intervals until relative viscosity <4 times that of water.

• Maintenance plasmapheresis alone may be sufficient to control the disease; viscosity need not be restored to normal.

Prognosis

• The disease is not curable.

• Median survival is 4 years in patients who respond to treatment, 2 years in non-responders; the peripheral neuropathy is frequently unresponsive.

Follow-up and management

• Patients should be followed up at regular intervals.

• Full blood count and IgM concentrations should be monitored.

• Plasma viscosity indicates whether plasmapheresis is indicated.

• No large controlled trials are available to guide the physician. By analogy with other low-grade lymphomas, it is reasonable to withhold treatment in asymptomatic patients.

Key reference

1. Kantarjian HM, *et al.*: Fludarabine therapy in macroglobulinaemic lymphoma. *Blood* 1990, **75**:1928–1931.

Wolff–Parkinson–White syndrome

Diagnosis

Definition

• Myocardial activation from atrial to ventricular myocardium occurs over an accessory connection (accessory to the normal His-Purkinje system).
• If conduction occurs in sinus rhythm, pre-excitation is apparent on the ECG.
• The substrate for atrioventricular re-entry tachycardia is present; conduction in tachycardia from ventricle to atrium over the accessory connection is orthodromic (90%) or from atrium to ventricle is antidromic.

Symptoms

• Most patients who are found to have the Wolff–Parkinson–White syndrome are asymptomatic; the only feature is the presence of pre-excitation on the surface ECG.

Palpitation: most common symptom; caused by re-entry tachycardia (sudden onset and termination, regular, rapid - often >200 beats/min); may also be caused by paroxysmal atrial fibrillation (in ~5% of patients).
Chest pain: during tachycardia; pain or discomfort similar to angina; rarely indicates coronary artery disease.
Impaired consciousness: dizziness or faintness common; syncope less frequent (5%) and usually follows vasodilatation occurring as a secondary response to tachycardia.
Polyuria: accompanying sustained episodes of tachycardia.

Signs

• In sinus rhythm, no clinical signs indicate the presence of the condition; during tachycardia, clinical signs associated with the impaired circulation and abnormal cardiac action may be found, principally the following:

Rapid pulse.
Hypotension.
Alteration in the venous pulse wave form.

Investigations

Pre-excitation ECG: pre-excitation is the QRS configuration generated by fusion of ventricular activation wave fronts from normal His-Purkinje system and accessory atrioventricular connection; myocardium activated through accessory connection gives rise to delta wave (slurred initial QRS); precise delta wave pattern depends on location of accessory connection on atrioventricular ring, and QRS configuration may be subtly or dramatically changed from normal; pre-excitation ceases with temporary cessation of anterograde conduction through accessory connection, or pre-excitation changes may vary depending on balance of activation between normal conduction system and accessory connection, (both influenced by autonomic tone); PR interval shortening results from myocardial activation through the accessory connection, which lacks decremental conduction properties.
ECG during tachycardia: usually (90%) narrow complex tachycardia; retrograde atrial activation may be seen as P waves of altered configuration inscribed in ST segments; rate-related bundle branch block (aberrancy) or antidromic tachycardia results in broad QRS complex tachycardia.
Ambulatory monitoring: paroxysms of tachycardia may be seen on 24-h or 48-h monitoring; usually too infrequent for capture of tachycardia to be probable; self-activated recording devices (cardiac memo/wrist recorder) with transtelephonic transmission to a recording center may be more useful.
Electrophysiological study: cardiac extrastimulation techniques and recording of endocardial ECG allows diagnosis and characterization of the condition in almost all cases; complex studies rarely done for diagnosis alone but used as prelude to radiofrequency catheter ablation of accessory connection; single wire study determines ventricular response rate through accessory connection conduction during atrial fibrillation to assess risk of malignant arrhythmias secondary to rapid ventricular activation; this is an imprecise means of assessing the risk of sudden death.
Exercise stress testing: no role in defining connection conduction properties.

Complications

Atrial fibrillation.
Sudden cardiac death: rare.

Differential diagnosis

Atrioventricular nodal re-entry tachycardia: tachycardia due to dual atrioventricular node physiology allowing re-entry within the atrioventricular node; other types of supraventricular tachycardia (*e.g.*, atrial flutter, fibrillation, ectopic atrial tachycardia, Mahaim re-entry).

Ventricular tachycardia: broad QRS complexes (due to antidromic tachycardia or aberrant conduction) may be misdiagnosed as tachycardia arising from a ventricular focus; algorithms are available to aid ECG differentiation.

Etiology

• Wolff–Parkinson–White syndrome is not inherited.

• During early cardiac development, direct physical continuity exists between ventricular and atrial myocardium; in growth of atrioventricular sulcus, tissue at a later stage in cardiac development interrupts this, but defects may persist into neonatal and subsequently adult life.

• Term infants have frequently been found to have these connections, but they are presumed to be nonfunctional in most.

• Accessory connections appear microscopically to be normal myocardial muscle bundles bridging atrial and ventricular myocardium; they may have subepicardial or subendocardial locations; they are multiple in ~10% of patients with the condition.

• Ebstein's anomaly is associated with their presence, and multiple pathways are more common in these patients.

Epidemiology

• Early studies have suggested that ECG evidence of pre-excitation can be found in 0.3% of the population; probably only a few of such patients are symptomatic, but the evidence is conflicting.

• Depending on the nature of the population studies, documentation of tachycardia has varied from 5% to 90% of patients.

Treatment

Diet and lifestyle

• In patients with frequent symptoms, lifestyle is restricted by the occurrence of palpitations (often apparently related to stress or exertion) or by the side effects of drug treatment.

Pharmacological treatment

• Drugs are now considered second-line treatment for the Wolff–Parkinson–White syndrome.

• Asymptomatic patients need no drug treatment unless their occupation demands removal of all risk of tachycardia (*e.g.*, airline pilots, certain military, police, and fire-brigade personnel).

• Symptomatic patients who need treatment but who do not wish to have radiofrequency catheter ablation can be given antiarrhythmic drugs; these exert their effect by altering atrioventricular nodal conduction or accessory connection conduction, or both, so that re-entry tachycardia will less probably be sustained.

• Drugs that slow atrioventricular nodal conduction but enhance accessory pathway conduction (*e.g.*, digoxin) should not be used in isolation.

• Antiarrhythmic drugs often have unacceptable side effects, and some have been shown to have dangerous proarrhythmic effects.

• Drugs must be taken continuously, and not on an ad-hoc basis, to give optimal control of symptoms; even then, abolition of symptoms is rare.

• Adenosine can be used as an i.v. bolus to abort an episode of atrioventricular re-entry tachycardia.

Nonpharmacological treatment

Catheter ablation

• Catheter ablation is technically demanding but is associated with very low mortality and morbidity in skilled hands [1].

• Apposition of an ablation electrode to the endocardial location nearest the accessory connection results in cessation of accessory connection conduction on delivery of radiofrequency energy through the electrode.

• This is a low-voltage, high-frequency energy source, which results in heating of the electrode tip, in turn producing a small endocardial lesion (5–7 mm) that extends into the myocardium.

• Primary success is >90%.

• Failure to achieve complete abolition of accessory connection conduction leads to a small recurrence rate after apparently successful procedures.

• Radiofrequency catheter ablation is the treatment of choice because it is curative; other energy sources are available but are associated with various disadvantages.

Surgery

• Although curative, surgical division of accessory connections needs major cardiac surgery and so is associated with higher morbidity and mortality than catheter ablation.

• It should be reserved for patients in whom catheter ablation has been a repeated failure.

Treatment aims

To abolish accessory connection conduction and therefore risk of tachycardia and palpitation.

To remove risk of sudden cardiac death.

To assess risk in asymptomatic patients.

Prognosis

• The prognosis is probably that of the normal population after successful catheter ablation.

• Lesions induced by radiofrequency catheter ablation have not been associated with impairment of ventricular function or arrhythmogenic complications except in infant hearts, when lesions may grow with heart size.

• Untreated asymptomatic Wolff–Parkinson–White syndrome carries a good prognosis; the risk of sudden death in asymptomatic patients is probably very small.

Follow-up and management

• Recurrence of pre-excitation may occur early after a primarily successful catheter ablation (within 6 weeks) in as many as 10% of patients; occasionally, recurrence is not accompanied by symptom recurrence because of modification of the connection conduction properties.

• Late recurrence after successful catheter ablation (>3 months) is rare; patients usually experience short-lived episodes of palpitation or rhythm irregularity for some months after successful ablations, which may relate to a learning effect through which individuals have become sensitized to any short-lived change in heart rhythm (*e.g.*, ectopic activity) because, before treatment, these heralded onset of tachycardia; these symptoms resolve with time and reassurance.

• After surgical treatment, standard follow-up is needed.

• Follow-up of patients treated by antiarrhythmic drugs is determined by their symptoms and drug side effects.

Key reference

1. Jackman WM, *et al.*: Catheter ablation of accessory atrioventricular pathways (Wolff–Parkinson–White syndrome) by radiofrequency current. *N Engl J Med* 1991, **324**:1605–1611.

Diagnosis

Symptoms

Presentations include the following.

Simple duodenal ulcer: especially if multiple or delayed healing, also if patient has neither *Helicobacter pylori* infection nor history of NSAID ingestion.

Recurrent peptic ulcer: after surgery.

Esophagitis and duodenal ulcer: in the same patient.

Symptoms of peptic ulcer and diarrhea or malabsorption.

Diarrhea or malabsorption alone.

Signs

• No typical physical signs are manifest, apart from those of complicated duodenal ulceration (hemorrhage, perforation, pyloric stenosis).

• Rarely, signs of hypercalcemia or pituitary adenoma in multiple endocrine neoplasia syndrome may be seen.

Investigations

Fasting plasma gastrin measurement: ideally when the patient has not taken antisecretory drugs for 48 h: normal concentration <150 pg/mL; Zollinger-Ellison syndrome (ZES) is probable if hypergastrinemia occurs with increased gastric acid secretion [1].

Basal acid output: ≥15 mEq/h or a basal acid output/maximal acid output (after pentagastrin infusion) ratio > 0.6 is highly suggestive of ZES.

Secretin test: a rise in serum gastrin of >200 pg/mL following an i.v. bolus of secretin has a sensitivity and specificity exceeding 90% for the diagnosis of ZES.

Gastric pH measurement: fasting pH >3.5 indicates hypergastrinemia due to hypo- or achlorhydria not to ZES.

CT of pancreas or arteriography: to check for primary tumor or metastases (only 40% and 20% positive, respectively, in ZES).

Transhepatic portal-vein sampling: to localize gastrin release (rarely used).

Endoscopic ultrasonography: of growing importance in tumor localization.

An islet cell tumor secreted gastrin and adrenocorticotrophic hormone. Postmortem examination showed hyperplastic adrenals and liver metastases. The patient died from perforated jejunal peptic ulceration before omeprazole treatment.

Complications

• Complications are those of severe peptic ulceration, often manifest as the following:

Nonhealing ulceration.

Surgical problems: after emergency ulcer surgery.

Widespread metastatic disease.

Differential diagnosis

Severe or refractory peptic ulceration.

Hypergastrinemia due to pernicious anemia, *Helicobacter pylori* infection, or profound hypoacidity secondary to acid antisecretory drugs (especially proton pump blockers: omeprazole, lansoprazole).

Retained gastric antrum after Billroth II partial gastrectomy (now extremely rare).

Etiology

• Zollinger–Ellison syndrome is caused by uncontrolled gastric acid hypersecretion, driven by plasma gastrin released by a gastrinoma (50% malignant).

• 75% of gastrinomas are localized in a triangle defined by the junction of the cystic and common bile ducts, the junction of the second and third parts of the duodenum, and the head and body of the pancreas.

• 15% of gastrinomas occur in the wall of the duodenum, 10% in extraintestinal locations.

Epidemiology

• Hypercalcemia, due to hyperparathyroidism in the multiple endocrine neoplasia syndrome type I, accounts for 25% of patients.

• Zollinger–Ellison syndrome can coexist with pheochromocytoma or ectopic corticotropic hormone production from tumor.

Treatment

Diet and lifestyle

• No special precautions are necessary.

Pharmacological treatment

• As soon as Zollinger–Ellison syndrome is suspected, blood must be taken for fasting plasma gastrin concentration, ideally when the patient is not on antisecretory treatment.

Emergency control of gastric acid secretion

Standard dosage Ranitidine, 300 mg, or omeprazole, 20 mg orally 4 times daily; if patient cannot take oral treatment, ranitidine, 100 mg i.v. as slow bolus and infusion of 0.5 mg/kg/h [2].

Contraindications Hypersensitivity.

Special points Medications should be adjusted to maintain basal acid output at <10 mEq/h (5 mEq/h in patients post-partial gastrectomy).

Main drug interactions None.

Main side effects None.

Long-term control of gastric acid secretion

• Omeprazole, 20–120 mg daily, is the treatment of choice (titrated to control basal acid secretion rate <10 mmol/h).

• Large doses of H_2-blockers may be needed because they are competitive antagonists.

• Lansoprazole, 30–120 mg daily is an alternative proton-pump inhibitor.

Treatment aims

To control gastric acid secretion and thereby heal aggressive peptic ulceration.

To identify and remove primary tumor, if possible.

Other treatments

For hyperparathyroidism: parathyroidectomy may decrease gastrin release and acid secretion.

For localized tumors: laparotomy to search for primary tumor; if no hepatic metastases detected on CT or arteriogram, after initial control of acid secretion by drugs [3].

Partial gastrectomy or vagotomy: no longer recommended.

Prognosis

• All complications of peptic ulceration should be avoided by pharmacological control of gastric acid secretion.

• ~20% of patients may be cured by surgical resection of the primary tumor.

• Death is usually from metastatic tumor, with survival prolonged by the usual chemotherapy for disseminated adenocarcinoma.

Follow-up and management

• Fasting plasma gastrin concentration should be measured and basal acid secretion assessed.

Causes of treatment failure

Hypercalcemia associated with multiple endocrine neoplasm syndrome type I.

Insufficient dose of medication.

Spread of the primary tumor.

Key references

1. Yamada T: *Textbook of Gastroenterology*. Philadelphia: JB Lippincott; 1995:1430–1445.
2. Maton PN: The management of Zollinger–Ellison syndrome. *Aliment Pharmacol Ther* 1993, **7**:467–475.
3. Norton J, Jensen R: Unresolved surgical issues in the management of patients with Zollinger–Ellison syndrome. *World J Surg* 1991, **15**:151–159.

Page numbers followed by *f* indicate figures; page numbers followed by *t* indicate tables.

A

ABCM chemotherapy
  for multiple myeloma, 261
Abdominal distension
  in acute lymphoblastic leukemia
    in children, 230
  in ascites, 46–47
  in cystic fibrosis, 58
  in diverticular disease of colon, 116
  with gastric ulcer, 150
  in irritable bowel syndrome, 222
  in myeloproliferative disorders, 268
  in polycystic kidney disease, 320
  in thalassemia, 388
  in typhoid fever, 406
Abdominal pain
  with acute pancreatitis, 294
  in AIDS-related lymphoma, 16
  with bacterial overgrowth of small
      intestine, 56
  with chronic fatigue syndrome, 76
  with chronic pancreatitis, 296
  with colorectal cancer, 82
  with Crohn's disease, 88
  with cystic fibrosis, 58
  with diabetes mellitus, 100, 104, 108
  with diverticular disease of colon, 116
  with duodenal ulcer, 118
  with dyslipoproteinemia, 120
  with fulminant liver failure, 238
  with gallstones, 146
  with gastric cancer, 148
  with gastric ulcer, 150
  with gram-negative septicemia, 158
  with granulomatous lung disease, 160
  with Henoch-Schönlein purpura, 174
  with hepatocellular carcinoma, 182
  with infectious diarrhea, 216
  with irritable bowel syndrome, 222
  Kaposi's sarcoma in AIDS and, 224
  with leptospirosis, 226
  with Lyme disease, 242
  with multiple myeloma, 260
  with *Mycobacterium* infection in AIDS,
      266
  with myeloproliferative disorders, 268
  with polycystic kidney disease, 320
  with primary biliary cirrhosis, 80
  with primary sclerosing cholangitis, 74
  with pulmonary tuberculosis, 404
  with sickle cell disease, 362
Abscess
  cerebral
    encephalitis *vs.*, 126
    in toxoplasmosis in AIDS, 394
    tumor *vs.*, 72
  peritonsillar
    in pharyngitis, 308
  skin, 364–365
  in typhoid fever, 406
ABVD chemotherapy
  for Hodgkin's disease, 189
Acanthosis nigricans
  in polycystic ovarian disease, 322
Acarbose
  for diabetes mellitus, 103
Acetaminophen
  for chronic fatigue syndrome, 77
  fulminant liver failure and, 238
  for measles, 247
  for osteoarthritis, 289
  for parvovirus B19 infection, 303
  for rubella, 355
  for sickle cell disease, 363
Acetylcysteine
  for cystic fibrosis, 59
  for fulminant liver failure, 239
Achalasia, 2f, 2–3
  esophageal carcinoma *vs.*, 136
Achilles tendon
  psoriatic arthritis and, 40
Acne, 4f, 4–5
  in Cushing's syndrome, 90
  in polycystic ovarian disease, 322
  pubertal abnormalities and, 334
Acquired immunodeficiency syndrome
      (AIDS), 14–15. *See also* Human
      immunodeficiency virus (HIV)
  acute pancreatitis *vs.*, 294
  buccal and esophageal candidiasis in,
      64f–65f, 64–65
  cryptococcal meningitis in, 250–251
  invasive fungal infections and, 142
  Kaposi's sarcoma in, 224f, 224–225
  lymphoma and, 16–17
  pericarditis and, 304
  Pneumocystis carinii infection in,
      316–317
  toxoplasmosis in, 394f, 394–395
Acrochordon
  viral warts *vs.*, 420
Acrodermatitis
  eczema *vs.*, 122
  in Lyme disease, 242
Acromegaly, 6f, 6–7
  diabetes mellitus in, 102
  hypertension and, 200
  in hypopituitarism, 210
  osteoarthritis and, 288
  polycystic ovarian disease *vs.*, 322
Acupuncture
  for postherpetic neuralgia, 277
Acyclovir
  for chickenpox, 187
  for eczema, 123
  for encephalitis, 127
  for erythema multiforme, 133
  for herpes simplex infection, 185
  for herpes zoster infection, 187
  for shingles, 187
Adams-Stokes attack, 168
Addison's disease, 10–11
  inappropriate antidiuresis syndrome *vs.*, 376
  primary biliary cirrhosis and, 80
Adenosine
  for supraventricular tachycardia, 383
  for Wolff-Parkinson-White syndrome, 425
Adhesions
  colorectal cancer *vs.*, 82
Adrenal cancer
  in Cushing's syndrome, 90–91
Adrenal hyperplasia
  in testicular disorders, 386–387
Adrenal insufficiency
  acromegaly and, 6
  in Addison's disease, 10
Adrenaline
  for cardiopulmonary resuscitation, 69
Adrenocorticotropic hormone (ACTH)
  in Addison's disease, 10
  in Cushing's syndrome, 90
  hypokalemia and, 194
  in hypopituitarism, 210
Advanced life support, 69
Agoraphobia
  in panic and anxiety disorder, 298
Airway
  in basic life support, 68
Albendazole
  for diarrhea and HIV infection, 113
  for infectious diarrhea, 217
Albumin gradient
  serum-ascites, 46–47
Albuterol
  for asthma, 49
  for chronic obstructive pulmonary
      disease, 79

Index

Alcohol dependence
acute pancreatitis in, 294
in attempted suicide, 55
in bulimia nervosa, 60
chronic pancreatitis and, 296
coma and, 84
definition of, 18
dementia *vs.*, 94
dyslipoproteinemia and, 120
hepatic encephalopathy *vs.*, 176
megaloblastic anemia *vs.*, 24
in panic and anxiety disorder, 298
in personality disorder, 306
Alcohol intake
gout and, 156–157
Alcohol withdrawal, 18–19
hepatic encephalopathy *vs.*, 176
hyperthyroidism *vs.*, 202
variceal bleeding and, 414
"Allergic shiners"
eczema and, 122
Allopurinol
for gout, 157
for non-Hodgkin's lymphoma, 283
All-*trans*-retinoic acid
for acute myeloid leukemia, 233
Alopecia, 20f, 20–21
in acute lymphoblastic leukemia
in children, 230
in Cushing's syndrome, 90
in female hypogonadotropic hypogonadism, 140
fungal nail infection *vs.*, 144
in systemic lupus erythematosus, 378
Alpha-1 antitrypsin deficiency
chronic obstructive pulmonary disease and, 78
Alpha blockers
for hypertension, 201
Alprazolam
for panic and anxiety disorder, 299
Alveolitis
fibrosing
rheumatoid arthritis and, 42
Alzheimer's disease
dementia in, 94–95
Amaurosis fugax
in cranial arteritis, 86
in transient ischemic attacks, 398
Amebiasis. *See also Entamoeba histolytica*
Crohn's disease *vs.*, 88
Amenorrhea. *See also* Puberty
in female hypogonadotropic hypogonadism, 140
in hypopituitarism, 210
ovarian failure and, 290
Amikacin
for infection, 215, 267
Aminocaproic acid
for coagulation disorders, 173
for platelet disorders, 313
Aminoglutethimide
for Cushing's syndrome, 91
Aminoglycoside
for pneumonia, 319
Amiodarone
for cardiac failure and dilated cardiomyopathy, 67
for cardiopulmonary resuscitation, 69
for hypertrophic cardiomyopathy, 205
interstitial lung diseases and, 218
for ventricular tachycardia, 385
Amitriptyline
for chronic fatigue syndrome, 77
for migraine, 253
for postherpetic neuralgia, 277
Amlodipine
for angina pectoris, 29, 31
Amoxicillin
for duodenal ulcer, 119
for gram-negative septicemia, 159
for infectious diarrhea, 217
for leptospirosis, 227
for Lyme disease, 243
for pneumonia, 319
for sickle cell disease, 363
for typhoid fever, 407
for urinary tract infection, 411
Amphotericin
for cryptococcal meningitis in AIDS, 251
for endocarditis, 129
for infection in hematological malignancy, 215
for invasive fungal infections, 143
for pulmonary complications, 337
Ampicillin
for endocarditis, 129
for leptospirosis, 227
for primary sclerosing cholangitis, 75
Amyloidosis
with dialysis, 110
glomerulonephritis *vs.*, 154
in multiple myeloma, 260
psoriatic arthritis and, 40
restrictive cardiomyopathy and, 350
rheumatoid arthritis and, 42
in Waldenström's macroglobulinemia, 422
Amyotrophic lateral sclerosis, 258
Anacastic personality disorder, 306
Anaphylactic shock
in urticaria, 412
Anemia
in acute hepatitis, 178
acute lymphoblastic leukemia and, 228, 230
in acute myeloid leukemia, 232
aplastic, 22f, 22–23
in bacterial overgrowth of small intestine, 56
in cardiac failure and dilated cardiomyopathy, 66
in celiac disease, 70
in chronic lymphocytic leukemia, 234
in chronic pancreatitis, 296
in chronic renal failure, 344
in colorectal cancer, 82
in diverticular disease of colon, 116
with duodenal ulcer, 118
in esophageal carcinoma, 136
hemolytic
chickenpox and, 186
in hypothyroidism, 212
in infectious diarrhea, 216
iron-deficiency
in platelet disorders, 312
in malaria, 244
megaloblastic, 24f, 24–25
microangiopathic hemolytic
hemolytic uremic syndrome and, 170–171
in multiple myeloma, 260
in parvovirus B19 infection, 302
pernicious, 26–27
Pneumocystis carinii in AIDS *vs.*, 316
in thalassemia, 388
in variceal bleeding, 414
Angina
in aortic regurgitation, 36
in aortic stenosis, 38
with dyslipoproteinemia, 120
Eisenmenger's complex and, 124
in hypothyroidism, 212
pheochomocytoma *vs.*, 310
stable, 28–29
unstable, 30–31
pericarditis *vs.*, 304
Angioedema of lips
in urticaria, 412
Angioplasty
for angina pectoris, 29, 31
for myocardial infarction, 271
Angiotensin-converting enzyme inhibitors
acute renal failure and, 342
for cardiac failure and dilated cardiomyopathy, 67
for chronic renal failure, 345
for hypertension, 201

for mitral regurgitation, 255
for systemic sclerosis, 381
Angular cheilitis
with *Candida* infection, 64, 142
Ankylosing spondylitis, 32–33
aortic regurgitation and, 36
with psoriasis, 40, 332
Ann Arbor Scheme
for staging Hodgkin's disease, 188
Anorexia. *See also* Anorexia nervosa
in acute lymphoblastic leukemia
in children, 230
with acute pancreatitis, 294
in chronic hepatitis, 180
in chronic renal failure, 344
in Crohn's disease, 88
diabetes mellitus *vs.,* 100
in endocarditis, 128
with gastric ulcer, 150
in hepatocellular carcinoma, 182
in hyponatremia, 196
Kaposi's sarcoma in AIDS and, 224
in malaria, 244
in *Mycobacterium* infection in AIDS, 266
in pancreatic cancer, 292
in sarcoidosis, 356
in typhoid fever, 406
Anorexia nervosa
aplastic anemia *vs.,* 22
bulimia nervosa *vs.,* 60
hypopituitarism *vs.,* 210
Anosmia
in female hypogonadotropic hypogonadism, 140
Antacids
for duodenal ulcer, 119
for esophagitis, 139
for gastric ulcer, 151
Anthracycline
for acute myeloid leukemia, 233
Antidiuretic hormone
syndrome of inappropriate secretion of, 376–377
bacterial meningitis and, 348
hyponatremia and, 196
in lung cancer, 240
Antilymphocyte globulin (ALG)
for aplastic anemia, 23
Antithymocyte globulin (ATG)
for aplastic anemia, 23
Antitoxin
for diphtheria, 309
Anxiety
chronic
major depression *vs.,* 96
chronic fatigue syndrome and, 76
in Cushing's syndrome, 90
dementia *vs.,* 94
generalized disorder, 298f, 298–299
in Guillain-Barré syndrome, 166
with hypoglycemia, 208
in Parkinson's disease, 300
in pheochromocytoma, 310
Aortic dissection, 34–35
aortic regurgitation and, 36
endocarditis *vs.,* 128
gastric ulcer *vs.,* 150
myocardial infarction *vs.,* 270
Aortic graft
in aortic dissection, 35
Aortic regurgitation, 36–37
in aortic dissection, 34
in rheumatic fever, 352
Aortic root dilatation
aortic regurgitation and, 36
Aortic rupture
with aortic dissection, 34
cranial arteritis *vs.,* 86
Aortic sclerosis
aortic stenosis *vs.,* 38
Aortic stenosis, 38–39
heart block and, 168
Aortic valve
in endocarditis, 128–129
hypertrophic cardiomyopathy and, 204
replacement of
for aortic regurgitation, 37
for aortic stenosis, 39
surgical repair of
in aortic dissection, 35
Aplasia cutis congenita
alopecia and, 20
Aplastic crisis
in parvovirus B19 infection, 302
Appendicitis
acute pancreatitis *vs.,* 294
diverticular disease *vs.,* 116
in infectious diarrhea, 216
Arachnodactyly
growth abnormalities and, 164
Arginine vasopressin
for diabetes insipidus, 98f, 98–99
for platelet disorders, 313
Arrhythmias
angina pectoris and, 28, 31
aortic regurgitation and, 36
in aortic stenosis, 38
in atrial septal defect, 52
in cardiac failure and dilated cardiomyopathy, 66
in constrictive pericarditis, 350
Eisenmenger's complex and, 124
epilepsy and, 130
in Guillain-Barré syndrome, 166
with hypokalemia, 194
in myocardial infarction, 270
with polymyositis, 326
sarcoidosis and, 356
in stroke, 374
Arsenic
lung cancer and, 240
Arsenical keratosis
viral warts *vs.,* 420
Arteriovenous malformation
colorectal cancer *vs.,* 82
Arteritis. *See also* Vasculitis
cranial, 86–87
giant cell, 324–325
systemic vasculitis and, 418
Takayasu's
renal artery stenosis and, 340
systemic vasculitis and, 418
temporal, 86
dementia in, 94
migraine *vs.,* 252
multiple myeloma *vs.,* 260
Arthralgia. *See also* Arthritis
in endocarditis, 128
in granulomatous lung disease, 160
in Henoch-Schönlein purpura, 174
in leptospirosis, 226
in Lyme disease, 242
in polymyositis, 326
primary biliary cirrhosis and, 80
rheumatic fever and, 352
in Stevens-Johnson syndrome, 132
with systemic lupus erythematosus, 378
in systemic sclerosis, 380
in tubulointerstitial nephropathy, 274
in urticaria, 412
Arthritis
in bacterial meningitis, 248
in bronchiectasis and cystic fibrosis, 58
in Crohn's disease, 88
with hemophilia, 172
in infectious diarrhea, 216
in Lyme disease, 242
in parvovirus B19 infection, 302
psoriatic, 40–41, 332
rheumatic fever and, 352
rheumatoid, 42–43
cutaneous vasculitis lesions in, 416
erythema nodosum *vs.,* 134
gout *vs.,* 156

Arthritis, rheumatoid *(continued)*
heart block and, 168
Lyme disease *vs.*, 242
pericarditis and, 304
pleural effusion *vs.*, 314
polymyalgia rheumatica *vs.*, 324
polymyositis *vs.*, 326
Stevens-Johnson syndrome and, 132
systemic vasculitis and, 418
in rubella, 354
septic, 44–45
acute crystal synovitis *vs.*, 8
gout *vs.*, 156
osteoarthritis and, 288
rheumatoid arthritis and, 42
systemic vasculitis and, 418
Arthropathy. *See also* Arthralgia; Arthritis
acromegaly and, 6
acute crystal syhovitis and, 8f, 8–9
ankylosing spondylitis and, 32
in chronic fatigue syndrome, 76
gout and, 156f, 156–157
in osteoarthritis, 288
in peripheral neuropathy, 280
Arthroplasty
for osteoarthritis, 289
Asbestos
lung cancer and, 240
Ascaris infection
bacterial overgrowth of small intestine *vs.*, 56
Ascites, 46–47
in chronic hepatitis, 180
in chronic pancreatitis, 296
with fulminant liver failure, 238
with gastric cancer, 148
with hepatocellular carcinoma, 182
in pancreatic cancer, 292
in primary biliary cirrhosis, 80
in primary sclerosing cholangitis, 74
in restrictive cardiomyopathy, 350
variceal bleeding and, 414
Asherman's syndrome
female hypogonadotropic hypogonadism *vs.*, 140
Asparaginase
in acute lymphoblastic leukemia, 229, 231
Aspergillus infection
in acquired immunodeficiency syndrome, 14
bronchiectasis and, 58
endocarditis and, 128–129
granulomatous lung disease *vs.*, 160
in hematological malignancy, 214
with immunosuppression, 336
invasive infection by, 142–143
Pneumocyctis carinii pneumonia *vs.*, 316
Aspirin
for angina pectoris, 29, 31
for chronic fatigue syndrome, 77
duodenal ulcer and, 118
for pericarditis, 305
for prothrombotic states, 331
for rheumatic fever, 352
for rheumatoid arthritis, 42
for stroke, 375
for transient ischemic attacks, 398
Astemizole
for urticaria, 413
Asterixis
in acute hepatitis, 178
in hepatic encephalopathy, 176
Asthma, 48–49
bronchiectasis *vs.*, 58
chronic obstructive pulmonary disease *vs.*, 78
in esophagitis, 138
in granulomatous lung disease, 160
occupational, 50–51
Pneumocystis carinii in AIDS *vs.*, 316
Astrocytoma, 72
Ataxia. *See also* Ataxia telangiectasia
in encephalitis, 126
in Guillain-Barré syndrome, 166
in peripheral neuropathy, 280
in toxoplasmosis in AIDS, 394
in Waldenström's macroglobulinemia, 422
Ataxia telangiectasia
acute lymphoblastic leukemia in children and, 230
pancreatic cancer and, 292
Atenolol
for hypertrophic cardiomyopathy, 205
for myocardial infarction, 271
for supraventricular tachycardia, 383
Atherosclerosis
aortic dissection and, 34
in cardiac failure and dilated cardiomyopathy, 66
chronic renal failure and, 344
with dyslipoproteinemia, 120
renal artery stenosis and, 340, 340f
transient ischemic attacks and, 398
unstable angina and, 30–31
Atopic triad, 122
Atrial septal defect, 52f, 52–53
Atrioventricular block, 168–169
with acute hypotensive shock, 361
in Lyme disease, 242
in rheumatic fever, 352
Atriventricular node
Wolff-Parkinson-White syndrome and, 424
Atropine
for cardiopulmonary resuscitation, 69
for heart block, 169
Attempted suicide, 54–55
Aura in migraine, 252
Austin Flint murmur
in aortic regurgitation, 36
Autoimmune disorders
acute lymphoblastic leukemia in children *vs.*, 230
acute viral hepatitis *vs.*, 178
adrenalitis
Addison's disease and, 10
ankylosing spondylitis and, 32
chronic hepatitis and, 180–181
in chronic lymphocytic leukemia, 234
cranial arteritis and, 86
diabetes mellitus and, 100
fulminant liver failure and, 238
in hepatocellular carcinoma, 182
hypothyroidism and, 212
non-Hodgkin's lymphoma and, 282
ovarian failure and, 290
pericarditis and, 304
platelet disorders and, 312
ulcerative colitis and, 408
Avascular necrosis
osteoarthritis and, 288
in sickle cell disease, 362
Avoidant personality disorder, 306
Azathioprine
for bullous disorders, 63
for chronic hepatitis, 181
for cranial arteritis, 87
for Crohn's disease, 89
for inflammatory myositis, 273
for myasthenia gravis, 265
for polymyositis, 327
for psoriatic arthritis, 41
for systemic vasculitis, 419
Azidothymidine
for acquired immunodeficiency syndrome, 15
Azithromycin
for diarrhea and HIV infection, 113
for Lyme disease, 243
AZT
for acquired immunodeficiency syndrome, 15

B

Babinski response
in motor neuron disease, 258
Bacillary angiomatosis
Kaposi's sarcoma *vs.*, 224
vasculitis *vs.*, 416

Baclofen
for multiple sclerosis, 263
for trigeminal neuralgia, 279
Bacterial overgrowth of small intestine, 56–57
celiac disease *vs.,* 70
Bacteroides
bacterial overgrowth of small intestine and, 56
Balanitis
in diabetes mellitus, 102
Balloon tamponade
for bleeding varices, 153
Balloon valvuloplasty
for aortic stenosis, 39
Barbiturate withdrawal
alcohol withdrawal syndrome *vs.,* 18
Barrett's esophagus
esophageal carcinoma and, 136
in esophagitis, 138
Bartter's syndrome
hypokalemia and, 194
Basic life support, 68, 68f
Beclomethasone
for asthma, 49, 51
for chronic obstructive pulmonary disease, 79
for obstructive sleep apnea, 369
Behavior disorders
growth abnormalities and, 164
Behavior therapy
for obsessive-compulsive disorder, 287
for panic and anxiety disorder, 299
for personality disorder, 307
Behçets syndrome
herpes simplex infection *vs.,* 184
Bell's palsy
in Lyme disease, 242
Benoxaprofen
primary biliary cirrhosis and, 80
Benzamycin
for acne, 5
Benzodiazepines
alcohol withdrawal syndrome and, 18, 19
for attempted suicide, 55
for chronic fatigue syndrome, 77
for insomnia, 371
for mania, 97
for panic and anxiety disorder, 299
for personality disorder, 307
Benzoyl peroxide
for acne, 5
Benztropine
for schizophrenia, 359
Bernard-Soulier disease
platelet disorders and, 312
Beta agonists
for asthma, 49
for cardiac failure and dilated cardiomyopathy, 67
for chronic obstructive pulmonary disease, 79
Beta blockers
for angina pectoris, 29, 31
for cardiac failure and dilated cardiomyopathy, 67
for hypertension, 201
for hyperthyroidism, 203
for hypertrophic cardiomyopathy, 205
for intracerebral hemorrhage, 221
Betamethasone
for eczema, 123
Biguanide
for diabetes mellitus, 103
Bile duct
duodenal ulcer and, 118
gallstone disease and, 146
primary sclerosing cholangitis and, 74, 74f
Biliary colic
with gallstones, 146
Binswanger's disease
dementia in, 94
"Bird-beak" esophagus
achalasia and, 2
Bismuth subsalicylate
for duodenal ulcer, 119
for infectious diarrhea, 217
Bites
insect
bullous disorders *vs.,* 62
Bladder obstruction
dialysis and, 110
"Blast" transformation
in myeloproliferative disorders, 268
Bleeding. *See also* Hemorrhage; Variceal bleeding
in acute lymphoblastic leukemia, 228, 230
in acute myeloid leukemia, 232
in acute renal failure, 342
in chronic lymphocytic leukemia, 234
in colorectal cancer, 82
with dialysis, 110
in disseminated intravascular coagulation, 114f, 114–115
in esophagitis, 138
gastrointestinal, 152f, 152–153
bulimia nervosa and, 60
in diverticular disease of colon, 116
in pancreatic cancer, 292
in hairy cell leukemia, 236
in myeloproliferative disorders, 268
in non-Hodgkin's lymphoma, 282
in platelet disorders, 312
in systemic lupus erythematosus, 378
with von Willebrand's disease, 172
in Waldenström's macroglobulinemia, 422
Bleomycin
for Hodgkin's disease, 189
interstitial lung diseases and, 218
for Kaposi's sarcoma in AIDS, 225
for pleural effusion, 314
Blind loop syndrome, 56
in megaloblastic anemia, 24
pernicious anemia *vs.,* 26
Blindness. *See also* Vision or eye disorders
cerebral tumor and, 72
in cranial arteritis, 86
with hypertension, 200
in Stevens-Johnson syndrome, 132
Blisters
bullous disorders and, 62, 62f
Bloom's syndrome
acute lymphoblastic leukemia in children and, 230
Boils, 364–365
Bone disorders. *See also* Arthritis; Arthropathy
in acute lymphoblastic leukemia, 228, 230
in congenital rubella, 354
in multiple myeloma, 260, 260f
in sarcoidosis, 356
Bone marrow
in aplastic anemia, 22f, 22–23
in myeloproliferative disorders, 269
in non-Hodgkin's lymphoma, 282
platelet disorders and, 313
transplantation
for multiple myeloma, 261
transplantation of
for acute myeloid leukemia, 233
for non-Hodgkin's lymphoma, 283
for thalassemia, 389
"Boozer's elbow"
gout and, 156
Borborygmi
with infectious diarrhea, 216
Borderline personality disorder, 306–307
Borrelia burgdorferi
Lyme disease and, 242–243
Botulism
Guillain-Barré syndrome *vs.,* 166
Bouchard's nodes
in osteoarthritis, 288
Bowen's disease
viral warts and, 420

Index

Bradykinesia
in Parkinson's disease, 300
Breathing. *See* Dyspnea; Respiration
Bretylium tosylate
for cardiopulmonary resuscitation, 69
Broadbent's sign
in constrictive pericarditis, 350
Bromocriptine
for acromegaly, 7
for pituitary macroadenoma, 198f, 199
Bronchiectasis, 58–59
Brown-Sequard's syndrome
in spinal cord compression, 372
Brucella
endocarditis and, 128
Brudzinski's sign
in bacterial meningitis, 248
Bruxism
with parasomnias, 370
Budd-Chiari syndrome
ascites *vs.*, 46
fulminant liver failure and, 238
variceal bleeding *vs.*, 414
Bulimia nervosa, 60f, 60–61
Bullous disorders, 62f, 62–63
Stevens-Johnson syndrome and, 132, 132f
Bullous pemphigoid, 62f, 62–63
Bumetanide
for acute tubular necrosis, 343
for hyperkalemia, 195
for renal tubular acidosis, 348
Bundle branch block
sarcoidosis and, 356
Burkitt's lymphoma
non-Hodgkin's lymphoma and, 283
Burns
adult respiratory distress syndrome and, 12
hyponatremia and, 196
Bursitis
gout and, 156
rheumatoid arthritis and, 42
Buspirone
for panic and anxiety disorder, 299
Busulfan
for myeloproliferative disorders, 269
Butterfly rash
in systemic lupus erythematosus, 378, 378f

C

Cachexia
in pancreatic cancer, 292
Calciferol
for hypocalcemia, 207
Calcipotriene
for psoriasis, 332
Calcitonin
for hypercalcemia, 191
Calcitriol
for hypocalcemia, 207
Calcium antagonists
for angina pectoris, 29, 31
for hypertension, 201
for hypertrophic cardiomyopathy, 205
Calcium channel blockers
heart block and, 168
Calcium chloride
for cardiopulmonary resuscitation, 69
Calcium gluconate
for hyperkalemia, 195
for hypocalcemia, 207
Calcium pyrophosphate dihydrate crystals
acute crystal synovitis and, 8
Campylobacter infection
bacterial overgrowth of small intestine *vs.*, 56
Crohn's disease *vs.*, 88
with diarrhea and HIV infection, 112
Campylobacter jejuni
in Guillain-Barré syndrome, 166
Cancer. *See also* Carcinoma; Lymphoma(s); Neoplasm(s); specific kinds
of colon
ulcerative colitis and, 408
colorectal, 82–83
gastric, 148–149
gastrointestinal bleeding and, 152
lung, 240–241
obesity and, 284
pancreatic, 292–293, 293f
Candida infection
in AIDS, 14
buccal and esophageal, 64f–65f, 64–65, 266
endocarditis and, 128–129
in hematological malignancy, 214–215
invasive infection by, 142–143
in nail infections, 144
Capsaicin
for osteoarthritis, 289
for postherpetic neuralgia, 277, 281
Capsulotomy
for obsessive-compulsive disorder, 287
Captopril
for aortic regurgitation, 37
for cardiac failure and dilated cardiomyopathy, 67
for myocardial infarction, 271
for systemic sclerosis, 381
Caput medusae
chronic hapatitis and, 180
Carbamazepine
for epilepsy, 131
with cerebral tumor, 73
for major depression, 97
for personality disorder, 307
for trigeminal neuralgia, 279
Carbuncle, 364
Carcinoid
gastric
pernicious anemia and, 26
Carcinoma. *See also* Cancer; Neoplasm(s); specific kinds
basal cell
acne treatment and, 4
cervical
in acquired immunodeficiency syndrome, 14
colonic
Crohn's disease *vs.*, 88
diverticular disease of colon *vs.*, 116
endocarditis and, 128
duodenal ulcer *vs.*, 118
esophageal, 136–137
achalasia and, 2
gastric
in megaloblastic anemia, 24
pernicious anemia and, 26
hepatocellular, 182f, 182–183
in chronic hepatitis, 180
in primary biliary cirrhosis, 80
pulmonary
bronchiectasis *vs.*, 58
in chronic obstructive pulmonary disease, 78
thyroid, 390f, 390–391
acne treatment and, 4
viral warts and, 420
Cardia
myotomy of
for achalasia, 3
Cardiac arrest
in hyperglycemia, 192
with hyperkalemia, 194
in ventricular tachycardia, 384
Cardiac failure. *See* Heart failure
Cardiac tamponade, 304f, 304–305
in aortic dissection, 34
pulmonary embolism *vs.*, 338
Cardiomyopathy
dilated, 66–67
hypertrophic, 204f, 204–205
in pheochromocytoma, 310
restrictive, 350–351

tamponade *vs.,* 304
in thalassemia, 388
Cardiopulmonary resuscitation
advanced life support, 69
basic life support, 68, 68f
Carotid artery
in cranial arteritis, 86
in dyslipoproteinemia, 120
in life support monitoring, 68
in stroke, 375
Carpal tunnel syndrome
in acromegaly, 6
in hypothyroidism, 212
Cauda equina
ankylosing spondylitis and, 32
compression of, 372–373
CD4 lymphocytes
in acquired immunodeficiency syndrome, 14, 16f, 16–17
Cefotaxime
for gram-negative septicemia, 159
for septic arthritis, 45
for urinary tract infection, 411
Cefotetan
for diverticulitis, 117
Ceftazidine
for gram-negative septicemia, 159
in hematological malignancy, 215
for urinary tract infection, 411
Ceftriaxone
for bacterial meningitis, 249
for gram-negative septicemia, 159
for Lyme disease, 243
for typhoid fever, 407
Cefuroxime
for pneumonia, 319
for urinary tract infection, 411
Celiac disease, 70–71
bacterial overgrowth of small intestine *vs.,* 56
cystic fibrosis *vs.,* 58
infectious diarrhea *vs.,* 216
primary biliary cirrhosis and, 80
Cellulitis, 364–365
bullous disorders *vs.,* 62
Cephalexin
for urinary tract infection, 411
Cephalosporin
for primary sclerosing cholangitis, 75
Cerebral abscess
in Eisenmenger's complex, 124
Cerebral edema. *See* Edema, cerebral
Cerebral thrombosis
in hypernatremia, 196
Cerebral tumor, 72–73
migraine *vs.,* 252
Cerebrovascular accident. *See* Stroke
Charcot's arthropathy
osteoarthritis *vs.,* 288
Chenodeoxycholic acid
for gallstone disease, 147
Chest
barrel-shaped
in chronic obstructive pulmonary disease, 78
Chest pain
in acute hypotensive shock, 360
with angina pectoris, 28–29, 30
in aortic dissection, 34
in bronchiectasis and cystic fibrosis, 58
in granulomatous lung disease, 160
with hypertrophic cardiomyopathy, 204
immunosuppression and, 336
in lung cancer, 240
in Lyme disease, 242
in myocardial infarction, 270
in panic disorder, 298
in pericarditis, 304
in pheochromocytoma, 310
pleural effusion and, 314
in pneumonia, 318
with pulmonary embolism, 338
retrosternal
achalasia and, 2
rheumatic fever and, 352
in Stevens-Johnson syndrome, 132
in supraventricular tachycardia, 382
in tamponade, 304
in Wolff-Parkinson-White syndrome, 424
Chest-wall disease
in central sleep apnea, 366–367, 367f
Cheyne-Stokes respiration
in central sleep apnea, 366–367, 367f
in hyponatremia, 196
Chickenpox, 186–187
Chlamydia psittaci
endocarditis and, 128
Chlorambucil
for chronic lymphocytic leukemia, 235
for glomerulonephritis, 155
for Hodgkin's disease, 189
for non-Hodgkin's lymphoma, 283
in Waldenström's macroglobulinemia, 423
Chloramphenicol
for infectious diarrhea, 217
for typhoid fever, 407
Chlordiazepoxide
for alcohol withdrawal syndrome, 19
2-Chlorodeoxyadenosine, 237
for chronic lymphocytic leukemia, 235
Chloroquine
for malaria, 245
for sarcoidosis, 357
Chlorpheniramine
for erythema multiforme, 133
Chlorpromazine
primary biliary cirrhosis and, 80
Chlorpropamide
for diabetes mellitus, 109
Cholangiocarcinoma
primary sclerosing cholangitis and, 74
Cholangitis
acute, 146
in acute pancreatitis, 294
in pancreatic cancer, 292
AIDS-related sclerosing, 112
primary sclerosing, 74f, 74–75
acute pancreatitis and, 294
chronic hepatitis *vs.,* 180
primary biliary cirrhosis *vs.,* 80
Cholecystectomy
for gallstone disease, 147
Cholecystitis
acute, 146
sickle cell disease and, 362
Cholelithiasis. *See* Gallstone disease
Cholestyramine
for primary biliary cirrhosis, 81
for primary sclerosing cholangitis, 75
Cholinergic crisis, 264
Chondrocalcinosis
polyarticular. *See also* Pseudogout
acute crystal synovitis and, 8
CHOP chemotherapy
for chronic lymphocytic leukemia, 235
for non-Hodgkin's lymphoma, 283
Chorea
tremor *vs.,* 400
Chronic fatigue syndrome, 76f, 76–77
myasthenia gravis *vs.,* 264
Chronic lymphocytic leukemia, 234f, 234–235
Chronic obstructive pulmonary disease (COPD), 78–79
sleep apnea *vs.,* 368
Churg-Strauss syndrome, 160–161
systemic vasculitis and, 418
Chvostek's sign
with hypocalcemia, 206
Cicatricial alopecia, 20
Cimetidine
for duodenal ulcer, 119
for gastric ulcer, 151
Ciprofloxacin
for bacterial meningitis, 249

Index

Ciprofloxacin *(continued)*
for bacterial overgrowth of small intestine, 57
for diverticulitis, 117
for gram-negative septicemia, 159
for infectious diarrhea, 217
for *Mycobacterium* infection in AIDS, 267
for primary sclerosing cholangitis, 75
for *Staphylococcus* infection, 365
for typhoid fever, 407
for urinary tract infection, 411
Circadian sleep disorders, 370
Cirrhosis
alcoholic
acute viral hepatitis *vs.,* 178
ascites *vs.,* 46
biliary
in cystic fibrosis, 58
primary, 80–81, 81f
primary sclerosing cholangitis *vs.,* 74
in chronic hepatitis, 180
glomerulonephritis *vs.,* 154
hepatic encephalopathy and, 176–177
with hepatocellular carcinoma, 182
inappropriate antidiuresis syndrome *vs.,* 376
Cisapride
for esophagitis, 139
for gastric cancer, 149
for systemic sclerosis, 381
Cisplatin
for hepatocellular carcinoma, 183
Clarithromycin
for duodenal ulcer, 119
for Lyme disease, 243
for *Mycobacterium* infection in AIDS, 267
Claudication
in cranial arteritis, 86
with dyslipoproteinemia, 120
Clavulanate
for gram-negative septicemia, 159
Clindamycin
for acne, 5
for pneumonia, 319
Clobetasol
for alopecia, 21
for eczema, 123
Clomiphene
for polycystic ovarian disease, 323
Clomipramine
for narcolepsy, 371
for obsessive-compulsive disorder, 287
Clonazapam
for epilepsy, 131
Clostridium
bacterial overgrowth of small intestine and, 56
erysipelas and, 364
in infectious diarrhea, 217
CLOtest
for *Helicobacter pylori,* 118f, 118–119
Clotrimazole
for buccal and esophageal candidiasis, 65
Clozapine
for schizophrenia, 359
Clubbing
in bronchiectasis and cystic fibrosis, 58
in Eisenmenger's complex, 124
in endocarditis, 128
in interstitial lung diseases, 218
in lung cancer, 240
Coagulation factors
for acute myeloid leukemia, 233
in disseminated intravascular coagulation, 114–115
in hemophilia and von Willebrand's disease, 172–173
prothrombotic states and, 330–331
Coal tar
for psoriasis, 332
for psoriatic arthritis, 41
Co-amoxiclav
for urinary tract infection, 411
Coarctation of aorta
with aortic stenosis, 38
Cognitive therapy
for obsessive-compulsive disorder, 287
for panic and anxiety disorder, 299
for personality disorder, 307
Colchicine
for acute crystal synovitis, 9
for gout, 157
Cold agglutination syndrome
in Waldenström's macroglobulinemia, 422
Colestipol
for primary biliary cirrhosis, 81
Colitis. *See* Crohn's disease; Inflammatory bowel disease; Irritable bowel syndrome; Ulcerative colitis
"Collapsing pulse"
in aortic regurgitation, 36
Colon
diverticular disease of. *See* Diverticular disease of the colon
Colorectal cancer, 82–83
Coma, 84f, 84–85
in acute renal failure, 342
in chronic renal failure, 344
in cryptococcal meningitis in AIDS, 250
in cytomegalovirus infection in AIDS, 92
in diabetes mellitus, 100, 102, 104
in encephalitis, 126
hemolytic uremic syndrome and, 170
in hepatic encephalopathy, 176
in herpes simplex infection, 184
in hypernatremia, 196
in hyponatremia, 196
in hypothyroidism, 212
with inappropriate antidiuresis syndrome, 376
in intracerebral hemorrhage, 220
in malaria, 244
in Stevens-Johnson syndrome, 132
in toxic shock syndrome, 392
Complete heart block, 168f, 168–169
Condyloma acuminatum, 420–421
Conn's syndrome
hypertension and, 200
Consciousness. *See also* Coma
anatomy of, 84f
Convulsions. *See* Epilepsy; Seizures
Cor pulmonale
in bronchiectasis and cystic fibrosis, 58
central sleep apnea and, 366
in interstitial lung diseases, 218
Corigan's sign
in aortic regurgitation, 36
Coronary artery bypass surgery
for angina pectoris, 29, 31
Corticosteroids. *See also* specific agents
for asthma, 49, 51
for Henoch-Schönlein purpura, 175
for osteoarthritis, 289
Corynebacterium diphtheriae
pharyngitis and, 308
Cotrimoxazole
for *Pneumocystis carinii* in AIDS, 317
for typhoid fever, 407
for urinary tract infection, 411
Cough
achalasia and, 2
with asthma, 48
in atrial septal defect, 52
in bronchiectasis and cystic fibrosis, 58–59
in chronic obstructive pulmonary disease, 78
in cranial arteritis, 86
in cryptococcosis, 142
in cytomegalovirus infection in AIDS, 92
in esophagitis, 138
in extrapulmonary tuberculosis, 402
with gram-negative septicemia, 158
in granulomatous lung disease, 160
in Guillain-Barré syndrome, 166

immunosuppression and, 336
in interstitial lung diseases, 218
in lung cancer, 240
in malaria, 244
in measles, 246
in pharyngitis, 308
in *Pneumocystis carinii* in AIDS, 316
in pneumonia, 318
in polymyositis, 326
in pulmonary tuberculosis, 404
in sarcoidosis, 356
in Stevens-Johnson syndrome, 132
in systemic sclerosis, 380
in tamponade, 304
in typhoid fever, 406
Coumadin
for stroke, 375
Courvoisier's sign
in pancreatic cancer, 292
Coxiella burnetti
endocarditis and, 128
Coxsackie A virus
pharyngitis and, 308
Cranial arteritis, 86–87
Craniopharyngioma
diabetes insipidus and, 98
female hypogonadotropic hypogonadism and, 140
CREST syndrome, 380
primary biliary cirrhosis and, 80
Crohn's disease, 88–89. *See also* Inflammatory bowel disease
acute pancreatitis *vs.,* 294
bacterial overgrowth of small intestine and, 56
duodenal ulcer *vs.,* 118
irritable bowel syndrome *vs.,* 222
in megaloblastic anemia, 24
pernicious anemia *vs.,* 26
pubertal abnormalities and, 334
sarcoidosis *vs.,* 356
tuberculosis *vs.,* 402
ulcerative colitis *vs.,* 408
Cryoglulinemia
cutaneous vasculitis and, 416
Cryoprecipitate
for disseminated intravascular coagulation, 115
Cryotherapy
for viral warts, 421
Cryptococcosis
in AIDS, 14, 250
invasive infection by, 142–143
Cryptosporidia infection
in AIDS, 14, 92, 112–113
Cullen's sign
in acute pancreatitis, 294
Cushing's disease or syndrome, 90–91
diabetes mellitus in, 102
with hypertension, 200
hypokalemia and, 194
in lung cancer, 240
obesity *vs.,* 284
polycystic ovarian disease *vs.,* 322
Cyanosis
in acute hypotensive shock, 360
adult respiratory distress syndrome and, 12
with asthma, 48
in central sleep apnea, 366
in chronic obstructive pulmonary disease, 78
immunosuppression and, 336
in interstitial lung diseases, 218
in pneumonia, 318
in tamponade, 304
Cyclophosphamide
for bullous disorders, 63
for chronic lymphocytic leukemia, 235
for cranial arteritis, 87
for glomerulonephritis, 155, 343
for granulomatous lung disease, 161
for interstitial lung disease, 219
for multiple myeloma, 261
for polymyositis, 327
for systemic lupus erythematosus, 379
for systemic vasculitis, 419
Cyclospora
with diarrhea and HIV infection, 112–113
Cyclosporin
for aplastic anemia, 23
for glomerulonephritis, 155
hypertension and, 200
for polymyositis, 327
for psoriasis, 332
for psoriatic arthritis, 41
for systemic sclerosis, 381
Cyclothymia
mania *vs.,* 96
Cypionate
for hypopituitarism, 211
Cyproheptadine
for urticaria, 413
Cyproterone
for pubertal abnormalities, 335
Cystic fibrosis, 58–59
celiac disease *vs.,* 70
chronic pancreatitis and, 296
sarcoidosis *vs.,* 356
Cystitis
with urinary tract infection, 410
Cytarabine
for acute lymphoblastic leukemia, 229, 231
Cytomegalovirus infection
acute viral hepatitis and, 178
in AIDS, 14, 92f, 92–93
buccal and esophageal candidiasis *vs.,* 64
duodenal ulcer *vs.,* 118
Guillain-Barré syndrome and, 166
Lyme disease *vs.,* 242
parvovirus B19 infection *vs.,* 302
Pneumocystis carinii in AIDS *vs.,* 316
rubella *vs.,* 354
toxoplasmosis *vs.,* 394
ulcerative colitis *vs.,* 408
Cytosine arabinoside
for acute myeloid leukemia, 233

D

Da Costa's syndrome
angina pectoris *vs.,* 28
Dacarbazine
for Hodgkin's disease, 189
Dactylitis
psoriatic arthritis and, 40
Danazol
for testicular disorders, 387
Dapsone
for bullous disorders, 63
for cutaneous vasculitis, 416
Daunorubicin
in acute lymphoblastic leukemia, 229, 231
for Kaposi's sarcoma in AIDS, 225
DDAVP
for coagulation disorders, 173
for diabetes insipidus, 98–99
for platelet disorders, 313
Deafness
platelet disorders and, 312
rubella and, 354
in Wegener's granulomatosis, 160
DeBakey classification of aortic dissection, 34
Defibrillation
in cardiopulmonary resuscitation, 69
Dehydration
in diabetes insipidus, 98
in diabetes mellitus, 100, 102, 104, 106
in hypercalcemia, 190
in hyperglycemia, 192
with infectious diarrhea, 216
in HIV infection, 112
migraine and, 252

Index

Delirium tremens, 18
  variceal bleeding and, 414
Delirum
  dementia *vs.*, 94
Delusion
  in schizophrenia, 358
Demeclocyline
  inappropriate antidiuresis syndrome and, 377
Dementia, 94–95
  in acquired immunodeficiency syndrome, 14
  major depression *vs.*, 96
  in motor neuron disease, 258
Dengue fever
  hemolytic uremic syndrome *vs.*, 170
Dennie-Morgan line
  eczema and, 122
Dental management
  endocarditis and, 128
2′Deoxycoformycin
  for hairy cell leukemia, 237
Dependent personality disorder, 306
Depression
  attempted suicide and, 54–55
  in bulimia nervosa, 60
  chronic fatigue syndrome and, 76
  in cranial arteritis, 86
  in Cushing's syndrome, 90
  in dementia, 94
  "double," 96–97
  in Guillain-Barré syndrome, 166
  herpes simplex infection and, 184
  herpes zoster infection and, 186
  with inappropriate antidiuresis syndrome, 376
  major, 96–97, 97f
  in motor neuron disease, 258
  with obsessive-compulsive disorder, 286
  in Parkinson's disease, 300
  in pernicious anemia, 26
  polymyalgia rheumatica *vs.*, 324
  in postherpetic neuralgia, 276
  puerperal pyschosis and, 328–329
  in schizophrenia, 358
  with sleep disorders, 370
  in trigeminal neuralgia, 278
Dermatitis
  acne *vs.*, 4
Dermatitis herpetiformis, 62–63
  eczema *vs.*, 122
Dermatofibroma
  Kaposi's sarcoma *vs.*, 224
Dermatomyositis
  in inflammatory myositis, 272, 272f
  polymyositis *vs.*, 272, 326
Desferrioxamine
  for thalassemia, 388
Desmopressin. *See also* DDAVP
  for diabetes insipidus, 98–99
  for hypopituitarism, 211
Desoximetasone
  for eczema, 123
Desquamation
  acute crystal synovitis and, 8
  gout and, 156
Dexamethasone
  for Addison's disease, 11
  for cerebral tumor, 73
  suppression test
    for Cushing's syndrome, 90
  for typhoid fever, 407
Dextroamphetamine
  for narcolepsy, 371
Diabetes insipidus, 98f, 98–99
  hypernatremia and, 196
  hypokalemia and, 194
Diabetes mellitus
  in acromegaly, 6–7
  acute pancreatitis and, 295
  in angina pectoris, 28
  bacterial overgrowth of small intestine with, 56
  in chronic pancreatitis, 296
  chronic renal failure and, 344
  coma and, 84
  in Cushing's syndrome, 90
  in cystic fibrosis, 58
  dyslipoproteinemia and, 120
  glomerulonephritis *vs.*, 154
  hyperglycemic emergency in, 192
  insulin-dependent, 100–101
  management of
    in children, 104–105
    in pregnancy, 106f, 106–107
    in surgery, 108–109
  myocardial infarction and, 270
  noninsulin-dependent, 102–103
    in obesity, 284
  in pancreatic cancer, 292
  peripheral neuropathy in, 280
  with pheochromocytoma, 310
  polycystic ovarian disease and, 322
  prothrombotic states and, 330
  in renal tubular acidosis, 348
  sarcoidosis and, 356
  transient ischemic attacks and, 398
Dialysis, 110–111
  for acute pancreatitis, 295
  for hemolytic uremic syndrome, 171
  for hypernatremia, 196
  megaloblastic anemia and, 24
  for multiple myeloma, 261
  for polycystic kidney disease, 321
  for renal failure, 343, 345
Diarrhea
  in acquired immunodeficiency syndrome, 14
  bacterial overgrowth of small intestine and, 56
  in celiac disease, 70
  in chronic pancreatitis, 296
  in chronic renal failure, 344
  in Crohn's disease, 88
  in cystic fibrosis, 58
  in cytomegalovirus infection in AIDS, 92
  with gram-negative septicemia, 158
  hemolytic uremic syndrome and, 170
  hepatic encephalopathy and, 176
  HIV infection and, 112–113
  infectious, 216–217
  in malaria, 244
  in *Mycobacterium* infection in AIDS, 266
  in peripheral neuropathy, 280
  in pneumonia, 318
  in Stevens-Johnson syndrome, 132
  in systemic sclerosis, 380
  in thalassemia, 388
  in toxic shock syndrome, 392
  in tuberculosis, 404
  in typhoid fever, 406
  in ulcerative colitis, 408
  with Zollinger-Ellison syndrome, 426
Diazepam
  for alcohol withdrawal syndrome, 19
  for attempted suicide, 55
  for panic and anxiety disorder, 299
  for seizures, 221
Diclofenac
  for rheumatoid arthritis, 42
Dicloxacillin
  for erysipela, 365
Dicyclomine
  for irritable bowel syndrome, 223
Didanosine
  for acquired immunodeficiency syndrome, 15
Dideoxycytosine
  for acquired immunodeficiency syndrome, 15
Digoxin
  for cardiac failure and dilated cardiomyopathy, 67
  for Eisenmenger's complex, 125
  heart block and, 168
  for mitral regurgitation, 255
  for mitral stenosis, 257
  for supraventricular tachycardia, 383

Dihydrocodeine
for chronic fatigue syndrome, 77
Diltiazem
for angina pectoris, 29, 31
Diphenoxylate and atropine
for irritable bowel syndrome, 223
Diphtheria
pharyngitis and, 308
Dipyridamole
for hemolytic uremic syndrome, 171
for prothrombotic states, 331
Disopyramide
for ventricular tachycardia, 385
Disseminated intravascular coagulation, 114f, 114–115
in acute myeloid leukemia, 233
in acute pancreatitis, 294
adult respiratory distress syndrome and, 12
in bacterial meningitis, 248
coma and, 84
gram-negative septicemia and, 158
hemolytic uremic syndrome and, 170
in malaria, 244
platelet disorders and, 312
septic arthritis and, 44
Dissocial personality disorder, 306–307
Distal intestinal obstruction syndrome
in cystic fibrosis, 58
Disulfiram
for alcohol withdrawal syndrome, 19
Diuretics
for cardiac failure and dilated cardiomyopathy, 67
gout and, 8, 156
for hypernatremia, 196
Diverticular disease of the colon, 116–117
colorectal cancer *vs.*, 82
gastrointestinal bleeding and, 152
irritable bowel syndrome and, 222
Diverticulitis, 116–117
Diverticulosis. *See also* Diverticular disease of colon
in bacterial overgrowth of small intestine, 56
Dizziness
with Addison's disease, 10
in chronic fatigue syndrome, 76
in hypertrophic cardiomyopathy, 204
in hypoglycemia, 208
in panic disorder, 298
in ventricular tachycardia, 384
in Waldenström's macroglobulinemia, 422
DNAase
for cystic fibrosis, 59
Donor criteria
for renal transplantation, 346
L-Dopa
for Parkinson's disease, 300–301
for tremor, 400
Dopamine
for acute hypotensive shock, 361
for acute tubular necrosis, 343
Dothiepin
for chronic fatigue syndrome, 77
"Double depression," 96–97
Down syndrome
acute lymphoblastic leukemia in children and, 230
alopecia and, 20
Doxepin
for chronic fatigue syndrome, 77
for urticaria, 413
Doxorubicin
for hepatocellular carcinoma, 183
for Hodgkin's disease, 189
for Kaposi's sarcoma in AIDS, 225
Doxycycline
for Lyme disease, 243
for malaria, 245
for pleural effusion, 314
Droperidol
for attempted suicide, 55
Drug abuse. *See* Substance abuse
Duckett-Jones criteria
for rheumatic fever, 352
Dukes' classification
for colorectal cancer, 82
Duroziez's sign
in aortic regurgitation, 36
Dysentery
with infectious diarrhea, 216
Dysgerminoma
diabetes insipidus and, 98
Dyskeratosis congenita
aplastic anemia and, 22
Dyslipoproteinemia, 120–121
Dysphagia
achalasia and, 2
in buccal and esophageal candidiasis, 64
in esophageal carcinoma, 136
in esophagitis, 138
with gastric cancer, 148
in motor neuron disease, 258
in polymyositis, 326
in tamponade, 304
in thyroid carcinoma, 390f, 390–391
Dysphasia
cerebral tumor and, 72
in dementia, 94
Dyspnea
in acute lymphoblastic leukemia, 228, 230
in adult respiratory distress syndrome, 12
in aortic dissection, 34
in aortic regurgitation, 36
in aortic stenosis, 38
in ascites, 46
in asthma, 48, 50
in atrial septal defect, 52
in bronchiectasis and cystic fibrosis, 58
cardiac failure and dilated cardiomyopathy with, 66
in central sleep apnea, 366
in chronic obstructive pulmonary disease, 78
in cryptococcosis, 142
in cytomegalovirus infection in AIDS, 92
Eisenmenger's complex and, 124
in esophagitis, 138
in granulomatous lung disease, 160
in Guillain-Barré syndrome, 166
in hyperthyroidism, 202
with hypertrophic cardiomyopathy, 204
in hypothyroidism, 212
immunosuppression and, 336
in interstitial lung diseases, 218
in megaloblastic anemia, 24
in mitral regurgitation, 254
in mitral stenosis, 256
in motor neuron disease, 258
in myocardial infarction, 270
with obesity, 284
in pericarditis, 304
in pernicious anemia, 26
in pheochromocytoma, 310
in *Pneumocystis carinii* in AIDS, 316
in pneumonia, 318
in polymyositis, 326
with pulmonary embolism, 338
renal artery stenosis and, 340
in restrictive cardiomyopathy, 350
in sarcoidosis, 356
in tamponade, 304
in thyroid carcinoma, 390
with ventricular tachycardia, 384
Dysthymia, 96
Dysuria
in gram-negative septicemia, 158

E

Ebstein's anomaly
Wolff-Parkinson-White syndrome and, 424
Ecthyma gangrenosum
in hematological malignancy, 214, 214f

Index

Eczema, 122–123
fungal nail infection *vs.*, 144
psoriasis *vs.*, 332
Eczema herpeticum, 122, 184
Edema
in acute renal failure, 342
ankle
cardiac failure and dilated cardiomyopathy with, 66
in central sleep apnea, 366
Eisenmenger's complex and, 124
cerebral
in diabetes mellitus, 104
in dialysis, 110
in encephalitis, 126
in extrapulmonary tuberculosis, 402, 402f
fulminant liver failure and, 238
in chronic renal failure, 344
pulmonary
adult respiratory distress syndrome and, 12
embolism *vs.*, 338
pheochromocytoma and, 310
in ventricular tachycardia, 384
in restrictive cardiomyopathy, 350
in systemic lupus erythematosus, 378
Effort syndrome, 76
Ehlers-Danlos syndrome
aortic regurgitation and, 36
gastrointestinal bleeding and, 152
platelet disorders *vs.*, 312
Eisenmenger's complex, 124–125
in atrial septal defect, 52
Electroconvulsive therapy
for major depression, 97
for puerperal psychosis, 329
for schizophrenia, 359
Electrodessication
for viral warts, 421
Embolism. *See also* Thromboembolism
amniotic fluid
adult respiratory distress syndrome and, 12
in atrial septal defect, 52
in Eisenmenger's complex, 124
in endocarditis, 128
Guillain-Barré syndrome and, 166
with hypertrophic cardiomyopathy, 204
in motor neuron disease, 258
peripheral
in cardiac failure and dilated cardiomyopathy, 66
pulmonary, 338–339
in acute hypotensive shock, 360
aortic dissection *vs.*, 34
asthma *vs.*, 48
in pneumonia, 318
unstable angina and, 30–31
systemic
in aortic stenosis, 38
in mitral regurgitation, 254
in mitral stenosis, 256
in transient ischemic attacks, 398
Empyema
in bronchiectasis and cystic fibrosis, 58
in pneumonia, 318
Enalapril
for cardiac failure and dilated cardiomyopathy, 67
for mitral regurgitation, 255
for systemic sclerosis, 381
Enanthema
in measles, 246
Encainide
for ventricular tachycardia, 385
Encephalitis, 126–127. *See also* Encephalopathy
cerebral tumor *vs.*, 72
chickenpox and, 186
coma and, 84
cytomegalovirus infection in AIDS *vs.*, 92
diabetes insipidus and, 98
epilepsy and, 130
Guillain-Barré syndrome *vs.*, 166
with herpes simplex infection, 184
in herpes zoster infection, 186
in Lyme disease, 242
malaria *vs.*, 244
in measles, 246
in rubella, 354
in toxoplasmosis in AIDS, 394
Encephalopathy
in ascites, 46
in chronic hepatitis, 180
in cranial arteritis, 86
encephalitis *vs.*, 126
with fulminant liver failure, 238
hepatic, 176–177
with hypertension, 200
in primary biliary cirrhosis, 80
variceal bleeding and, 414
Endocarditis, 128–129
in aspergillosis, 142
with *Candida* infection, 142
infective
aortic regurgitation and, 36–37
in aortic stenosis, 38
atrial septal defect and, 52–53
Eisenmenger's complex and, 124
heart block and, 168
with hypertrophic cardiomyopathy, 204
hypertrophic cardiomyopathy and, 205
septic arthritis and, 44
in mitral regurgitation, 254
in mitral stenosis, 256
subacute bacterial
granulomatous lung disease *vs.*, 160
Henoch-Schönlein purpura *vs.*, 174
systemic vasculitis *vs.*, 418
type of, 128
Endometrial cancer
in polycystic ovarian disease, 322
Endometriosis
diverticular disease of colon *vs.*, 116
irritable bowel syndrome *vs.*, 222
Entamoeba histolytica
with diarrhea and HIV infection, 112–113
in infectious diarrhea, 216–217
Enterobacter
gram-negative septicemia and, 158
Enterobius vermicularis
in infectious diarrhea, 216–217
Enterocytozoon bienusi
with diarrhea and HIV infection, 112–113
Enteropathy
gluten sensitive
in bullous disorders, 62
megaloblastic anemia and, 24
Enuresis
in diabetes insipidus, 98
Epidermolysis bullosa
bullous disorders *vs.*, 62
Epidermophyton
in nail infections, 144
Epilepsy, 130–131. *See also* Seizures
cerebral tumor and, 72–73
hyperprolactinemia *vs.*, 198
with hypocalcemia, 206
hypoglycemia *vs.*, 208
in hypopituitarism, 210
in systemic lupus erythematosus, 378
Epinephrine
for acute hypotensive shock, 361
Epiphyseal fusion
growth abnormalities and, 162–163
Epipodophyllotoxin
complications of
in acute lymphoblastic leukemia, 229, 231
Epirubicin
for hepatocellular carcinoma, 183
Epstein-Barr virus
in acute hepatitis, 178
aplastic anemia and, 22
chronic fatigue syndrome *vs.*, 76
in encephalitis, 126
Guillain-Barré syndrome and, 166

non-Hodgkin's lymphoma and, 282
parvovirus B19 infection *vs.,* 302
pharyngitis and, 308
rubella *vs.,* 354
Ergotamine
for migraine, 253
Erysipelas, 364f, 364-365
Erythema
acute crystal synovitis and, 8
in herpes simplex infection, 184
palmar
chronic hapatitis and, 180
in primary sclerosing cholangitis, 74
in pharyngitis, 308
septic arthritis and, 44
Erythema chronicum migrans
in Lyme disease, 242, 242f
Erythema infectiosum, 302
Erythema marginatum
Lyme disease *vs.,* 242
in rheumatic fever, 352
Erythema multiforme, 132f, 132-133. *See also* Stevens-Johnson syndrome
with herpes simplex infection, 184
herpes zoster infection *vs.,* 186
Lyme disease *vs.,* 242
Mycoplasma pneumoniae and, 308
urticaria *vs.,* 412
Erythema nodosum, 134f, 134-135
in Crohn's disease, 88
in infectious diarrhea, 216
Lyme disease *vs.,* 242
pharyngitis and, 308
in pulmonary tuberculosis, 404
in sarcoidosis, 356
Erythrocytes
for disseminated intravascular coagulation, 115
transfusion of, 396-397
Erythroderma
exfoliative
eczema and, 122
in psoriasis, 332
Erythromycin
for acne, 5
for boils and abscesses, 365
for erythema multiforme, 133
for leptospirosis, 227
for Lyme disease, 243
for pneumonia, 319
for rheumatic fever, 352
Erythropoietin
for chronic renal failure, 345
Escherichia coli
bacterial overgrowth of small intestine and, 56
endocarditis and, 128
gram-negative septicemia and, 158
hemolytic uremic syndrome and, 170
pneumonia and, 318
in urinary tract infection, 410
Esophageal stricture
esophageal carcinoma and, 136
in esophagitis, 138
Esophagitis, 138-139
gallstone disease *vs.,* 146
reflux
angina pectoris *vs.,* 28
Esophagus
achalasia and, 2f, 2-3
bleeding varices of. *See* Variceal bleeding
candidiasis of
in AIDS, 64f-65f, 64-65
carcinoma of, 136-137
spasm of
angina pectoris *vs.,* 28
Estradiol
for female hypogonadotropic hypogonadism, 141
for growth abnormalities, 163, 165
for hypopituitarism, 211
for ovarian failure, 291
for pubertal abnormalities, 335
Estrogen
for female hypogonadotropic hypogonadism, 140
Ethambutol
for *Mycobacterium* infection, 267, 403, 405
Ethosuximide
for epilepsy, 131
Etidronate
for hypercalcemia, 191
Etoposide
for acute myeloid leukemia, 233
for Hodgkin's disease, 189
Etretinate
dyslipoproteinemia and, 120
for psoriatic arthritis, 41
EVAP chemotherapy
for Hodgkin's disease, 189
Eye disorders. *See* Vision or eye disorders

F

Famcyclovir
for herpes simplex infection, 185
Familial hypercholesterolemia
dyslipoproteinemia and, 121
Familial polyposis
colorectal cancer and, 82
Famotidine
for duodenal ulcer, 119
for gastric ulcer, 151
Fanconi's anemia
acute lymphoblastic leukemia in children and, 230
aplastic anemia and, 22
Fanconi's syndrome
renal tubular acidosis and, 348
with tubulointerstitial nephropathy, 274
Fansidar
for malaria, 245
Fatigue
in acute lymphoblastic leukemia, 228
in acute myeloid leukemia, 232
with Addison's disease, 10
in anxiety disorder, 298
in aortic regurgitation, 36
aplastic anemia and, 22
cardiac failure and dilated cardiomyopathy with, 66
chronic syndrome of, 76f, 76-77
in cranial arteritis, 86
in dementia, 94
in extrapulmonary tuberculosis, 402
in Guillain-Barré syndrome, 166
in hairy cell leukemia, 236
in hypercalcemia, 190
in hyperglycemia, 192
in hyperthyroidism, 202
with hypokalemia, 194
in hypothyroidism, 212
in megaloblastic anemia, 24
in mitral regurgitation, 254
in mitral stenosis, 256
in myasthenia gravis, 264
in pernicious anemia, 26
in *Pneumocystis carinii* in AIDS, 316
in postherpetic neuralgia, 276
in primary sclerosing cholangitis, 74-75
in restrictive cardiomyopathy, 350
in sarcoidosis, 356
in systemic sclerosis, 380
in Waldenström's macroglobulinemia, 422
Female hypogonadotropic hypogonadism, 140-141, 141f
Fertile eunuch syndrome, 387
Fetal implant therapy
for Parkinson's disease, 301
Fetor hepaticus, 176, 178
Fever
in acquired immunodeficiency syndrome, 14
in acute crystal synovitis, 8
in acute hepatitis, 178

Fever *(continued)*
in acute lymphoblastic leukemia
in children, 230
in AIDS-related lymphoma, 16
in aortic dissection, 34
aplastic anemia and, 22
in ascites, 46
in aspergillosis, 142
in bacterial meningitis, 248
in bronchiectasis and cystic fibrosis, 58
in chickenpox, 186
in chronic lymphocytic leukemia, 234
in coma, 84
in cranial arteritis, 86
in cryptococcosis, 142
in AIDS, 14, 250
in cytomegalovirus infection in AIDS, 92
with dialysis, 110
in diverticular disease of colon, 116
in encephalitis, 126
in endocarditis, 128
in erythema nodosum, 134
in extrapulmonary tuberculosis, 402
with gallstones, 146
in granulomatous lung disease, 160
in hematological malignancy
infections and, 214
in Henoch-Schönlein purpura, 174
with hepatocellular carcinoma, 182
with herpes simplex infection, 184
in Hodgkin's disease, 188
immunosuppression and, 336
with infectious diarrhea, 216
in leptospirosis, 226
in Lyme disease, 242
in malaria, 244
in measles, 246
in *Mycobacterium* infection in AIDS, 266
in myocardial infarction, 270
in parvovirus B19 infection, 302
in pericarditis, 304
in pharyngitis, 308
in pheochromocytoma, 310
pleural effusion and, 314
in *Pneumocystis carinii* in AIDS, 316
in pneumonia, 318
in primary sclerosing cholangitis, 74
in pulmonary tuberculosis, 404
in renal transplantation, 347
in rubella, 354
in sarcoidosis, 356
in septic arthritis, 44
in Stevens-Johnson syndrome, 132
in systemic lupus erythematosus, 378
systemic vasculitis and, 418
in thalassemia, 388
in toxic shock syndrome, 392
in toxoplasmosis in AIDS, 394
in tubulointerstitial nephropathy, 274
in typhoid fever, 406
in ulcerative colitis, 408
in urinary tract infection, 410
Fibrates
for dyslipoproteinemia, 121
Fibrosis
pulmonary
primary biliary cirrhosis and, 80
Fifth disease, 302
urticaria *vs.*, 412
Filariasis
ascites *vs.*, 46
Fish oil
for dyslipoproteinemia, 121
for glomerulonephritis, 155
Fistulas
in colorectal cancer, 82
Flecainide
for ventricular tachycardia, 385
Flegel's disease
viral warts *vs.*, 420
Floxacillin
for boils and abscesses, 365
for septic arthritis, 45
Flucloxacillin
for urinary tract infection, 411
Fluconazole
for buccal and esophageal candidiasis, 65
for cryptococcal meningitis in AIDS, 251
for invasive fungal infections, 143
for nail infections, 145
Flucytosine
for cryptococcal meningitis in AIDS, 251
for invasive fungal infections, 143
Fludarabine
for chronic lymphocytic leukemia, 235
Fludrocortisone
for Addison's disease, 11
for renal tubular acidosis, 348
Flumazenil
for hepatic encephalopathy, 177
Fluocinolone
for eczema, 123
5-Fluorouracil
for colorectal cancer, 83
for viral warts, 421
Fluoxetine
for bulimia nervosa, 61
for chronic fatigue syndrome, 77
for irritable bowel syndrome, 223
for major depression, 97
for obsessive-compulsive disorder, 287
for panic and anxiety disorder, 299
Fluphenazine
for schizophrenia, 359
Flurandrenolide
for eczema, 123
Fluvastatin
for dyslipoproteinemia, 121
Fluvoxamine
for obsessive-compulsive disorder, 287
Folate deficiency
in megaloblastic anemia, 24–25
Folic acid
for megaloblastic anemia, 25
Follicle-stimulating hormone
in hypopituitarism, 210
for polycystic ovarian disease, 323
Folliculitis
gram-negative
acne *vs.*, 4
Folliculitis decalvans
alopecia *vs.*, 20
Foscarnet
for cytomegalovirus infection in AIDS, 92
for pulmonary complications, 337
Fulminant liver failure, 238–239
encephalopathy and, 176
malaria *vs.*, 244
Fungal infections
invasive, 142–143
nail, 144f, 144–145
Furosemide
for ascites, 47
for hyperkalemia, 195
inappropriate antidiuresis syndrome and, 377
for increased intracranial pressure
with intracerebral hemorrhage, 221
for mitral regurgitation, 255
for mitral stenosis, 257
Fusidic acid
for *Staphylococcus* infection, 365

G

Gabapentin
for epilepsy, 131
Gait
in dementia, 94
in Parkinson's disease, 300
Galactorrhea
in female hypogonadotropic hypogonadism, 140
with hyperprolactinemia, 198
in hypopituitarism, 210

Gallbladder disease
duodenal ulcer *vs.*, 118
Gallstone disease
acute pancreatitis and, 294
cholesterol, 146–147
in cystic fibrosis, 58
esophagitis *vs.*, 138
irritable bowel syndrome *vs.*, 222
with obesity, 284
Ganciclovir
cytomegalovirus infection in AIDS *vs.*, 92
for encephalitis, 127
for pulmonary complications, 337
Gastric cancer, 148–149
gastric ulcer *vs.*, 150
Gastric ulcer. *See* Ulcer
Gastritis
gastric ulcer *vs.*, 150
pernicious anemia and, 26
Gastroesophageal reflux
duodenal ulcer *vs.*, 118
in esophagitis, 138
Gastrointestinal bleeding, 152f, 152–153
in pancreatic cancer, 292
Gaucher's disease
myeloproliferative disorders *vs.*, 268
"Gelling"
in osteoarthritis, 288
Genetic mutation
in cystic fibrosis, 58
Genital herpes, 184–185
Genital warts, 420–421
Gentamicin
for bronchiectasis, 59
for endocarditis, 129
for gram-negative septicemia, 159
for urinary tract infection, 411
German measles, 354f, 354–355
Gestational diabetes, 106–107
Giant cell arteritis. *See* Arteritis, giant cell
Giardia infection
bacterial overgrowth of small intestine *vs.*, 56
celiac disease *vs.*, 70
with diarrhea and HIV infection, 112–113
in infectious diarrhea, 216–217
Gigantism
acromegaly and, 6
Gingivitis
buccal and esophageal candidiasis *vs.*, 64
herpes simplex infection *vs.*, 184
pemphigus vulgaris and, 62
Glanzmann's disease
platelet disorders and, 312
Glasgow coma scale, 84
Glaucoma
migraine *vs.*, 252
Glipizide
for diabetes mellitus, 103, 109
Glomerulonephritis, 154–155
acute renal failure and, 342–343
chronic renal failure and, 344
endocarditis and, 128
in Henoch-Schönlein purpura, 174
pharyngitis and, 308
primary biliary cirrhosis and, 80
Glomerulosclerosis, 154
Glossitis
in megaloblastic anemia, 24
in pernicious anemia, 26
Glucagon
for hypoglycemia, 209
Glucose
for hypoglycemia, 209
Glucose tolerance test
for diabetes mellitus, 102, 106
Gluten sensitivity
celiac disease and, 70–71
Glyburide
for diabetes mellitus, 103, 109
Goiter
acromegaly and, 6
in hyperthyroidism, 202
in hypothyroidism, 212
in thyroid carcinoma, 390
Gold sodium thiomalate
for bullous disorders, 63
Gonadotropin-releasing hormone
for pubertal abnormalities, 335
for testicular disorders, 387
Goodpasture's syndrome
glomerulonephritis and, 154–155
granulomatous lung disease *vs.*, 160
systemic vasculitis *vs.*, 418
Gottron's papules
in inflammatory myositis, 272
Gout, 156f, 156–157. *See also* Synovitis, acute crystal
in myeloproliferative disorders, 268
osteoarthritis *vs.*, 288
rheumatoid arthritis *vs.*, 42
Graft dysfunction
renal transplantation and, 347
Gram-negative infections
ankylosing spondylitis and, 32
septicemia in, 158–159
Granuloma annulare
Lyme disease *vs.*, 242
Granulomatous lung disease, 160–161, 161f
Graves' ophthalmopathy, 202
Green nail syndrome, 144
Griseofulvin
for nail infections, 145
Group therapy
for personality disorder, 307
Growth abnormalities
in celiac disease, 70
pubertal abnormalities and, 334, 386
short stature, 162–163
in female hypogonadotropic hypogonadism, 140
in hypopituitarism, 210
tall stature, 164–165
in thalassemia, 388
Growth hormone
in acromegaly, 6–7
for growth abnormalities, 162–163
hypopituitarism and, 210–211
Guillain-Barré syndrome, 166–167
Lyme disease *vs.*, 242
spinal cord compression *vs.*, 372
Gynecomastia
testicular disorders and, 386

H

Haemophilus influenzae
in bacterial meningitis, 249
in septic arthritis, 44
Haemophilus parainfluenzae
endocarditis and, 128
Hair loss. *See* Alopecia
Hairy cell leukemia, 236f, 236–237
Hairy leukoplakia
in *Pneumocystis carinii* in AIDS, 316
Hallucination
with alcohol withdrawal, 18
puerperal psychosis and, 328
in schizophrenia, 358
in systemic lupus erythematosus, 378
Haloperidol
for attempted suicide, 55
for mania, 97
for personality disorder, 307
for puerperal psychosis, 329
for schizophrenia, 359
Hand, foot, and mouth disease
pharyngitis and, 308
Hantavirus
hemolytic uremic syndrome *vs.*, 170
Hashimoto's thyroiditis, 212, 212f
Headache
in acute hepatitis, 178

Headache *(continued)*
in acute lymphoblastic leukemía
in children, 230
in AIDS-related lymphoma, 16
in aplastic anemia, 22
in bacterial meningitis, 248
cerebral tumor and, 72
in chickenpox, 186
in chronic fatigue syndrome, 76
cluster, 252–253
with parasomnias, 370
in cranial arteritis, 86
in cryptococcosis, 142, 250
in cytomegalovirus infection in AIDS, 92
in dementia, 94
in encephalitis, 126
in extrapulmonary tuberculosis, 402
in female hypogonadotropic hypogonadism, 140
in giant-cell arteritis, 324
with gram-negative septicemia, 158
in herpes simplex infection, 184
with hypoglycemia, 208
in hypopituitarism, 210
with inappropriate antidiuresis syndrome, 376
in intracerebral hemorrhage, 220
in leptospirosis, 226
in lung cancer, 240
in Lyme disease, 242
in megaloblastic anemia, 24
migraine, 252–253
in mucormycosis, 142
in pharyngitis, 308
in pheochromocytoma, 310
platelet disorders and, 312
in stroke, 374
tension
cranial arteritis *vs.*, 86
migraine *vs.*, 252
in toxoplasmosis in AIDS, 394
in typhoid fever, 406
in Waldenström's macroglobulinemia, 422
Heart block, 168f, 168–169
in hyperkalemia, 194
Heart disease. *See also* specific diseases
ascites with, 46
ischemic
esophagitis *vs.*, 138
in hypothyroidism, 212
Heart failure, 66–67
in acromegaly, 6
with acute hypotensive shock, 361
aortic regurgitation and, 36
in aortic stenosis, 38
in central sleep apnea, 366
in constrictive pericarditis, 350
dialysis for, 110
in endocarditis, 128
glomerulonephritis *vs.*, 154
with heart block, 168
with hypertension, 200
in hyperthyroidism, 202
with hypertrophic cardiomyopathy, 204
in mitral regurgitation, 254
in mitral stenosis, 256
in multiple myeloma, 260
pernicious anemia and, 26
pleural effusion and, 314
with pulmonary embolism, 338
with rheumatic fever, 352
in stroke, 374
in systemic sclerosis, 380
in thalassemia, 388
in Wolff-Parkinson-White syndrome, 424
Heart sounds
in aortic regurgitation, 36
in aortic stenosis, 38
in atrial septal defect, 52
in cardiac failure and dilated cardiomyopathy, 66
in constrictive pericarditis, 350
in Eisenmenger's complex, 124
in hypertension, 200
in mitral regurgitation, 254
in mitral stenosis, 256
in myocardial infarction, 270
in pericarditis, 304
Heart transplantation
for hypertrophic cardiomyopathy, 205
for restrictive cardiomyopathy, 351
Heartburn
in esophagitis, 138
Heart-lung transplantation
for Eisenmenger's complex, 125
Heberden's nodes
in osteoarthritis, 288
Helicobacter pylori infection
duodenal ulcer caused by, 118–119
in gastric cancer, 148
gastric ulcer and, 150–151
with gastrointestinal bleeding, 152
Hemarthroses
with hemophilia, 172
septic arthritis *vs.*, 44
Hematemesis
with duodenal ulcer, 118
with gastric cancer, 148
with gastric ulcer, 150
with gastrointestinal bleeding, 152
in variceal bleeding, 414
Hematological malignancy
infections in, 214f, 214–215
Hematoma
brain stem, 220
with hemophilia, 172
Hematuria
in polycystic kidney disease, 320
Hemiparesis
cerebral tumor and, 72
in encephalitis, 126
Hemiplegic migraine, 252
Hemochromatosis
chronic hepatitis *vs.*, 180
in restrictive cardiomyopathy, 351
Hemodialysis. *See* Dialysis
Hemofiltration
for dialysis, 111
Hemoglobin A_1c
in diabetes mellitus, 102, 106, 108
Hemolytic uremic syndrome, 170f, 170–171
acute renal failure and, 343
glomerulonephritis *vs.*, 154
Hemophilia, 172–173
in Waldenström's macroglobulinemia, 422
Hemoptysis
Eisenmenger's complex and, 124
immunosuppression and, 336
in pneumonia, 318
Hemorrhage. *See also* Bleeding; Variceal bleeding
in acute hypotensive shock, 360
adult respiratory distress syndrome and, 12
aplastic anemia and, 22
in disseminated intravascular coagulation, 114–115
with gastric ulcer, 150
with hemophilia, 172–173
intracerebral, 220f, 220–221
pleural effusion and, 314
in typhoid fever, 406
in ulcerative colitis, 408
Henoch-Schönlein purpura, 174f, 174–175
pharyngitis and, 308
platelet disorders *vs.*, 312
rheumatic fever *vs.*, 352
systemic vasculitis and, 418
Heparin
for disseminated intravascular coagulation, 115
for hyperglycemia, 193
for prothrombotic states, 331
for pulmonary embolism, 339
for stroke, 375
Hepatic encephalopathy, 176–177
in acute hepatitis, 178

Hepatitis
acute, 178f, 178–179
aplastic anemia and, 22
chronic, 180–181
chronic fatigue syndrome *vs.*, 76
in congenital rubella, 354
dialysis and, 110
fulminant liver failure and, 238
gallstone disease *vs.*, 146
glomerulonephritis and, 154
leptospirosis *vs.*, 226
malaria *vs.*, 244
pancreatic cancer *vs.*, 292
pharyngitis and, 308
primary biliary cirrhosis *vs.*, 80
renal transplantation and, 346
rheumatic fever *vs.*, 352
systemic vasculitis and, 418
transfusion and, 172, 397
vasculitis and, 416
Hepatomegaly
in colorectal cancer, 82
in congenital rubella, 354
in esophageal carcinoma, 136
in hairy cell leukemia, 236
in Lyme disease, 242
in primary biliary cirrhosis, 80
in primary sclerosing cholangitis, 74
in sarcoidosis, 356
in thyroid carcinoma, 390
in Waldenström's macroglobulinemia, 422
Hepatosplenomegaly
in acute lymphoblastic leukemia in children, 230
Herpes simplex infection, 184–185
cytomegalovirus infection in AIDS *vs.*, 92
in encephalitis, 126–127
Herpes virus infection. *See also* Herpes simplex infection; Herpes zoster infection; Varicella
in AIDS, 14
cytomegalovirus infection in AIDS *vs.*, 92
in hematological malignancy, 214
Herpes zoster infection, 186–187
bullous disorders *vs.*, 62
cytomegalovirus infection in AIDS *vs.*, 92
in Hodgkin's disease, 188
peripheral neuropathy and, 280
postherpetic neuralgia and, 276
Hexachlorophene
for *Staphylococcus aureus* infection, 365
Hiatal hernia
in esophagitis, 138
with obesity, 284
Hirsutism
in Cushing's syndrome, 90
in polycystic ovarian disease, 322
Histoplasmosis
in AIDS, 14
invasive, 142–143
Pneumocytis carinii pneumonia *vs.*, 316
Histrionic personality disorder, 306
HIV. *See* Human immunodeficiency virus (HIV)
Hodgkin's lymphoma, 188–189
sarcoidosis *vs.*, 356
toxoplasmosis in AIDS *vs.*, 394
Horner's syndrome
lung cancer and, 240
Hot flushes
ovarian failure and, 290
in panic disorder, 298
Human chorionic gonadotropin
for polycystic ovarian disease, 323
Human immunodeficiency virus (HIV). *See also* Acquired immunodeficiency syndrome (AIDS)
in acquired immunodeficiency syndrome, 14
Addison's disease and, 10
bacterial overgrowth of small intestine with, 56
buccal and esophageal candidiasis and, 64–65
dementia in, 94
dialysis and, 110
diarrhea and, 112–113
eczema *vs.*, 122
glomerulonephritis and, 154
Guillain-Barré syndrome and, 166
hemolytic uremic syndrome and, 170
herpes zoster infection and, 186
in megaloblastic anemia, 24
non-Hodgkin's lymphoma and, 282
peripheral neuropathy and, 280
platelet disorders and, 312
psoriatic arthritis and, 40
pulmonary complications of, 336
renal transplantation and, 346
systemic vasculitis *vs.*, 418
transfusion-transmitted, 172
viral warts and, 420
Humulin, 101
Huntington's disease
dementia in, 94
Hürthle cell cancer
thyroid carcinoma and, 390
Hydralazine
for mitral regurgitation, 255
Hydramnios
gestational diabetes and, 106
Hydrocephalus
in hypopituitarism, 210
in intracerebral hemorrhage, 220
normal-pressure
dementia in, 94
with pituitary macroadenoma, 198
pubertal abnormalities and, 334
in toxoplasmosis in AIDS, 394
Hydrocortisone
for Addison's disease, 11
for celiac disease, 71
for eczema, 123
for hypopituitarism, 211
for testicular disorders, 387
Hydrops fetalis
in parvovirus B19 infection, 302
Hydroxocobalamin
for megaloblastic anemia, 25
for pernicious anemia, 26–27
Hydroxychloroquine
for rheumatoid arthritis, 42
for systemic lupus erythematosus, 379
Hydroxyurea
for myeloproliferative disorders, 269
Hydroxyzine
for urticaria, 413
Hyperaldosteronism
hypokalemia and, 194
Hypercalcemia, 190–191
acromegaly and, 6
in Addison's disease, 10
chronic pancreatitis and, 296
in hepatocellular carcinoma, 182
in lung cancer, 240
in multiple myeloma, 260
with pheochromocytoma, 310
sarcoidosis and, 356
Hypercalciuria
acromegaly and, 6
Hyperglycemia, 192–193
acute pancreatitis and, 294
Hyperglycemic nonketotic coma
in diabetes mellitus, 102
"Hyperinfection syndrome"
in infectious diarrhea, 216
Hyperkalemia, 194–195
in acute renal failure, 342
in Addison's disease, 10
with diabetes mellitus, 104
renal tubular acidosis and, 348
Hyperlipidemia
in angina pectoris, 28
hyponatremia *vs.*, 196
in hypothyroidism, 212
myocardial infarction and, 270
primary biliary cirrhosis and, 80

Index

Hypernatremia, 196–197
Hyperostosis
  psoriatic arthritis and, 40
Hyperparathyroidism
  hypercalcemia and, 190–191
  osteoarthritis and, 288
  primary
    renal tubular acidosis and, 348
Hyperprolactinemia, 198f, 198–199
  acromegaly and, 6
  female hypogonadotropic hypogonadism and, 140
  in hypothyroidism, 212
  with pubertal abnormalities, 335
Hypertension, 200–201
  in acromegaly, 6
  in acute renal failure, 342
  in angina pectoris, 28
  in aortic dissection, 34
  in cardiac failure and dilated cardiomyopathy, 66
  in chronic renal failure, 344
  in coma, 84
  in Cushing's syndrome, 90
  with fulminant liver failure, 238
  with glomerulonephritis, 154
  hemolytic uremic syndrome and, 170
  hypertrophic cardiomyopathy *vs.*, 204
  intracerebral hemorrhage and, 220–221
  malignant
    hemolytic uremic syndrome and, 170
  in myeloproliferative disorders, 268
  myocardial infarction and, 270
  in obesity, 284
  in pheochromocytoma, 310
  portal
    myeloproliferative disorders *vs.*, 268
    in primary biliary cirrhosis, 80
  pulmonary
    in atrial septal defect, 52
    in chronic obstructive pulmonary disease, 78
    Eisenmenger's complex and, 124
    in interstitial lung diseases, 218
    in mitral regurgitation, 254
    in mitral stenosis, 256
    with pulmonary embolism, 338
  pulmonary embolism *vs.*, 338
  in renal artery stenosis, 340
  in renal transplantation, 347
  stroke and, 374
  in systemic lupus erythematosus, 378
  systemic vasculitis and, 418
  transient ischemic attacks and, 398
Hyperthyroidism, 202f, 202–203
  growth abnormalities and, 162
  renal tubular acidosis *vs.*, 348
Hypertrophic cardiomyopathy, 204f, 204–205
  aortic stenosis *vs.*, 38
  mitral regurgitation *vs.*, 254
Hyperuricemia
  Eisenmenger's complex and, 124
  gout and, 157
Hyperventilation
  in hepatic encephalopathy, 176
  pulmonary embolism *vs.*, 338
Hyperviscosity syndrome
  in acute lymphoblastic leukemia, 228
  in multiple myeloma, 260
  in myeloproliferative disorders, 268
  prothrombotic states *vs.*, 330
  in Waldenström's macroglobulinemia, 422
Hypnosis
  for panic and anxiety disorder, 299
Hypocalcemia, 206–207
  in acute pancreatitis, 294
  gestational diabetes and, 106
Hypochlorhydria
  bacterial overgrowth of small intestine with, 56
Hypochondriasis
  in panic and anxiety disorder, 298
Hypoglycemia, 208f, 208–209
  in Addison's disease, 10
  alcohol withdrawal syndrome *vs.*, 18
  fulminant liver failure and, 238
  hepatic encephalopathy and, 176
  in hepatocellular carcinoma, 182
  insulin therapy and, 101, 104, 106
  pheochromocytoma *vs.*, 310
Hypogonadism. *See also* Puberty
  female hypotropic, 140–141, 141f
  testicular disorders and, 386
Hypokalemia, 194–195
  with diabetes mellitus, 104
  renal tubular acidosis and, 348
Hypomagnesemia
  hypocalcemia and, 206–207
Hyponatremia, 196–197
  in Addison's disease, 10
  inappropriate antidiuresis syndrome and, 376
Hypoparathyroidism
  with hypocalcemia, 206–207
Hypophosphatemia
  with diabetes mellitus, 104
Hypopituitarism, 210–211
  acromegaly and, 6
  hypoglycemia and, 208
  with pituitary macroadenoma, 198
  pubertal abnormalities and, 334
  in toxoplasmosis in AIDS, 394
Hypotension
  in acute hypotensive shock, 360
  in acute renal failure, 342
  in Addison's disease, 10–11
  in aortic dissection, 34
  in coma, 84
  in constrictive pericarditis, 350
  in diabetes mellitus, 104, 108
  with dialysis, 110
  fulminant liver failure and, 238
  with gallstones, 146
  with gastrointestinal bleeding, 152
  with gram-negative septicemia, 158
  in hyperglycemia, 192
  with hypokalemia, 194
  in hypopituitarism, 210
  in pneumonia, 318
  postural
    in peripheral neuropathy, 280
  in tamponade, 304
  in toxic shock syndrome, 392
  in Wolff-Parkinson-White syndrome, 424
Hypo-thalamo-pituitary axis
  growth abnormalities and, 162–163
Hypothermia
  in coma, 84
  in hypothyroidism, 212
Hypothyroidism, 212f, 212–213
  acromegaly and, 6
  chronic fatigue syndrome *vs.*, 76
  dementia and, 94
  dyslipoproteinemia and, 120
  female hypogonadotropic hypogonadism and, 140
  obesity *vs.*, 284
  in obstructive sleep apnea, 368
  peripheral neuropathy in, 280
  polycystic ovarian disease *vs.*, 322
  polymyalgia rheumatica *vs.*, 324
  pubertal abnormalities and, 334
Hypovolemia
  acute hypotensive shock and, 360
  dialysis and, 110
  hepatic encephalopathy and, 176
  with inappropriate antidiuresis syndrome, 376
  pulmonary embolism *vs.*, 338

I

Ibuprofen
  for chronic fatigue syndrome, 77
  for rheumatoid arthritis, 42
Ichthyosis
  eczema *vs.*, 122

Ileus
in bacterial overgrowth of small intestine, 56
in hyperkalemia, 194
paralytic
in acute hypotensive shock, 360
in diverticular disease of colon, 116
pheochromocytoma and, 310
Imipramine
for major depression, 97
for narcolepsy, 371
for panic and anxiety disorder, 299
Immune disorders. *See also* Acquired immunodeficiency syndrome (AIDS); Autoimmune disorders; specific disorders
glomerulonephritis and, 154
tubulointerstitial nephropathy and, 274
Immunization. *See* Vaccination
Immunosuppression
pulmonary complications of, 336f, 336-337
renal transplantation and, 347
Impetigo, 364, 364f
eczema and, 122
Impotence
in Cushing's syndrome, 90
with hyperprolactinemia, 198
in hypopituitarism, 210
in multiple sclerosis, 262
in obstructive sleep apnea, 368
in peripheral neuropathy, 280
Indomethacin
for ankylosing spondylitis, 33
for cutaneous vasculitis, 416
for gout, 157
for pericarditis, 305
for rheumatoid arthritis, 42
for sarcoidosis, 357
Infanticide
puerperal psychosis and, 328
Infantile digital fibroma
viral warts *vs.*, 420
Infection(s). *See also* specific infectious agents
in acute lymphoblastic leukemia, 228
in acute myeloid leukemia, 232-233
fulminant liver failure and, 238
in hairy cell leukemia, 236
in hematological malignancy, 214f, 214-215
in multiple myeloma, 260
in non-Hodgkin's lymphoma, 282
in polycystic kidney disease, 320
with pulmonary embolism, 338
skin, 364f, 364-365
in stroke, 374
Infectious mononucleosis
Lyme disease *vs.*, 242
pharyngitis and, 308, 308f
sarcoidosis *vs.*, 356
Infertility
in female hypogonadotropic hypogonadism, 140
in megaloblastic anemia, 24
in obesity, 284
ovarian failure and, 290
in polycystic ovarian disease, 322
pubertal abnormalities and, 334
testicular disorders and, 386
Inflammatory bowel disease. *See also* Crohn's disease; Ulcerative colitis
ankylosing spondylitis *vs.*, 32
celiac disease *vs.*, 70
colorectal cancer *vs.*, 82
diverticular disease of colon *vs.*, 116
erythema nodosum and, 134
herpes simplex infection *vs.*, 184
infectious diarrhea *vs.*, 216
irritable bowel syndrome *vs.*, 222
primary sclerosing cholangitis and, 74
Influenza
interstitial lung diseases and, 218
Lyme disease *vs.*, 242
polymyositis *vs.*, 326
Insomnia, 370-371
Insulin
for diabetes mellitus, 100-101, 103, 104-109
for hyperglycemia, 193
hypoglycemia and, 208f, 208-209
Insulin resistance
in gestational diabetes, 106
Insulinoma
hypoglycemia and, 208
Interferon
for chronic hepatitis, 181
for hairy cell leukemia, 237
for Kaposi's sarcoma in AIDS, 225
for multiple myeloma, 261
for multiple sclerosis, 263
for myeloproliferative disorders, 269
for non-Hodgkin's lymphoma, 283
for viral warts, 421
Interstitial lung disease(s), 218-219
bronchiectasis *vs.*, 58
with polymyositis, 326
Intertrigo
with *Candida* infection, 142
Intestinal obstruction
in Crohn's disease, 88
in diverticular disease of colon, 116
Kaposi's sarcoma in AIDS and, 224
Intracerebral hemorrhage, 220f, 220-221
Intracranial pressure
increased
cerebral tumor and, 72-73
coma and, 84
in encephalitis, 126
in epilepsy, 130
in hepatic encephalopathy, 176
in hyponatremia, 196
in intracerebral hemorrhage, 220
Intussusception
in Henoch-Schönlein purpura, 174
Ipratropium bromide
for chronic obstructive pulmonary disease, 79
Iron overload
transfusion and, 397
Irritable bowel syndrome, 222-223
celiac disease *vs.*, 70
chronic fatigue syndrome and, 76
colorectal cancer *vs.*, 82
duodenal ulcer *vs.*, 118
gallstone disease *vs.*, 146
gastric ulcer *vs.*, 150
ulcerative colitis *vs.*, 408
Islet cell tumor
in Zollinger-Ellison syndrome, 426, 426f
Isoniazid
for extrapulmonary tuberculosis, 403
for pulmonary tuberculosis, 405
Isoproterenol
for acute hypotensive shock, 361
for heart block, 169
Isospora infection
in diarrhea, 216-217
and HIV infection, 112-113
Isotretinoin
for acne, 5
Itching. *See* Pruritus
Itraconazole
for buccal and esophageal candidiasis, 65
for invasive fungal infections, 143
for nail infections, 145
for pulmonary complications, 337

J

Jaundice
in acute hepatitis, 178
in acute pancreatitis, 294
in aplastic anemia, 22
in chronic hepatitis, 180
in chronic pancreatitis, 296
in cystic fibrosis, 58

Jaundice *(continued)*
with fulminant liver failure, 238
with gallstones, 146
with hepatocellular carcinoma, 182
in leptospirosis, 226
in malaria, 244
in non-Hodgkin's lymphoma, 282
in pancreatic cancer, 292
in primary biliary cirrhosis, 80
in primary sclerosing cholangitis, 74
in thalassemia, 388
in typhoid fever, 406
Joint disease. *See* Arthralgia; Arthritis; Arthropathy
Juguloperitoneal shunt
for ascites, 47

K

Kallmann's syndrome
in female hypogonadotropic hypogonadism, 140
pubertal abnormalities and, 334
testicular disorders and, 386, 386f
Kaposi's sarcoma
in acquired immunodeficiency syndrome, 14, 224f, 224–225
AIDS-related lymphoma *vs.*, 16
buccal and esophageal candidiasis *vs.*, 64
cutaneous vasculitis *vs.*, 416
cytomegalovirus infection in AIDS *vs.*, 92
with diarrhea and HIV infection, 112
with gastrointestinal bleeding, 152
with *Mycobacterium* infection in AIDS, 266
in *Pneumocystis carinii* in AIDS, 316
pulmonary complications of, 336
Kaposi's varicelliform eruption
eczema and, 122
Kawasaki syndrome
Stevens-Johnson syndrome *vs.*, 132
systemic vasculitis and, 418
Keloids
acne and, 4
Kennedy's syndrome
motor neuron disease *vs.*, 258
Keratosis
eczema and, 122
Kerion
alopecia and, 20
Kernig's sign
in bacterial meningitis, 248
in coma, 84
with herpes meningitis, 184
Ketoacidosis, 192–193
in diabetes mellitus, 100
alcohol withdrawal syndrome *vs.*, 18
hypoglycemia *vs.*, 208
Ketoconazole
for Cushing's syndrome, 91
for gastric cancer, 149
for invasive fungal infections, 143
Klebsiella
gram-negative septicemia and, 158
Klinefelter's syndrome
growth abnormalities and, 164, 165
pubertal abnormalities and, 334
testicular disorders and, 386
Kogenate
for coagulation disorders, 173
Koplik's spots
in measles, 246, 246f
Korsakoff's psychosis
with alcohol withdrawal syndrome, 18
in celiac disease, 70
dementia *vs.*, 94
Kussmaul's respiration
in chronic renal failure, 344
in constrictive pericarditis, 350
in diabetes mellitus, 100
in ketoacidosis, 192
Kyphosis
in Cushing's syndrome, 90

L

Labetalol
for intracerebral hemorrhage, 221
Lactic acidosis
in malaria, 244
Lactitol
for fulminant liver failure, 239
Lactose intolerance
infectious diarrhea *vs.*, 216
Lactulose
for cystic fibrosis, 59
for fulminant liver failure, 239
for hepatic encephalopathy, 177
for irritable bowel syndrome, 223
Lambert-Eaton syndrome
myasthenia gravis and, 264
polymyositis *vs.*, 326
Lamotrigine
for epilepsy, 131
Lansoprazole
for esophagitis, 139
for Zollinger-Ellison syndrome, 427
Laryngitis
with pharyngitis, 308
Larynx
viral warts in, 420
Lazarus mnemonic
for behavioral assessment, 286
Lead poisoning
gout and, 156
Left ventricular dysfunction
in angina pectoris, 28
cardiac failure and dilated cardiomyopathy with, 66–67
chronic obstructive pulmonary disease *vs.*, 78
Left ventricular failure
in aortic regurgitation, 36
asthma *vs.*, 48
in myocardial infarction, 270
in supraventricular tachycardia, 382
Legionella infection
pneumonia and, 318
Leishmaniasis
acute lymphoblastic leukemia in children *vs.*, 230
typhoid fever *vs.*, 406
Lennert classification
for non-Hodgkin's lymphoma, 282
Lente insulin, 101
Leprosy
erythema nodosum *vs.*, 134
peripheral neuropathy in, 280–281
Leptospirosis, 226–227
hemolytic uremic syndrome *vs.*, 170
Leukemia
acute lymphoblastic
in adults, 228–229
in children, 230–231, 231f
acute myeloid, 232–233
aplastic anemia and, 22
chronic lymphocytic, 234f, 234–235
chronic myeloid, 268–269
hairy cell, 236f, 236–237
aplastic anemia *vs.*, 22
chronic lymphocytic leukemia *vs.*, 234
polymyalgia rheumatica *vs.*, 324
prolymphocytic
chronic lymphocytic leukemia and, 234
Leukodystrophy
progressive multifocal
toxoplasmosis in AIDS *vs.*, 394
Leukoplakia
buccal and esophageal candidiasis *vs.*, 64
hairy
in acquired immunodeficiency syndrome, 14

Levamisole
for colorectal cancer, 83
Lewy bodies
dementia and, 94
in Parkinson's disease, 300
Libman-Sacks endocarditis, 128
Lichen planopilaris
alopecia and, 20
Lichen planus
fungal nail infection *vs.*, 144
psoriasis *vs.*, 332
Lidocaine
for cardiopulmonary resuscitation, 69
for postherpetic neuralgia, 277
for ventricular tachycardia, 385
Limbic leukotomy
for obsessive-compulsive disorder, 287
Lipidemia retinalis
with dyslipoproteinemia, 120
Lipiodol computed tomography
for hepatocellular carcinoma, 182, 182f
Listeria monocytogenes
in bacterial meningitis, 248
Lithium
acneiform eruptions of, 4
inappropriate antidiuresis syndrome and, 377
for mania, 97
for migraine, 253
for personality disorder, 307
for puerperal psychosis, 329
for schizophrenia, 359
Livedo reticularis
cutaneous vasculitis and, 416
in systemic lupus erythematosus, 378
Liver disease. *See also* Cirrhosis; Hepatitis; Hepatomegaly
ascites and, 46–47
in cardiac failure and dilated cardiomyopathy, 66
in colorectal cancer, 82
in hepatic encephalopathy, 176
Liver failure
in constrictive pericarditis, 350
fulminant, 238–239
in acute hepatitis, 178
gram-negative septicemia and, 158
Liver transplantation
for chronic hepatitis, 181
for variceal bleeding, 415
Lobar collapse
in lung cancer, 240
Locked-in syndrome
coma *vs.*, 84
Loperamide
for irritable bowel syndrome, 223
LOPP chemotherapy
for Hodgkin's disease, 189
Loratadine
for urticaria, 413
Lorazepam
for mania, 97
for schizophrenia, 359
Lormetazepam
for chronic fatigue syndrome, 77
Lovastatin
for dyslipoproteinemia, 121
Lukes-Collins classification
for non-Hodgkin's lymphoma, 282
Lung cancer, 240–241
interstitial lung disease and, 218
pneumonia *vs.*, 318
in systemic sclerosis, 380
Lung disease(s). *See also* Lung cancer; specific diseases; Tuberculosis
chronic obstructive pulmonary disease, 78–79
complications of immunosuppression and, 336f, 336–337
granulomatous, 160–161, 161f
interstitial, 218–219
pulmonary edema. *See* Edema
pulmonary embolism, 338–339
pulmonary hypertension. *See* Hypertension
Lupus erythematosus
cutaneous
psoriasis *vs.*, 332
discoid
alopecia and, 20
systemic, 378f, 378–379
heart block and, 168
hemolytic uremic syndrome and, 170
interstitial lung diseases and, 218
pericarditis and, 304
primary biliary cirrhosis and, 80
prothrombotic states and, 330
renal tubular acidosis and, 348
rheumatic fever *vs.*, 352
rheumatoid arthritis *vs.*, 42
systemic vasculitis and, 418
Luteinizing hormone
in hypopituitarism, 210
Luteinizing-hormone releasing hormone
for infertility, 141, 141f
Lyme disease, 242f, 242–243
chronic fatigue syndrome *vs.*, 76
in Guillain-Barré syndrome, 166
heart block and, 168
multiple sclerosis *vs.*, 262
polymyositis *vs.*, 326
Lymphadenopathy
in acquired immunodeficiency syndrome, 14
in acute lymphoblastic leukemia, 228
in acute myeloid leukemia, 232
in chronic lymphocytic leukemia, 234
in esophageal carcinoma, 136
in extrapulmonary tuberculosis, 402, 402f
in Hodgkin's disease, 188
Kaposi's sarcoma in AIDS and, 224
in lung cancer, 240
in non-Hodgkin's lymphoma, 282
in pharyngitis, 308
in *Pneumocystis carinii* in AIDS, 316
in pulmonary tuberculosis, 404
in rubella, 354
in sarcoidosis, 356
in systemic lupus erythematosus, 378
in thyroid carcinoma, 390
in toxoplasmosis in AIDS, 394
with tubulointerstitial nephropathy, 274
in Waldenström's macroglobulinemia, 422
Lymphangitis
skin infections and, 364
Lymphoma(s)
acute lymphoblastic leukemia *vs.*, 228, 230
AIDS-related, 14, 16–17
ascites *vs.*, 46
buccal and esophageal candidiasis *vs.*, 64
in bullous disorders, 62
Crohn's disease *vs.*, 88
cytomegalovirus infection in AIDS *vs.*, 92
with diarrhea and HIV infection, 112
duodenal ulcer *vs.*, 118
extrapulmonary tuberculosis *vs.*, 402
gastrointestinal bleeding and, 152
in granulomatous lung disease, 160
high-grade
chronic lymphocytic leukemia and, 234
Hodgkin's disease, 188–189
invasive fungal infections *vs.*, 142
Lyme disease *vs.*, 242
Mediterranean
infectious diarrhea *vs.*, 216
non-Hodgkin's, 282–283
rheumatoid arthritis and, 42
polymyalgia rheumatica *vs.*, 324
postherpetic neuralgia and, 276
small-intestinal
in celiac disease, 70
Lyphadenosis benigna cutis
in Lyme disease, 242

Index

M

Macrolide
for erythema multiforme, 133
Malaria, 244–245
glomerulonephritis and, 154
hemolytic uremic syndrome *vs.*, 170
myeloproliferative disorders *vs.*, 268
typhoid fever *vs.*, 406
Mallory-Weiss tear
with gastrointestinal bleeding, 152
variceal bleeding *vs.*, 414
Malnutrition
bacterial overgrowth of small intestine with, 56
in Crohn's disease, 88
with dialysis, 110
in esophageal carcinoma, 136
with infectious diarrhea, 216
Mania, 96–97
Manic-depressive psychosis
puerperal, 328–329
Mannitol
for coma, 85
for increased intracranial pressure
with intracerebral hemorrhage, 221
Mantoux test
in pericarditis, 304
for tuberculosis, 402, 402f
Marfan syndrome
aortic dissection and, 34
aortic regurgitation and, 36
growth abnormalities and, 164
Mazindol
for narcolepsy, 371
McArdle's disease
inflammatory myositis *vs.*, 272
McCune-Albright syndrome
pubertal abnormalities and, 334
Measles, 246f, 246–247
Crohn's disease and, 88
German, 354f, 354–355
parvovirus B19 infection *vs.*, 302
Mechlorethamine
for Hodgkin's disease, 189
Meckel's diverticulum
gastrointestinal bleeding and, 152
Meclocyline
for acne, 5
Medroxyprogesterone
for pubertal abnormalities, 335
Mefloquine
for malaria, 245
Meformin
for diabetes mellitus, 103, 109
Megulumine diatrizoate
for cystic fibrosis, 59
Melanoma
Kaposi's sarcoma *vs.*, 224
Melena
drug ingestion and, 152
in gastric cancer, 148
with gastrointestinal bleeding, 152
Melphalan
for multiple myeloma, 261
Memory
in chronic fatigue syndrome, 76
"Meningeal cry," 248
Meningioma
cranial arteritis *vs.*, 86
Meningitis
bacterial, 248f, 248–249
coma and, 84
cranial arteritis *vs.*, 86
cryptococcal
in AIDS, 250–251
cytomegalovirus infection in AIDS *vs.*, 92
diabetes insipidus and, 98
encephalitis *vs.*, 126
epilepsy and, 130
in extrapulmonary tuberculosis, 402, 402f
hepatic encephalopathy *vs.*, 176
with herpes simplex infection, 184
hypoglycemia *vs.*, 208
in leptospirosis, 226
in Lyme disease, 242
malaria *vs.*, 244
sarcoidosis and, 356
Meningococcus infection
hemolytic uremic syndrome *vs.*, 170
Menkes' kinky hair syndrome
alopecia and, 20
Menstruation
in Cushing's syndrome, 90
in polycystic ovarian disease, 322
pubertal abnormalities and, 334
Mental illness. *See also* specific disorders
attempted suicide and, 54–55
Mental retardation
testicular disorders and, 386
Mepacrine
for diarrhea and HIV infection, 113
Mercaptopurine
in acute lymphoblastic leukemia, 229, 231
Mesalamine
for Crohn's disease, 89
for ulcerative colitis, 409
Mesothelioma
pleural effusion *vs.*, 314
^{131}I-Metaiodobenzylguanidine
for pheochromocytoma, 311
Metaproterenol
for chronic obstructive pulmonary disease, 79
Methimazole
for hyperthyroidism, 203
Methotrexate
in acute lymphoblastic leukemia, 229, 231
for inflammatory myositis, 273
interstitial lung diseases and, 218
for polymyositis, 327
for psoriasis, 332
for psoriatic arthritis, 41
for rheumatoid arthritis, 42
for sarcoidosis, 357
for systemic sclerosis, 381
Methyl tert-butyl ether (MTBE)
for gallstone disease, 147
Methylphenidate
for narcolepsy, 371
Methylprednisolone
for acute crystal synovitis, 9
for cranial arteritis, 87
for glomerulonephritis, 155
for granulomatous lung disease, 161
for multiple sclerosis, 263
for systemic lupus erythematosus, 379
Methysergide
for migraine, 253
Metoclopramide
for gastric cancer, 149
Metolazone
for cardiac failure and dilated cardiomyopathy, 67
Metoprolol
for myocardial infarction, 271
Metronidazole
for bacterial overgrowth of small intestine, 57
for Crohn's disease, 89
for diarrhea and HIV infection, 113
for diverticulitis, 117
for duodenal ulcer, 119
for hepatic encephalopathy, 177
for infectious diarrhea, 217
Metyrapone
for Cushing's syndrome, 91
Microsporidia infection
in AIDS, 14
alopecia and, 20
with diarrhea and HIV infection, 112–113
Migraine, 252–253
cranial arteritis *vs.*, 86
epilepsy and, 130
pheochromocytoma *vs.*, 310
transient ischemic attacks *vs.*, 398
Milk-alkali syndrome
hypercalcemia and, 190

Miller-Fisher syndrome
Guillain-Barré syndrome and, 166
Minocycline
for pleural effusion, 314
for rheumatoid arthritis, 43
Minoxidil
for alopecia, 21
Misoprostol
for gastric ulcer, 151
Mitotane
for Cushing's syndrome, 91
Mitoxantrone
for hepatocellular carcinoma, 183
Mitral regurgitation, 254–255
aortic stenosis *vs.*, 38
in cardiac failure, 66
in myocardial infarction, 270
Mitral stenosis, 256–257
Mitral valve
in endocarditis, 128–129
in rheumatic fever, 352, 353t
"Mixed crystal deposition"
acute crystal synovitis and, 8
Mobitz atrioventricular block, 168–169
Mollaret's meningitis
bacterial meningitis *vs.*, 248
Molluscum contagiosum
eczema and, 122
viral warts *vs.*, 420
Monilethrix
alopecia and, 20
Monoamine oxidase inhibitors
for personality disorder, 307
Monosodium urate crystals
acute crystal synovitis and, 8
"Moon face"
in Cushing's syndrome, 90
MOPP chemotherapy
for Hodgkin's disease, 189
Morphine
for acute pancreatitis, 295
for esophageal carcinoma, 137
for myocardial infarction, 271
for pancreatic cancer, 293
for sickle cell disease, 363
Motor neuron disease, 258f, 258–259
multiple sclerosis *vs.*, 262
Mouth
in aplastic anemia, 22
candidiasis of, 142
in AIDS, 64f–65f, 64–65, 266
in Crohn's disease, 88
in herpes simplex infection, 184
Kaposi's sarcoma in AIDS and, 224, 224f
in megaloblastic anemia, 24
in Stevens-Johnson syndrome, 132, 132f
Mucormycosis
invasive, 142–143
Multiple endocrine neoplasia syndrome
acromegaly and, 6
Multiple myeloma, 260f, 260–261
acute renal failure and, 342
polymyalgia rheumatica *vs.*, 324
systemic vasculitis *vs.*, 418
Multiple sclerosis, 262f, 262–263
dementia in, 94
Lyme disease *vs.*, 242
spinal cord compression *vs.*, 372
transient ischemic attacks *vs.*, 398
tremor and, 400
Mumps
bacterial meningitis *vs.*, 348
ovarian failure and, 290
Munich checklist for ICD-10
for personality disorder, 306
Mupirocin
for *Staphylococcus* infection, 365
Murphy's sign
with gallstones, 146
Muscle twitches
in hypernatremia, 196
with hypocalcemia, 206
Muscular dystrophy
inflammatory myositis *vs.*, 272
Musset's sign
in aortic regurgitation, 36
Myalgia
in chronic fatigue syndrome, 76
in cranial arteritis, 86
Myalgic encephalomyelitis, 76
Myasthenia gravis, 264–265
Guillain-Barré syndrome *vs.*, 166
motor neuron disease *vs.*, 258
Myasthenic crisis, 264
Mycobacterium infection. *See also* Tuberculosis
in AIDS, 14, 266f, 266–267
lymphoma *vs.*, 16
in bacterial meningitis, 248
with diarrhea and HIV infection, 112–113
in hematological malignancy, 214
Mycoplasma
hemolytic uremic syndrome *vs.*, 170
Mycoplasma pneumoniae
in Guillain-Barré syndrome, 166
Stevens-Johnson syndrome and, 132–133
Mycosis fungoides
urticaria *vs.*, 412
Myelitis
cytomegalovirus infection in AIDS *vs.*, 92
Myelodysplastic syndrome
aplastic anemia and, 22
Myelofibrosis
primary, 268–269
Myelopathy
in acquired immunodeficiency syndrome, 14
Myeloproliferative disorders, 268–269
Myocardial infarction, 270–271, 271f
acute hypotensive shock and, 360–361
acute pancreatitis *vs.*, 294
angina pectoris and, 28, 30
with aortic dissection, 34
cranial arteritis *vs.*, 86
diabetes mellitus and, 108
duodenal ulcer *vs.*, 118
with dyslipoproteinemia, 120
gastric ulcer *vs.*, 150
with heart block, 169
hyperglycemia and, 192
with obesity, 284
pericarditis and, 304
in pheochromocytoma, 310
polycystic ovarian disease and, 322
pulmonary embolism and, 338
restrictive cardiomyopathy *vs.*, 350
in stroke, 374
supraventricular tachycardia *vs.*, 382
systemic vasculitis and, 418
transient ischemic attacks and, 398
ventricular tachycardia and, 384
Myocarditis
with diphtheria, 308
in typhoid fever, 406
Myositis
inflammatory, 272f, 272–273
Myxedema
ascites *vs.*, 46
erythema nodosum *vs.*, 134
"Myxedema madness," 212
Myxoma
left atrial
mitral stenosis and, 256

N

Nafcillin
for endocarditis, 129
for septic arthritis, 45
for toxic shock syndrome, 393
Naproxen
for erythema multiforme, 133
for erythema nodosum, 135
for Henoch-Schönlein purpura, 175
for rheumatoid arthritis, 42

Index

Narcolepsy, 370–371
central sleep apnea and, 366
obstructive sleep apnea *vs.*, 368
Nasal continuous positive airway pressure
for obstructive sleep apnea, 369
Nasal polyps
in cystic fibrosis, 59
Nausea
in aortic dissection, 34
in hemolytic uremic syndrome, 170
in hyponatremia, 196
in pheochomocytoma, 310
Neck rigidity
in bacterial meningitis, 248
Neisseria
endocarditis and, 128
gram-negative septicemia and, 158
Neisseria gonorrhoeae
pharyngitis and, 308
in septic arthritis, 44
Neisseria meningitidis
in bacterial meningitis, 249
Neoplasm(s). *See also* Cancer; Carcinoma; Lymphoma(s); specific kinds
cerebral, 72–73
dementia in, 94
endocarditis *vs.*, 128
gonadal
with ovarian failure, 290
hematological
infections in, 214f, 214–215
inappropriate antidiuresis syndrome and, 376
with inflammatory myositis, 272
malignant
ascites with, 46–47
bronchiectasis and, 58
in bullous disorders, 62
chronic fatigue syndrome *vs.*, 76
diabetes mellitus *vs.*, 100
pericarditis and, 304
pheochromocytoma and, 310
spinal cord compression and, 372
Stevens-Johnson syndrome and, 132
testicular disorders and, 386
Nephritis
acute interstitial
acute renal failure and, 343
Henoch-Schönlein purpura and, 174
hypokalemia and, 194
Nephrocalcinosis
renal tubular acidosis and, 348
Nephrolithiasis
acromegaly and, 6
in hypercalcemia, 190
in polycystic kidney disease, 320
renal tubular acidosis and, 348
Nephromegaly
in polycystic kidney disease, 320
Nephrotic syndrome
with glomerulonephritis, 154
hyponatremia and, 196
Netherton's syndrome
eczema *vs.*, 122
Neuralgia
postherpetic, 276–277
trigeminal, 278–279
Neuritis
in rubella, 354
Neurodermatitis
eczema *vs.*, 122
Neurofibromatosis
pheochomocytoma and, 310
Neuropathy
autonomic, 280–281
in bacterial overgrowth of small intestine, 56
in diabetes mellitus, 100, 102, 104, 106
infectious diarrhea *vs.*, 216
with dialysis, 110
in multiple myeloma, 260
peripheral, 280–281
in chronic renal failure, 344
in dementia, 94
sarcoidosis and, 356
systemic vasculitis and, 418
in Waldenström's macroglobulinemia, 422
Nevus
spider
with gastrointestinal bleeding, 152
in primary biliary cirrhosis, 80
in primary sclerosing cholangitis, 74
Nifedipine
for aortic regurgitation, 37
for mitral regurgitation, 255
for systemic sclerosis, 381
Nitrates
for angina pectoris, 29, 31
for myocardial infarction, 271
Nitrofurantoin
for urinary tract infection, 411
Nitroglycerin
for angina pectoris, 29, 31
Nitrosurea
for cerebral tumor, 73
Nizatidine
for duodenal ulcer, 119
for gastric ulcer, 151
Nocturnal ventilatory support
for central sleep apnea, 367, 367f
Nodules
in cutaneous vasculitis, 416
in erythema nodosum, 134, 134f
in rheumatoid arthritis, 42
subcutaneous
in rheumatic fever, 352
Nodulocystic acne, 4
Non-Hodgkin's lymphoma, 282–283. *See also* Lymphoma(s)
Nonketotic hyperosmolar coma
hypoglycemia *vs.*, 208
Noonan's syndrome
testicular disorders and, 386
Norepinephrine
for acute hypotensive shock, 361
Nortriptyline
for migraine, 253
Novolin, 101
NPH insulin, 101
NSAIDs
for acute crystal synovitis, 9
for ankylosing spondylitis, 33
duodenal ulcer and, 118
for erythema nodosum, 135
gastric ulcer and, 150
glomerulonephritis and, 154
for gout, 157
for Henoch-Schönlein purpura, 175
hypertension and, 200
for osteoarthritis, 289
for parvovirus B19 infection, 303
for psoriatic arthritis, 41
for rheumatoid arthritis, 42
for sarcoidosis, 357
Nystatin
for buccal and esophageal candidiasis, 65
for gastric cancer, 149
for invasive fungal infections, 143

O

Obesity, 284f, 284–285
angina pectoris and, 28
in bulimia nervosa, 60
in Cushing's syndrome, 90
gout and, 8, 156–157
with hypocalcemia, 206
myocardial infarction and, 270
in obstructive sleep apnea, 368
osteoarthritis and, 288
in polycystic ovarian disease, 322
pulmonary embolism and, 338
testicular disorders and, 386
Obsessive-compulsive disorder, 286–287

Occipital neuralgia
 cranial arteritis *vs.*, 86
Octreotide
 for acromegaly, 7
 for diarrhea and HIV infection, 113
 for gastrointestinal bleeding, 153
 for variceal bleeding, 415
Odynophagia
 in esophagitis, 138
"Oil spots"
 in psoriasis, 332
Oliguria
 in hemolytic uremic syndrome, 170
Olsalazine
 for Crohn's disease, 89
 for ulcerative colitis, 409
Omeprazole
 for duodenal ulcer, 119
 for esophagitis, 139
 for gastric ulcer, 151
 for gastrointestinal bleeding, 153
 for systemic sclerosis, 381
 for Zollinger-Ellison syndrome, 427
Onychodystrophy
 alopecia and, 20
Onycholysis, 144
Onychomycosis, 144f, 144–145
Ophthalmic disorders. *See* Vision or eye disorders
Ophthalmoplegic migraine, 252
Opiates
 for gastric cancer, 149
Orchitis
 testicular disorders and, 386
Organic affective syndrome
 depression and mania *vs.*, 96
Osler-Weber-Rendu syndrome
 gastrointestinal bleeding and, 152
Osmotic demyelination syndrome, 377
Osteoarthritis, 288f, 288–289. *See also* Arthritis
 growth abnormalities and, 164
 with obesity, 284
 polymyalgia rheumatica *vs.*, 324
Osteoarthropathy
 hypertrophic
  lung cancer and, 240
Osteodystrophy
 renal
  in chronic renal failure, 344
Osteolysis
 acne fulminans and, 4
Osteomalacia
 in celiac disease, 70
 inflammatory myositis *vs.*, 272
Osteomyelitis
 psoriatic arthritis and, 40
 septic arthritis and, 44–45
Osteoporosis
 ankylosing spondylitis and, 32
 in celiac disease, 70
 cranial arteritis and, 87
 with hyperprolactinemia, 198
 in hyperthyroidism, 202
 with ovarian failure, 290
 in primary biliary cirrhosis, 80
Ostium primum defect, 52–53
Ostium secundum defect, 52–53
Otitis media
 in aspergillosis, 142
Ovarian failure, 290–291
Oxacillin
 for endocarditis, 129
Oxazepam
 for alcohol withdrawal syndrome, 19
Oxybutynin
 for multiple sclerosis, 263
Oxygen
 for central sleep apnea, 367, 367f
 for chronic obstructive pulmonary disease, 79
Oxymetholone
 for aplastic anemia, 23

P

PACEBOM chemotherapy
 for non-Hodgkin's lymphoma, 283
Pacemaker implantation
 for heart block, 169
 for hypertrophic cardiomyopathy, 205
Paget's disease
 cranial arteritis *vs.*, 86
Pain. *See also* Abdominal pain; Chest pain
 with acne, 4
 with acute crystal synovitis, 8
 in esophageal carcinoma, 136
 in extrapulmonary tuberculosis, 402
 in herpes zoster infection, 186
 in multiple sclerosis, 262
 with obesity, 284
 in osteoarthritis, 288
 in pancreatic cancer, 292
 in peripheral neuropathy, 280
 in polymyalgia rheumatica, 324
 in postherpetic neuralgia, 276
 in renal tubular acidosis, 348
 with septic arthritis, 44
 in sickle cell disease, 362
 in spinal cord compression, 372
 in trigeminal neuralgia, 278
Pallidotomy
 for Parkinson's disease, 301
Pallor
 in myocardial infarction, 270
 in pheochromocytoma, 310
 in thalassemia, 388
Palpitations
 in mitral stenosis, 256
 in panic disorder, 298
 in pheochromocytoma, 310
 in supraventricular tachycardia, 382
 with ventricular tachycardia, 384
 in Wolff-Parkinson-White syndrome, 424–425
Pamidronate
 for hypercalcemia, 191
 for multiple myeloma, 261
Pancreatic cancer, 292–293, 293f
 chronic pancreatitis and, 296
Pancreatitis
 acute, 294–295
  adult respiratory distress syndrome and, 12
  with gallstones, 146
 cancer and, 292
 chronic, 296–297
  bacterial overgrowth of small intestine *vs.*, 56
  celiac disease *vs.*, 70
 diabetes mellitus *vs.*, 100
 duodenal ulcer *vs.*, 118
 with dyslipoproteinemia, 120
 gastric ulcer *vs.*, 150
 hypercalcemia and, 190
 with hypocalcemia, 206
 pleural effusion *vs.*, 314
Panic attacks
 in obstructive sleep apnea, 368
Panic disorder, 298f, 298–299
Paralysis
 in aortic dissection, 34
 in Guillain-Barré syndrome, 166
 in hepatic encephalopathy, 176
 in herpes zoster infection, 186
 with hyperkalemia, 194
Paramomycin
 for diarrhea and HIV infection, 113
Paranoid personality disorder, 306–307
Parasomnias, 370
Paratyphoid fever, 406f, 406–407
Paresthesia
 in chronic fatigue syndrome, 76
 in multiple sclerosis, 262
 in panic disorder, 298
 in peripheral neuropathy, 280
 in spinal cord compression, 372

Index

Parkinsonism, 300-301
dementia and, 94
polymyalgia rheumatica *vs.,* 324
tremor in, 400
Parkinson's disease, 300-301
Paronychia
with *Candida* infection, 142
Paroxetine
for obsessive-compulsive disorder, 287
Parvovirus B19 infection, 302f, 302-303
sickle cell disease and, 362
Patent ductus arteriosus
with aortic stenosis, 38
in congenital rubella, 354
Pelvic inflammatory disease
diverticular disease of colon *vs.,* 116
Pemoline
for narcolepsy, 371
Pemphigus vulgaris, 62-63
Penicillamine
for rheumatoid arthritis, 42
for systemic sclerosis, 381
Penicillin
for bacterial meningitis, 249
for endocarditis, 129
for erysipelas, 365
for leptospirosis, 227
for Lyme disease, 243
for pharyngitis, 309
for rheumatic fever, 352
for septic arthritis, 45
Peppermint oil
for irritable bowel syndrome, 223
Peptic ulcer. *See* Ulcer
Perforation
gastrointestinal
in Crohn's disease, 88
in cytomegalovirus infection in AIDS, 92
in diverticular disease of colon, 116
in duodenal ulcer, 118
in Henoch-Schönlein purpura, 174
in infectious diarrhea, 216
in typhoid fever, 406
in ulcerative colitis, 408
Pericarditis, 304f, 304-305
aortic dissection *vs.,* 34
in chronic renal failure, 344
constrictive, 350-351
Peristalsis
esophageal
achalasia and, 2
Peritoneal dialysis, 111
Peritonitis
in acute pancreatitis, 294
bacterial
with ascites, 46-47
hepatic encephalopathy and, 176
with *Candida* infection, 142
in colorectal cancer, 82
with dialysis, 110
with duodenal ulcer, 118
with gastric ulcer, 150
Personality disorders, 306-307
dysthymia *vs.,* 96
in schizophrenia, 358
Petechiae
in acute myeloid leukemia, 232
aplastic anemia and, 22
Peutz-Jeghers disease
pancreatic cancer and, 292
Pharyngitis, 308f, 308-309
rheumatic fever and, 352
Phenobarbitol
for epilepsy, 131
Phenoxybenzamine
for pheochromocytoma, 311
Phenoxymethylpenicillin
for pharyngitis, 309
Phenylketonuria
eczema *vs.,* 122
Phenytoin
acneiform eruptions of, 4
for epilepsy, 131
with cerebral tumor, 73
inappropriate antidiuresis syndrome and, 377
for seizures
with intracerebral hemorrhage, 221
for trigeminal neuralgia, 279
Pheochromocytoma, 310f, 310-311
with hypertension, 200
hyperthyroidism *vs.,* 202
infectious diarrhea *vs.,* 216
panic and anxiety disorder *vs.,* 298
Philadelphia chromosome
in myeloproliferative disorders, 268-269
Phosphodiesterase inhibitors
for cardiac failure and dilated cardiomyopathy, 67
Physical therapy
for adult respiratory distress syndrome, 11
for ankylosing spondylitis, 33
for cystic fibrosis, 59
for rheumatoid arthritis, 42, 43
Pick's disease
dementia in, 94
Pigmentation
in Addison's disease, 10
café-au-lait
in endocarditis, 128
in chronic renal failure, 344
in primary biliary cirrhosis, 80
pubertal abnormalities and, 334
Pili torti
alopecia and, 20
"Pill-rolling" tremor
in Parkinson's disease, 300, 400
Piperacillin
for gram-negative septicemia, 159
for infections in hematological malignancy, 215
"Pistol-shot femorals"
in aortic regurgitation, 36
Pitressin
for diabetes insipidus, 99
Pituitary disorders and tumors
acromegaly and, 6-7
in Cushing's syndrome, 90-91
in female hypogonadotropic hypogonadism, 140
hyperprolactinemia and, 198, 198f
hypopituitarism and, 210, 211
ovarian failure *vs.,* 290
pubertal abnormalities and, 334-335
testicular disorders and, 386
Pityriasis alba
eczema and, 122
Pityriasis rosea
psoriasis *vs.,* 332
Plantar wart, 420-421
Plaques
psoriatic, 332, 332f
Plasma
for disseminated intravascular coagulation, 115
for hemolytic uremic syndrome, 171
transfusion of, 396-397
Plasma exchange
for Guillain-Barré syndrome, 167
Plasmapheresis
for inflammatory myositis, 273
for systemic vasculitis, 419
Plasmodium species
in malaria, 244-245
Platelet disorders, 312f, 312-313
Platelet transfusions, 396-397
for disseminated intravascular coagulation, 115
Pleural effusion, 314-315
with ascites, 46
in chronic pancreatitis, 296
with gastric cancer, 148
immunosuppression and, 336
in lung cancer, 240
with pulmonary embolism, 338

Pleurisy
  rheumatoid arthritis and, 42
Pleurodesis
  for pleural effusion, 314
Pneumococcus infection
  in AIDS, 14
  in bacterial meningitis, 249
  hemolytic uremic syndrome *vs.,* 170
Pneumocystis carinii infection
  in AIDS, 14, 316-317
    cytomegalovirus infection, 92
  in hematological malignancy, 214
  with immunosuppression, 336
Pneumonia, 318-319
  with *Candida* infection, 142
  central sleep apnea and, 366
  chickenpox and, 186
  in dementia, 94
  in esophagitis, 138
  in hyperglycemia, 192
  in lung cancer, 240
  in measles, 246
  pleural effusion and, 314
  pneumococcal
    chronic lymphocytic leukemia and, 234
  pulmonary embolism *vs.,* 338
  in Stevens-Johnson syndrome, 132
Pneumonitis
  in cytomegalovirus infection in AIDS, 92
Pneumothorax
  with adult respiratory distress syndrome, 12
  with asthma, 48
  in bronchiectasis and cystic fibrosis, 58
  in chronic obstructive pulmonary disease, 78
  pleural effusion and, 314
  in *Pneumocystis carinii* in AIDS, 316
Podophyllin
  for viral warts, 421
Poisoning
  dialysis for, 110
Poliomyelitis
  Guillain-Barré syndrome *vs.,* 166
Polyarteritis
  in hairy cell leukemia, 236
Polyarteritis nodosa
  cutaneous vasculitis and, 416
  Henoch-Schönlein purpura *vs.,* 174
  peripheral neuropathy and, 280
  pleural effusion *vs.,* 314
  systemic vasculitis and, 418
Polycystic kidney disease, 320-321
  renal failure and, 344
Polycystic ovarian disease, 322f, 322-323
  Cushing's syndrome *vs.,* 90
  with hyperprolactinemia, 198
  ovarian failure *vs.,* 290
Polycythemia
  in Eisenmenger's complex, 124
  in hepatocellular carcinoma, 182
  in polycystic kidney disease, 320
  transient ischemic attacks and, 398
Polycythemia vera, 268-269
Polydipsia
  in diabetes insipidus, 98
  in diabetes mellitus, 100, 102, 104, 108
Polymyalgia rheumatica, 324-325, 325f
  polymyositis *vs.,* 326
Polymyositis, 326-327
  dermatomyositis *vs.,* 272
  interstitial lung diseases and, 218
  polymyalgia rheumatica *vs.,* 324
Polyradiculoneuropathy
  chronic inflammatory demyelinating,
    280-281
Polyuria
  in diabetes mellitus, 100, 102, 104, 108
  in polycystic kidney disease, 320
  in Wolff-Parkinson-White syndrome, 424
Porphyria cutanea tarda
  bullous disorders *vs.,* 62
Post poliomyelitis syndrome
  motor neuron disease *vs.,* 258
Postherpetic neuralgia, 276-277
Postpartum mental illness, 328-329
Postviral fatigue syndrome, 76
Potassium
  for hyperglycemia, 193
  for hypokalemia, 194
  for renal tubular acidosis, 348
Pouchitis
  in bacterial overgrowth of small intestine,
    56
Prader-Willi syndrome
  testicular disorders and, 386
Pravastatin
  for dyslipoproteinemia, 121
Praziquantel
  for infectious diarrhea, 217
Precordial thump
  for cardiopulmonary resuscitation, 69
Prednisolone
  for Addison's disease, 11
  for chronic lymphocytic leukemia, 235
  complications of
    in acute lymphoblastic leukemia, 229,
      231
  for cranial arteritis, 87
  for cutaneous vasculitis, 416
  for erythema nodosum, 135
  for giant-cell arteritis, 325
  for Henoch-Schönlein purpura, 175
  for migraine, 253
  for pericarditis, 305
  for platelet disorders, 313
  for polymyalgia rheumatica, 325
  for rheumatic fever, 352
  for Stevens-Johnson syndrome, 133
  for systemic sclerosis, 381
  for systemic vasculitis, 419
  for tubulointerstitial nephropathy, 275
Prednisone
  for asthma, 49
  for bullous disorders, 63
  for celiac disease, 71
  for chronic hepatitis, 181
  for chronic obstructive pulmonary disease,
    79
  for Crohn's disease, 89
  for granulomatous lung disease, 161
  for Hodgkin's disease, 189
  for hypercalcemia, 191
  for inflammatory myositis, 273
  for interstitial lung disease, 219
  for multiple myeloma, 261
  for myasthenia gravis, 265
  for polymyositis, 327
  for sarcoidosis, 357
  for systemic lupus erythematosus, 379
  for ulcerative colitis, 409
  for urticaria, 413
  for vasculitis, 281
Pre-eclampsia
  adult respiratory distress syndrome and,
    12
  gestational diabetes and, 106
  glomerulonephritis *vs.,* 154
  hypertension and, 200
Pregnancy
  acute pancreatitis *vs.,* 294
  aortic dissection and, 34
  female hypogonadotropic hypogonadism
    and, 140
  with fulminant liver failure, 238
  hemolytic uremic syndrome *vs.,* 170
  hyperthyroidism and, 203
  hyponatremia and, 196
Primaquine
  for malaria, 245
Primary biliary cirrhosis, 80-81, 81f
Primidone
  for tremor, 400
Prion disease
  dementia in, 94
Probucol
  for dyslipoproteinemia, 121

Procarbazine
for cerebral tumor, 73
for Hodgkin's disease, 189
Progestogen
for female hypogonadotropic hypogonadism, 141
for ovarian failure, 291
Progressive bulbar palsy, 258
Progressive multifocal leukoencephalopathy, 14, 92, 126
Progressive muscular atrophy, 258
Prolactinoma, 198, 198f
Propafenone
for ventricular tachycardia, 385
Propantheline
for myasthenia gravis, 265
Propionibacterum acnes
acne development and, 4
Propranolol
for hyperthyroidism, 203
for hypertrophic cardiomyopathy, 205
for migraine, 253
for panic and anxiety disorder, 299
for pheochromocytoma, 311
for schizophrenia, 359
for tremor, 400
for variceal bleeding, 415
Propylthiouracil
for hyperthyroidism, 203
Prostacyclin
for hemolytic uremic syndrome, 171
Prostaglandins
for gastric ulcer, 151
Prostatitis
with urinary tract infection, 410
Prosthetic joints
septic arthritis and, 44-45
Prosthetic valves
endocarditis and, 128-129
Proteus
gram-negative septicemia and, 158
Prothrombotic states, 330-331
Proton-pump inhibitors
for duodenal ulcer, 119
for esophagitis, 139
for gastric ulcer, 151
for systemic sclerosis, 381
Protriptyline
for obstructive sleep apnea, 369
Pruritus
in acute hepatitis, 178
in acute renal failure, 342
with *Candida* infection, 142
in chickenpox, 186
chronic renal failure and, 344
in dermatitis herpetiformis, 62
in eczema, 122
erythema multiforme and, 132
in Hodgkin's disease, 188
in multiple myeloma, 260
in myeloproliferative disorders, 268
in pancreatic cancer, 292
in primary biliary cirrhosis, 80-81
in primary sclerosing cholangitis, 74-75
in psoriasis, 332
in urticaria, 412
Pruritus vulvae
in diabetes mellitus, 102
Pseudocysts
in acute pancreatitis, 294
in chronic pancreatitis, 296
"Pseudodementia"
dementia *vs.*, 94
Pseudogout
acute crystal synovitis and, 8-9
gout *vs.*, 156
Pseudomembranous colitis
Crohn's disease *vs.*, 88
Pseudomonas
endocarditis and, 128
gram-negative septicemia and, 158
in hematological malignancy, 214, 214f
Pseudoxanthoma elasticum
gastrointestinal bleeding and, 152
Psittacosis
hemolytic uremic syndrome *vs.*, 170
pneumonia and, 318
Psoriasis, 332f, 332-333
ankylosing spondylitis and, 32
arthritis and, 41-42
eczema *vs.*, 122
fungal nail infection *vs.*, 144
spondylitis and, 32
Psychogenic coma, 84
Psychosis
attempted suicide and, 54-55
puerperal, 328-329
Psychotherapy
for bulimia nervosa, 61
for irritable bowel syndrome, 222
for major depression, 97
for obesity, 285
for obsessive-compulsive disorder, 287
for panic and anxiety disorder, 299
for personality disorder, 307
Puberty
abnormalities of, 334-335
delayed, 334-335
growth abnormalities and, 162
in hypothyroidism, 212
ovarian failure and, 290
precocious, 334-335
growth abnormalities and, 164-165
testicular disorders and, 386
Puerperal pyschosis, 328-329
Pugh's grading of liver disease, 414
Pulmonary complications of immunosuppression, 336f, 336-337
Pulmonary edema
pneumonia *vs.*, 318
Pulmonary stenosis
in congenital rubella, 354
Pulse
in aortic regurgitation, 36
in aortic stenosis, 38
in atrial septal defect, 52
in basic life support, 68
with dyslipoproteinemia, 120
in Eisenmenger's complex, 124
in myocardial infarction, 270
in renal artery stenosis, 340
in supraventricular tachycardia, 382
Pulsus paradoxus
with asthma, 48, 50
in tamponade, 304
Purine intake
gout and, 156-157
Purpura
in cutaneous vasculitis, 416
in platelet disorders, 312, 312f
in systemic lupus erythematosus, 378
Purpura fulminans
in disseminated intravascular coagulation, 114f, 114-115
Pustules
in acne, 4, 4f
Pyelonephritis
diverticular disease of colon *vs.*, 116
with urinary tract infection, 410
Pyoderma faciale
acne *vs.*, 4
Pyoderma gangrenosum
in Crohn's disease, 88
Pyrazinamide
for extrapulmonary tuberculosis, 403
for pulmonary tuberculosis, 405
Pyridostigmine
for myasthenia gravis, 265
Pyridoxine
for extrapulmonary tuberculosis, 403

Q

Q fever
chronic hepatitis *vs.*, 180
pneumonia and, 318

Quincke's sign
in aortic regurgitation, 36
Quinidine
for malaria, 245
Quinine
for malaria, 245
Quinolones
for gram-negative septicemia, 159

R

Radioiodine
for hyperthyroidism, 203
for thyroid carcinoma, 391
Ramsey Hunt syndrome
in herpes zoster infection, 186
Ranitidine
for duodenal ulcer, 119
for esophagitis, 139
for fulminant liver failure, 239
for gastric ulcer, 151
for Zollinger-Ellison syndrome, 427
Rappaport classification
for non-Hodgkin's lymphoma, 282
Rash
in acquired immunodeficiency syndrome, 14
in bacterial meningitis, 248, 248f
in chickenpox, 186
in endocarditis, 128
with gram-negative septicemia, 158
in granulomatous lung disease, 160
in Henoch-Schönlein purpura, 174f, 174–175
in herpes zoster infection, 186
in infectious diarrhea, 216
in infectious pharyngitis, 308
in inflammatory myositis, 272
in leptospirosis, 226
in Lyme disease, 242, 242f
in measles, 246, 246f
in parvovirus B19 infection, 302, 302f
in rheumatic fever, 352
in rubella, 354, 354f
in sarcoidosis, 356
in systemic lupus erythematosus, 378, 378f
systemic vasculitis and, 418
in toxic shock syndrome, 392
in tubulointerstitial nephropathy, 274
in typhoid fever, 406
in urticaria, 412, 412f
Raynaud's phenomenon
with inflammatory myositis, 272
polymyositis and, 326
in primary biliary cirrhosis, 80
in systemic lupus erythematosus, 378
in systemic sclerosis, 380–381
Reaven's syndrome
diabetes mellitus and, 102
Recombinate
for coagulation disorders, 173
Reed-Sternberg cells
in Hodgkin's disease, 188
Refsum's disease
heart block and, 168
Regurgitation. *See* Aortic regurgitation; Mitral regurgitation
Reitan trail test
for hepatic encephalopathy, 176
Reiter's syndrome
ankylosing spondylitis *vs.,* 32
aortic regurgitation and, 36
heart block and, 168
in infectious diarrhea, 216
psoriasis *vs.,* 40, 332
Relaxation training
for panic and anxiety disorder, 299
Renal artery stenosis, 340f, 340–341
Renal disease
analgesic, 274–275
ascites and, 46–47
cutaneous vasculitis and, 416
in diabetes mellitus, 100, 102, 104, 106
gout and, 8, 156
in leptospirosis, 226
tubulointerstitial, 274f, 274–275
with urinary tract infection, 410
in Wegener's granulomatosis, 160
Renal failure
acute, 342–343
in acute hypotensive shock, 360
hemolytic uremic syndrome and, 170f, 170–171
myeloma and, 343
in acute pancreatitis, 294
bulimia nervosa and, 60
in cardiac failure and dilated cardiomyopathy, 66
chronic, 344–345
hyponatremia and, 196
dialysis for, 110–111
fulminant liver failure and, 238
with glomerulonephritis, 154
gram-negative septicemia and, 158
in Henoch-Schönlein purpura, 174
in hyperglycemia, 192
hyperkalemia and, 194
with hypertension, 200
with hypocalcemia, 206–207
in infectious diarrhea, 216
in malaria, 244
in multiple myeloma, 260
in pneumonia, 318
in polycystic kidney disease, 320, 344
renal artery stenosis and, 340
in restrictive cardiomyopathy, 350
in Stevens-Johnson syndrome, 132
systemic vasculitis and, 418
in tamponade, 304
in toxic shock syndrome, 392
in variceal bleeding, 414
Renal stones. *See* Nephrolithiasis
Renal transplantation, 344–345
Renal tubular acidosis, 348–349
Resins
for dyslipoproteinemia, 121
Respiration. *See also* Dyspnea; Respiratory failure
in basic life support, 68
Cheyne-Stokes
in central sleep apnea, 366–367, 367f
in hyponatremia, 196
in chronic obstructive pulmonary disease, 78
in coma, 84
Kussmaul's
in diabetes mellitus, 100
pleural effusion and, 314
Respiratory distress syndrome
adult, 12f, 12–13
in acute renal failure, 342
in disseminated intravascular coagulation, 114–115
in extrapulmonary tuberculosis, 402
gram-negative septicemia and, 158
in hematological malignancy, 214
in leptospirosis, 226
in *Pneumocystis carinii* in AIDS, 316
in pneumonia, 318
in toxic shock syndrome, 392
hyperglycemia and, 193
neonatal
gestational diabetes and, 106
Respiratory failure
fulminant liver failure and, 238
immunosuppression and, 336
Kaposi's sarcoma in AIDS and, 224
in obstructive sleep apnea, 368
in systemic sclerosis, 380
Restlessness
in anxiety disorder, 298
Restrictive cardiomyopathy, 350–351
Retinal migraine, 252
Retinoids
for psoriasis, 332

Reye's syndrome
chickenpox and, 186
fulminant liver failure *vs.*, 238
Rhabdomyolysis
in hyperglycemia, 192
Rheumatic disease
mitral stenosis and, 256
Rheumatic fever, 352f, 352–353
endocarditis and, 128
heart block and, 168
pericarditis and, 304
pharyngitis and, 308
skin infections and, 364
Rheumatoid arthritis. *See* Arthritis, rheumatoid
Rhinitis
with asthma, 50
Ribavirin
for measles, 247
Richter's syndrome
chronic lymphocytic leukemia and, 234
Rifabutin
for *Mycobacterium* infection in AIDS, 267
Rifampicin
for bacterial meningitis, 249
Rifampin
for extrapulmonary tuberculosis, 403
for pulmonary tuberculosis, 405
for *Staphylococcus* infection, 365
Right ventricular failure
in Eisenmenger's complex, 124
Rigidity
in Parkinson's disease, 300
Rigors
in malaria, 244
Riluzole
for motor neuron disease, 259
Risperidone
for puerperal psychosis, 329
for schizophrenia, 359
Rosacea
acne *vs.*, 4
Rose spots
in typhoid fever, 406
Royal Free disease, 76
rt-PA
for myocardial infarction, 271
for pulmonary embolism, 339
Rubella, 354f, 354–355
measles *vs.*, 246
parvovirus B19 infection *vs.*, 302
rheumatic fever *vs.*, 352
Rubral tremor, 400
Russell's sign
in bulimia nervosa, 60, 60f

S

Sacroilitis
psoriatic arthritis and, 40
Salicylic acid
for viral warts, 421
Salivary glands
in bulimia nervosa, 60, 60f
Salmonella infection
in AIDS, 14
Crohn's disease *vs.*, 88
with diarrhea and HIV infection, 112
in infectious diarrhea, 216–217
sickle cell disease and, 362
typhoid fever and, 406
Sarcoid
dementia in, 94
systemic vasculitis *vs.*, 418
Sarcoidosis, 356–357
Addison's disease and, 10
alopecia and, 20
with hypercalcemia, 191
hypercalcemia and, 190
primary biliary cirrhosis *vs.*, 80
Sarcoma
Kaposi's. *See* Kaposi's sarcoma
Saturnine gout, 156
"Sausage digits"
psoriatic arthritis and, 40, 332
Savary-Miller endoscopic classification of esophagitis, 138
Scabies
eczema *vs.*, 122
Scarlatina
toxic shock syndrome *vs.*, 392
Scarlet fever
parvovirus B19 infection *vs.*, 302
skin infections and, 364
Schatzki's ring
esophageal carcinoma *vs.*, 136
Schistosoma mansoni
in infectious diarrhea, 216–217
Schizoaffective disorder
mania *vs.*, 96
Schizoid personality disorder, 306–307
Schizophrenia, 358–3599
major depression *vs.*, 96
panic and anxiety disorder *vs.*, 298
Scleredema of Buschke
systemic sclerosis *vs.*, 380
Sclerodactyly
primary biliary cirrhosis and, 80
in systemic sclerosis, 380
Scleroderma
pericarditis and, 304
Sclerotherapy
for variceal bleeding, 153, 415
Scoliosis
central sleep apnea and, 366
growth abnormalities and, 164
obstructive sleep apnea *vs.*, 368
Seborrheic dermatitis
psoriasis *vs.*, 332
Seizures. *See also* Epilepsy
in acute renal failure, 342
with alcohol abuse, 18
in bacterial meningitis, 248
in cryptococcal meningitis in AIDS, 250
in cytomegalovirus infection in AIDS, 92
in dementia, 94
in encephalitis, 126
in epilepsy, 130
hemolytic uremic syndrome and, 170
in hepatic encephalopathy, 176
in hypernatremia, 196
hypoglycemia and, 208
with inappropriate antidiuresis syndrome, 376
in intracerebral hemorrhage, 220
with pituitary macroadenoma, 198
in schizophrenia, 358
in stroke, 374
in toxoplasmosis in AIDS, 394
Selegiline
for Parkinson's disease, 301
Sepsis
in adult respiratory distress syndrome, 12
Septata intestinalis
with diarrhea and HIV infection, 112–113
Septicemia
acute hypotensive shock and, 360
gram-negative, 158–159
skin infections and, 364
Sequestration syndromes
in sickle cell disease, 362
Seroconversion illness
in acquired immunodeficiency syndrome, 14
Serratia
gram-negative septicemia and, 158
Sertraline
for obsessive-compulsive disorder, 287
Sézary syndrome
chronic lymphocytic leukemia *vs.*, 234
Sheehan's syndrome
diabetes insipidus and, 98
female hypogonadotropic hypogonadism and, 140
hypopituitarism and, 210

Shigella infection
Crohn's disease *vs.,* 88
in infectious diarrhea, 217
and HIV infection, 112
Shingles, 186–187
in chronic lymphocytic leukemia, 234
Shock. *See also* Toxic shock syndrome
acute hypotensive, 360–361
in acute renal failure, 342
in adult respiratory distress syndrome, 12
cardiogenic
in myocardial infarction, 270
in ventricular tachycardia, 384
in diabetes mellitus, 100
in diverticular disease of colon, 116
gram-negative bacterial, 158–159
in hypopituitarism, 210
in malaria, 244
septic
in bacterial meningitis, 248
Shwachman syndrome
celiac disease *vs.,* 70
Sicca syndrome
primary biliary cirrhosis and, 80
Sickle cell disease, 362f, 362–363
bacterial meningitis and, 348
diabetes insipidus and, 98
Simvastatin
for dyslipoproteinemia, 121
Sinus venosus atrial septal defect, 52, 52f
Sinusitis
in bronchiectasis and cystic fibrosis, 58
Sister Joseph's nodule
with gastric cancer, 148
Sjögren's syndrome
polymyositis *vs.,* 326
in primary biliary cirrhosis, 80
renal tubular acidosis and, 348
sarcoidosis *vs.,* 356
Skin
in Cushing's syndrome, 90
eczema of, 122–123
in female hypogonadotropic hypogonadism, 140
in Henoch-Schönlein purpura, 174f, 174–175
in herpes simplex infection, 184
in hypothyroidism, 212
infections of, 364f, 364–365
Kaposi's sarcoma in AIDS and, 224
in psoriasis, 332, 332f
in systemic sclerosis, 380
Slapped cheek syndrome, 302, 302f
Sleep apnea
central, 366–367, 367f
obstructive, 368–369, 370
Sleep disorders, 370–371. *See also* Sleep apnea
in anxiety disorder, 298
in chronic fatigue syndrome, 76
Smoking
chronic obstructive pulmonary disease and, 78, 79
lung cancer and, 240–241
pancreatic cancer and, 292
Snoring
in obstructive sleep apnea, 368
Sodium aurothiomalate
for psoriatic arthritis, 41
Sodium bicarbonate
for cardiopulmonary resuscitation, 69
for hyperglycemia, 193
for hyperkalemia, 195
for renal tubular acidosis, 348
Sodium polystyrene sulfonate
for hyperkalemia, 195
Sorbitol
for hepatic encephalopathy, 177
Sore throat
in pharyngitis, 308
Sotalol
for ventricular tachycardia, 385
Sotos' syndrome
growth abnormalities and, 164
Spasticity
in motor neuron disease, 258
in stroke, 374
Speech
in stroke, 374
Spinal cord compression, 372–373
in thyroid carcinoma, 390
Splenomegaly
in endocarditis, 128
with gastrointestinal bleeding, 152
in hairy cell leukemia, 236
with infectious diarrhea, 216
in Lyme disease, 242
in myeloproliferative disorders, 268
platelet disorders and, 312
in *Pneumocystis carinii* in AIDS, 316
in primary biliary cirrhosis, 80
in primary sclerosing cholangitis, 74
in Waldenström's macroglobulinemia, 422
Sprionolactone
for ascites, 47
Sprue
tropical
celiac disease *vs.,* 70
Squamous cell carcinoma
viral warts and, 420
Stanford classification of aortic dissection, 34
Staphylococcus aureus
chickenpox and, 186
eczema and, 122
endocarditis and, 128–129
hemolytic uremic syndrome *vs.,* 170
methicillin-resistant
skin infections and, 364–365
in septic arthritis, 44
in toxic shock syndrome, 392
Staphylococcus infection
in hematological malignancy, 214
Stature. *See* Growth abnormalities
Status epilepticus
coma and, 84
in encephalitis, 126
epilepsy and, 130
Stavudine
for acquired immunodeficiency syndrome, 15
Steatorrhea
in bacterial overgrowth of small intestine, 56
in celiac disease, 70
in cystic fibrosis, 58
Steroid acne, 4
Steroids. *See also* specific agents
for bronchiectasis, 59
for bullous disorders, 63
for coma, 85
for glomerulonephritis, 155
for psoriatic arthritis, 41
for rheumatoid arthritis, 42
Stevens-Johnson syndrome, 132f, 132–133. *See also* Erythema multiforme
Stomatitis
herpes simplex infection *vs.,* 184
Streptococcus infection
in bacterial meningitis, 248–249
endocarditis and, 128–129
erysipelas and, 364
in hematological malignancy, 214
pharyngitis and, 308, 308f
rheumatic fever and, 352f, 352–353
in septic arthritis, 44
sickle cell disease and, 362
Streptococcus viridans
endocarditis and, 128
Streptokinase
Henoch-Schönlein purpura and, 174
for myocardial infarction, 271
for pulmonary embolism, 339
Stroke, 374–375
in acute hypotensive shock, 360
with aortic dissection, 34
central sleep apnea and, 366

Stroke *(continued)*
in cranial arteritis, 86
with dyslipoproteinemia, 120
in endocarditis, 128
epilepsy and, 130
with hypertension, 200
with migraine, 252
pheochromocytoma and, 310
polycystic ovarian disease and, 322
pulmonary embolism and, 338
in sickle cell disease, 362
transient ischemic attacks and, 398
in Waldenström's macroglobulinemia, 422
Strongyloides infection
bacterial overgrowth of small intestine *vs.*, 56
in infectious diarrhea, 216–217
Subarachnoid hemorrhage
coma and, 84
Subdural hematoma
dementia in, 94
stroke *vs.*, 374
Substance abuse. *See also* Alcohol dependence
in attempted suicide, 55
coma and, 84
panic and anxiety disorder *vs.*, 298
in personality disorder, 306
in schizophrenia, 358
"Succussion splash"
with duodenal ulcer, 118
with gastric cancer, 148
Sucralfate
for duodenal ulcer, 119
for esophagitis, 139
for fulminant liver failure, 239
Suicide
attempted, 54–55
depression and, 96
in personality disorder, 306
puerperal psychosis and, 328
in schizophrenia, 358
Sulfasalazine
for ankylosing spondylitis, 33
for Crohn's disease, 89
for psoriatic arthritis, 41
for rheumatoid arthritis, 42
for ulcerative colitis, 409
Sulfonylureas
for diabetes mellitus, 103
Sumatriptan
for migraine, 253
"Superficial white onychomycosis," 144–145
Sweating
in AIDS-related lymphoma, 16
in angina pectoris
unstable, 30
in anxiety disorder, 298
in aortic dissection, 34
in extrapulmonary tuberculosis, 402
in gram-negative septicemia, 158
hypernatremia and, 196
in hyperthyroidism, 202
with hypoglycemia, 208
in malaria, 244
in myocardial infarction, 270
in panic disorder, 298
in pheochromocytoma, 310
in pulmonary tuberculosis, 404
in tamponade, 304
Sympathomimetic agents
for cardiac failure and dilated cardiomyopathy, 67
Syncope
with Addison's disease, 10
in aortic dissection, 34
in aortic stenosis, 38
in atrial septal defect, 52
Eisenmenger's complex and, 124
with heart block, 168
with hypertrophic cardiomyopathy, 204
in myocardial infarction, 270
with pulmonary embolism, 338
in supraventricular tachycardia, 382
in toxic shock syndrome, 392
Syndenham's chorea
with rheumatic fever, 352
Syndrome of inappropriate antidiuresis. *See* Antidiuretic hormone
Syndrome X
diabetes mellitus and, 102
Synovial fluid analysis
in acute crystal synovitis, 8, 8f
for septic arthritis, 44
Synovitis
acute crystal, 8f, 8–9. *See also* Gout
osteoarthritis and, 288
septic arthritis *vs.*, 44
in polymyalgia rheumatica, 324
rheumatoid arthritis and, 42
Syphilis
aortic regurgitation and, 36
cytomegalovirus infection in AIDS *vs.*, 92
dementia in, 94
psoriasis *vs.*, 332
sarcoidosis *vs.*, 356
Stevens-Johnson syndrome *vs.*, 132
Systemic sclerosis, 380–381

T

Tachycardia
in acute hypotensive shock, 360
in acute pancreatitis, 294
in angina pectoris
unstable, 30
in anxiety disorder, 298
with asthma, 48, 50
in cardiac failure, 66
diabetes mellitus and
surgery and, 108
gastrointestinal bleeding and, 152
with gram-negative septicemia, 158
with heart block, 168
in rheumatic fever, 352
supraventricular, 382–383
in tamponade, 304
ventricular, 384–385
Wolff-Parkinson-White syndrome *vs.*, 424
Tachypnea
in bronchiectasis and cystic fibrosis, 58
immunosuppression and, 336
in *Pneumocystis carinii* in AIDS, 316
with pulmonary embolism, 338
Tacrine
for dementia, 95
Takayasu's arteritis. *See* Arteritis, Takayasu's
Tamponade. *See* Cardiac tamponade
Target lesions
in erythema multiforme, 132f, 132–133
Teicoplanin
for *Staphylococcus* infection, 365
Telangiectasia
with gastrointestinal bleeding, 152
Telogen effluvium
alopecia and, 20
Temazepam
for chronic fatigue syndrome, 77
for insomnia, 371
Temporal arteritis. *See* Arteritis, temporal
Temporomandibular joint disease
cranial arteritis *vs.*, 86
Tenesmus
in Crohn's disease, 88
Tenosynovitis
rheumatoid arthritis and, 42
Terbinafine
for nail infections, 145
Terbutaline
for asthma, 49
for chronic obstructive pulmonary disease, 79
Terfenadine
for urticaria, 413

Testicular disorders, 386f-387f, 386-387
  in chronic hepatitis, 180
Testolactone
  for pubertal abnormalities, 335
Testosterone
  for growth abnormalities, 163, 165
  for hypopituitarism, 211
  for testicular disorders, 387
Tetany
  in acute pancreatitis, 294
  with hypocalcemia, 206
Tetracycline
  for acne, 5
  for bacterial overgrowth of small intestine, 57
  for duodenal ulcer, 119
  for erythema multiforme, 133
Tetrahydroaminoacridine
  for dementia, 95
Tetralogy of Fallot
  Eisenmenger's complex *vs.*, 124
Thalassemia, 388-389
  myeloproliferative disorders *vs.*, 268
  pubertal abnormalities and, 334
Theophylline
  for asthma, 49
  for chronic obstructive pulmonary disease, 79
Thermocoagulation gangliolysis
  for trigeminal neuralgia, 279
Thiabendazole
  for infectious diarrhea, 217
Thiamine
  for alcohol withdrawal syndrome, 19
  for hepatic encephalopathy, 177
Thiazide diuretics
  for cardiac failure and dilated cardiomyopathy, 67
  for hypertension, 201
Thioguanine
  for acute myeloid leukemia, 233
  complications of
    in acute lymphoblastic leukemia, 229, 231
Thionamides
  for hyperthyroidism, 203
Thioridazine
  for personality disorder, 307
Thirst
  in Cushing's syndrome, 90
  in hyperglycemia, 192
Thrombocythemia
  essential, 268-269
Thrombocytopenia
  cutaneous vasculitis *vs.*, 416
  in measles, 246
  in non-Hodgkin's lymphoma, 282
  platelet disorders and, 312-313, 321f
  in rubella, 354
Thromboembolism, 330-331. *See also* Embolism
  in hyperglycemia, 192
  in stroke, 374
Thrombosis, 330-331
  ascites with, 46
  in platelet disorders, 312
  pulmonary embolism and, 338
  in systemic lupus erythematosus, 378
Thrombotic thrombocytopenic purpura, 330
  acute renal failure and, 343
  in congenital rubella, 354
  hemolytic uremic syndrome and, 170-171
  platelet disorders and, 313
Thymoma
  in myasthenia gravis, 264
Thyroid carcinoma, 390f, 390-391
Thyroid disease. *See also* Hyperthyroidism; Hypothyroidism
  erythema nodosum and, 134
  hypopituitarism and, 211
  irritable bowel syndrome *vs.*, 222
  in primary biliary cirrhosis, 80
Thyroiditis
  hyperthyroidism and, 202
Thyroid-stimulating hormone
  in hypopituitarism, 210
Thyrotoxicosis
  diabetes mellitus and, 100, 102
  growth abnormalities and, 164
  hypercalcemia and, 190
  panic and anxiety disorder *vs.*, 298
  pheochromocytoma *vs.*, 310
  in thyroid carcinoma, 390
Thyroxine
  for growth abnormalities, 163
  for hyperprolactinemia, 141
  for hypopituitarism, 211
  for hypothyroidism, 213
Tick bites
  in Lyme disease, 242-243
Ticlopidine
  for stroke, 375
Tinea capitis
  alopecia and, 20
Tinea corporis
  psoriasis *vs.*, 332
Tinidazole
  for diarrhea and HIV infection, 113
Toe
  gout and, 156, 156f
Tongue
  geographic
    in psoriasis, 332
  plaques of
    in buccal and esophageal candidiasis, 64, 64f
  "strawberry"
    in scarlet fever, 308
    in toxic shock syndrome, 392
Tonsils
  in pharyngitis, 308, 308f
Tooth (teeth)
  in bulimia nervosa, 60, 60f
  endocarditis and, 129
Tophi
  gout and, 156
Toxemia
  gestational diabetes and, 106
Toxic shock syndrome, 392f, 392-393
  gram-negative septicemia and, 158
Toxoplasmosis
  in AIDS, 394f, 394-395
  cerebral
    AIDS-related lymphoma *vs.*, 16
  chronic fatigue syndrome *vs.*, 76
  cytomegalovirus infection in AIDS *vs.*, 92
  in hematological malignancy, 214
  Lyme disease *vs.*, 242
  parvovirus B19 infection *vs.*, 302
  Pneumocystis carinii in AIDS *vs.*, 316
  polymyositis *vs.*, 326
  tuberculosis *vs.*, 402
Tranexamic acid
  for platelet disorders, 313
Tranquillizers
  for attempted suicide, 55
Transcutaneous electrical nerve stimulation
  for postherpetic neuralgia, 277
Transfusion medicine, 396-397
  for disseminated intravascular coagulation, 115
  for hemophilia and von Willebrand's disease, 172-173
Transient ischemic attacks, 398f, 398-399
  in cranial arteritis, 86
  with dyslipoproteinemia, 120
  Eisenmenger's complex and, 125
  epilepsy and, 130
  with hypertension, 200
Transplantation. *See* specific organ
Transposition of great vessels
  Eisenmenger's complex and, 124
Trauma
  adult respiratory distress syndrome and, 12
  alopecia and, 20
  coma and, 84
  epilepsy and, 130
Travelers' diarrhea, 217

Tremor, 400–401
with alcohol abuse, 18
in hyperthyroidism, 202
in Parkinson's disease, 300
in pheochromocytoma, 310
Tretinoin
for acne, 5
Triamcinolone
for acute crystal synovitis, 9
for alopecia, 21
for eczema, 123
for urticaria, 413
Trichophyton infection
alopecia and, 20
in nail infections, 144
Trichorrhexis
alopecia and, 20
Trichotillomania
alopecia and, 20, 20f
Tricuspid regurgitation
in cardiac failure, 66
Tricyclic antidepressants
for irritable bowel syndrome, 223
for major depression, 97
for obstructive sleep apnea, 369
for puerperal psychosis, 329
Trigeminal neuralgia, 278–279
Triiodothyronine
for hypothyroidism, 213
Trimethoprim
for acne, 5
for bacterial overgrowth of small intestine, 57
for diverticulitis, 117
for infectious diarrhea, 217
for pulmonary complications, 337
for urinary tract infection, 411
Trousseau's sign
with hypocalcemia, 206
Trousseau's syndrome
in pancreatic cancer, 292
Trypanosomiasis
typhoid fever *vs.*, 406
Tuberculosis
Addison's disease and, 10
ascites and, 46
constrictive pericarditis and, 350
Crohn's disease *vs.*, 88
endocarditis *vs.*, 128
epilepsy and, 130
extrapulmonary, 402f, 402–403
in Hodgkin's disease, 188
hypopituitarism and, 210
invasive fungal infections *vs.*, 142
lung cancer *vs.*, 240
pleural effusion and, 314–315
Pneumocystis carinii in AIDS *vs.*, 316
pulmonary, 404–405
restrictive cardiomyopathy and, 350
sarcoidosis *vs.*, 356
spinal cord compression and, 372
tubulointerstitial nephropathy and, 274
Tuberous sclerosis
acne *vs.*, 4
polycystic kidney disease *vs.*, 320
Tubular necrosis
acute
acute renal failure and, 342–343
renal transplantation and, 347
Tumor lysis syndrome
in acute lymphoblastic leukemia
in children, 230
Turner's sign
in acute pancreatitis, 294
Turner's syndrome
growth abnormalities and, 162–163
ovarian failure and, 290
pubertal abnormalities and, 334
testicular disorders and, 386
Typhoid fever, 406f, 406–407
Tzanck test
for herpes virus infection, 184, 186

U

Ulcerative colitis, 408f, 408–409. *See also* Inflammatory bowel disease
Crohn's disease *vs.*, 88
Ulcers
aphthous
AIDS-related lymphoma *vs.*, 16
herpes simplex infection *vs.*, 184
duodenal, 118f, 118–119
bleeding from, 152, 152f
in chronic pancreatitis, 296
with Zollinger-Ellison syndrome, 426
gastric, 150–151
bleeding, 152, 152f
duodenal ulcer *vs.*, 118
neuropathic, 280
oral
in aplastic anemia, 22
in herpes simplex infection, 184
in pemphigus vularis, 62
peptic
angina pectoris *vs.*, 28
diverticular disease of colon *vs.*, 116
esophagitis *vs.*, 138
gallstone disease *vs.*, 146
gastrointestinal bleeding and, 152–153
in myeloproliferative disorders, 268
variceal bleeding *vs.*, 414
with Zollinger-Ellison syndrome, 426
in peripheral neuropathy, 280
in pharyngitis, 308
rectal
colorectal cancer *vs.*, 82
skin
bullous disorders and, 62
cutaneous vasculitis and, 416
Unstable angina, 28, 30–31
Uremia
in acute pancreatitis, 294
in acute renal failure, 342
cardiac tamponade and, 304
Urethral obstruction
chronic renal failure and, 344
Urethritis
with *Candida* infection, 142
Uric acid production
gout and, 156
Urinary tract infection, 410–411
Urokinase
for pulmonary embolism, 339
Ursodeoxycholic acid
in acute hepatitis, 178
for gallstone disease, 147
for primary biliary cirrhosis, 81, 81f
for primary sclerosing cholangitis, 75
Urticaria, 412f, 412–413
bullous disorders *vs.*, 62
Stevens-Johnson syndrome *vs.*, 132
Uterine malformation
female hypogonadotropic hypogonadism *vs.*, 140

V

Vaccination
for diphtheria, 309
Guillain-Barré syndrome and, 166
for hepatitis, 179, 181
for influenza, 309
pneumonia and, 319
for measles, 247
for platelet disorders, 313
for pneumonia, 319
for rubella, 355
VAD chemotherapy
for multiple myeloma, 261
Valproate
for epilepsy, 131

Vancomycin
for endocarditis, 129
for infection
in hematological malignancy, 215
for infectious diarrhea, 217
for septic arthritis, 45
for *Staphylococcus* infection, 365
Variceal bleeding, 414–415
in chronic hepatitis, 180
gastrointestinal, 152–153
with hepatocellular carcinoma, 182
in primary biliary cirrhosis, 80
in primary sclerosing cholangitis, 74
Varicella, 186–187
Varices
in chronic pancreatitis, 296
Vasculitis. *See also* Arteritis
granulomatous
Crohn's disease and, 88
rheumatoid arthritis and, 42
skin manifestations of, 416f, 416–417
systemic, 418–419
Vasopressin
in diabetes insipidus, 98
inappropriate antidiuresis syndrome and, 377
VBMCP chemotherapy
for multiple myeloma, 261
Vegetative state
coma *vs.*, 84
Ventricular septal defect
aortic stenosis *vs.*, 38
in congenital rubella, 354
Eisenmenger's complex and, 124
in myocardial infarction, 270
Verapamil
for angina pectoris, 29
for hypertrophic cardiomyopathy, 205
for supraventricular tachycardia, 383
Verruca vulgaris, 420–421
Vertigo
in transient ischemic attacks, 398
Vibrio cholerae
in infectious diarrhea, 216–217
Vinblastine
for Kaposi's sarcoma in AIDS, 225
Vincristine
in acute lymphoblastic leukemia, 229, 231
for Hodgkin's disease, 189
for Kaposi's sarcoma in AIDS, 225
Vinyl chloride disease
systemic sclerosis *vs.*, 380
Virilization
in polycystic ovarian disease, 322
pubertal abnormalities and, 334
testicular disorders and, 386
Vision or eye disorders
acromegaly and, 6
ankylosing spondylitis and, 32
cerebral tumor and, 72
in coma, 84
in congenital rubella, 354
in cranial arteritis, 86
in Crohn's disease, 88
in cytomegalovirus infection in AIDS, 92, 92f
in diabetes mellitus, 100, 102, 104, 106
with dyslipoproteinemia, 120
in female hypogonadotropic hypogonadism, 140
in giant-cell arteritis, 324
in Guillain-Barré syndrome, 166
in herpes simplex infection, 184
in herpes zoster infection, 186
in hypercalcemia, 190
in hyperthyroidism, 202, 202f
with hypocalcemia, 206
in hypoglycemia, 208
in intracerebral hemorrhage, 220
in leptospirosis, 226
in measles, 246, 246f
in multiple sclerosis, 262
in myasthenia gravis, 264
with pituitary macroadenoma, 198
platelet disorders and, 312
psoriatic arthritis and, 40
rheumatoid arthritis and, 42
in sarcoidosis, 356
sickle cell disease and, 362
in stroke, 374
in transient ischemic attacks, 398
Vitamin B_{12}
dementia and, 94
Vitamin deficiencies
in bacterial overgrowth of small intestine, 56
with hypocalcemia, 206–207
hypocalcemia and, 206
in measles, 246–247
in megaloblastic anemia, 24–25
megaloblastic anemia and, 22
in pernicious anemia, 26–27
primary biliary cirrhosis and, 81
in primary sclerosing cholangitis, 75
Vomiting
in acute lymphoblastic leukemia in children, 230
with acute pancreatitis, 294
in acute renal failure, 342
in aortic dissection, 34
in bacterial meningitis, 248
in bulimia nervosa, 60
in celiac disease, 70
cerebral tumor and, 72
in cryptococcal meningitis in AIDS, 250
with duodenal ulcer, 118
in extrapulmonary tuberculosis, 402
with fulminant liver failure, 238
with gallstones, 146
with gastric cancer, 148
with gastric ulcer, 150
with gram-negative septicemia, 158
hepatic encephalopathy and, 176
in hypercalcemia, 190
in hypopituitarism, 210
with inappropriate antidiuresis syndrome, 376
in intracerebral hemorrhage, 220
in leptospirosis, 226
in malaria, 244
in myocardial infarction, 270
in peripheral neuropathy, 280
in pneumonia, 318
in Stevens-Johnson syndrome, 132
in toxic shock syndrome, 392
von Hippel-Lindau disease
pancreatic cancer and, 292
pheochomocytoma and, 310
von Willebrand's disease, 172–173
platelet disorders *vs.*, 312

W

Waldenström's macroglobulinemia, 422f, 422–423
multiple myeloma *vs.*, 260
Warfarin
for Eisenmenger's complex, 125
for mitral regurgitation, 255
for mitral stenosis, 257
for prothrombotic states, 331
for pulmonary embolism, 339
for transient ischemic attacks, 398
for vasculitis, 416
Warts
viral, 420f, 420–421
Waterhouse-Friderichsen's syndrome
in bacterial meningitis, 248
Weakness
with Addison's disease, 10
in AIDS-related lymphoma, 16
in central sleep apnea, 366–367, 367f
in Guillain-Barré syndrome, 166
in hairy cell leukemia, 236
in hepatocellular carcinoma, 182

Weakness *(continued)*
in hypercalcemia, 190
with hyperkalemia, 194
in hyperthyroidism, 202
with hypoglycemia, 208
with hypokalemia, 194
in inflammatory myositis, 272
in motor neuron disease, 258
in multiple sclerosis, 262
in myasthenia gravis, 264
in peripheral neuropathy, 280
in pheochromocytoma, 310
in polymyalgia rheumatica, 324
in polymyositis, 326
in postherpetic neuralgia, 276
in renal tubular acidosis, 348
in spinal cord compression, 372
systemic vasculitis and, 418
in transient ischemic attacks, 398
Wegener's granulomatosis, 160–161, 161f
peripheral neuropathy and, 280
systemic vasculitis and, 418
Weight gain
in Cushing's syndrome, 90
in hypopituitarism, 210
in hypothyroidism, 212
Weight loss
in achalasia, 2
with Addison's disease, 10
in AIDS-related lymphoma, 16
in celiac disease, 70
in chronic lymphocytic leukemia, 234
in chronic obstructive pulmonary disease, 78
in chronic pancreatitis, 296
in colorectal cancer, 82
in cranial arteritis, 86
in Crohn's disease, 88
in cytomegalovirus infection in AIDS, 92
in diabetes mellitus, 100, 102, 104, 108
with diarrhea, 216
HIV infection and, 112–113
in endocarditis, 128
in esophageal carcinoma, 136
in extrapulmonary tuberculosis, 402
in female hypogonadotropic hypogonadism, 140
with gastric cancer, 148
in granulomatous lung disease, 160
in hairy cell leukemia, 236
with hepatocellular carcinoma, 182
in Hodgkin's disease, 188
in hyperglycemia, 192
in hyperthyroidism, 202
immunosuppression and, 336
in lung cancer, 240
in multiple myeloma, 260
in *Mycobacterium* infection in AIDS, 266
in myeloproliferative disorders, 268
in pancreatic cancer, 292
in pheochromocytoma, 310
in *Pneumocystis carinii* in AIDS, 316
in primary sclerosing cholangitis, 74
in pulmonary tuberculosis, 404
in sarcoidosis, 356
in systemic sclerosis, 380
testicular disorders and, 386
in tuberculosis, 404
in Waldenström's macroglobulinemia, 422
Weight:height ratio
in obesity, 284, 284f
Wenckebach heart block, 168
Wernicke-Korsakoff syndrome
variceal bleeding and, 414
Wernicke's encephalopathy
with alcohol withdrawal syndrome, 18–19
in celiac disease, 70
dementia *vs.*, 94
hepatic encephalopathy *vs.*, 176
Whipple's disease
dementia in, 94
Wilm's tumor
acute viral hepatitis *vs.*, 178
Wilson's disease
chronic hepatitis and, 180
Parkinson's disease *vs.*, 300
renal tubular acidosis and, 348
Wiskott-Aldrich syndrome
eczema *vs.*, 122
lymphoma and, 16
Wolff-Parkinson-White syndrome, 424–425

X

Xanthelasma
in primary biliary cirrhosis, 80
Xanthines
for asthma, 49
Xanthoma
with dyslipoproteinemia, 120
gout *vs.*, 156
in primary biliary cirrhosis, 80
Xerosis
eczema and, 122

Y

Yeast infection(s)
vaginal
acne treatment and, 4
Yersinia infection
bacterial overgrowth of small intestine *vs.*, 56
Crohn's disease *vs.*, 88
in infectious diarrhea, 217

Z

Zidovudine
for acquired immunodeficiency syndrome, 15
for encephalitis, 127
Zollinger-Ellison syndrome, 426f, 426–427
celiac disease *vs.*, 70
duodenal ulcer *vs.*, 118
gastric ulcer and, 151
Zoster. *See* Herpes zoster infection; Varicella
Zygomycosis
invasive, 142–143